New Frontiers in Ovarian Research

New Frontiers in Ovarian Research

Editor: Margaret Booth

FOSTER
ACADEMICS
www.fosteracademics.com

www.fosteracademics.com

FOSTER ACADEMICS

Cataloging-in-Publication Data

New frontiers in ovarian research / edited by Margaret Booth.
p. cm.
Includes bibliographical references and index.
ISBN 978-1-63242-945-2
1. Ovaries--Diseases. 2. Ovaries--Abnormalities. 3. Ovaries--Research. I. Booth, Margaret.
RG441 .N49 2020
618.11--dc23

Foster Academics,
118-35 Queens Blvd., Suite 400,
Forest Hills, NY 11375, USA

ISBN 978-1-63242-945-2 (Hardback)

Contents

Preface

In my initial years as a student, I used to run to the library at every possible instance to grab a book and learn something new. Books were my primary source of knowledge and I would not have come such a long way without all that I learnt from them. Thus, when I was approached to edit this book; I became understandably nostalgic. It was an absolute honor to be considered worthy of guiding the current generation as well as those to come. I put all my knowledge and hard work into making this book most beneficial for its readers.

The ovaries are female reproductive organs that produce ovum. They play a crucial role in women fertility and the menstrual cycle. The ovaries progress through different stages of development that start in the prenatal period all through menopause. Disorders of the ovaries can also be classified as endocrine or reproductive disorders. Small ovarian cysts are a common occurrence in women. This occurs when the egg does not release from the follicle in the ovary. When women have more follicles than usual, a condition called the polycystic ovary syndrome may develop that can cause cycle irregularities. Some ovarian disorders are ovarian neoplasms, ovaritis, ovarian cancer, germ cell tumor, teratoma, ovarian apoplexy, follicular cyst of ovary, etc. Ovarian research seeks to build an understanding of these conditions and the genetic processes that predispose individuals to these conditions. Such research allows the development of drugs that can prevent and treat these. The objective of this book is to give a general view of the different disorders of the ovary and their management strategies. It contains some path-breaking studies in ovarian research. Coherent flow of topics, student-friendly language and extensive use of examples make this book an invaluable source of knowledge.

I wish to thank my publisher for supporting me at every step. I would also like to thank all the authors who have contributed their researches in this book. I hope this book will be a valuable contribution to the progress of the field.

Editor

1

Neurofibroma involving obturator nerve mimicking an adnexal mass

Wei-Ting Chao[1,3], Chia-Hao Liu[2,3], Yi-Jen Chen[2,3], Hua-Hsi Wu[2,3], Chi-Mu Chuang[2,3,4*] and Peng-Hui Wang[2,3,5*]

Abstract

Background: Pelvic masses are a common gynecologic problem, and majority of them are diagnosed as ovarian tumors finally. Sometimes, it is hard to distinguish the origin of these pelvic masses. The following case is a solitary neurofibroma arising from the right-side obturator nerve, which was impressed as a right-side ovarian tumor initially. We reported this case, and also performed a PRISMA-driven systematic review to summary the similar cases in the literature. This review includes image, molecular and pathological findings and outcome of neurofibroma.

Case presentation: A 33-year-old woman with a regular menstrual period denied any symptoms or signs. During her physical check-up, image examination revealed a right-side heterogeneous pelvic mass; it was suggestive of a complex of right-side ovarian tumor. A provisional diagnosis of retroperitoneal pelvic mass, probably a benign ovarian tumor, was made. Excision of the right-side pelvic mass was performed. We sent the specimens for frozen pathology, which indicated neurofibroma and lipomatous tumor and that the possibility of liposarcoma cannot be excluded. A segment of the obturator nerve was attached to the tumor and was severed. A right-side obturator nerve tear during tumor excision was observed, and a neurosurgeon was consulted for obturator nerve grafting and repair. The patient complained of mild weakness and paresthesia affecting the right leg, and we consulted a rehabilitation doctor for neuron injury. The patient's recovery was uneventful, and she was discharged eight days after the drain was removed. Further rehabilitation treatment was arranged.

Conclusion: A neurofibroma is an uncommon pelvic retroperitoneal tumor, and it can be misdiagnosed as an adnexal mass. To our knowledge, this is a rare case of a solitary neurofibroma arising from the obturator nerve. It usually does not have any neurological deficit. We present this case to demonstrate that pelvic neurofibroma can be mistaken for an adnexal mass. This fact should be borne in mind during the diagnosis process.

Keywords: Neurofibroma, Ovarian cancer, Retroperitoneal, Solitary

Background

A neurofibroma is a benign soft tissue tumor arising from Schwann cells. Neurofibromas have been classically associated with neurofibromatosis type I (NF-1, Von Recklinghausen's disease). They are found in diverse anatomical locations but seldom in the retroperitoneal location [1]. We report this case of a pelvic neurofibroma in a 33-year-old woman, which mimicked an adnexal mass on presentation. A systematic review was conducted to identify published relevant reports.

* Correspondence: cmjuang@gmail.com; phwang@vghtpe.gov.tw; phwang@ym.edu.tw; pongpongwang@gmail.com
[2]Faculty of Medicine, School of Medicine, National Yang-Ming University, Taipei, Taiwan
Full list of author information is available at the end of the article

Case presentation

A 33-year-old woman (gravida 2, para 0) with a regular menstrual period denied any symptoms or signs such as abdominal pain, dysmenorrhea, or menorrhagia. During a routine physical examination, ultrasonography revealed two right-side adnexal masses. One measuring 3.7 cm × 3.0 cm was suggestive of a right-side chocolate cyst. The other one measured 6.9 cm × 4.1 cm with vascularity on color-flow Doppler study. A computed tomography scan revealed a right-side heterogeneous pelvic mass posterior to the urinary bladder pushing the uterus to the left side (Fig. 1); it was suggestive of a complex of right-side ovarian tumor. A provisional diagnosis of retroperitoneal pelvic mass, probably a benign ovarian tumor, was made.

Excision of the right-side pelvic mass and a right-side ovarian cystectomy were performed. The uterus was normal in size. One 3-cm right-side chocolate cyst (Fig. 2a) was visualized, and cystectomy was performed. The other 4-cm right-side pelvis mass (Fig. 2b) was identified, and tumor excision was performed. We sent the specimens for frozen pathology, which indicated (a) a spindle cell tumor and compatible with neurofibroma and (b) lipomatous tumor and that the possibility of liposarcoma cannot be excluded. A segment of the obturator nerve was attached to the tumor and was severed. A right-side obturator nerve tear during tumor excision was observed, and a neurosurgeon was consulted for obturator nerve grafting and repair. A Jackson–Pratt drain was kept on the right side of the abdomen, and the patient stood for the duration of the entire procedure—7 h and 30 min. The patient complained of mild weakness and paresthesia affecting the right leg, and we consulted a rehabilitation doctor for neuron injury. The patient's recovery was uneventful, and the drain was removed on postoperative day 7, and she was discharged eight days after the drain was removed. Further rehabilitation treatment was arranged.

The surgical pathology report included a picture of the neurofibroma (Fig. 3a), which comprised oval to eel-like spindle nuclei on a background of generally wavy, arranged collagenous fibers and myxoid matrixes. Many areas contained schwannoma-like features, characterized by a biphasic pattern with compact areas of spindle cells alternating with loosely arranged foci containing collections of foamy histiocytes. The tumor was diffusely positive for S100 (Fig. 3b) and SOX-10. Several axons within the tumor were demonstrated with NF immunostain (Fig. 3c).

Methods

PRISMA-driven systematic review for solitary retroperitoneal neurofibroma

Search strategy of systemic reviews

An extensive literature review was performed in accordance with the guidelines published for PRISMA [2]. An expansive computerized systemic review of published reports, including meta-analysis, randomized controlled trials, cohort studies, and case reports, was performed by searching the following databases: PubMed, Ovid Medline, EMBASE, Cochrane Database of Systematic Reviews, Cochrane Central Register of Controlled Trials, and Google Scholar. The key search terms included "neurofibroma," "retroperitoneal," and "solitary". The search was limited to human studies and full-text published in English from January 1960 to July 2017.

Screening and data extraction

The aforementioned searching strategy was completed by July 2017. Two independent reviewers (W.T.C. and C.M.C.) reviewed the relevance of all titles and abstracts identified from the computerized database. Full articles were further assessed when the abstracts appeared to meet the inclusion criteria. The reviewed data were obtained and entered onto an ad hoc standardized data entry form by each reviewer. We compared the inclusion data for the origin (continent/country), year of publication, case report text and discussion, length of recruitment period, and source of information.

Assessment of methodological quality

The quality of observational studies (e.g., database analysis, case report, and cohort study) was scored in

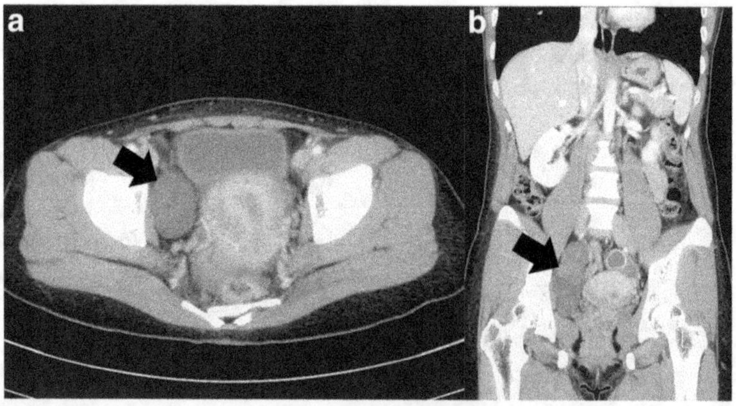

Fig. 1 Computed tomography (**a**) axial and (**b**) sagittal view showing a right-side heterogeneous pelvic mass posterior to the urinary bladder pushing the uterus to the left side

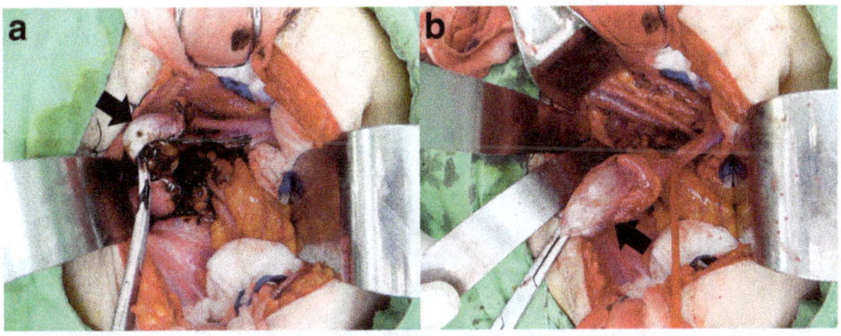

Fig. 2 **a** A 3-cm right-side chocolate cyst. **b** Neurofibroma, 4 cm, attached to the right-side obturator nerve

accordance with the Newcastle–Ottawa Quality Assessment Scale, which ranges from 1 (*poor*) to 9 (*excellent*) [3]. Because no regular descriptions for this scale exist except for the lowest and highest scores, we classified studies with a total score equal to or greater than 7 as high-quality studies.

Results

Our search yielded 20 citations. After reviewing the title and abstract and reviewing the entire text, 12 were discarded as they did not meet the criteria proposed. In total, eight papers were identified for review, as illustrated in the PRISMA flow diagram (Fig. 4). The clinical characteristics of the eight included papers [4–11], associated with our case report, were summarized (total cases = 45) (Table 1).

Of these eight citations, the gender was female in seven cases and unknown in thirty-eight cases. Age varied from young to old. Tumor location was focused on the retroperitoneal space, presacral space, and pelvic cavity, and symptoms were dependent on the location of organic compression. Surgical intervention was included in laparoscopic-assisted tumor excision ($n = 2$) or surgical exploratory total or subtotal tumor excision ($n = 6$). The prognosis in most cases ($n = 7$) was uneventful without neurological deficit but one was under physical therapy; it improved after 7 months of surgery. Computed tomography, magnetic resonance imaging, and ultrasound are screening imaging tools, but diagnosis depends on pathologic reports and immunochemistry staining. Genetic analysis of four citations showed no neurofibromatosis gene, and the other was not mentioned. Immunochemistry staining of four cases showed positive S-100, and that of two cases showed negative S-100.

Discussion

The lifetime risk is approximately 5%–10% for women undergoing surgery for a suspected ovarian neoplasm [12]. An adnexal mass may be found in females of all ages; it is a common gynecologic problem. Borgfeldt et al. investigated 335 woman between 25 and 40 years old who underwent transvaginal ultrasound examinations. The prevalence of adnexal mass lesions determined through ultrasound examination was 7.8% [13]. We present the case of a pelvic neurofibroma in a 33-year-old woman, which mimicked an adnexal mass. Topsakal et al. presented a case who was initially considered to have a giant ovarian mass, but was referred to a neurosurgeon for a solitary giant neurofibroma [4].

Neurofibromatosis is hereditary, and the clinical presentation could vary in the bones, nervous system, eyes, skin, gastrointestinal tract, and other body parts [14]. It is classified into two types. NF-1 is an autosomal-dominant inheritable syndrome because of genetic mutations in the coding of the neurofibromin [7], which is characterized by peripheral manifestations. Neurofibromas are benign tumors of the peripheral nerves and are usually considered pathognomonic of neurofibromatosis type 1 (NF-1). NF-1 is a disease that results from spontaneous or familial transmitted mutations in the NF-1

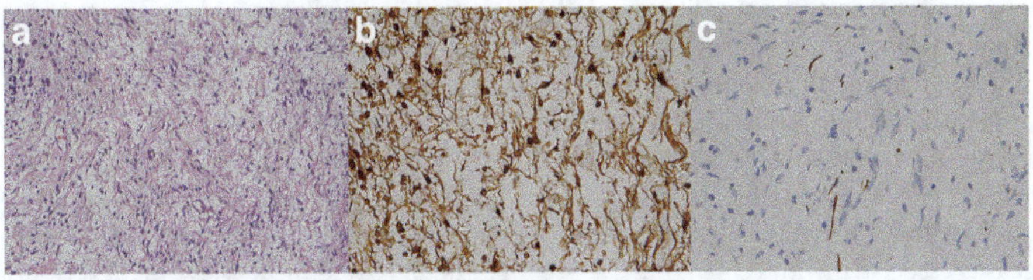

Fig. 3 **a** Hematoxylin–eosin stain. Under the microscope, the neurofibroma is characterized by interlacing bundles of elongated cells with wavy, hyperchromatic nuclei. The tumor has a myxoid background with strands of collagen mimicking shredded carrots, × 200. **b** Stain of S-100. Part of the tumor cells is immunoreactive for S-100, × 400, (**c**) Stain of neurofilaments. Axons within the neurofibroma are demonstrated with neurofilaments, × 400

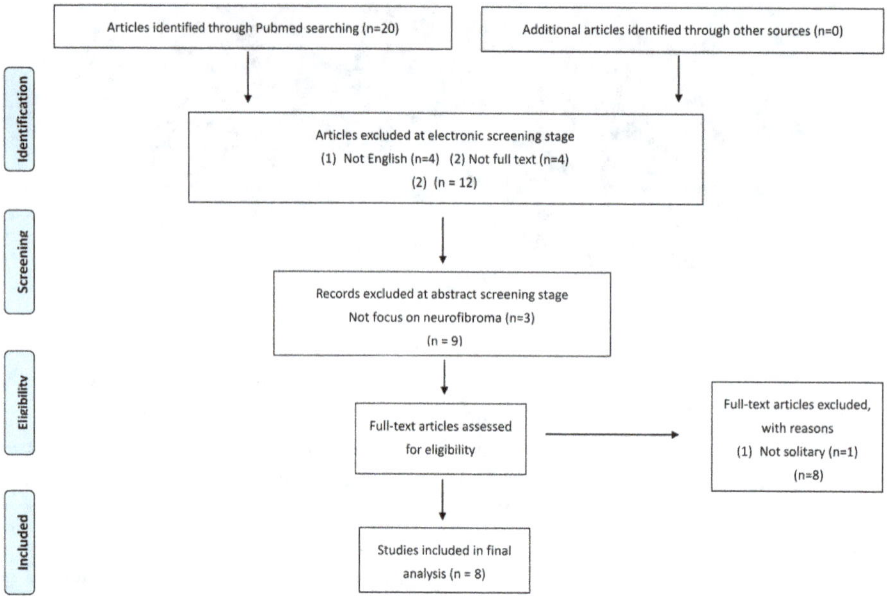

Fig. 4 PRISMA flow diagram

gene located on chromosome 17q11.2. These mutations cause a loss-of-function in the protein neurofibromin, which typically functions as a tumor suppressor. However, diagnosis of NF-1 was depending on clinical symptoms and criteria for diagnosis was established by the NIH in 1988 and is listed in Table 2. Our patient was found to lack the typical signs of NF-1 with absence of Lisch nodules, cafe'-au-lait spots, optic gliomas, multiple other neurofibromas or axillary/inguinal freckling. Computed tomography did not showed other mass lesion of spinal cord or central nervous system. With clinical exclusion of NF-1, she was determined to have a solitary neurofibroma. Type II neurofibromatosis has alternative presentations of the central nervous system [14]. Solitary neurofibromas are solid and nonencapsulated tumors that tend to grow slowly in the skin of people aged 20–30 years and is present without sex differences. Neurofibromas rarely arise from other parts of the body [14]. Most patients with retroperitoneal pelvic neurofibroma have associated neurofibromatosis/Von Recklinghausen's disease [1, 15, 16]. Our patient did not have any hereditary disorder. The present case of pelvic retroperitoneal neurofibroma indicates that these tumors can arise de novo with neither genetic disorder nor other particular organ involvement. A patient with a single neurofibroma represents a true sporadic case or carries the defective gene with only mild clinical presentation [17]. It may become malignant [15, 16]; however, malignant transformation was rare, except in the 4%–11% of cases associated with NF-1 [18].

Patients with neurofibroma usually do not have any neurological symptoms [1]. These tumors, unlike other peripheral nerve tumors, may grow to a considerable size and occupy an unusual position, compressing the neighboring structures and causing severe pain. The most common symptom of retroperitoneal tumors is inadequately localized pain that may be present in the genitalia or lower extremities, often accompanied by numbness, tingling, and, occasionally, urinary symptoms [4]. Other studies have reported that the other clinical manifestations of solitary neurofibromas depend on their location. Shen et al. presented a case of a 45-year-old-female who underwent surgical intervention for a giant, retroperitoneal neurofibroma that compressed the visceral and genitoanal organs [7]. Topsakal et al. presented a 35-year-old woman with a solitary presacral neurofibroma without neurofibromatosis manifesting as bilateral chronic sciatica for 2 years [4] who was initially diagnosed with a giant right ovarian mass.

If a case has no cutaneous neurofibromatosis, diagnosis of pelvic neurofibroma is made only on histology of the excised specimen [1]. When a diagnosis of solitary neurofibroma is made, other subclinical forms of neurofibromatosis must be excluded. The mass must be confirmed as solitary [14]. Computed tomography is a useful preoperative diagnostic imaging tools. A neurofibroma arising from the presacral location may displace the uterus and rectum [4]. However, a neurofibroma arising from the obturator nerve did not displace the visceral organs and it made making the correct diagnosis—either ovarian mass or neural sheath tumor—more difficult. Systemic review of description of image study of solitary neurofibroma was also analyzed (Table 3). Computed tomography scan revealed hypodense lesion with intermediate contrast-enhancement, it was easily

Table 1 The included papers

Author	Year of publication	Gender	Age	Tumor location	Symptoms	Surgical intervention	Prognosis	Image study/Genetic analysis	Immunohistochemistry stain
Topsakal et al. [4]	2001	female	35	Right pre-sacral solitary neurofibroma	Bilateral sciatica radiating to the right inguinal and lumbar area for 2 years	Extra-peritoneal approach through a right J incision with complete resection	Uneventful without neurological deficit	Transvaginal ultrasound, Computed Tomography / Without gene of neurofibromatosis	Vimentin (+), Fibronectin(+), S-100(−), Cytokeratin(−), Desmin(−)
Kim et al. [5]	2013	female	72	Early gastric cancer with a 1.6-cm sized neurofibroma posterior to duodenum	Epigastric discomfort for 2 months	Laparoscopic assisted distal gastrectomy and retro-pancreatic nodal dissection	Uneventful without neurological deficit	Abdominal Computed Tomography / Without gene of neurofibromatosis	S-100 (+)
Dafford et al. [6]	2007	Total 38 patients	Total 38 patients	Pelvic retroperitoneal region	Pelvic pain, paresthesia or weakness, palpable pelvic mass	Total or subtotal resection	Moderate pain reduction	Magnetic resonance imaging, Computed Tomography / Without gene of neurofibromatosis	S-100 (+)
Shen et al. [7]	2016	female	45	Giant neurofibroma involving the pelvic cavity, retroperitoneal space and right buttock	Compressive displacement of abdominal and pelvic organs	En-bloc abdominopelvic tumor removal	Uneventful without neurological deficit	Computed Tomography / Not mention	Vimentin (+), CD-34(+), S-100(−), smooth muscle actin(−), desmin(−), cytokeratin(−)
Ishikawa et al. [8]	1989	female	56	Retro-vesical space	Dysuria for 2 years, traction pain in the left lower limb	Exploratory laparotomy	Uneventful without neurological deficit	Computed Tomography / Not mention	S-100 (+), neuron specific enolase(NSE) (+)
Hunter et al. [9]	1988	female	34	Pulsatile mass at the right pelvic side-wall	Right lower pelvic pain with sharp radiation into the right lower extremity for 3 years	Total tumor excision, right side J incision with extra-peritoneal approach	Loss of range of motion in the right foot, receiving physical therapy and improvement after 7 month of surgery	Intravenous pyelogram, cystoscopy / Not mention	Not mention
Cowles et al. [10]	1987	female	25	Soft mass extending from pubo-coccygeus muscle and para-vaginal space	Mild pelvic discomfort for one year exacerbated by prolong sitting	Surgical exploration and total excision	Uneventful without neurological deficit	Not mention / Not mention	Not mention
Gupta et al. [11]	2015	female	51	Over the left adrenal gland	Upper abdominal pain for 2 years	Laparoscopic left adrenalectomy	Uneventful without neurological deficit	Computed Tomography / Without gene of neurofibromatosis	S-100 (+)

Table 2 Gives NIH consensus guidelines for type I neurofibromatosis diagnostic criteria

NIH consensus guidelines: diagnostic criteria for neurofibromatosis I. Two or more of the following
1. Six or more cafe'-au-lait macules that are (in greatest diameter) > 5 mm in pre-pubertal individuals > 15 mm in post-pubertal individuals
2. Two or more neurofibromas of any type, or one plexiform neurofibroma
3. Axillary/inguinal freckling
4. Optic glioma
5. Two or more Lisch nodules
6. Distinctive osseous lesion (i.e. sphenoid dysplasia or thinning of long bone cortex with or without pseudoarthrosis)
7. First degree relative with NF-1

confused with benign ovarian tumor if the location of lesion was close to adnexa. Our patient did not receive Magnetic resonance imaging, however, it could differentiate ovarian tumor and neurofibroma. According to our systemic review, neurofibroma was high intensity with a well-circumscribed low intensity center or low intensity surrounding under T2-weighted image and T1-weighted image was intermediate intensity. We strongly advised patient to receive Magnetic resonance imaging for correct provisional diagnosis to differentiate.

Complete surgical resection is the only treatment for these tumors [14]. The neurofibroma can recur after surgical intervention [19], but a complete resection is preferred to prevent local recurrence and malignant transformation [4]. Malignant transformation and recurrence are unusual [14]. Nerve root sacrifice is often required to achieve total tumor excision, but resection does not always result in a postoperative neurological deficit [4]. Levy et al. analyzed 66 spinal neurofibromas and determined that nerve fibers involved in a neurofibroma can usually be resected. This suggests that these nerve roots retained no function and would not degenerate further [20].

The exact pathogenesis of solitary neurofibroma remains unclear and genetic studies of neurofibromas in the literature are scarce. Systemic review of genetic analysis of solitary neurofibroma was also analyzed (Table 4). Beert et al. identified a bi-allelic NF inactivation as the cause of solitary neurofibroma in a 13-year-old boy without other NF diagnostic criteria [21]. Bi-allelic inactivation leading to the development of neurofibroma seems to occur in embryonic cells, which have the potential of cells carrying a NF second-hit mutation. Jungmann et al. identified p.P733L mutation in exon 15 of the *KIT* gene in a 22-year-old man with solitary neurofibroma on the left flank [22]. Sawyer et al. revealed reciprocal translocation t(4;9)(q31;p22) in a 29-year-old woman with solitary neurofibroma on her left arm [23]. Sugiyama et al. presented abnormal gains in NF-1 gene (17q11.2) by the single nucleotide polymorphism identification method in a 33-year-old man with solitary epicranial neurofibroma [24]. Solitary neurofibromas in "clinically" non-NF-1 patients are benign tumors and the identification of genetic aberrations in these tumors are not expected to play a role in diagnosis. However, it was believed that genetic sporadic mutation or familial germline mutation were essential for pathogenesis and further genetic investigation

Table 3 Description of image study

Author	Year of publication	Description of Image study	
		Computed Tomography	Magnetic resonance imaging
Topsakal et al. [4]	2001	Smooth-contoured hypodense lesion with intermediate contrast-enhancement	T1-weighted image: intermediate intensity T2-weighted image: high intensity with a well-circumscribed low intensity center. It was also partially enhanced with contrast-medium
Kim et al. [5]	2013	A well-defined, 1.6 cm sized ovoid retroperitoneal mass with intermediate contrast-enhancement	Not mention
Dafford et al. [6]	2007	Low attenuating and hypodense mass lesion	T2-weighted image: High signal intensity with a low intensity surrounding. Hypointense septations have also been reported
Shen et al. [7]	2016	Hypodense lesion and with partially contrast-enhancement	Not mention
Ishikawa et al. [8]	1989	Well encapsulated homogeneous and hypodense mass lesion	Not mention
Hunter et al. [9]	1988	Not mention	Not mention
Cowles et al. [10]	1987	Not mention	Not mention
Gupta et al. [11]	2015	Heterogeneously intermediate enhancing mass lesion with calcification	Not mention

Table 4 Genetic analysis

Author	Year of publication	Family history	Genetic analysis of mutation
Beert et al. [21]	2012	No	Insertion of chromosomal bands 1p36-p35 at 17q11.2, in 11 of 18 analyzed cells (Biallelic *NF1* inactivation).
Jungmann et al. [22]	2016	Yes	p.P733L mutation in exon 15 of the *KIT* gene, while wild-type sequences were found in *KIT* exons 8, 9, 11, 13, 14 and 17.
Sawyer et al. [23]	2004	Yes	Reciprocal translocation t(4;9)(q31;p22)
Sugiyama et al. [24]	2014	No	Abnormal gains in NF1 gene (17q11.2)

combined with more case experience can provide more information of pathogenic mechanism.

A solitary retroperitoneal neurofibroma is rare, and it can be misdiagnosed as an adnexal mass. A neurofibroma can be associated with NF-1; however, a solitary pelvic neurofibroma probably arises de novo without other organ involvement. It usually does not have any neurological deficit. Inadequately localized pain is the most common symptom, and the other clinical symptoms depend on the tumor location. Histology of the excised tumor specimen is the only diagnostic tool. Computed tomography could facilitate preoperative diagnosis. Complete surgical resection is the only treatment for such tumors—it is preferred because it prevents local recurrence and malignant transformation. We present this case to demonstrate that pelvic neurofibroma can be mistaken for an adnexal mass. This fact should be borne in mind during the diagnosis process.

Abbreviations

NF: Neurofibromatosis; NF-1: Neurofibromatosis type I; *NIH*: National Institutes of Health; *PRISMA*: Preferred Reporting Items for *Systematic* Reviews and Meta-Analyses; *SOX-10*: SRY-related HMG-box-10

Acknowledgements

This work was supported by grants from the Ministry of Science and Technology, Executive Yuan (MOST 103-2314-B-010-043-MY3 and MOST 106-2314-B-075-061-MY3), and Taipei Veterans General Hospital (V105C-096, V106C-129; V107C-136; and 106D23-001-MY2-1).No external funding was received for this study. The authors thank the Medical Science & Technology Building of Taipei Veterans General Hospital for providing experimental space and facilities.

Authors' contributions

WTC collected the clinical data, carried out the manual microdissection and drafted the manuscript. WTC and CMC participated in the treatment and reviewed the manuscript. CHL, YJC and HHW carried out the pathological diagnosis and immunohistochemical staining. PHW conceived of the study and wrote and revised the manuscript. All authors read and approved the final manuscript.

Competing interests

The authors declare that they have no competing interests.

Author details

[1]Faculty of Medicine, College of Medicine, Fu-Jen Catholic University, Taipei, Taiwan. [2]Faculty of Medicine, School of Medicine, National Yang-Ming University, Taipei, Taiwan. [3]Section of Gynecologic Oncology, Department of Obstetrics and Gynecology, Taipei Veterans General Hospital, No. 201, Section 2, Shih-Pai Road, Taipei 112, Taiwan. [4]Department of Midwifery and Women Health Care, National Taipei University of Nursing and Health Sciences, Taipei, Taiwan. [5]Department of Medical Research, China Medical University Hospital, Taichung, Taiwan.

References

1. Bakhshi GD, Tayade MB, Yadav RB, Jadhav KV, Shenoy SS, Amin MV. Pelvic neurofibroma. Clin Pract. 2014;4:660.
2. Moher D, Liberati A, Tetzlaff J, Altman DG, PRISMA Group. Reprint–preferred reporting items for systematic reviews and meta-analyses: the PRISMA statement. Phys Ther. 2009;89:873–80.
3. Lo CK, Mertz D, Loeb M. Newcastle-Ottawa scale: comparing reviewers' to authors' assessments. BMC Med Res Methodol. 2014;14:45.
4. Topsakal C, Erol FS, Ozercan I, Murat A, Gurates B. Presacral solitary giant neurofibroma without neurofibromatosis type 1 presenting as pelvic mass–case report. Neurol Med Chir (Tokyo). 2001;41:620–5.
5. Kim S, Kim YS, Kim JH, Min YD, Hong R. Early gastric cancer with neurofibroma mimicking a metastatic node: a case report. J Gastric Cancer. 2013;13:185–7.
6. Dafford K, Kim D, Reid N, Kline D. Pelvic plexus tumors. Neurosurg Focus. 2007;22:E10.
7. Shen XQ, Shen H, Wu SC, Lv Y, Lu H, Lin XJ. Surgically treated solitary giant gluteal and retroperitoneal neurofibroma: a case report. World J Surg Oncol. 2016;14:125.
8. Ishikawa J, Kamidono S, Maeda S, et al. Solitary retroperitoneal neurofibroma: a case report. Hinyokika Kiyo. 1989;35:1157–60.
9. Hunter VP, Burke TW, Crooks LA. Retroperitoneal nerve sheath tumors: an unusual cause of pelvic mass. Obstet Gynecol. 1988;71:1050–2.
10. Cowles T, Schwartz PE. A suprapubic retroperitoneal operative approach to solitary paravaginal tumors. Obstet Gynecol. 1987;69:420–2.
11. Gupta P, Aggarwal R, Sarangi R. Solitary neurofibroma of the adrenal gland not associated with type-1 neurofibromatosis. Urol Ann. 2015;7:124–6.
12. National Institutes of Health Consensus Development Conference Statement. Ovarian cancer: screening, treatment, and follow-up. Gynecol Oncol. 1994;55:S4–14.
13. Borgfeldt C, Andolf E. Transvaginal sonographic ovarian findings in a random sample of women 25-40 years old. Ultrasound Obstet Gynecol. 1999;13:345–50.
14. Barajas-Gamboa JS, Florez-Salamanca L. Solitary neurofibroma in the abdominal wall of a patient without neurofibromatosis: case report. Biomedica. 2009;29:501–5.
15. Bequet D, Labauge P, Larroque P, Renard JL, Goasguen J. Peripheral neurofibromatosis and involvement of lumbosacral nerves. Value of imaging. Rev Neurol (Paris). 1990;146:757–61.
16. Erlandson RA, Woodruff JM. Peripheral nerve sheath tumors: an electron microscopic study of 43 cases. Cancer. 1982;49:273–87.
17. Seppala MT, Haltia MJ, Sankila RJ, Jääskeläinen JE, Heiskanen O. Long-term outcome after removal of spinal neurofibroma. J Neurosurg. 1995;82:572–7.
18. Zimmerman RA, Bilaniuk LT. Imaging of tumors of the spinal canal and cord. Radiol Clin N Am. 1988;26:965–1007.
19. Lu H, Chen Q, Shen H. Hamartoma compress medial and radial nerve in neurofibromatosis type 1. Int J Clin Exp Med. 2015;8:15313–6.
20. Levy WJ, Latchaw J, Hahn JF, Sawhny B, Bay J, Dohn DF. Spinal neurofibromas: a report of 66 cases and a comparison with meningiomas. Neurosurgery. 1986;18:331–4.
21. Beert E, Brems H, Renard M, Ferreiro JF, Melotte C, Thoelen R, et al. Biallelic inactivation of NF1 in a sporadic plexiform neurofibroma. Genes Chromosomes Cancer. 2012;51:852–7.

22. Jungmann J, Heydt C, Bohle R, Pfohler C, Vogt T, Muller CS. Genetic basis of a solitary familial plexiform neurofibroma without verified associated neurofibromatosis. J Dtsch Dermatol Ges. 2016;14:525–7.
23. Sawyer JR, Parr LG, Gokden N, Nicholas RW. A reciprocal t(4;9)(q31;p22) in a solitary neurofibroma. Cancer Genet Cytogenet. 2005;156:172–4.
24. Sugiyama N, Tsutsumi S, Akiba C, Nakanishi H, Ogino I, Yasumoto Y, et al. Solitary epicranial neurofibroma with NF1-related germline mutation: case report. Neurol Med Chir (Tokyo). 2014;54:310–3.

2

Characterization of ovarian cancer cells and tissues by Fourier transform infrared spectroscopy

Lei Li[1], Xiaoning Bi[1], Hengzi Sun[1], Simiao Liu[1], Mei Yu[1], Ying Zhang[1], Shifu Weng[2], Limin Yang[3], Yanan Bao[2], Jinguang Wu[2], Yizhuang Xu[2*] and Keng Shen[1*]

Abstract

Background: Ovarian cancer is the most lethal of gynecological malignancies. Fourier Transform Infrared (FTIR) spectroscopy has gradually developed as a convenient, inexpensive and non-destructive technique for the study of many diseases. In this study, FTIR spectra of normal and several heterogeneous ovarian cancer cell lines as well as ovarian cancer tissue samples were compared in the spectral region of 4000 cm^{-1} - 600 cm^{-1}.

Methods: Cell samples were collected from human ovarian surface epithelial cell line (HOSEpiC) and five ovarian cancer cell lines (ES2, A2780, OVCAR3, SKOV3 and IGROV1). Validation spectra were performed on normal and cancerous tissue samples from 12 ovarian cancer patients. FTIR spectra were collected from a NICOLET iN10 MX spectrometer and the spectral data were analyzed by OMNIC 8.0 software.

Results: Spectral features discriminating malignant tissues from normal tissues were integrated by cell line data and tissue data. In particular changes in cancerous tissues, the decrease in the amount of lipids and nucleic acids were observed. Protein conformation and composition were also altered in some cancer cells. The band intensity ratio of 1454/1400 was higher in normal cells/tissues and lower in cancer cells/tissues.

Conclusion: The spectral features revealed the important molecular characteristics about ovarian cancer cells/ tissues. These findings demonstrate the possible diagnostic use of FTIR spectroscopy, providing the research model and evidences, and supporting the future study on more tissue samples to establish a data bank of spectra features for the possible discrimination of ovarian cancers.

Keywords: Ovarian cancer, Fourier transform infrared (FTIR) spectroscopy, Tumor heterogeneity, Clinical diagnosis

Background

Ovarian cancer is associated with the worst prognosis among gynecological malignancies, accounting for more than 150,000 deaths annually worldwide [1]. Most patients with advanced stages of ovarian cancer result in five-year survival rates less than 30% [2]. Ovarian cancer includes several heterogeneous subtypes with different clinical phenotypes, molecular features and prognosis. About 90 % are epithelial ovarian cancers (EOC) [3], which is traditionally subtyped as serous, endometrioid, clear cell and mucinous. Among them, serous ovarian cancer accounts for about 70% of EOC [4]. High-grade serous ovarian cancer (HGSOC), the most malignant subtype, is responsible for 90% of serous tumors [5]. Developing methods for detecting ovarian cancer at the early stage and illuminating the molecular mechanism underlying this tumor heterogeneity would provide us new insights into ovarian cancer and lead to more effective diagnostic approaches.

Currently, there are two approaches available for diagnosing ovarian cancer patients. One is the detection of the blood-derived biomarkers. The frequently used

* Correspondence: xuyzh_peking@sina.com; kengshen_pumch@sina.com
[2]Beijing National Laboratory for Molecular Sciences, State Key Laboratory for Rare Earth Materials Chemistry and Applications, College of Chemistry and Molecular Engineering, Peking University, No. 202 Chengfu Road, Haidian District, Beijing 100871, China
[1]Department of Obstetrics and Gynecology, Peking Union Medical College Hospital, Chinese Academy of Medical Sciences & Peking Union Medical College, No. 1 Shuai Fu Yuan, Eastern District, Beijing 100730, China
Full list of author information is available at the end of the article

biomarker is serum Cancer Antigen 125 (CA-125) [6]. However, limited specificity exists in this method as CA-125 level also rises in some other types of cancers and also fluctuates in premenopausal women during menstrual cycle [7]. The other method is to provide detailed images of ovaries through imaging techniques such as Magnetic Resonance Imaging (MRI), Doppler Ultrasound and Computed Tomography (CT). However, ultrasound shows a poor accuracy in diagnosing diseases at early stages [8]. It is obvious that these current methods have some limitations. Therefore new insights are needed to identify novel methods for detecting and categorizing ovarian cancer patients.

Vibrational spectroscopy is one kind of the bio-analytical methods that increasingly shows significant potential to provide a novel diagnostic tool to distinguish normal and pathological tissues [9]. Fourier-transform infrared (FTIR) spectroscopy, in particular, has been utilized in the past several decades [10–12]. It has the advantage of convenience and non-destruction to detect tumors with minimal sample preparations, and also allows the investigation of both qualitative and quantitative assesses of certain components [13, 14].

Many studies by this technique have been focused on several cancer cells or tissues, such as endometrial [15], cervical [16], breast [17], lung [18] and brain cancers [19]. Few studies have screened ovarian cancer by FTIR. Gajjar et al. [20], Owens et al [21] and Lima et al [22] have respectively examined blood plasma or serum of ovarian cancer by attenuated total reflection Fourier-transform infrared (ATR-FTIR) spectroscopy coupled with other selection methods. Mehrotra et al [23] analyzed FTIR data of the post surgical tissue sections of ovarian cancer and discovered some particular changes in the spectral regions of protein, nucleic acid and lipid, using 12 samples without classifying the cancer subtype. Theophilou et al [24] provided a novel approach in discriminating normal, borderline and malignant ovarian tissues. The authors used ATR-FTIR spectroscopy combined with three chemometric methods followed by linear discriminant analysis. However, there were little common insights in these few studies, as they explored on different aspects. In the present study, we fundamentally focused on EOC with respect to its normal and several heterogeneous cancer cell line models using FTIR technique and confirmed the results by several tissue samples, providing proof of principal that there were differences between EOC and healthy donor epithelium and supporting the future study to move to more clinical tissue samples to establish a data bank of spectra features.

Methods

Cell culture

The normal cell line used in this study was human ovarian surface epithelial cell line (HOSEpiC) obtained from ScienCell Research Laboratories (San Diego, CA). The ovarian cancer cell lines used in this study were ES2, A2780, OVCAR3, SKOV3 and IGROV1. Among them, ES2, A2780 and SKOV3 were purchased from the Cell Support Center, Institute of Basic Medical Science, Chinese Academy of Medical Sciences; OVCAR3 and IGROV1 were purchased from the NIH cell bank. OVCAR3 originates from the malignant ascites of a patient with ovarian adenocarcinoma [25], possesses characteristics of HGSOC [26]. ES2 is a recognized ovarian clear cell carcinoma cell line [27]. IGROV1, originating from an ovarian carcinoma of a 47-year-old woman, is an ovarian adenocarcinoma cell line with multiple differentiations, and endometrioid is its major part [28]. A2780 and SKOV3 both have been widely used as models for HGSOC. However, recent studies demonstrated that they carried some characteristics of endometrioid/clear cell ovarian carcinomas [26].

HOSEpiC, A2780, IGROV1 and OVCAR3 cells were incubated in Roswell Park Memorial Institute (RPMI)-1640 medium (HyClone, Logan, Utah, USA) supplemented with 15, 10, 10 and 20% heat-inactivated fetal bovine serum (FBS; Gibco, Carlsbad, CA, USA), respectively, at 37 °C in 5% carbon dioxide. ES2 and SKOV3 cells were cultured in McCoy's 5A medium (HyClone) containing 10% FBS at 37 °C in 5% carbon dioxide. The cells were subcultured when they reached approximately 80% confluence, and harvested at almost the same life time after two passages.

Cell preparation for spectroscopy

Cells were trypsinized and washed twice in saline, suspended and centrifuged at 1000 rpm for 5 min. Supernatant was then removed gently and cells were stored at − 80 °C until removal for experiments.

Tissue collection and preparation for spectroscopy

Tissue specimens from 12 cases of EOC were obtained from Peking Union Medical College Hospital, Chinese Academy of Medical Sciences & Peking Union Medical College. Informed consents have been taken before surgery. Cancer tissue and their corresponding normal tissue samples were collected respectively from 10 histologically serous cancer and 2 clear cell cancer patients. Tissue samples were frozen at − 80 °C until removal for spectral scanning.

FTIR spectroscopy

FTIR spectra of cell and tissue samples were collected using a NICOLET iN10 MX (Thermo Scientific, Waltham, MA, USA) spectrometer, equipped with a KBr/Ge beam splitter and a mercury cadmium telluride (MCT) detector. For each spectrum, 16 scans were performed at the resolution of 4 cm^{-1} between 4000 cm^{-1} and 600 cm^{-1}. The spectrum was then baseline corrected and normalized from 0 to 1 so as to have better comparison for the intensity.

Analysis of FTIR data

Second Derivative (DII) and Curve Fitting (Gaussian algorithm) procedures were performed to identify the precise position and absorbance of specific bands. By using OMNIC 8.0 software (Thermo Fisher Scientific), Curve Fitting was conducted on spectra in the range of 1700–1600 cm^{-1} after two points baseline linear fitted. In order to determine the underlying component bands, the number of peaks as well as their positions was identified based on DII results, resulting in the optimal reconstructed curve (residual close to zero). Positions and percentages of band areas were obtained for every component peak.

Subtraction spectra

In order to further identify spectral variations between normal cells and ovarian cancer cells, the spectrum of ovarian surface epithelial cell line (HOSEpiC) was subtracted by the spectrum of each of the ovarian cancer cell lines, respectively. Thus we obtained the "subtraction spectra". All of the subtraction spectra were calculated using fully preprocessed spectra, that were baseline corrected and normalized from 0 to 1.

Statistical analysis

The percentages of band areas are presented as mean ± SEM. For statistical comparisons among multiple cell lines, one-way ANOVA test was used by SPSS 17.0 software (Chicago, Illinois, USA) with a significance set at $P < 0.05$ for at least three times. For statistical comparisons of spectra intensities between normal and malignant tissues at specific bands, a Wilcoxon paired signed-rank test with a significant level of 0.05 was used by SPSS 17.0 software.

Results

FTIR spectral analysis for normal and ovarian cancer cell lines

This study first focused on the biochemical differences between several heterogeneous ovarian cancer cell lines (ES2, A2780, OVCAR3, SKOV3 and IGROV1) and the normal human ovarian surface epithelial cell line (HOSEpiC) by FTIR spectroscopy. For each cell line, a typical spectrum was presented (Fig. 1). The apparent spectral differences were observed, above all in the C-H stretching region of fatty acids in cell membranes (3000–2800 cm^{-1}), in the ester C = O stretching of phospholipids (1800–1700 cm^{-1}) and in the C-H bending vibrations of amino acid side chains and some lipids (1500–1300 cm^{-1}) [29]. Relative band intensities, which could be considered as spectral features for normal and cancer cells, were calculated. Second Derivative (DII) and Curve Fitting procedures of 1700–1600 cm^{-1} were used to investigate Amide I of protein, and subtraction spectra were performed in the region of 4000–600 cm^{-1} for additional comparison of each ovarian cancer cells versus normal cells.

Comparison of the relative intensities of the specific bands for normal and ovarian cancer cell lines

Several spectral markers for cancer cell lines differed considerably from normal cell line, as shown in Fig. 2. The band signals at 2958 cm^{-1} and 2925 cm^{-1} (ν_{asym} CH_3 and CH_2), 2872 cm^{-1} and 2854 cm^{-1} (ν_{sym} CH_3 and CH_2) are characteristics of alkyl chains mainly present in lipids [30]. After analyzing the relative band intensities, lower amounts of the relative intensities of 2925 cm^{-1} and 2854 cm^{-1} were found in the five cancer cells as compared to HOSEpiC cells, respectively (Fig. 2a, b), consisting with their corresponding FTIR spectra in the region of 3000–2800 cm^{-1} (Fig. 3a). The differences were significant for ES2, A2780, OVCAR3 and IGROV1 vs. HOSEpiC, respectively, indicating a lower amount of lipids present in the four cancer cells. Moreover, ovarian cancer cell lines also showed heterogeneous characteristics between themselves. ES2 showed lower relative intensity at 2925 cm^{-1} than that of OVCAR3, SKOV3 and IGROV1, respectively. The relative intensity at 2925 cm^{-1} in A2780 was significantly lower from that in SKOV3, while the relative intensity at 2854 cm^{-1} in ES2 was significantly lower from that in SKOV3 (Fig. 2a, b).

The absorption bands at 1242 cm^{-1} ($\nu_{as}PO_2^-$) and 1086 cm^{-1} ($\nu_sPO_2^-$) were attributed to asymmetric and symmetric phosphodiester vibrations of nucleic acids [31]. The relative intensity at 1242 cm^{-1} in OVCAR3 was lower than that in HOSEpiC, A2780, SKOV3 and IGROV1, respectively (Fig. 2d). A2780 showed lower relative intensity at 1086 cm^{-1} than that of OVCAR3, SKOV3 and IGROV1, while ES2 showed lower relative intensity at 1086 cm^{-1} than that of SKOV3 and IGROV1 (Fig. 2e). The differences were all significant. These findings also suggested heterogeneous characteristics between ovarian cancer cells.

In the absorption signals between 1800 and 1700 cm^{-1}, the prominent band intensity difference was found around 1741 cm^{-1}, which was attributed to ester C = O stretching of phospholipids [32, 33]. It is obvious that the signal at 1741 cm^{-1} was enhanced in HOSEpiC cells than in all of the ovarian cancer cells (Fig. 2c, Fig. 3b), indicating increased lipids and esterified components in cell membranes in normal ovarian cells than in cancerous cells. This result was in corroboration with the previous finding in breast cancer cells that the peak at 1741 cm^{-1} increased progressively with the increasing

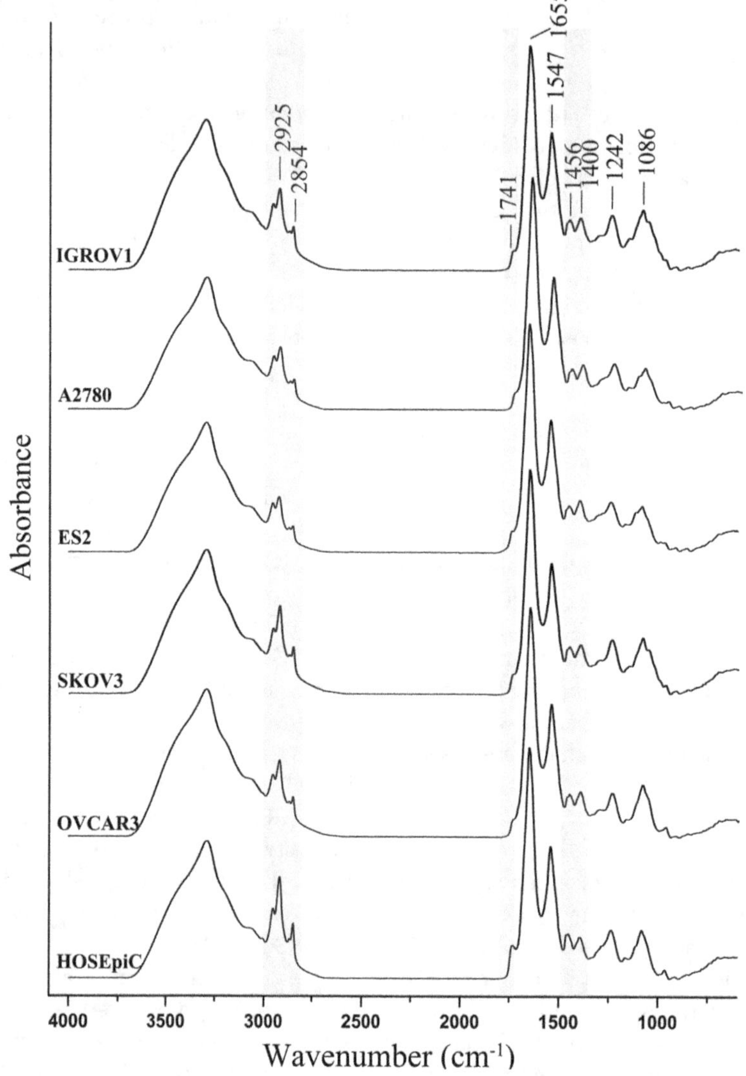

Fig. 1 Representative FTIR spectra of ovarian cancer cells and normal cells. FTIR spectra of the five ovarian cancer cell lines (IGROV1, A2780, ES2, SKOV3 and OVCAR3) and the normal human ovarian surface epithelial cell line (HOSEpiC) were presented in the region 4000–600 cm^{-1}. The apparent differences were indicated in blue box

5-fluorouracil dose in MCF-7 cells (human breast adenocarcinoma cell line) [34]. As 5-fluorouracil overtly inhibited tumor cell proliferation in a concentration dependent manner, cells with the high level of proliferation showed the lower peak at 1741 cm^{-1}, correspondence with our result that the malignant ovarian cancer cells exhibited lower intensities at 1741 cm^{-1} than normal ovarian cells.

The bands at 1454 and 1400 cm^{-1} usually attribute to the C-H bending vibrations of various amino acid side chains and some lipids, etc. [29]. They are critical bands to distinguish normal and malignant tissues, and the precise assignments are not clear [35]. It is obvious to see that the band height at 1454 cm^{-1} was always lower than that at 1400 cm^{-1} in all of the ovarian cancer cell lines ($I_{1454}/I_{1400} < 1$). In HOSEpiC cells, comparison of the heights of the two bands were apparently opposite ($I_{1454}/I_{1400} > 1$). Besides, ES2 exhibited the lowest ratio of 1454/1400 among other cells (Fig. 2f, Fig. 3c).

Curve fitting of protein amide I in normal and ovarian cancer cell lines

The region between 1700 cm^{-1} and 1500 cm^{-1} was usually assigned to protein absorption with dominant bands at ~ 1655 cm^{-1} (Amide I) and ~ 1547 cm^{-1} (Amide II) [36]. After the Curve Fitting procedure, Amide I of the cells was analyzed respectively and split into a series of bands. In general for Amide I, α-helical structures have a band at 1653 ± 4 cm^{-1}; β-sheet structures occurs between 1620 and 1640 cm^{-1}; β-turn structures are usually found at 1660–1680 cm^{-1} [37]. The percentage of

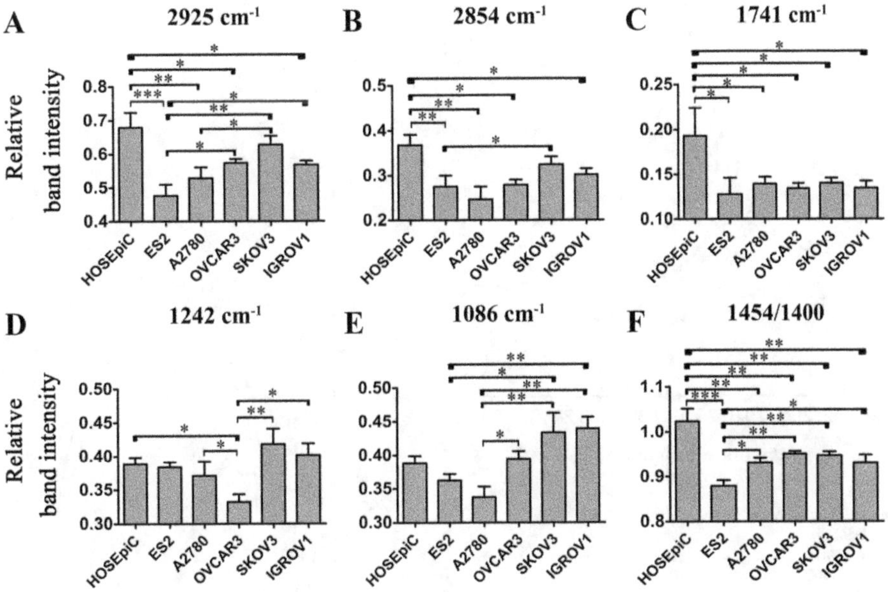

Fig. 2 Relative band intensitie of normal cells and ovarian cancer cells. Error bars represent the SEM, $n = 3$ (*: $P < 0.05$. **: $P < 0.01$. ***: $P < 0.001$)

the component band areas, representative of their relative amounts, was calculated (Table 1). The band areas of β-sheet structures in HOSEpiC were significantly lower than that in ES2 and higher than that in SKOV3 [(25.45 ± 0.07) % vs. (26.55 ± 0.36) %, (25.45 ± 0.07) % vs. (23.71 ± 0.35) %], while the band areas of α-helical structures in HOSEpiC were significantly higher than that in ES2 and lower than that in SKOV3 [(16.39 ± 0.04) % vs. (15.51 ± 0.04) %, (16.39 ± 0.04) % vs. (18.09 ± 0.23) %]. HOSEpiC also had a higher band area of β-turn structures than ES2 [(50.92 ± 0.17) % vs. (50.09 ± 0.37) %]. There also seemed significant differences between normal and some cancer cells and differences among the different types of ovarian cancer cells (Fig. 4, Table 1). These findings indicated that the secondary structure of protein had been altered in some but not all types of cancer cells, probably attributed to cell specificity.

Subtraction spectrum of the ovarian cancer cells vs. normal cells

In order to further indentify the differences between normal cells and ovarian cancer cells, subtraction spectrum was performed for each of the cancer cell line vs. HOSEpiC, respectively. In subtraction spectra, the differences between the two samples in details were observed visibly. For example, if we have A and B spectra, adjusting subtraction factor using subtraction spectrum is performed, and the positive and negative bands were clearly observed. A-B, the same components of A and B were subtracted out; positive bands represent the part A > B, while negative bands represent the part B > A [38, 39]. As showing in Fig. 5, positive bands, indicating higher amounts, were seen in the region 3600–3000 cm^{-1} ($\nu_{N\text{-}H}$ of protein) as well as at the bands around 1655 cm^{-1}, 1548 cm^{-1} and 1406 cm^{-1} in all of the ovarian cancer cells. Negative bands, indicating lower amounts, were seen at the bands around 2922 cm^{-1}, 2852 cm^{-1} and 1741 cm^{-1} in ES2, A2780, OVCAR3 and IGROV1; negative bands for the subtraction spectrum of SKOV3 vs. HOSEpiC were seen at 2958 cm^{-1}, 2852 cm^{-1} and 1741 cm^{-1}. These were consistent with our above results that lower amounts in lipids (3000–2800 cm^{-1}) were found in ovarian cancer cells as compared to HOSEpiC cells, and that the signal at 1741 cm^{-1} was enhanced in HOSEpiC cells than in ovarian cancer cells. Increased amount at the band ~ 1406 cm^{-1} also indicated decreased ratio of 1454/1400 in ovarian cancer cells. These findings also suggested that ovarian cancer cells might have higher amount of protein (3600–3000 cm^{-1}, 1655 cm^{-1} and 1548 cm^{-1}) than normal cells. As proteins play crucial role in the physiological processes, the alteration of conformation and content of proteins in cancer cells may indicate a diversified and impending energy demands for the metabolism of malignant cells.

FTIR spectra analysis of normal and ovarian cancer tissues

To further confirm the data derived from ovarian cancer cell lines vs. HOSEpiC cell line, the FTIR spectra of normal and ovarian cancer tissues from 12 patients were analyzed. There were significant differences between normal and cancerous tissues identified in the regions 3000–2800 cm^{-1}, 1500–1300 cm^{-1} and 1300–900 cm^{-1} (Fig. 6).

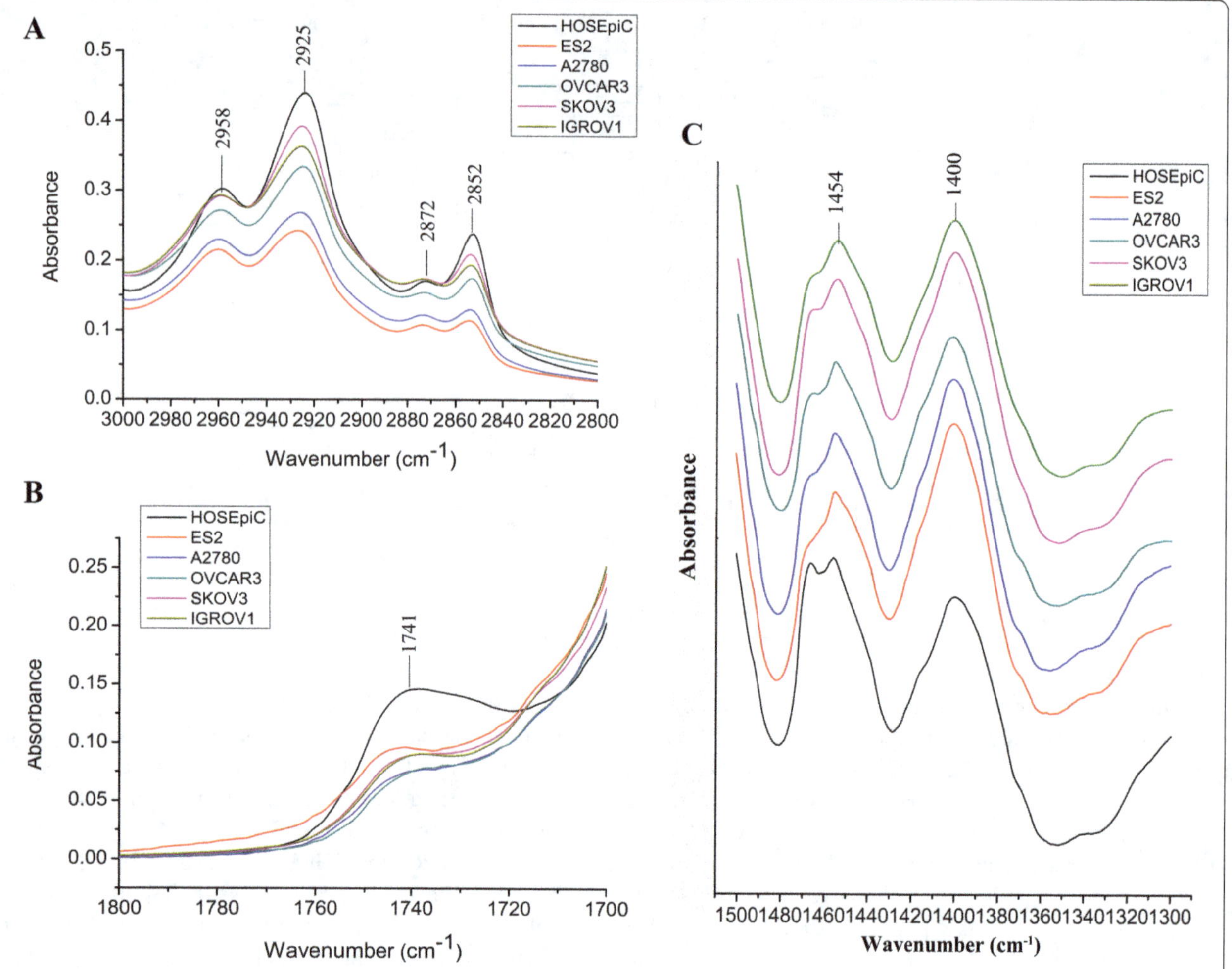

Fig. 3 FTIR spectra in the region 3000–2800 cm^{-1} (**a**), 1800–1700 cm^{-1} (**b**) and 1500–1300 cm^{-1} (**c**)

Table 1 Percentage of component band areas after Curve Fitting procedure in the region 1700–1600 cm^{-1}

Position	Area (%)						Assignment
	HOSEpiC	ES2	A2780	OVCAR3	SKOV3	IGROV1	
1629	9.46 ± 0.12	9.45 ± 0.02	9.66 ± 0.15	9.40 ± 0.04	8.91 ± 0.17	9.43 ± 0.12	β-sheet
1639	15.99 ± 0.18	17.10 ± 0.35	15.67 ± 0.28	15.18 ± 0.47	14.80 ± 0.17	16.16 ± 0.17	β-sheet
β-sheet SUM	**25.45 ± 0.07**	**26.55 ± 0.36**	**25.33 ± 0.43**	**24.58 ± 0.50**	**23.71 ± 0.35**	**25.59 ± 0.06**	**β-sheet SUM**
1649	**16.39 ± 0.04**	**15.51 ± 0.04**	**16.46 ± 0.25**	**16.89 ± 0.29**	**18.09 ± 0.23**	**16.58 ± 0.17**	**α-helical**
1657	22.86 ± 0.30	21.09 ± 0.35	22.34 ± 0.06	22.44 ± 0.24	23.46 ± 0.11	23.64 ± 0.11	β-turn
1667	9.38 ± 0.16	9.82 ± 0.29	9.66 ± 0.08	9.53 ± 0.09	9.60 ± 0.15	9.35 ± 0.15	β-turn
1674	5.13 ± 0.10	5.66 ± 0.06	5.31 ± 0.15	5.05 ± 0.05	4.70 ± 0.05	4.77 ± 0.04	β-turn
1681	13.55 ± 0.13	13.52 ± 0.25	13.32 ± 0.58	14.32 ± 0.44	13.15 ± 0.06	13.26 ± 0.07	β-turn
β-turn SUM	**50.92 ± 0.17**	**50.09 ± 0.37**	**50.63 ± 0.41**	**51.34 ± 0.24**	**50.91 ± 0.07**	**51.02 ± 0.06**	**β-turn SUM**
1693	7.24 ± 0.20	7.85 ± 0.03	7.58 ± 0.23	7.19 ± 0.03	7.29 ± 0.05	6.81 ± 0.18	

Bold texts indicate the area percentages of β-sheet, α-helical and β-turn structures, respectively

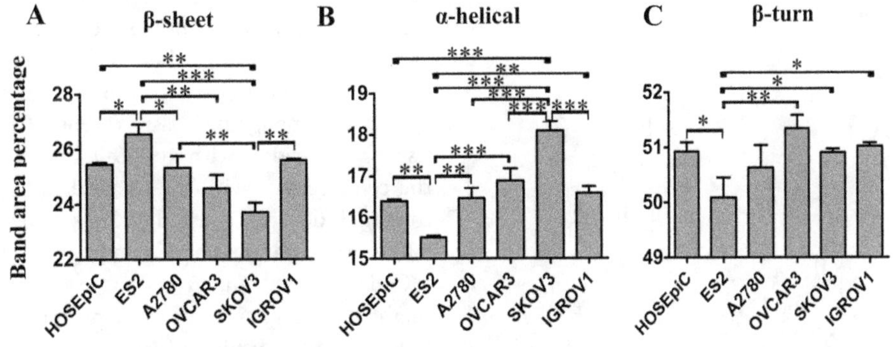

Fig. 4 Percentage of secondary structures of protein Amide I in normal and ovarian cancer cells. (**a**) β-sheet, (**b**) α-helix, (**c**) β-turn structures. Error bars represent the SEM, $n = 3$ (*: $P < 0.05$. **: $P < 0.01$. ***: $P < 0.001$)

Malignant tissues showed lower absorption signals in 3000–2800 cm^{-1}. The relative intensities of 2925 cm^{-1} and 2854 cm^{-1} were lower in malignant tissues and higher in normal tissues (Fig. 6); the differences were significant ($P = 0.010$, 0.023, respectively). Moreover, ten and eight ovarian cancer patients respectively showed lower absorption levels of 2925 cm^{-1} and 2854 cm^{-1} in malignant tissues (Fig. 7a, b), suggesting a decreased amount of lipids in malignant tissues. These results were consistent with the above cell line data.

For the absorption signal at around 1741 cm^{-1}, there was no significant difference ($P = 0.239$) between normal and malignant tissues, although there were still 9 in 12 patients showed lower signals at this peak in malignant tissues (Fig. 7c). Cell line data showed no significant differences between HOSEpiC and other five cancer cell lines at the band intensities of 1242 cm^{-1} and 1086 cm^{-1}, however, malignant tissues showed significantly lower intensities at 1242 cm^{-1} and 1086 cm^{-1} than normal tissues ($P = 0.003$, 0.002), and almost all the cancerous samples had the same decrease (11/12, 12/12; Fig. 7d, e). These findings indicated lower amount of nucleic acids in malignant tissues, and 1242 cm^{-1} and 1086 cm^{-1} might have been new spectra signatures to distinguish normal and ovarian cancer tissues.

The relative band intensity ratios of 1454/1400 were significantly lower in malignant tissues than normal tissues in all of the ovarian cancer patients ($P = 0.002$;

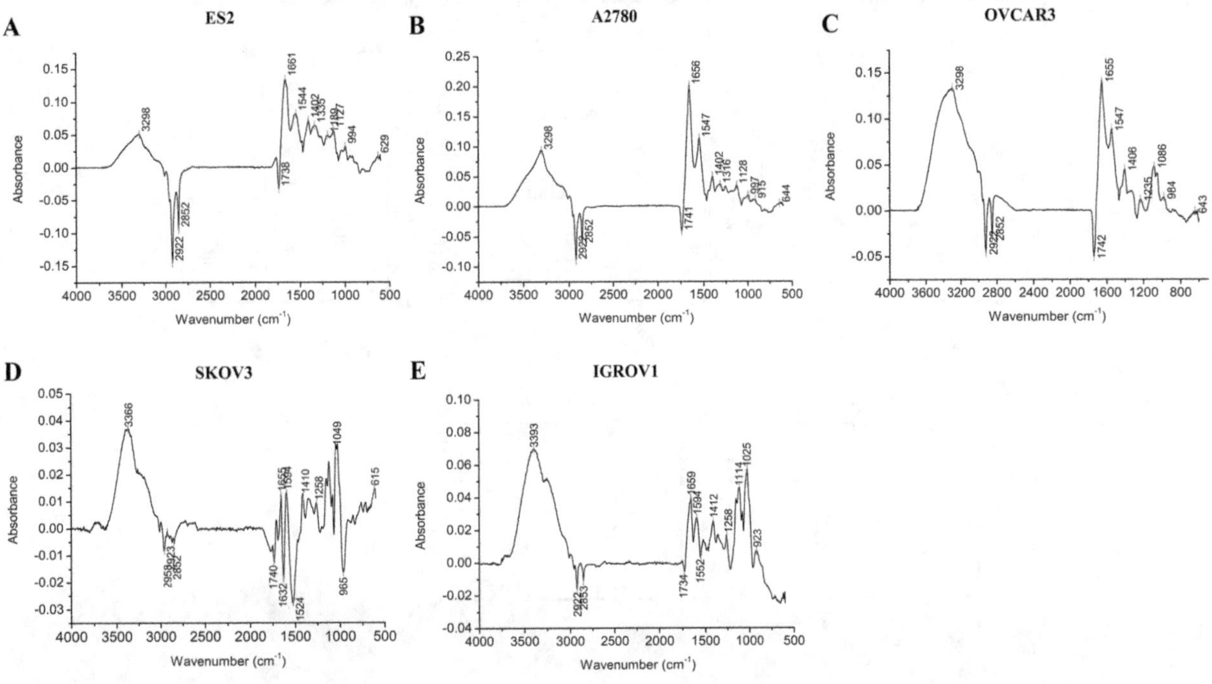

Fig. 5 Subtraction spectra of each of the ovarian cancer cells vs. normal cells. **a** ES2 vs. HOSEpiC, (**b**) A2780 vs. HOSEpiC, (**c**) OVCAR3 vs. HOSEpiC, (**d**) SKOV3 vs. HOSEpiC, (**e**) IGROV1 vs. HOSEpiC

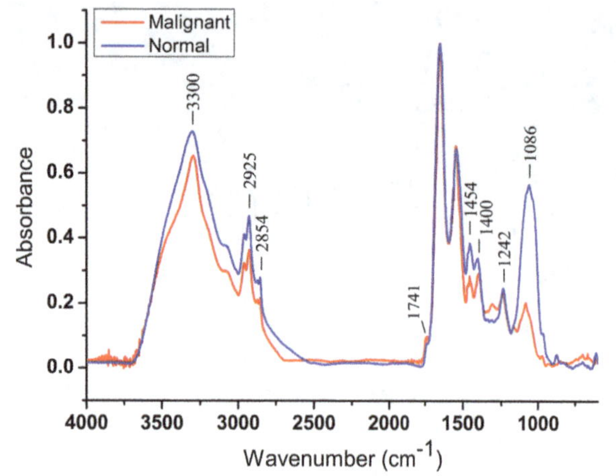

Fig. 6 Representative FTIR spectra of normal and malignant ovarian tissue

12/12). Cell line data above concluded that the ratios were $I_{1454}/I_{1400}>1$ for normal cells and $I_{1454}/I_{1400}<1$ for cancer cells, however, there were 9 patients with $I_{1454}/I_{1400} \geq 1$ in normal tissues and 11 patients with $I_{1454}/I_{1400}<1$ in malignant tissues (Fig. 7f). Not all of the tissues coincided with the cell line results. Integrating the cell line data with the tissue data, it was undoubtedly to conclude that normal tissues showed higher 1454/1400 ratios than its corresponding malignant tissues.

Cell line data analyzed that ovarian cancer cell lines might have higher amount of protein than normal cells, however, the results of the tissue samples were the opposite. Most patients exhibited lower signal levels of 3300 cm^{-1} and 1544 cm^{-1} in malignant tissues (Fig. 7g, h), indicating that the spectra feature of protein was debatable and needed further investigation.

Discussion

This study investigated the spectroscopic method to the identification of ovarian cancer. FTIR spectra were first analyzed on normal human ovarian surface epithelial cell line (HOSEpiC) and ovarian cancer cell lines (ES2,

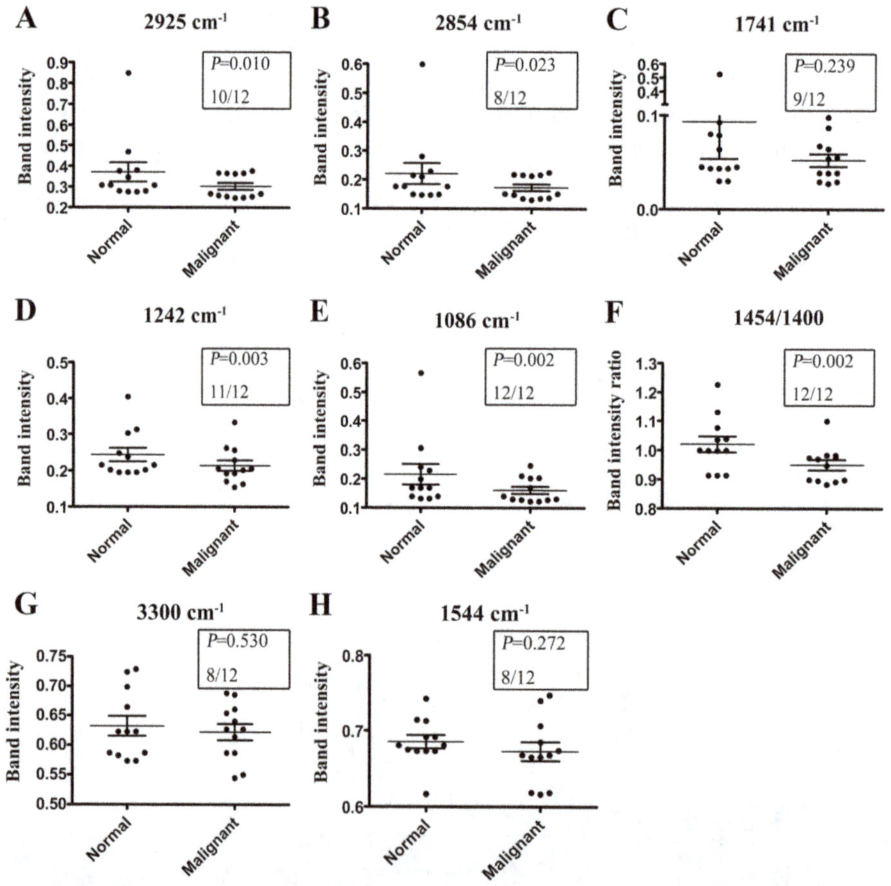

Fig. 7 Comparison of the specific band intensities for normal and malignant ovarian tissues. Error bars represent the SEM. *P* value and the numbers of patients with $I_{normal} > I_{malignant}$ at each specific bands (n/12) were indicated in boxes

A2780, OVCAR3, SKOV3 and IGROV1) at the molecular level in order to a better understanding of their ingredients and contents. The analysis was performed on the spectral ranges of CH_2, CH_3 and C = O stretching modes of lipids, Amide I band, and $\nu_{as}PO_2^-$ and $\nu_sPO_2^-$ of nucleic acids. The differences between normal cells and ovarian cancer cells were highlighted including (1) a decrease in lipid synthesis (3000–2800 cm^{-1}) in ovarian cancer cells; (2) lower amount of phospholipids in cell membrane (1741 cm^{-1}) in cancer cells; (3) the different proportion of the band intensity of ~ 1454 and ~ 1400 cm^{-1} in normal cells and in cancer cells, usually $I_{1454}/I_{1400} \geq 1$ for normal cells and $I_{1454}/I_{1400}<1$ for cancer cells; (4) an increase in protein amount (Amide I, Amide II and $\nu_{N\text{-}H}$ of proteins) in cancer cells.

These results were then verified by tissue samples from 12 ovarian cancer patients. FTIR spectra were compared and analyzed between normal tissues and the corresponding cancer tissues. However, there was no significant difference between normal and malignant tissues at the band intensity of 1741 cm^{-1}. The spectra features of protein (3300 cm^{-1} and 1544 cm^{-1}) were also not consistent with the cell line results. The intensity ratios of 1454/1400 were still lower in malignant tissues and higher normal tissues; however, $I_{1454}/I_{1400}>1$ or <1 was not the accurate criterion to distinguish normal and cancerous tissues. In addition, lower levels of nucleic acids (1242 cm^{-1} and 1086 cm^{-1}) were observed in malignant tissues; however, this result was not summarized by cell line data. To integrate cell line data with tissue sample data, we can conclude that the differences between normal and ovarian cancer tissues were included (1) a decrease in lipid synthesis in malignant tissues; (2) lower amount of nucleic acids in malignant tissues; (3) normal tissues showed higher 1454/1400 ratios than malignant tissues. These results have shown the remarkable spectra differences between normal and ovarian cancer cells/tissues with respect to their intensities of the prominent bands of cellular molecules, reflecting changes in the contents of proteins, nucleic acids and lipids. Cell line data also showed heterogeneity existing between different types of ovarian cancer cells. They differed in the synthesis of lipids and nucleic acids. The secondary structure of protein had also been altered between different types of cancer cells, indicating the appearance of new proteins and the alterations in their conformation and composition [23]. As for the data from tissue samples from 12 ovarian cancer patients, there were 10 serous and 2 clear cell cancer. However, no spectra differences were observed between the two types. This may because the sample size was quite small, and it might not be able to summarize the differences.

Conclusions

Although the results have considerable significance, more reliable evidences from tissue samples with heterogeneous subtypes are necessary to establish the specific and accurate spectral features that could classify malignant ovarian tissues from the normal tissues, as well as identify the precise type and status of malignant tissues. Spectral absorption modes of several heterogeneous ovarian cancer cell lines and some tissue samples primarily provide a research model and proof of principal that there are differences between EOC and healthy donor epithelium, and that this forms the evidences that further investigation is justified. Based on this, in the further study the FTIR spectrum, or prospectively in combination with other assistant methods, would be a useful diagnostic approach for ovarian cancer.

Abbreviations

ATR-FTIR: Attenuated total reflection Fourier-transform infrared; CA-125: Serum Cancer Antigen 125; CT: Computed Tomography; DII: Second Derivative; EOC: Epithelial ovarian cancer; FTIR: Fourier Transform Infrared; HGSOC: High-grade serous ovarian cancer; HOSEpiC: Human ovarian surface epithelial cell line; MRI: Magnetic Resonance Imaging

Funding

This study was supported by the National Natural Science Foundation of China (NO. 81502254) and the Chinese Academy of Medical Sciences Initiative for Innovative Medicine (CAMS-2017-I2M-1-002).

Authors' contributions

Conception and design: LL, JW, YX, KS; Funding acquisition: LL, KS; Data Acquisition: LL, JW, XB, HS, SW; Data analysis: LL, JW, SW, LY, YB; Project administration: LL, JW, KS; Investigation: LL, JW, LY; Writing original draft: LL, JW; Revising and editing: MY, YZ, JW, SL. All authors read and approved the final manuscript.

Competing interests

The authors declare that they have no competing interests.

Author details

[1]Department of Obstetrics and Gynecology, Peking Union Medical College Hospital, Chinese Academy of Medical Sciences & Peking Union Medical College, No. 1 Shuai Fu Yuan, Eastern District, Beijing 100730, China. [2]Beijing National Laboratory for Molecular Sciences, State Key Laboratory for Rare Earth Materials Chemistry and Applications, College of Chemistry and Molecular Engineering, Peking University, No. 202 Chengfu Road, Haidian District, Beijing 100871, China. [3]State Key Laboratory of Nuclear Physics and Technology, Institute of Heavy Ion Physics, School of Physics, Peking University, No. 202 Chengfu Road, Haidian District, Beijing 100871, China.

References

1. Ferlay J, Soerjomataram I, Dikshit R, Eser S, Mathers C, Rebelo M, Parkin DM, Forman D, Bray F. Cancer incidence and mortality worldwide: sources, methods and major patterns in GLOBOCAN 2012. Int J Cancer. 2015;136(5): E359–86.
2. Pierredon S, Ribaux P, Tille JC, Petignat P, Cohen M. Comparative secretome of ovarian serous carcinoma: gelsolin in the spotlight. Oncol Lett. 2017;13(6): 4965–73.
3. Chuaqui RF, Cole KA, Emmert-Buck MR, Merino MJ. Histopathology and molecular biology of ovarian epithelial tumors. Ann Diagn Pathol. 1998;2(3): 195–207.
4. Seidman JD, Horkayne-Szakaly I, Haiba M, Boice CR, Kurman RJ, Ronnett BM. The histologic type and stage distribution of ovarian carcinomas of surface epithelial origin. Int J Gynecol Pathol. 2004;23(1):41–4.
5. Gershenson DM, Sun CC, Lu KH, Coleman RL, Sood AK, Malpica A, Deavers MT, Silva EG, Bodurka DC. Clinical behavior of stage II-IV low-grade serous carcinoma of the ovary. Obstet Gynecol. 2006;108(2):361–8.
6. Fritsche HA, Bast RC. CA 125 in ovarian cancer: advances and controversy. Clin Chem. 1998;44(7):1379–80.
7. Togashi K. Ovarian cancer: the clinical role of US, CT, and MRI. Eur Radiol. 2003;13(Suppl 4):L87–104.
8. O'Rourke J, Mahon SM. A comprehensive look at the early detection of ovarian cancer. Clin J Oncol Nurs. 2003;7(1):41–7.
9. Martin FL. Shining a new light into molecular workings. Nat Methods. 2011; 8(5):385–7.
10. Baker MJ, Trevisan J, Bassan P, Bhargava R, Butler HJ, Dorling KM, Fielden PR, Fogarty SW, Fullwood NJ, Heys KA, Hughes C, Lasch P, Martin-Hirsch PL, Obinaju B, Sockalingum GD, Sule-Suso J, et al. Using Fourier transform IR spectroscopy to analyze biological materials. Nat Protoc. 2014;9(8):1771–91.
11. Jackson M, Sowa MG, Mantsch HH. Infrared spectroscopy: a new frontier in medicine. Biophys Chem. 1997;68(1–3):109–25.
12. Taillandier E, Liquier J. Infrared spectroscopy of DNA. Methods Enzymol. 1992;211:307–35.
13. Andrus PG, Strickland RD. Cancer grading by Fourier transform infrared spectroscopy. Biospectroscopy. 1998;4(1):37–46.
14. Wood BR, Quinn MA, Tait B, Ashdown M, Hislop T, Romeo M, McNaughton D. FTIR microspectroscopic study of cell types and potential confounding variables in screening for cervical malignancies. Biospectroscopy. 1998;4(2):75–91.
15. Taylor SE, Cheung KT, Patel II, Trevisan J, Stringfellow HF, Ashton KM, Wood NJ, Keating PJ, Martin-Hirsch PL, Martin FL. Infrared spectroscopy with multivariate analysis to interrogate endometrial tissue: a novel and objective diagnostic approach. Br J Cancer. 2011;104(5):790–7.
16. Sindhuphak R, Issaravanich S, Udomprasertgul V, Srisookho P, Warakamin S, Sindhuphak S, Boonbundarlchai R, Dusitsin N. A new approach for the detection of cervical cancer in Thai women. Gynecol Oncol. 2003;90(1):10–4.
17. Kelly JG, Ahmadzai AA, Hermansen P, Pitt MA, Saidan Z, Martin-Hirsch PL, Martin FL. A biospectroscopic interrogation of fine needle aspirates points towards segregation between graded categories: an initial study towards diagnostic screening. Anal Bioanal Chem. 2011;401(3):957–67.
18. Das RM, Ahmed MK, Mantsch HH, Scott JE. FT-IR spectroscopy of methylmercury-exposed mouse lung. Mol Cell Biochem. 1995;145(1):75–9.
19. Gajjar K, Heppenstall LD, Pang W, Ashton KM, Trevisan J, Patel II, Llabjani V, Stringfellow HF, Martin-Hirsch PL, Dawson T, Martin FL. Diagnostic segregation of human brain tumours using Fourier-transform infrared and/or Raman spectroscopy coupled with discriminant analysis. Anal Methods. 2012;5:89–102.
20. Gajjar K, Trevisan J, Owens G, Keating PJ, Wood NJ, Stringfellow HF, Martin-Hirsch PL, Martin FL. Fourier-transform infrared spectroscopy coupled with a classification machine for the analysis of blood plasma or serum: a novel diagnostic approach for ovarian cancer. Analyst. 2013;138(14):3917–26.
21. Owens GL, Gajjar K, Trevisan J, Fogarty SW, Taylor SE, Da Gama-Rose B, Martin-Hirsch PL, Martin FL. Vibrational biospectroscopy coupled with multivariate analysis extracts potentially diagnostic features in blood plasma/serum of ovarian cancer patients. J Biophotonics. 2014;7(3–4):200–9.
22. Lima KM, Gajjar KB, Martin-Hirsch PL, Martin FL. Segregation of ovarian cancer stage exploiting spectral biomarkers derived from blood plasma or serum analysis: ATR-FTIR spectroscopy coupled with variable selection methods. Biotechnol Prog. 2015;31(3):832–9.
23. Mehrotra R, Tyagi G, Jangir DK, Dawar R, Gupta N. Analysis of ovarian tumor pathology by Fourier transform infrared spectroscopy. J Ovarian Res. 2010;3:27.
24. Theophilou G, Lima KM, Martin-Hirsch PL, Stringfellow HF, Martin FL. ATR-FTIR spectroscopy coupled with chemometric analysis discriminates normal, borderline and malignant ovarian tissue: classifying subtypes of human cancer. Analyst. 2016;141(2):585–94.
25. Hamilton TC, Young RC, McKoy WM, Grotzinger KR, Green JA, Chu EW, Whang-Peng J, Rogan AM, Green WR, Ozols RF. Characterization of a human ovarian carcinoma cell line (NIH:OVCAR-3) with androgen and estrogen receptors. Cancer Res. 1983;43(11):5379–89.
26. Domcke S, Sinha R, Levine DA, Sander C, Schultz N. Evaluating cell lines as tumour models by comparison of genomic profiles. Nat Commun. 2013;4:2126.
27. Lau DH, Lewis AD, Ehsan MN, Sikic BI. Multifactorial mechanisms associated with broad cross-resistance of ovarian carcinoma cells selected by cyanomorpholino doxorubicin. Cancer Res. 1991;51(19):5181–7.
28. Benard J, Da Silva J, De Blois MC, Boyer P, Duvillard P, Chiric E, Riou G. Characterization of a human ovarian adenocarcinoma line, IGROV1, in tissue culture and in nude mice. Cancer Res. 1985;45(10):4970–9.
29. Dong L, Sun X, Chao Z, Zhang S, Zheng J, Gurung R, Du J, Shi J, Xu Y, Zhang Y, Wu J. Evaluation of FTIR spectroscopy as diagnostic tool for colorectal cancer using spectral analysis. Spectrochim Acta A Mol Biomol Spectrosc. 2014;122:288–94.
30. Gioacchini G, Giorgini E, Vaccari L, Ferraris P, Sabbatini S, Bianchi V, Borini A, Carnevali O. A new approach to evaluate aging effects on human oocytes: Fourier transform infrared imaging spectroscopy study. Fertil Steril. 2014; 101(1):120–7.
31. Wood BR, Chiriboga L, Yee H, Quinn MA, McNaughton D, Diem M. Fourier transform infrared (FTIR) spectral mapping of the cervical transformation zone, and dysplastic squamous epithelium. Gynecol Oncol. 2004;93(1):59–68.
32. Derenne A, Van Hemelryck V, Lamoral-Theys D, Kiss R, Goormaghtigh E. FTIR spectroscopy: a new valuable tool to classify the effects of polyphenolic compounds on cancer cells. Biochim Biophys Acta. 2013;1832(1):46–56.
33. Gaigneaux A, Ruysschaert JM, Goormaghtigh E. Infrared spectroscopy as a tool for discrimination between sensitive and multiresistant K562 cells. Eur J Biochem. 2002;269(7):1968–73.
34. Wu BB, Gong YP, Wu XH, Chen YY, Chen FF, Jin LT, Cheng BR, Hu F, Xiong B. Fourier transform infrared spectroscopy for the distinction of MCF-7 cells treated with different concentrations of 5-fluorouracil. J Transl Med. 2015;13:108.
35. Gao Y, Huo X, Dong L, Sun X, Sai H, Wei G, Xu Y, Zhang Y, Wu J. Fourier transform infrared microspectroscopy monitoring of 5-fluorouracil-induced apoptosis in SW620 colon cancer cells. Mol Med Rep. 2015;11(4):2585–91.
36. Glassford SE, Byrne B, Kazarian SG. Recent applications of ATR FTIR spectroscopy and imaging to proteins. Biochim Biophys Acta. 2013; 1834(12):2849–58.
37. Susi H, Byler DM. Resolution-enhanced Fourier transform infrared spectroscopy of enzymes. Methods Enzymol. 1986;130:290–311.
38. Gezici O, Demir I, Demircan A, Unlu N, Karaarslan M. Subtractive-FTIR spectroscopy to characterize organic matter in lignite samples from different depths. Spectrochim Acta A Mol Biomol Spectrosc. 2012;96:63–9.
39. Derenne A, Verdonck M, Goormaghtigh E. The effect of anticancer drugs on seven cell lines monitored by FTIR spectroscopy. Analyst. 2012;137(14):3255–64.

3

Risk of synchronous endometrial disorders in women with endometrioid borderline tumors of the ovary

Shuang-zheng Jia[1†], Jun-ji Zhang[1†], Jun-jun Yang[1], Yang Xiang[1], Zhiyong Liang[2] and Jin-hua Leng[1*]

Abstract

Background: Synchronous endometrial disorders have been poorly studied in women with endometrioid borderline ovarian tumors (EBOT). The aims of this study were to investigate the risk of endometrial disorders among women with EBOT and associated factors, as well as their oncological and fertility outcomes.

Results: This retrospective study included 33 women with EBOT. Their mean age was 41.9 years, and endometria were evaluated in 25 of these patients. The prevalence of synchronous endometrial disorders was 52.0% ($n = 13/25$) and this incidence was 41.4% ($n = 46/111$) after systematic analysis. Univariable analysis showed that EBOT patients who were younger, nulliparous, and had experienced abnormal vaginal bleeding were more likely to have synchronous endometrial disorders. The median follow-up was 54 months (range: 14-250 months), and three patients (10.3%) developed recurrences. No deaths due to EBOT were recorded. Among the nine nulliparous women treated conservatively who were attempting to conceive, only one (11.1%) pregnancy resulted in a live birth.

Conclusions: Synchronous endometrial disorders are common in women with EBOT, especially in those who are younger, nulliparous, and have experienced abnormal vaginal bleeding. Thus, endometrial sampling should be performed in women with EBOT undergoing conservative surgery, and a hysterectomy should be performed in cases requiring radical treatment.

Keywords: Endometrioid borderline ovarian tumor, Endometrial disorder, Fertility, Risk factor

Background

Borderline ovarian tumors (BOT), indolent neoplasms characterized by the presence of cellular proliferation and nuclear atypia in the absence of destructive stromal invasion, account for 10-20% of all epithelial ovarian cancers [1, 2]. Over the past two decades, considerable work has been performed to investigate the clinicopathologic features of serous and mucinous BOTs, as well as the oncological and fertility outcomes of patients with BOTs [3–5]. However, due to its rare incidence, endometrioid BOTs (EBOTs), the third most common BOT, have been poorly studied [6]. Most studies on EBOTs have focused mainly on the pathological characteristics and included only brief descriptions of management and follow-up [6–10]. Additionally, only a few cases that were treated with conservative surgery have been reported; therefore, the fertility outcomes of these patients are unknown [6, 9].

Although approximately one-third of patients with EBOT have endometrial hyperplasia and/or carcinoma, to the best of our knowledge, no specific data are available that identify groups at high risk for EBOT [10]. Furthermore, staging surgery without endometrial biopsy remains the cornerstone for women with EBOT who hope to become pregnant. Thus, to better understand the course of EBOT and to improve the surveillance of these patients, a thorough exploration of the prevalence of synchronous endometrial disorders in women with EBOT and identification of potential risk factors is urgently needed.

The primary objective of our study was to investigate the risk of synchronous endometrial disorders among

* Correspondence: lengjenny@vip.sina.com
†Equal contributors
[1]Department of Obstetrics and Gynecology, Peking Union Medical College Hospital, Chinese Academy of Medical Science & Peking Union Medical College, Beijing 100730, People's Republic of China
Full list of author information is available at the end of the article

women with EBOT and to identify their risk factors. We also evaluated the oncological and fertility outcomes in these EBOT patients.

Methods

Patients

After obtaining approval from the Institutional Review Board at the Peking Union Medical College Hospital (approval No. S-K351), consecutive patients with EBOT who were treated or referred to our hospital were identified through a search of medical records between 1995 and 2015. Medical records, including patient charts and operative, pathological, and follow-up records, were comprehensively reviewed. All EBOT were diagnosed by two gynecologic pathologists at our institution, and the FIGO 2013 staging system for epithelial ovarian tumors was used for determining disease stage based on the operative descriptions and pathology records [11].

Surgical management

Conservative surgery was defined as fertility-sparing, wherein the uterus and at least part of one ovary are salvaged, whereas radical surgery was defined as bilateral salpingo-oophorectomy (BSO) with or without a hysterectomy. A proper staging surgery consisted of carefully inspecting all peritoneal surfaces with peritoneal washing, random or oriented multiple biopsies, and omentectomy [1]. For those patients referred to our hospital after EBOT diagnosis, a second surgery was offered. The extent of surgery was determined by the combination of previous surgeries and surgeries performed at our hospital. Pelvic lymphadenectomy and adjuvant platinum-based chemotherapy were performed according to the surgeon's preference.

Post-operative evaluation, including clinical examination, vaginal ultrasonography, and CA-125 measurements, was offered every 3 months during the first 2 years, every 6 months during the next 3 years, and yearly thereafter.

Literature review

We used MEDLINE and PubMed to perform a literature search. The following search terms were used: "borderline" OR "atypical" OR "low-malignant potential" OR "low malignant potential" AND "endometrioid" AND "tumor" AND "ovary" OR "ovarian". Only articles published in English were included.

Statistical analysis

Primary outcomes included coexisting endometrial disorders in women with EBOT, defined as endometrial cancer, atypical hyperplasia (AH), and endometrial hyperplasia without atypia, during primary surgery and/or follow-up. Data were expressed as mean ± standard deviation, median (range), or number (percentage). For inferential analysis, an independent t test and Fisher's exact test were used to compare study variables between cases (women with synchronous endometrial disorders) and controls (women with normal endometrium) when appropriate. Due to the small sample size, multivariable analyses were not performed. All data were analyzed using SPSS 23.0 and $p < 0.05$ was considered significant.

Results

Patient characteristics

A total of 590 BOTs were identified, of which 33 (5.6%) were diagnosed as EBOT. The mean age of the patients was 41.9 years (range: 23-81 years). More than two-thirds of the participants (69.7%) were premenopausal. Of the 16 nulliparous women, four were infertile prior to treatment of their ovarian tumor. Ovarian cysts were the most common indications for surgery (75.8%; 25/33) and elevated serum CA-125 values were found in more the half of the patients (56.7%; 17/30). The mean tumor diameter was 7.3 cm and bilateral tumors were present in 4 patients (including three recurring in the contralateral ovary). Demographic features and disease characteristics of the 33 patients are detailed in Table 1.

Approximately two-thirds of the patients were treated with laparotomy ($n = 21$), including five conversions from laparoscopy to laparotomy during a 2-step staging procedure. Among the 33 patients, 17 underwent conservative surgery and 16 underwent radical surgery after a one-step ($n = 12$) or a two-step procedure ($n = 4$). Staging surgery was performed for 18 patients, of which five were conservative. Fourteen patients underwent lymphadenectomy; no positive findings were recorded. Postoperatively, 10 women received chemotherapy and radiotherapy was prescribed to three women to treat synchronous endometrial cancer.

Pathological findings

Histological analysis revealed that 10 patients had coexisting peritoneal or ovarian endometriosis, including six that occurred in the ipsilateral ovary. Intraepithelial carcinoma (IEC) and stromal microinvasion were found in four and seven patients, respectively; all but two patients had stage I disease, including four patients with stage IC2. One patient with EBOT and microinvasion had an invasive implant of the sigmoid colon. Noninvasive implants of the omentum were seen in a 43-year-old woman with bilateral EBOT who had positive cytology as well as right ovarian IEC associated with EBOT.

Synchronous endometrial disorders

Twenty-five women had endometrial evaluations and 13 patients had synchronous endometrial disorders, including six women with endometrial cancer, five with

Table 1 Demographic features and disease characteristics of participants

Variable	n (%)	Mean ± SD	Median
Age (y)		41.9 ± 12.85	
Nulliparous	16 (48.48%)		
Preoperative serum CA-125 (*n* = 30)			39.9 (8-1037)
< 35 IU/L	13 (43.33%)		
> 35 IU/L	17 (56.67%)		
Tumor diameter (cm)		7.3 ± 4.56	
Surgical extent			
Conservative surgery	17 (51.52%)		
Radical	16 (48.48%)		
Staging surgery	18 (54.55%)		
Stage			
I	31[b] (93.94%)		
II-III	2 (6.06%)		
Histological feathers			
Stromal microinvasion	7 (21.21%)		
Intraepithelial carcinoma	4 (12.12%)		
Implants	2[c] (6.06%)		
Coexisting endometriosis	10 (30.30%)		
Endometrial evaluations	25 (75.76%)		
No lesions	12 (48.00%)		
Hyperplasia without atypia	2 (8.00%)		
EIN	5 (20.00%)		
Endometrial cancer	6 (24.00%)		
Additional treatment			
Chemotherapy	10[d] (30.30%)		
Radiotherapy	3 (9.09%)		

USO unilateral salpingo-oophorectomy; *EIN* endometrial intraepithelial neoplasia
[a]Including three recurrences in the contralateral ovary
[b]Including four patients with stage IC2
[c]Including one invasive and one non-invasive implant respectively
[d]Including one melphalan chemotherapy

Table 2 Risk factors of synchronous endometrial disorders in women with EBOT

Variables	Cases (*n* = 13)	Controls (*n* = 12)	*p*
Age (y)	39.1 ± 10.4	50.9 ± 13.1	0.02[a]
Menopausal			0.11[b]
No	10	5	
Yes	3	7	
AVB			0.001[b]
No	3	11	
Yes	10	1	
Nulliparous			0.03[b]
No	5	10	
Yes	8	2	
Tumor diameter	5.7 ± 2.1	8.2 ± 4.3	0.07[a]
CA-125			0.25[b]
< 35 IU/L	6	3	
> 35 IU/L	5	7	
Coexisting endometriosis			0.45[b]
No	10	8	
Yes	3	4	
Stage			0.28[b]
I-IC1	11	8	
IC2-III	2	4	
IEC			0.47[b]
No	12	10	
Yes	1	2	
Microinvasion			0.46[b]
No	11	9	
Yes	2	3	

[a]Independent sample *t* test assuming equal variance
[b]Fisher's Exact test

atypical hyperplasia (AH), and two with endometrial hyperplasia without atypia. The crude prevalence of endometrial disorders in the women with EBOT was 52.0% ($n = 13/25$).

Analyses of the data indicated that EBOT patients who were younger, nulliparous, and had abnormal vaginal bleeding (AVB) were more likely to have synchronous endometrial disorders ($P = 0.02$; $P = 0.03$; $P = 0.001$; respectively; Table 2). However, no histological variables were found to be significantly associated with endometrial disorders.

Oncological and fertility outcomes

Four patients were lost to follow-up after surgery. Among the remaining 29 patients, the median follow-up was 54 months (range: 14-250 months). Three patients (10.3%) developed recurrences but no women died of their disease. The time to recurrence among these 3 patients was 18 months, 100 months, and 180 months, respectively. These three women were young (23, 30, and 30 years old, respectively), nulliparous, and had co-existing endometrial disorders (two women with AH and one women with EC). Conservative surgeries without staging were performed at their initial treatment. Two women recurred on the residual contralateral ovary and one woman relapsed as bilateral recurrence (Table 3).

Among the 16 nulliparous women, 13 women were treated conservatively with a fertility-sparing procedure. One patient was lost to follow-up and three women had not attempted to conceive at the time of analysis. Of the nine patients who had attempted to conceive, only one (11.1%) pregnancy resulted in a live birth. Moreover, of these nine women, five had synchronous endometrial disorders and two experienced contralateral EBOT recurrence.

Table 3 Details of the three patients who experienced recurrence

Age	Initial surgery	Initial pathology	Time to recurrence	Secondary surgery	Secondary pathology	Coexisting endometrial disorders
30	Lap UC+Hys	EBOT	18 months	Lap BUC+D&C	Bilateral EBOT	EC
30	LSO+LN	EBOT	240 months	Lap RSO	EBOT	EIN II-III
23	RSO	EBOT	100 months	Lap UC	EBOT	EIN II-III

Lap laparoscopy; *Hys* hysteroscopy; *D&C* dilation & curettage; *UC* unilateral cystectomy; *EC* endometrial cancer; *LSO* left salpingo-oophorectomy; *RSO* right salpingo-oophorectomy; *EIN* endometrial intraepithelial neoplasia

Literature review

We identified 347 citations from 1981 to November 2015. After reviewing titles and abstracts, only five papers that described 147 patients were included in the final analysis. Of these 147 women, 86 were evaluated for endometrial status. Thirty-three of these women were diagnosed with synchronous endometrial disorders, including nine who had endometrial cancer. Together with the present study, a total of 111 women with EBOT underwent endometria sampling and 46 were diagnosed with endometrial disorders, indicating a crude prevalence of 41.4% (Fig. 1).

Discussion

EBOT is a rare tumor that represents 0.2% of all epithelial ovarian tumors. To our knowledge, this is the first study to evaluate risk factors for synchronous endometrial disorders in women with EBOT. Our results indicated that synchronous endometrial disorders are highly prevalent in women with EBOT, especially in those who are younger, nulliparous, and have AVB. Our study also demonstrated that, although women with EBOT have a favorable prognosis, their fertility outcomes are poor.

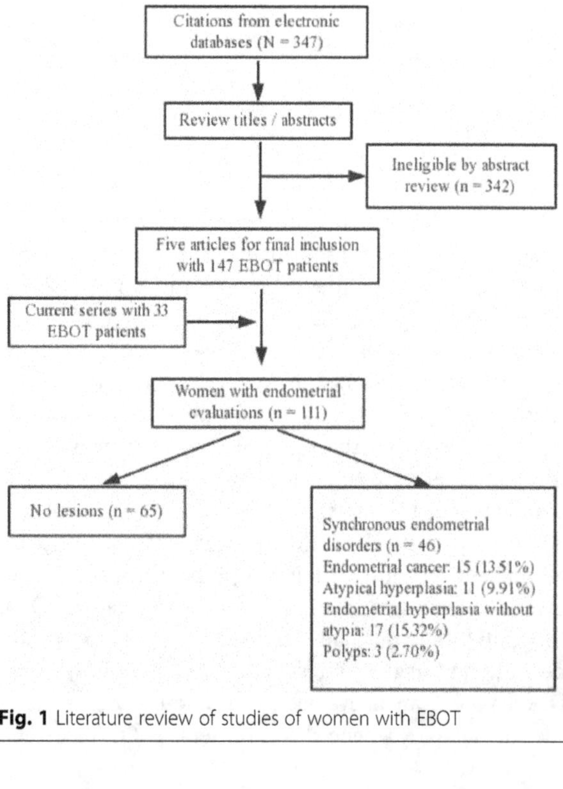

Fig. 1 Literature review of studies of women with EBOT

When treating EBOT patients, physicians must decide whether to include endometrial curettage as a therapeutic approach. Although few studies have evaluated the incidence of endometrial disorders in women with EBOT, studies by Bell and Kurman and Snyder et al. found that 12.5% (3/24) and 68.4% (13/19), respectively, of EBOT patients also had endometrial disorders [7, 9]. However, our study revealed that the prevalence of synchronous endometrial disorders was 52%; this incidence remained high (41.4%) following systematic analysis. Thus, as recommended by Uzan et al., endometrial sampling should be performed in women with EBOT undergoing conservative surgery; in addition, a hysterectomy should be performed in cases requiring radical treatment [6, 12].

The mechanisms underlying endometrial disorders in EBOT patients remain unclear. Although one study indicated that stromal luteinizations were more common in EBOT patients with concurrent endometrial disorders, to our knowledge, no other study has confirmed this result [8]. Analyses of our data showed that EBOT patients who were younger, nulliparous, and had AVB were more likely to experience endometrial disorders. To our knowledge, this is the first study to demonstrate this relationship.

Endometrioid carcinomas of the ovary tend to coexist with various forms of endometrial neoplasia, whereas mutations in several genes, including β-catenin and PTEN, have been demonstrated to occur concurrently with endometrial cancers and endometrioid ovarian cancers [13]. Furthermore, distinct clinical characteristics, including younger age, obesity, premenopausal status, and nulliparity were demonstrated in women with synchronous primary cancers of the endometrium and ovary [14].

The finding that women with AVB were more likely to have concurrent endometrial disorders was not surprising. Endometrial cancer or atypical hyperplasia occurs in 1.31% of premenopausal women with AVB, and this incidence can increase to 17.3% in menopausal women [15, 16]. However, 88.9% ($n = 10/11$) of women with EBOT and AVB also had endometrial disorders, and this incidence was significantly higher than that of the general population. Furthermore, uterine endometrioid adenocarcinomas can also be found in women who do not show uterine symptoms [6]. More than 60% (8/13) of our study participants were nulliparous, which is consistent with a study by Eifel et al., wherein 50% of the study participants who had synchronous endometrioid/endometrioid tumors were nulliparous [17]. Similarly, Herrinton et al. reported a lower than expected mean parity in women with synchronous endometrial and ovarian cancers [18].

In our study population, women with EBOT and synchronous endometrial disorders were approximately 12 years younger than those with EBOT alone. Similar findings were also reported in women with coexisting endometrial and ovarian carcinomas [19]. The combination of younger age, AVB, and nulliparity, as well as other characteristics, including obesity, in women with synchronous endometrioid/endometrial carcinomas suggests the involvement of a hormonal "field effect" in the development of these simultaneous tumors, particularly endometrioid cell-type tumors [14, 19]. In recent years, accumulating evidence has suggested that ovarian cancer arises from the pleiotropic interactions of the committed stem cells within the ovary, the surrounding microenvironment, and the infiltrating immune cells [20, 21]. Thus, whether these interactions may contribute to the development of synchronous endometrial and ovarian disorders needs further exploration.

With respect to oncological outcomes, over the past decade several studies have demonstrated the safety of fertility-sparing surgery in early stage epithelial ovarian cancer patients whose preservation of reproductive potential is pivotal to their quality of life [22–24]. Previous studies have found that women with EBOT have a favorable prognosis, with minimal recurrence and no EBOT-associated deaths [6–9]. However, in this study, three patients experienced recurrences, of which two recurred on the contralateral ovary and one relapsed as a bilateral recurrence. All three women were young (23, 30, and 30 years old, respectively), nulliparous, and had synchronous endometrial disorders. Uzan et al. reported a malignant transformation, wherein a 37-year old woman suffered an invasive relapse as endometrioid carcinoma after radical treatment for her first recurrence [6]. This unusual case, in combination with our three recurrences, emphasizes the importance of endometrial biopsy in women with EBOT and the need for an intensive postoperative follow-up, especially in younger patients.

Promising data have been reported for fertility outcomes in women with serous/mucinous BOTs after conservative management. One study reported a pooled estimated spontaneous pregnancy rate of 54% that increased to 80% after fertility treatment [4]. In women with advanced-stage serous BOTs, a long-term follow-up study reported a pregnancy rate of 57.1% [25]. For BOTs, conservative treatment, patient age, and BOT histologic subtype have been reported to influence fertility outcomes; however, for patients with EBOT, there is limited information about fertility outcomes [26–28].

In this study, we demonstrated for the first time that women with EBOT have poor fertility outcomes. Of the nine women who attempted conception, only one (11.1%) pregnancy was achieved that resulted in a live birth. We should note that five of these nine women developed endometrial disorders after their initial EBOT surgery, including two women with endometrial cancer. Only two women experienced AVB but endometrial sampling was not performed during the initial surgery (unpublished data). Thus, whether nulliparity itself contributes to the development of endometrial disorders or vice versa awaits further study. In addition, adherence and alterations in ovarian function following surgery could also contribute to poor fertility outcomes.

This study has several limitations. First, the present study is inherently limited by its retrospective design and small sample size; in addition, the data were collected from a single institution. As a result, the data in this study did not include all factors that could contribute to the etiology of EBOT tumors, such as body mass index. Women with obesity are at increased risk of endometrial disorders due to excess peripheral conversion of androstenedione to estrone in adipose tissue. However, to the best of our knowledge, due the rare incidence of this condition, this is the largest study to focus on endometrial sampling in women with EBOT. Second, pathological review of the specimens was not performed. The Peking Union Medical College Hospital is a major referral center and has the best gynecology and pathology department in the country. In addition, two gynecological pathologists reviewed original pathology reports. Finally, not all women included in this study underwent endometrial biopsies during their initial surgery (endometrial disorders were observed in six women during follow-up), which may have resulted in overestimation of the incidence of synchronous endometrial disorders. However, this incidence of was 41.4% following after systematic analysis.

Conclusions

In summary, the present study demonstrated that endometrial disorders are common in women with EBOT, especially in those who are younger, nulliparous, and have AVB. Thus, endometrial sampling should be performed in women with EBOT undergoing conservative surgery, and a hysterectomy should be performed in cases requiring radical treatment. Although there were no negative oncological outcomes, the fertility rates for these patients were poor, implying that a more active approach should be taken for EBOT patients who wish to become pregnant.

Abbreviations

AH: Atypical hyperplasia; AVB: Abnormal vaginal bleeding; BOT: Borderline ovarian tumors; BSO: Bilateral salpingo-oophorectomy; EBOT: Endometrioid borderline ovarian tumors; IEC: Intraepithelial carcinoma

Acknowledgements

We thank all of the patients for participating in our study.

Funding

This study was supported by the National Key R&D Program of China (2017YFC1001200).

Authors' contributions

SJ, JZ, and JL contributed substantially to the study conceptualization, and design, acquisition of data, analysis and interpretation of data, and manuscript writing. JY, YX, and ZL contributed to the interpretation of data and performed critical revisions of important intellectual content. All authors gave approval for the publication of the final version.

Competing interests

The authors declare that they have no competing interests.

Author details

[1]Department of Obstetrics and Gynecology, Peking Union Medical College Hospital, Chinese Academy of Medical Science & Peking Union Medical College, Beijing 100730, People's Republic of China. [2]Department of Pathology, Peking Union Medical College Hospital, Chinese Academy of Medical Science & Peking Union Medical College, Beijing, People's Republic of China.

References

1. Cadron I, Leunen K, Van Gorp T, Amant F, Neven P, Vergote I. Management of borderline ovarian neoplasms. J Clin Oncol. 2007;25:2928–37.
2. Ellenson LH, Carinelli SG, Cho KR, Kim KR, Kupryjanczyk J, Prat J, et al. Endometrioid tumours. In: Kurman RJ, Carcangiu ML, Herrington CS, Young RH, editors. WHO classification of Tumours of female reproductive organs. Lyon: IARC; 2014. p. 29–32.
3. Uzan C, Nikpayam M, Ribassin-Majed L, Gouy S, Bendifallah S, Cortez A, et al. Influence of histological subtypes on the risk of an invasive recurrence in a large series of stage I borderline ovarian tumor including 191 conservative treatments. Ann Oncol. 2014;25:1312–9.
4. Darai E, Fauvet R, Uzan C, Gouy S, Duvillard P, Morice P. Fertility and borderline ovarian tumor: a systematic review of conservative management, risk of recurrence and alternative options. Hum Reprod Update. 2013;19: 151–66.
5. Morice P, Uzan C, Fauvet R, Gouy S, Duvillard P, Darai E. Borderline ovarian tumour: pathological diagnostic dilemma and risk factors for invasive or lethal recurrence. Lancet Oncol. 2012;13:e103–15.
6. Uzan C, Berretta R, Rolla M, Gouy S, Fauvet R, Darai E, et al. Management and prognosis of endometrioid borderline tumors of the ovary. Surg Oncol. 2012;21:178–84.
7. Bell KA, Kurman RJ. A clinicopathologic analysis of atypical proliferative (borderline) tumors and well-differentiated endometrioid adenocarcinomas of the ovary. Am J Surg Pathol. 2000;24:1465–79.
8. Bell DA, Scully RE. Atypical and borderline endometrioid adenofibromas of the ovary. A report of 27 cases. Am J Surg Pathol. 1985;9:205–14.
9. Snyder RR, Norris HJ, Tavassoli F. Endometrioid proliferative and low malignant potential tumors of the ovary. A clinicopathologic study of 46 cases. Am J Surg Pathol. 1988;12:661–71.
10. Roth LM, Emerson RE, Ulbright TM. Ovarian endometrioid tumors of low malignant potential: a clinicopathologic study of 30 cases with comparison to well-differentiated endometrioid adenocarcinoma. Am J Surg Pathol. 2003;27:1253–9.
11. Prat J. Staging classification for cancer of the ovary, fallopian tube, and peritoneum. Int J Gynecol Obstet. 2014;124:1–5.
12. Harter P, Gershenson D, Lhomme C, Lecuru F, Ledermann J, Provencher DM, et al. Gynecologic Cancer InterGroup (GCIG) consensus review for ovarian tumors of low malignant potential (borderline ovarian tumors). Int J Gynecol Cancer. 2014;24:S5–8.
13. Kurman RJ, Shih I. Molecular pathogenesis and extraovarian origin of epithelial ovarian cancer–shifting the paradigm. Hum Pathol. 2011;42:918–31.
14. Soliman PT, Slomovitz BM, Broaddus RR, Sun CC, Oh JC, Eifel PJ, et al. Synchronous primary cancers of the endometrium and ovary: a single institution review of 84 cases. Gynecol Oncol. 2004;94:456–62.
15. Pennant ME, Mehta R, Moody P, Hackett G, Prentice A, Sharp SJ, et al. Premenopausal abnormal uterine bleeding and risk of endometrial cancer. BJOG. 2017;124:404–11.
16. Ozdemir S, Celik C, Gezginc K, Kiresi D, Esen H. Evaluation of endometrial thickness with transvaginal ultrasonography and histopathology in premenopausal women with abnormal vaginal bleeding. Arch Gynecol Obstet. 2010;282:395–9.
17. Eifel P, Hendrickson M, Ross J, Ballon S, Martinez A, Kempson R. Simultaneous presentation of carcinoma involving the ovary and the uterine corpus. Cancer. 1982;50:163–70.
18. Herrinton LJ, Voigt LF, Weiss NS, Beresford SA, Wingo PA. Risk factors for synchronous primary endometrial and ovarian cancers. Ann Epidemiol. 2001;11:529–33.
19. Caldarella A, Crocetti E, Taddei GL, Paci E. Coexisting endometrial and ovarian carcinomas: a retrospective clinicopathological study. Pathol Res Pract. 2008;204:643–8.
20. Giannakeas V, Sopik V, Narod SA. A model for ovarian cancer progression based on inherent resistance. Gynecol Oncol. 2016;142:484–9.
21. Laganà AS, Sofo V, Vitale SG, Triolo O. Epithelial ovarian cancer inherent resistance: may the pleiotropic interaction between reduced immunosurveillance and drug-resistant cells play a key role? Gynecologic Oncology Reports. 2016;18:57–8.
22. Wright JD, Shah M, Mathew L, Burke WM, Culhane J, Goldman N, et al. Fertility preservation in young women with epithelial ovarian cancer. Cancer. 2009;115:4118–26.
23. Kwon YS, Hahn HS, Kim TJ, Lee IH, Lim KT, Lee KH, et al. Fertility preservation in patients with early epithelial ovarian cancer. J Gynecol Oncol. 2009;20:44–7.
24. Vitale SG, Rosa VLL, Rapisarda AMC, Laganà AS. Fertility preservation in women with gynaecologic cancer: the impact on quality of life and psychological well-being. Hum Fertil. 2018;21:35–8.
25. Uzan C, Kane A, Rey A, Gouy S, Duvillard P, Morice P. Outcomes after conservative treatment of advanced-stage serous borderline tumors of the ovary. Ann Oncol. 2010;21:55–60.
26. Palomba S, Falbo A, Del NS, Rocca M, Russo T, Cariati F, et al. Ultra-conservative fertility-sparing strategy for bilateral borderline ovarian tumours: an 11-year follow-up. Hum Reprod. 2010;25:1966–72.
27. Kanat-Pektas M, Ozat M, Gungor T, Dikici T, Yilmaz B, Mollamahmutoglu L. Fertility outcome after conservative surgery for borderline ovarian tumors: a single center experience. Arch Gynecol Obstet. 2011;284:1253–8.
28. Fauvet R, Demblocque E, Morice P, Querleu D, Darai E. Behavior of serous borderline ovarian tumors with and without micropapillary patterns: results of a French multicenter study. Ann Surg Oncol. 2012;19:941–7.

4

Clinical study of a CT evaluation model combined with serum CA125 in predicting the treatment of newly diagnosed advanced epithelial ovarian cancer

Lu Qin, Huming Huang, Mengjie Chen, Yuejuan Liang and He Wang*

Abstract

Background: The treatment of newly diagnosed advanced epithelial ovarian cancer (EOC) was predicted by an ovarian cancer computed tomography (CT) evaluation model combined with serum CA125.

Methods: Clinical data for 194 patients with advanced EOC treated with neoadjuvant chemotherapy (NACT) combined with interval debulking surgery (IDS) or primary debulking surgery (PDS) were retrospectively analyzed, and the appropriate treatment was predicted by comparing the subgroup differences in intraoperative situations, postoperative situations and survival rates.

Results: There were no significant differences with respect to operation time, intraoperative blood loss, ideal tumor cytoreductive rate or postoperative complication rate between the NACT + IDS group and the PDS group with scores less than 5 (score < 5) ($p = 0.764$, $p = 0.504$, $p = 0.906$, $p = 0.176$). However, there was a statistically significant difference in overall survival rate between the two groups ($p = 0.029$), with better survival in the PDS group than in the NACT + IDS group. There were significant differences between the NACT + IDS group and the PDS group with scores greater than or equal to 5 (score ≥ 5). The former was better than the latter in terms of operation time, intraoperative blood loss, ideal tumor cytoreductive rate, and postoperative complication rate ($p = 0.002$, $p = 0.040$, $p = 0.014$, $p = 0.021$). However, there was no significant difference in overall survival rate between the two groups ($p = 0.383$).

Conclusions: According to the new evaluation system, for a score < 5, we suggest that patients with newly diagnosed advanced EOC undergo PDS; for a score ≥ 5, we recommend NACT + IDS.

Keywords: CA125, Advanced epithelial ovarian cancer, Neoadjuvant chemotherapy, Debulking surgery

Background

Ovarian cancer is one of the most common gynecological cancers and has the highest mortality of all gynecological cancers. Since ovarian cancer has no typical clinical manifestations or exact early screening methods, Siegel et al. [1] reported that 70% of ovarian cancer patients had advanced stage disease (stage III-IV) upon presentation and that the overall 5-year survival rate was only 27%. The prognosis of advanced ovarian cancer is closely related to the volume of postoperative residual tumor. Therefore, the ability to achieve ideal tumor cytoreduction becomes a pivotal prognostic factor for advanced ovarian cancer. The ideal tumor cytoreductive surgery standard is a maximum postoperative residual tumor diameter < 1 cm [2]. At present, there are two primary approaches to the treatment of advanced EOC: neoadjuvant chemotherapy combined with intermittent debulking surgery (NACT + IDS) and primary debulking surgery (PDS). To predict the treatment regimen of newly diagnosed EOC patients by an ovarian cancer CT evaluation model combined with serum CA125, clinical data for 194 newly diagnosed

* Correspondence: wanghe10430@126.com
Department of Gynecologic Oncology, Affiliated Tumor Hospital of Guangxi Medical University, 71 Hedi Road, Qingxiu District, Nanning, Guangxi 530021, People's Republic of China

advanced EOC patients who came to our hospital from March 2010 to July 2016 were retrospectively analyzed.

Methods

Patient selection

Data were collected for 194 patients who had been newly diagnosed with advanced EOC when they arrived at our hospital from March 2010 to July 2016. According to our hospital gynecologists' clinical experience, laboratory tests, imaging data and the patients' own wishes, 99 patients with advanced EOC were treated with NACT + IDS. Patients were 29 to 75 years old (mean 53.05 ± 9.74 years); 78 cases were in pathological stage III, and 21 were in stage IV. Preoperative chemotherapy was based on platinum-based chemotherapy, and tumor cells were destroyed by chemotherapy. These patients completed 1~ 2 courses of platinum-based NACT before undergoing tumor cytoreductive surgery. Ninety-five patients with advanced EOC were treated with PDS. They were 25 to 79 years old (mean 54.72 ± 10.59 years old) with pathological stage III (79 cases) or stage IV (16 cases) disease. According to their wishes, 176 patients underwent platinum-based systemic vein NACT, and 18 patients had no postoperative chemotherapy.

Measurement of CT evaluation model and CA125

We recorded the operation time, intraoperative blood loss, operative efficacy, postoperative recovery, postoperative complications, and postoperative follow-up of 194 patients with newly diagnosed advanced EOC. Based on the CT evaluation model of ovarian cancer patients that was established by Bristow et al. [3] in 2000, patients with a cumulative score ≥ 4 were not suitable for PDS. According to Vorgias et al. [4], when serum CA125 levels are higher than 500 U/ml, its accuracy is highest for predicting tumor cytoreductive surgery. Therefore, if at initial diagnosis the serum CA125 levels were ≥ 500 U/ml, we recorded 1 point. We now establish a New Scoring System based on a CT evaluation model combined with serum CA125 for patients with newly diagnosed advanced EOC. Five points will be designated as the demarcation point. One hundred ninety-four cases were divided into 4 groups by this New Scoring System: NACT + IDS group (score < 5, n = 49), PDS group (score < 5, n = 47), NACT + IDS group (score ≥ 5, n = 50) and PDS group (score ≥ 5, n = 48). In accordance with the intraoperative situation, postoperative situation and prognosis of patients in each group, appropriate treatment was predicted. The size of the residual tumor after surgery is an important prognostic factor. According to the 2014 National Comprehensive Cancer Network (NCCN) guidelines for ovarian cancer, non-ideal tumor cytoreductive surgery is indicated by postoperative residual ovarian cancer lesions ≥1 cm [5]. Four groups of patients were followed up until April 2017 (Table 1).

Table 1 New Scoring System based on a CT evaluation model combined with serum CA125

The initial diagnosis of serum CA125 levels (U/ml)	Point value
≥ 500	1
< 500	0
Predictive index parameter	Point value
Peritoneal thickening	2
Peritoneal implants ≥2 cm	2
Small bowel mesentery disease ≥2 cm	2
Large bowel mesentery disease ≥2 cm	2
Omentum extension to stomach, spleen, or lesser sac	2
Extension to pelvic sidewall, parametria, or hydroureter	2
Ascites-large volume (seen on all cuts)	2
Performance status ≥2	2
Suprarenal paraaortic lymph nodes ≥1 cm	2
Diaphragm or lung base disease ≥2 cm or confluent plaque	1
Inguinal canal disease or lymph nodes ≥2 cm	1
Liver lesion ≥2 cm on surface or any size parenchymal lesion	1
Porta hepatis or gallbladder fossa disease ≥1 cm	1
Infrarenal paraaortic lymph nodes ≥2 cm	1

Statistical analysis

SPSS 20.0 software was used for statistical analysis. Normally distributed data are presented as the mean ± standard deviation ($\bar{x} \pm S$). Skewed data are presented as M (P_{25} ~ P_{75}). The data were analyzed by t-test, χ^2 test, non-parametric test or survival analysis. For all comparisons, differences were considered significant when $p < 0.05$. All findings were confirmed in at least one additional independent experiment.

Results

Clinicopathological factors in patients

After statistical analysis, patients in the NACT + IDS group (score < 5) were 53.16 ± 9.40 years old, and patients in the PDS group (score < 5) were 53.64 ± 10.79 years old. There was no significant difference in age between the two groups (p = 0.818). There was also no significant difference in clinical stage, pathological type or histological grade between the two groups (p = 0.343, p = 0.970, p = 0.598). Patients in the NACT + IDS group (score ≥ 5) were 52.94 ± 10.16 years old, and patients in the PDS group (score ≥ 5) group were 55.77 ± 10.39 years old. There was no significant difference in age between the two groups (p = 0.176). There was also no significant difference in clinical stage, pathological type or histological grade between the two groups (p = 0.876, p = 0.819, p = 0.448) (Table 2).

Table 2 Clinicopathological factors in the NACT + IDS and PDS groups of patients grouped according to the New Scoring System

Clinicopathological factors	Groups with score < 5			Groups with score ≥ 5		
	NACT + IDS	PDS	*p*	NACT + IDS	PDS	*p*
Age (y)	(53.16 ± 9.40)	(53.64 ± 10.79)	0.818	(52.94 ± 10.16)	(55.77 ± 10.39)	0.176
Stage						
III	38	40	0.343	40	39	0.876
IV	11	7		10	9	
Histology						
Serous	42	41	0.970	44	41	0.819
Mucous	6	5		5	5	
Endometrioid	1	1		1	2	
Grade						
G1	15	19	0.598	16	19	0.448
G2	4	3		3	5	
G3	30	25		31	24	

NACT + IDS neoadjuvant chemotherapy and interval debulking surgery, *PDS* primary debulking surgery

Comparison of intraoperative and postoperative situations in the NACT + IDS and PDS groups (score < 5)

There were no significant differences in terms of operation time, intraoperative blood loss or ideal tumor cytoreductive rate between the two groups ($p = 0.764$, $p = 0.504$, $p = 0.906$). The incidence of complications in the NACT + IDS group was 12.24%, and that in the PDS group was 14.89%. There was no significant difference in the incidence of complications between the two groups after χ^2 tests ($p = 0.705$). On follow-up of the NACT + IDS group, 20 patients survived, 24 died, and 5 were lost to follow-up. On follow-up of the PDS group, 28 patients survived, 12 died, and 7 were lost to follow-up. There was a significant difference in overall survival between the two groups ($p = 0.029$) (Table 3, Fig. 1).

Comparison of intraoperative and postoperative situations in the NACT + IDS and PDS groups (score ≥ 5)

There were significant differences in operation time, intraoperative blood loss and ideal tumor cytoreductive rate between the two groups ($p = 0.002$, $p = 0.040$, $p = 0.014$). That is, the operation time and intraoperative blood loss of patients in the NACT + IDS group were lower than those of patients in the PDS group. In addition, the ideal rate of reduction in NACT + IDS patients was higher than that it was in PDS patients. The incidence of complications was 4.00% in the NACT + IDS group and 18.75% in the PDS group. There was an obvious and significant difference in the incidence of complications between the two groups after χ^2 tests ($p = 0.021$). We can conclude that the incidence of complications was lower in the NACT + IDS group than in the PDS group. On follow-up of the NACT + IDS group, 20 patients survived, 24 died, and 5 were lost to follow-up. On follow-up of the PDS group, 28 patients survived, 12 died, and 7 were lost to follow-up. There was no significant difference in overall survival between the two groups ($p = 0.383$) (Table 4, Fig. 2).

Comparative analysis of ideal tumor reduction at operation in the two PDS groups with scores < 5 and ≥ 5

According to case information, the two groups of patients with scores < 5 and ≥ 5 in terms of ideal tumor reduction were significantly different macroscopically. However, after statistical analysis, there was no statistically significant difference between the two groups of patients in terms of ideal tumor reduction rate ($p = 0.296$).

Discussion

Ovarian cancer not only is a serious threat to the health and life of women but also has the highest mortality rate of all gynecological cancers. Because there is no exact method of screening, 70% of patients have reached the

Table 3 Surgery parameters in the NACT + IDS and PDS groups of patients with score < 5

Index	NACT + IDS	PDS	*p*
Number of cases	49	47	/
Operation time (min)	285.04 ± 92.24	278.57 ± 116.32	0.764
Intraoperative blood loss (ml)	550 (340~1300)	700 (300~1200)	0.504
Ideal tumor cytoreductive surgery	37	35	/
Ideal tumor cytoreductive rate (%)	75.51	74.47	0.906

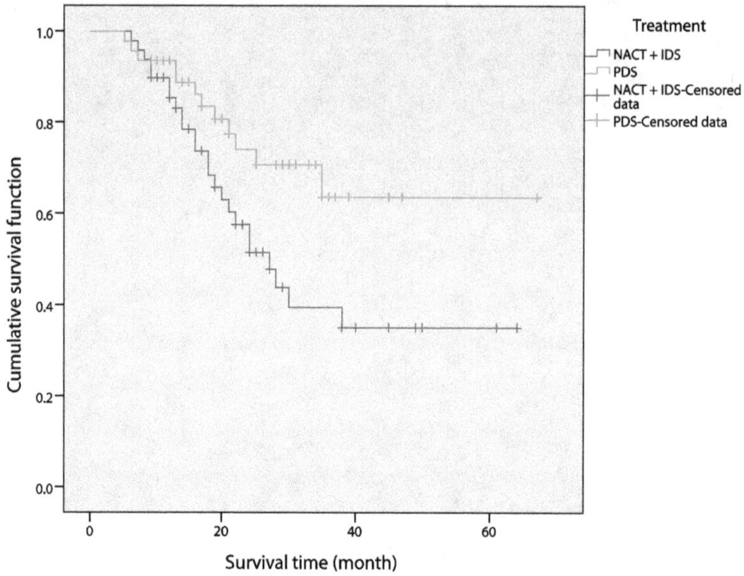

Fig. 1 Overall survival rates were compared between the NACT + IDS and PDS groups with a score < 5

advanced stage by the time of presentation and often have abdominal metastasis, organ metastasis, ascites and pleural effusion. At present, the treatment of newly diagnosed patients with advanced epithelial ovarian cancer (EOC) is divided into two types: neoadjuvant chemotherapy combined with interval debulking surgery (NACT + IDS) and primary debulking surgery (PDS). NACT, also known as primary chemotherapy, refers to systemic chemotherapy that is administered before local treatment (such as radiotherapy or surgery). This treatment is primarily administered when PDS cannot achieve ideal tumor cytoreduction and/or patients are in poor condition and cannot tolerate tumor cytoreductive surgery. The ideal tumor cytoreductive rate can be improved by NACT [6]. Ovarian cancer is very sensitive to chemotherapy drugs. About 70 to 80% of patients with ovarian cancer have a complete response after chemotherapy [7]. Studies have shown that NACT has the following advantages: it kills metastastic cells surrounding the lesion, loosens the adhesion of the tumor and surrounding tissue, reduces tumor volume, improves the ideal tumor cytoreductive rate, and reduces the difficulty and complications of surgery [8]; it controls ascites and pleural effusion to improve the overall condition of patients and improve their surgical tolerance; it shortens the operation time, reduces intraoperative blood loss, and improves patient quality of life [9]; and it puts the tumor cells into a "dormant state", reducing tumor spread and tumor cell seeding by surgery due to intraoperative squeezing and mechanical trauma stimulation, thereby reducing recurrence. However, the use of NACT for the treatment of patients with advanced ovarian cancer has been continuously controversial. For patients with advanced ovarian cancer who remain in good condition, studies have shown that PDS can achieve better tumor reduction and prognosis than NACT.

Based on the CT evaluation model of ovarian cancer patients that was established by Bristow et al. in 2000, patients with a cumulative score ≥ 4 (score ≥ 4) are not suitable for PDS. They noted that such patients should undergo NACT until the condition is under control prior to surgery. In addition, a large number of studies have shown that more than 85% of patients with ovarian cancer have a serum CA125 level higher than 35 U/mL, and serum CA125 levels are closely related to disease status in 93% of patients. Therefore, the level of serum CA125 is considered strong

Table 4 Surgery parameters in the NACT + IDS and PDS groups of patients with score ≥ 5

Index	NACT + IDS	PDS	*p*
Number of cases	50	48	/
Operation time (min)	270.64 ± 92.64	339.48 ± 119.04	0.002
Intraoperative blood loss (ml)	550 (275~1100)	950 (400~1675)	0.040
Ideal tumor cytoreductive surgery	43	31	/
Ideal tumor cytoreductive rate (%)	86.00	64.58	0.014

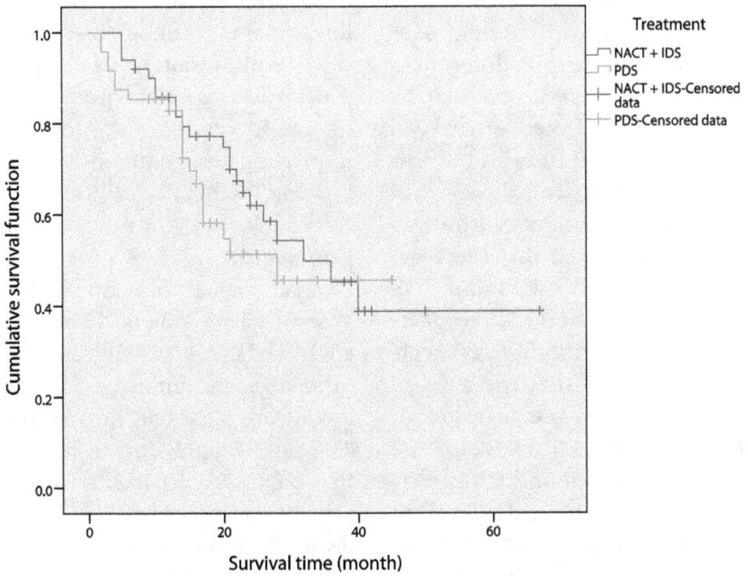

Fig. 2 Overall survival rates were compared between the NACT + IDS and PDS groups with a score ≥ 5

evidence in the evaluation of the ability of patients to achieve ideal tumor cytoreduction [10]. Vorgias et al. found that when serum CA125 levels were higher than 500 U/ml, the accuracy of its predictive ability was highest for patients undergoing tumor cytoreductive surgery to achieve the ideal standard, accounting for 84.2% in all observed ideal tumor cytoreductive surgeries. Obeidat et al. [11] supported this view and reported that a preoperative serum CA125 level of 500 U/ml was the most valuable indicator of whether ideal tumor cytoreductive surgery could be achieved. This indicator's sensitivity and specificity were 72 and 73%, respectively. The positive predictive value was 68%. However, some investigators believed that the negative predictive value of CA125 is poor and that this measure cannot be used independently as an index to predict surgery. Therefore, in order to predict more suitable treatment for patients, we have assessed patients with newly diagnosed advanced EOC by taking advantage of an ovarian cancer CT evaluation model established by Bristow et al. combined with serum CA125 levels.

By comparing two groups (NACT + IDS and PDS), we found that there was no significant difference in the operation time, intraoperative blood loss, the ideal tumor cytoreductive rate or postoperative complications between the two groups of patients with a score < 5 ($p = 0.764$, $p = 0.504$, $p = 0.906$, $p = 0.705$). However, the overall survival rate was significantly different between the two groups ($p = 0.029$), with the PDS group having superior survival to the NACT + IDS group. This finding suggests that PDS did not show any advantage in terms of intraoperative and postoperative complications compared with the NACT + IDS group for patients with newly diagnosed advanced EOC when the score was < 5, but the postoperative quality of life and long-term prognosis of these patients were significantly better than those of the NACT + IDS group. For scores < 5, there was no significant difference between the NACT + IDS and PDS groups in terms of operation time, intraoperative blood loss and ideal tumor cytoreduction. Therefore, in order to avoid side effects and adverse reactions brought on by unnecessary chemotherapy, as well as excessive treatment costs and lengths of treatment that may delay the optimal operation time, we support the notion that advanced EOC patients should undergo PDS. In the two groups of patients with a score ≥ 5, the operation time of the NACT + IDS group was significantly shorter than that of the PDS group ($p = 0.002$). The amount of blood loss during operation in the former was less than that in the latter, and the ideal cytoreductive rate was higher ($p = 0.040$, $p = 0.014$). This finding showed that for scores ≥ 5, patients undergoing NACT could significantly improve their condition prior to surgery to reduce surgical difficulty and risks. In addition, the incidence of postoperative complications in the NACT + IDS group was significantly lower than that in the PDS group ($p = 0.021$). This result suggested that NACT could significantly reduce the incidence of complications and improve the quality of life of patients who were newly diagnosed with severe illness. None of these patients could undergo PDS immediately. In terms of overall survival rate, we found no significant difference between the two groups of patients ($p = 0.383$). NACT + IDS did not appear to improve prognosis. This result was in line with that of many published reports. Lozzi et al. [12]

conducted a paired study of neoadjuvant chemotherapy with patients treated with standard treatment over the same period and showed no significant differences between the neoadjuvant chemotherapy group and the standard treatment group in terms of median survival time, median progression-free survival time and 3-year survival rate. Wright et al. [13] compared the efficacy of PDS and NACT + IDS in elderly patients with ovarian cancer using SEER data. They noted that the average survival of patients in the NACT + IDS and PDS groups was 15.8 months and 28.8 months, respectively, with 2-year survival rates of 36 and 56%, respectively. Fago-Olsen et al. [14] reported that the average overall survival of patients without residual tumor in the PDS group was better than that of those in the NACT + IDS group, at 55.5 and 36.7 months, respectively ($p = 0.002$). Simultaneously, patients in the NACT + IDS group had an increased risk of death after 2 years. We speculated that the reason for this analysis may be as follows: although NACT can reduce the difficulty and risk of surgery, the criterion for satisfactory tumor shrinkage in these studies was the same for patients with intermittent cytoreductive surgery following neoadjuvant chemotherapy as for direct cytoreductive surgery, namely, residual lesions less than 1 cm. The number of chemotherapy regimens after intermittent neoplastic cytoreductive surgery following neoadjuvant chemotherapy is fewer than the number after direct surgery, because neoadjuvant chemotherapy may increase the chemoresistance potential of ovarian cancer cells. However, NACT + IDS did not improve patient prognosis. By analyzing the ideal tumor cytoreductive rates of two PDS groups of patients who scored < 5 and ≥ 5, the difference in the ideal tumor cytoreductive rate of the two groups was approximately 10%, and the ideal surgical cytoreductive rate in patients in the PDS group and with a score < 5 was significantly higher than that of patients with a score ≥ 5. Although there was no statistically significant difference between the two groups ($p = 0.296$), we cannot conclude that there was no difference in the rate of reduction between the two groups. We believe the reason may stem from limitations in the collection of cases. For the treatment of patients with newly diagnosed advanced EOC, the choice of the re-established New Scoring System score cut-off point has substantial guiding significance. Whether there is a score < 5 or ≥ 5, patients with ovarian cancer can choose a relatively more favorable treatment. Therefore, we believe the choice of the cut-off point was reasonable. Taken together, we hypothesize that patients with newly diagnosed advanced EOC and score < 5 who can tolerate PDS at presentation may be better able to manage the optimal surgical treatment time, shorten the duration of patient treatment, reduce pain, reduce treatment costs and improve long-term outcomes. However, patients with a score ≥ 5 who were treated with NACT + IDS were more conducive to reducing the difficulty and risk of surgery, improving the reduction rate of tumor cells and improving the quality of life.

Conclusion

Ovarian cancer has the highest mortality rate of all gynecological tumors. Most patients are already in advanced stages when they present for care. Advanced ovarian cancer tumor cells are widely disseminated. Their lesions are large and heavily infiltrate surrounding tissue. They also suppress organ function. Relevant reports show that only 42% of patients with severe disease can achieve ideal tumor reduction [15]. To delay the progression of the disease and to improve the quality of life, it is very important to choose treatment modalities for patients with newly diagnosed advanced epithelial ovarian cancer (EOC). We have evaluated the treatment by establishing a new evaluation system (new ovarian cancer CT model combined with serum CA125 levels). When patients are newly diagnosed with advanced EOC and have a score < 5, we suggest primary debulking surgery because this approach is able to save treatment time and costs and to improve the long-term prognosis. When the score is greater than or equal to 5 points, we are more inclined to recommend NACT + IDS in order to reduce the difficulty and risk of surgery and to improve the quality of life. There remains space for improvement and refinement of treatment options for patients with newly diagnosed EOC under the New Scoring System. Although at this stage of our research we can only provide some treatment ideas, we have laid a solid foundation for future research and analysis. There remain statistics from studies in other countries that show that NACT failed to improve 5-year survival rate and median survival time in patients with advanced ovarian cancer [16]. Therefore, in the future, we also need to explore and verify the treatment modalities of NACT and to conduct additional research and analysis on the New Scoring System to further demonstrate the rationale and validity of the scoring system and to provide strong evidence to support the choice of treatment modality.

Abbreviations

EOC: Epithelial ovarian cancer; IDS: Interval debulking surgery; NACT: Neoadjuvant chemotherapy; PDS: Primary debulking surgery

Acknowledgements

Thanks for the corresponding author's guidance and other authors' assistance.

Funding

This study was funded by a special project on the prevention and control of major chronic noncommunicable diseases in Chongqing, China: a research project on ovarian cancer treatment programs and clinical pathway planning. The funding item number is 2016YFC1303702.

Authors' contributions

LQ made substantial contributions to conception and design, planned and ran the experiments, collected data, performed data analysis, interpreted the results, reviewed the literature and wrote the manuscript. HH contributed to data collection. MC contributed to the literature discussion and conclusion. YL supervised the statistical analysis. HW gave final approval of the version to be published. All authors read and approved the final manuscript.

Competing interests

The authors declare that they have no competing interests.

References

1. Siegel R, Ma J, Zou Z. Cancer statistics,2014. Cancer. 2014;64(1):9–29.
2. Ce B, Xia Z. Neoadjuvant chemotherapy in the treatment of advanced ovarian cancer. J Pract Obstet Gynecol. 2015;04:263–6.
3. Bristow RE, Duska LR, Lambrou NC, et al. A model for predicting surgical outcome in patients with advanced ovarian carcinoma using computed tomography. Cancer. 2000;89(7):1532–40.
4. Vorgias G, Iavazzo C, Savvopoulos P, et al. Can the preoperative ca-125 level predict optimal cytoreduction in patients with advanced ovarian carcinoma?A single institution cohort study. Gynecol Oncol. 2009;112(1):11–5.
5. Colombo N, Van Gorp T, Parma G, et al. Ovarian cancer. Oncol Hematol. 2006;60(2):159–79.
6. Kang S. Does neoadjuvant chemotherapy increase optimal cytoreduction rate in advanced ovarian cancer? Meta-analysis of 21 studies. Surg Oncol. 2009;16(8):2315–20.
7. McGuire WP, Hoskins WJ, Brady MF, et al. Cyclophosphamide and cisplatin compared with paclitaxel and cisplatin in patients with stage III and stage IV ovarian cancer. N Engl J Med. 1996;334(1):1–6.
8. Xuemei J, Huihua D, Shuyu W, Wei X, Zhihong Z. The effect of neoadjuvant chemotherapy in gynecologic malignancies. Jiangsu Med. 2010;09:1017–20.
9. Tongwei R. Application of neoadjuvant chemotherapy in the treatment of advanced ovarian cancer. Chinese and Foreign Medical. 2009;22:8–10.
10. Ying Z, Yingli Z, Ping Z. Progress in Neoadjuvant Chemotherapy for Advanced Ovarian Cancer. J Oncol. 2014;11:942–6.
11. Obeidat B, Latimer J. Can optimal primary cytoreduction be predicted in advanced stage epithelial ovarian cancer? Role of preoperative serum CA-125 level. Gynecol Obstet Investig. 2004;57(3):153–6.
12. Loizzi V, Cormio G, Resta L, et al. Neoadjuvant chemotherapy in advanced ovarian cancer:a case-control study[J]. Int J Gynecol Cancer. 2005;15(2):217–23.
13. Wright JD, Ananth CV, Tsui J, et al. Comparative effectiveness of upfront treatment strategies in elderly women with ovarian cancer[J]. Cancer. 2014;120(8):1246–54.
14. Fago-Olsen CL, Ottesen B, Kehlet H, et al. Dose neoadjuvant chemotherapy impair long-term survival for ovarian cancer patients?A nationwide Danish study[J]. Gynecol Oncol. 2014;132(2):292–8.
15. Bristow RE, Tomacruz RS, Armstrong DK, et al. Survival effect of maximal cytoreductive surgery for advanced ovarian carcinoma during the platinum era: a meta-analysis. J Clin Oncol. 2002;20(5):1248–59.
16. Schwart PE. Contemporary considerations for neoadjuvant chemotherapy in primary ovarian cancer[J].Gynecology. Cancers. 2009;11(6):457–65.

Establishment and molecular characterization of a human ovarian clear cell carcinoma cell line (FDOV1)

Wei Jiang[1,3†], Shuang Ye[1,3†], Libing Xiang[1,3], Wentao Yang[2,3], Tiancong He[1,3], Xuan Pei[1,3], Lin Guo[3,4] and Huijuan Yang[1,3*]

Abstract

Background: Ovarian clear cell carcinoma is a distinct histologic subtype with grave survival. The underlying molecular mechanism is not fully elucidated. However, we don't have many cell lines, which are useful experimental tools for research. We describe the establishment and characterization of a new ovarian clear cell carcinoma cell line from a Chinese patient.

Results: FDOV1 has been subcultured for more than 80 generations. Monolayer cultured cells are polygonal in shape, showing a transparent cytoplasm full of vacuoles. The number of chromosomes ranges from 45 to 90. FDOV1 cells produces CA-125, but not CA-199. The cells could be transplanted and produced tumors mimicking the donor tumor morphologically and immunohistochemically. Whole exome sequence showed both FDOV1 and tissue block harbored PIK3CA H1047R mutation and ARID1A frameshift mutations (p.L2106 fs, p.N201 fs). More interestingly, we observed SPOP mutation (p.D82H) and ZNF217 (chromosome 20q13) amplification in FDOV1, which are quite novel.

Conclusions: Only a few patient-derived ovarian clear cell carcinoma cell lines have been reported in the literature. FDOV1 is the very first one, to the best of our knowledge, from a Mainland Chinese patient. It showed infinite multiplication until now and tumorigenicity in vivo. FDOV1 has co-existing PIK3CA and ARID1A mutations. It also harbored SPOP mutation and ZNF217 amplification, which would probably be a good model for exploring the molecular mechanism of ovarian clear cell carcinoma.

Keywords: Ovarian clear cell carcinoma, Cell line, FDOV1, ARID1A, PIK3CA, SPOP, ZNF217 amplification

Background

Epithelial ovarian carcinoma is the most lethal gynecologic malignancy. Ovarian clear cell carcinoma (OCCC) is the second most common histologic subtype, accounting for 5–25% of all ovarian cancer depending on geographic location [1, 2]. It is well acknowledged that OCCC is more commonly seen in Asia women [3, 4]. OCCC represents a great challenge due to its disease aggressiveness and chemotherapy resistance. The grave survival and lack of effective treatment prompt us to investigate the underlying molecular mechanism of OCCC.

The two most widely reported gene mutations in OCCC are AT-Rich Interactive Domain-containing protein 1A (ARID1A) and Phosphoinositide-3-kinase Catalytic Alpha (PIK3CA), representing around 50% [5, 6] and 40% [7, 8] of all cases, respectively. Further studies supported that loss of ARID1A expression frequently coexisted with PIK3CA mutations [9]. What's more, coexistent ARID1A-PIK3CA mutations might promote ovarian clear cell tumorigenesis through synergic effects [10, 11]. The breakthrough finding of ARID1A mutation has renewed the interest in elucidating the molecular pathways of OCCC [2], which still remains less well-understood than that of high-grade serous carcinoma.

* Correspondence: huijuanyang@hotmail.com
†Wei Jiang and Shuang Ye contributed equally to this work.
[1]Department of Gynecologic Oncology, Fudan University Shanghai Cancer Center, Shanghai 200032, China
[3]Department of Oncology, Shanghai Medical College, Fudan University, Shanghai 200032, China
Full list of author information is available at the end of the article

Cancer cell lines are affordable models for genetic and molecular profiles, reflecting the characteristics of the origin tumor. According to documentations till now, 16 OCCC cell lines were established and their characteristics have been reported [12–25], added ES-2 and TOV-21G, two commercial available cell lines, which characteristics and genetic features were obtained from ATCC database (http://www.atcc.org) and COSMIC database (https://cancer.sanger.ac.uk/cell_-lines), respectively. The majority of the established cell lines were derived from Japanese patients. Besides, only one OCCC cell line TOV-21G was found with PIK3CA and ARID1A mutation. We describe here the establishment and characterization of a novel cell line (FDOV1) from a Chinese patient that harbors coexistent ARID1A-PIK3CA mutations.

Results

Morphology and growth characteristics

Up to now, more than 80 serial passages have been carried out successively. FDOV1 cells grew in the form of an adherent monolayer without contact inhibition (Fig. 1). Several types of cells were noted: small round cells, oval cells, polygonal spindle cells and irregular cells. The cytoplasm was characteristic of transparency and vacuolation.

The cell growth curve was shown in Fig. 2. The population doubling time was 37.4 h, which was consistent with the low proliferation rate of OCCC. On flow cytometry analysis (Fig. 3), the cell cycle was distributed as: G1 phase, 42.3%; G2 phase, 36.1%; S phase, 21.6%.

Chromosomal analysis

A total of 45 metaphase cells from FDOV1 were examined for chromosome analysis. Chromosome numbers ranged from 45 to 90 (Fig. 4). The following karyotypes

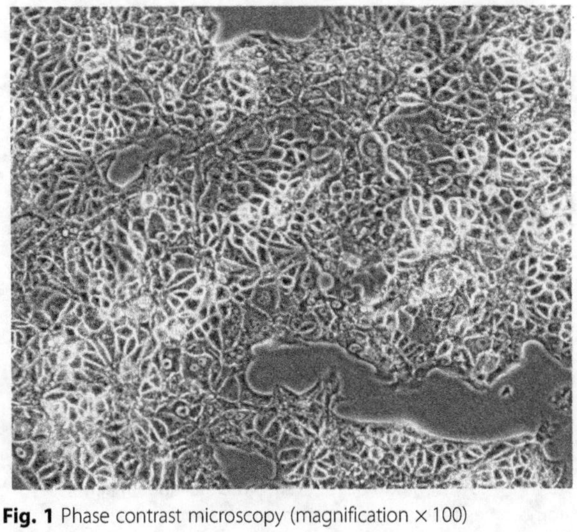

Fig. 1 Phase contrast microscopy (magnification × 100)

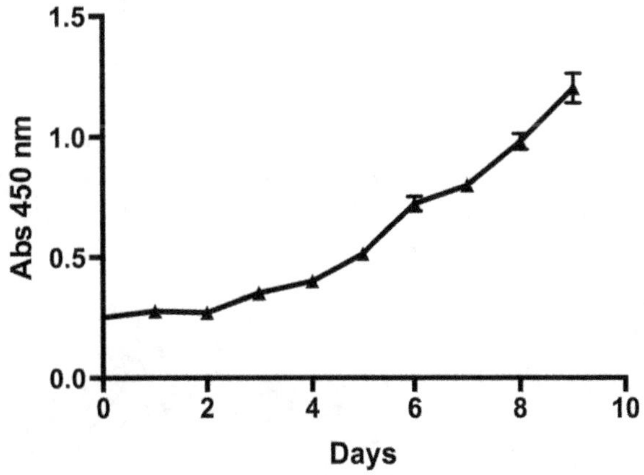

Fig. 2 Growth curve of FDOV1 (15th generation)

were observed: $2n = 45/46$ (35, 78%); $2n = 47$ (3, 7%); $4n = 86–90$ (6, 13%). Chromosomal aberrations including complex translocations and deletions were noted, which were consistent with that of malignant tumors.

Tumor markers

The results for tumor marker measurement were listed as follow: CA125, 33.7 U/ml; CA199, 0.78 U/ml; CA153, < 1.00 U/ml; CA724, 2.96 U/ml; AFP, < 0.61 ng/ml; CEA, 0.21 ng/ml; HE4, < 15 pmol/L.

Heterotransplantation

To determine tumorigenicity, FDOV1 cells were injected into the dorsal flanks of two mice. Both mice developed visible tumors 20 days after injection. Fig. 5 presents the magnetic resonance imaging (MRI) of transplanted tumors of two mice 40 days after transplantation.

Histopathology and immunohistochemical staining

As clearly seen from Fig. 6, the xenografts morphologically mimicked the primary tumor in HE staining. Both the transplant and donor tumors showed diffuse intensive positivity for HNF-1β and Pax-8. Besides, negative Napsin A, ER and PR were observed for both tumors (results not presented).

WES and sanger sequencing results

We performed WES on FDOV1 cell, patient's tissue block and peripheral blood. It was reported that the tumor purity of FDOV1 cells achieved 100% approximately, and that of the tumor block was 73%, which is fit for investigating the molecular aberrations, including single nucleotide variant (SNV), insertion and deletion (indel) and copy number variation (CNV). From the SNV related to cancer, it is shown that the tissue block and FDOV1 cell line shared some same somatic variations although diverse allele frequency (Fig. 7a). Interestingly, both tissue block and FDOV1 harbored PIK3CA

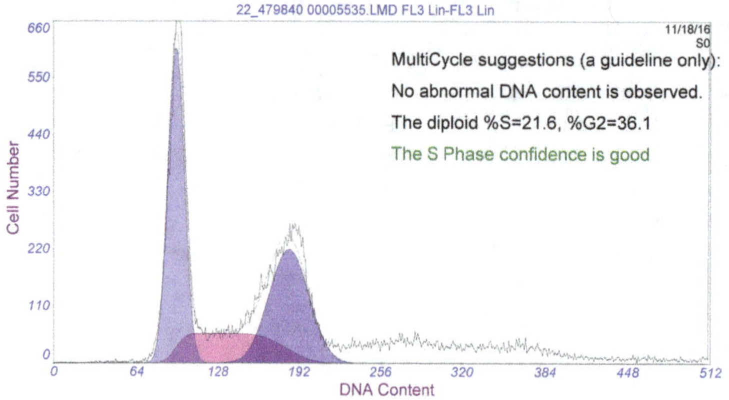

CELL CYCLE DATA

Mean G1= 96.108
CV G1 = 6.633
% G1 = 42.275

Mean G2=185.726
CV G2 = 8.185
% G2 = 36.101

% S = 21.623

G2/G1 = 1.932
Chi Sq.= 2.814
Cell No.=32138
% Debris= -1.000

Model	Chis	Dip S	Dip G2
S0	2.814	21.623	36.101
Sliced Bkgd	2.920	21.367	36.360
G2/G1 Fixed	4.219	25.561	32.464
Aggregates	2.902	21.381	36.351
S Order= 1	2.750	23.585	33.422
CVs Fixed	3.976	23.679	33.857
[S0 BADs]: Dip BAD= 0.00;			

Fig. 3 Cell cycle of FDOV1 by flow-cytometry analysis

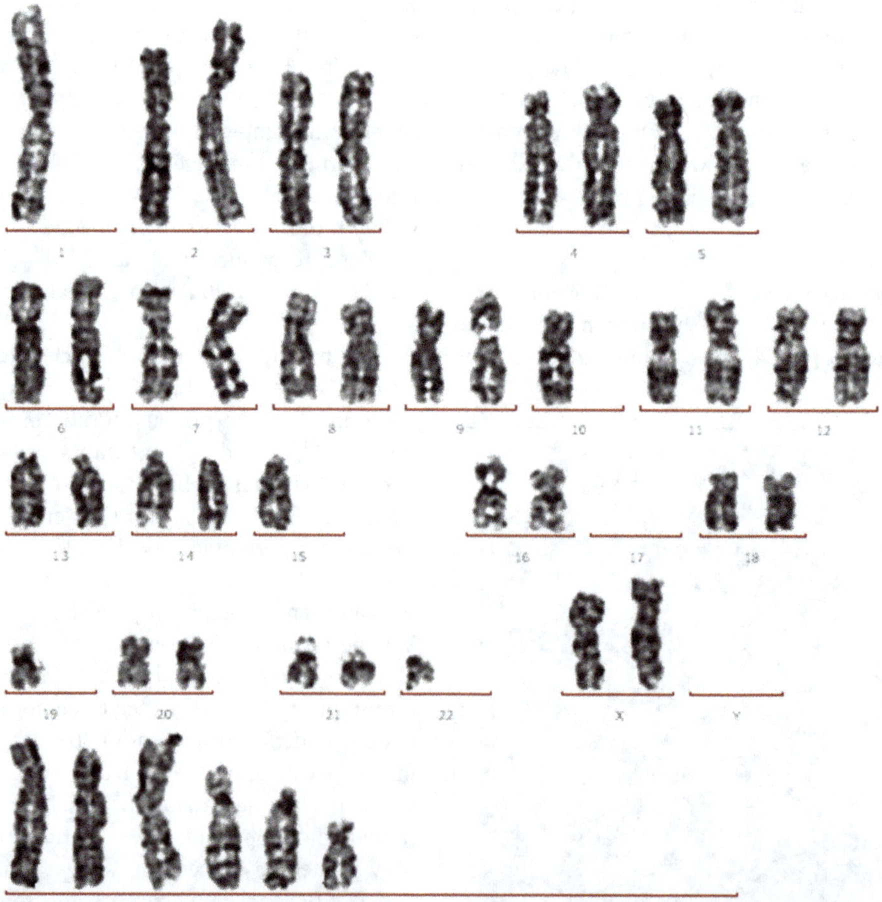

Fig. 4 Karyotype of FDOV1 (18th generation). The additional chromosomes listed in the lowest group have severe structural abnormality, including complex translocation and deletion. It is so difficult to identify the chromosomes that we present them in the lowest group

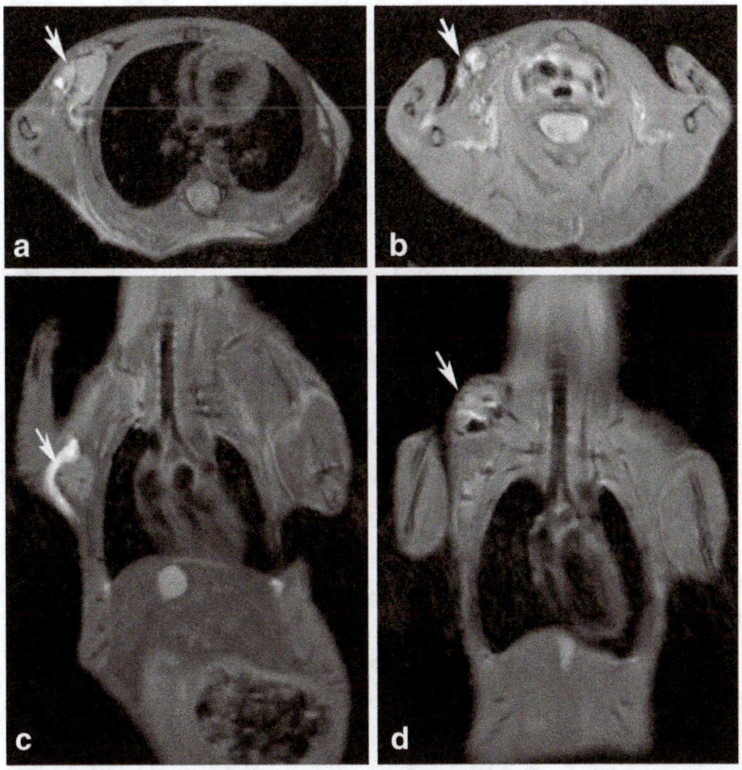

Fig. 5 Magnetic resonance imaging of two transplanted tumors. **a** and **c** showed the horizontal plane and coronal plane of one transplanted tumor, respectively, **b** and **d** showed the horizontal plane and coronal plane of the other transplanted tumor. The tumors in the dorsal flank were pointed out by arrows

H1047R mutation and ARID1A frameshift mutations (p.L2106 fs, p.N201 fs), which are viewed as the most important gene variations in OCCC. In addition, Both of them were found to carry SPOP (p.D82H, c.G244 T), ZNF217 (p.T985I, c.C2954T) and ARID1B (p.E1681X, c.G5041 T) mutations (Table 1), which were further validated by Sanger Sequencing (Fig. 8). Besides, Fig. 7b showed the CNV of tissue block and FDOV1. We observed that somatic copy number was increased in ZNF217(chr.20) and MYC(chr.8), which were reported as frequent amplifications in OCCC [26, 27], as well as MCL1(chr.1), RAD51(chr.15), DOT1L(chr.19), while copy number was decreased in TP53(chr.17), which was documented as a common copy number variant in OCCC [26], as well as NRAS(chr.1), AURKB(chr.17), STK11(chr.19) and CRLF2(chr.X) (Table 2).

Discussion

Ovarian clear cell carcinoma, as a subtype with distinct clinical behavior, is notorious for its poor survival and

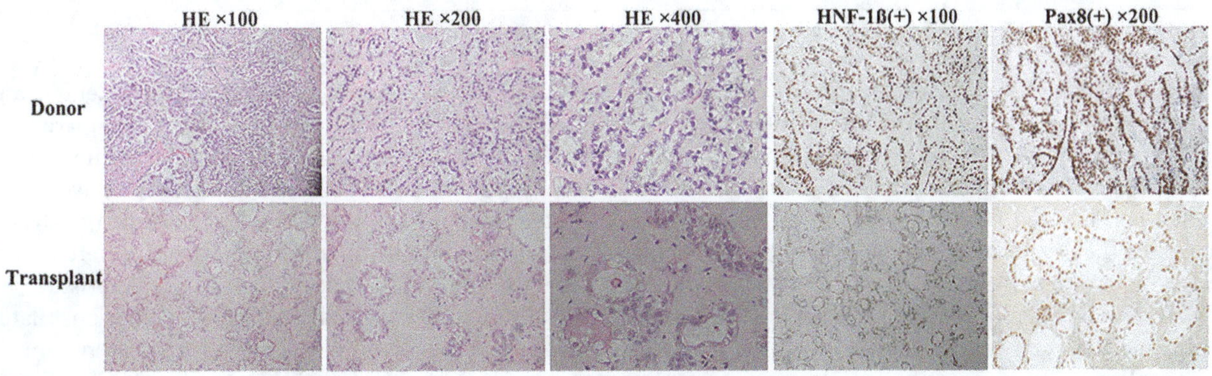

Fig. 6 Histology and immunohistochemistry of FDOV1 cell, donor tumor and transplanted tumor

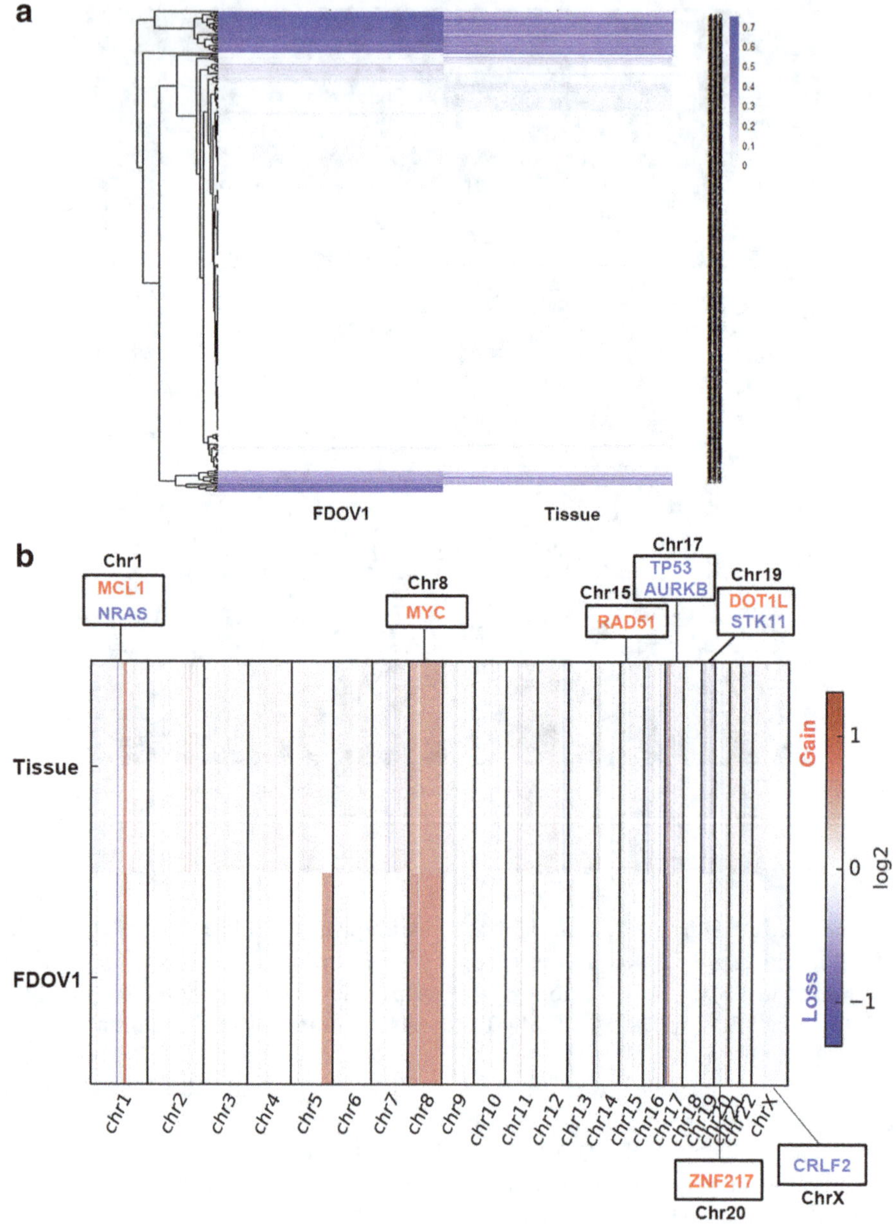

Fig. 7 The results of whole-exome sequencing of FDOV1 and patient's tumor tissue block. **a**. Somatic variation of FDOV1 and tumor tissue. **b**. Copy number analysis in FDOV1 and tissue. The genes in red mean copy number gain, the genes in blue mean copy number loss

resistance to conventional platinum-based chemotherapy. An international phase III clinical trial was conducted to investigate the addition of irinotecan as adjuvant chemotherapy for patients with advanced-stage [28]. Unfortunately, no significant survival benefit was found. Given the limited benefit from cytotoxic drugs, there is now great interest in the development of molecular targeted therapy, which requires investigation of a number of areas in the laboratory [3]. Better understanding of the underlying molecular mechanism is of importance.

According to documentations, there were 16 ovarian clear cell carcinoma cell lines reported so far, in addition, TOV-21G, ES-2, which are commercially available from American Tissue Culture Center, and FDOV1. Their characteristics were compared in Table 3. Firstly, most of the OCCC cell lines were from Japan, while FDOV1 is the only one derived from a Chinese mainland woman. It has been demonstrated that the same kind of carcinoma from different race even country tends to have distinct characteristics, especially genetic characteristics [29–31]. We postulated that genetic background might be partly the reason for the marked geographic difference in OCCC. Therefore, the establishment and characterization of a novel

Table 1 Single nucleotide variant (SNV) of FDOV1 by whole-exome sequencing(WES)

Gene	Pdot	Tissue	FDOV1
PIK3CA	p.H1047R	0.372	0.369
SPOP	p.D82H	0.36	0.5
ZNF217	p.T985I	0.329	0.46
ARID1A	p.L2106 fs	0.285	0.311
ARID1B	p.E1681X	0.277	0.588
ARID1A	p.N201 fs	0.271	0.339
FOXP1	p.S650delinsIS	0.081	
NOTCH2	p.P6fs	0.081	
KMT2C	p.K2797 fs	0.048	
MAP3K1	p.941_942del	0.039	
TGFBR2	p.E125fs	0.034	
KMT2C	p.T820I	0.033	
ABL1	p.605_605del	0.029	
ROCK2	p.R1295G	0.026	
KMT2D	c.8366 + 1G > T	0.02	
ERBB4	p.G565 V	0.017	
KMT2C	p.D319Y	0.014	
CTNNA1	p.M721 fs	0.013	
KMT2C	p.R4418S		0.028
KMT2D	p.3860_3861del		0.02
RNF43	p.R145L		0.018
KMT2A	p.A1253S		0.012

cell line derived from Chinese patients is of significance. Secondly, all cell lines were derived from ovary (10/19), ascites (6/19), and metastatic or recurrent site (3/19), which implied good materials for primarily culture. Lastly, as previously mentioned, ARID1A and PIK3CA mutations are the two most commonly reported. Interestingly, it is found that ARID1A–PIK3CA mutational co-occurrence (33%) is very high in ovarian CCC [11]. Research work by Chandler et al. supported that a genetic epistasis model wherein ARID1A and PIK3CA mutations cooperate and ovarian cancer can arise only when these genes are co-mutated in the mouse ovarian surface epithelium [11]. Coexistent ARID1A–PIK3CA mutations might be a major driver of OCCC in humans. Among 19 OCCC cell lines, only FDOV1 and TOV-21G carried coexistent ARID1A–PIK3CA mutations. The character of concurrent ARID1A–PIK3CA mutations of FDOV1 might help to better understand the underlying mechanism and even to explore the activity of dual inhibitors in vitro. However, the cell lines established before 2000 lack genetic information due to testing techniques. Besides, some new molecular features found by WES in FDOV1 requires more attentions.

Notably, SPOP, a relatively new gene regulating DNA damage repair, is the most frequently mutated gene in prostate carcinoma [32, 33]. Mutations in SPOP lead to genomics instability and are identified as driver events resulting in tumorigenesis of prostate carcinoma via coordination with PI3K/mTOR and AR (Androgen Receptor) pathway in mouse [34, 35]. Studies on SPOP mutation in other solid carcinomas is reported in follicular and papillary thyroid cancers [36, 37], endometrial clear cell carcinoma [38, 39], gynecological carcinosarcoma [40], lung cancer [41], and colorectal cancer [42]. What is worthy of mentioning is that SPOP mutation in gynecological malignant tumor is not uncommon (18% in endometrial clear cell carcinoma, 14% in carcinosarcoma) [38, 40]. In OCCC, the mutation rate of SPOP is 11.1% (1/9) according to COSMIC (Catalogue Of Somatic Mutations In Cancer) database. However, few relevant functional studies are documented in OCCC. Thus, FDOV1, a novel cell line harbored SPOP mutation, is an ideal tool for functional study. In addition, it is suggested that SPOP mutation might represent sensitivity to DNA damaging agents such as PARP inhibitor in prostate carcinoma [35]. Consequently, whether it is indicated a similar effect on OCCC still needs further investigation.

Chromosome 20q13 ZNF217 (Zinc Finger Protein 217) locus amplification, which has found in FDOV1, is one of common molecuclar genetic aberrations in OCCC [43]. The frequency is reported from 20 to 36% [10, 43, 44]. It is reported that ZNF217 amplification often coexisted with loss of ARID1A expression and PIK3CA mutation [10]. Importantly, ZNF217 amplification has a correlation with shorter worse survival outcome in OCCC, and multivariate analysis suggest it is an independent prognostic factor of PFS (Progression-Free Survival) and OS (Overall survival) [43]. Still, ZNF217 amplification has an adverse prognostic implication in breast and gastric cancer [45–47]. However, the underlying mechanism is still tensely studied. FDOV1 will be an good cell line for mechanism research in vitro.

Conclusions

An ovarian clear cell carcinoma cell line named FDOV1 was established from a Mainland Chinese patient. FDOV1 showed fast and unlimited multiplication until now and tumorigenicity in vivo. In addition, WES showed that it harbors concurrent ARID1A–PIK3CA mutations and SPOP mutation, also with ZNF217 amplification, which will be an ideal tool for mechanism research of ovarian clear cell carcinoma.

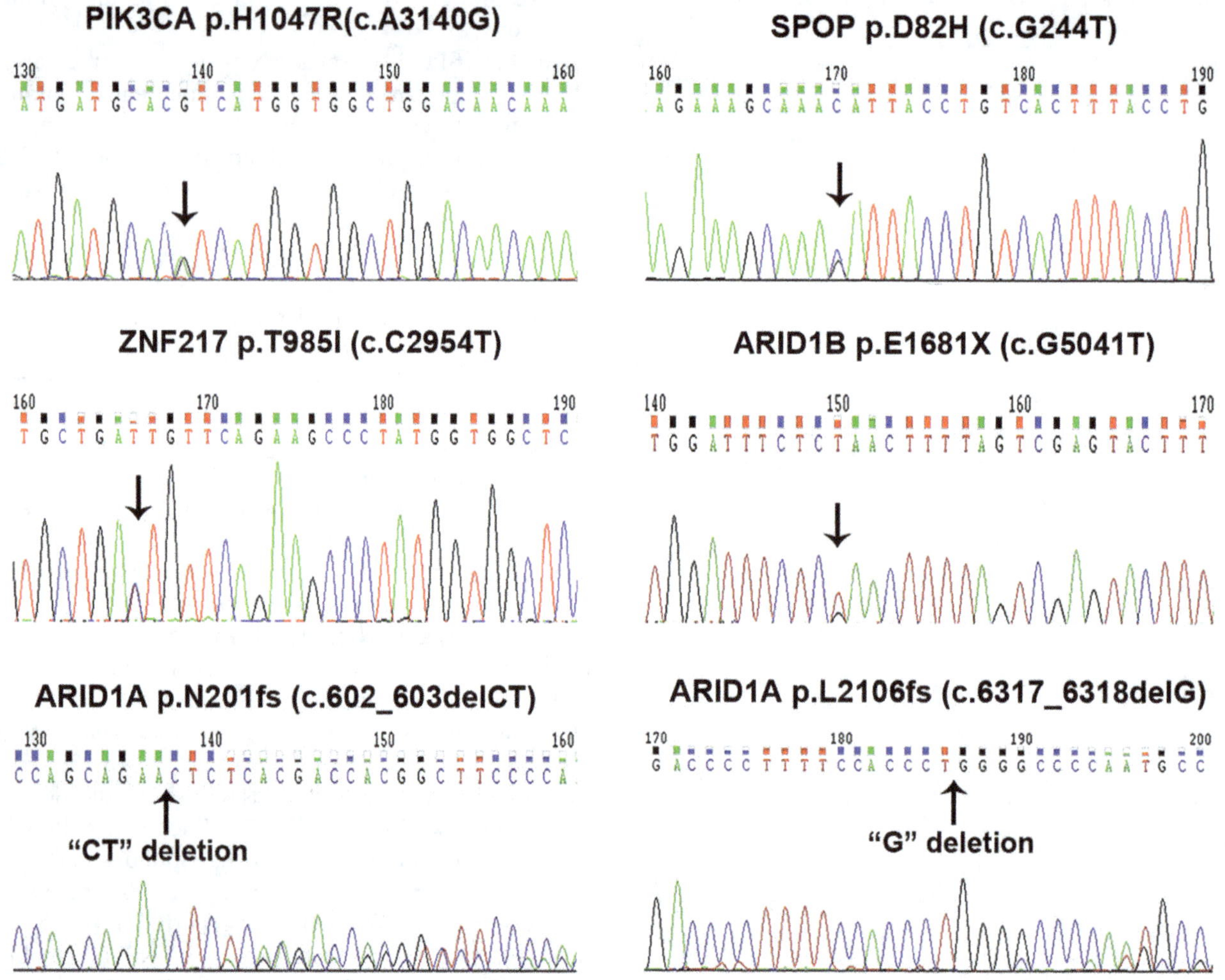

Fig. 8 Sanger sequencing of single nucleotide variant (SNV) in FDOV1

Table 2 Copy number variant (CNV) of FDOV1 by whole-exome sequencing (WES)

	Chr	Tissue	FDOV1
Upregulated Genes			
ZNF217	chr20	0.75	0.91
MYC	chr8	0.50	0.89
DOT1L	chr19	0.78	1.12
MCL1	chr1	0.48	0.77
RAD51	chr15	0.47	0.94
Downregulated Genes			
NRAS	chr1	−0.65	−1.01
TP53	chr17	−0.55	− 1.04
AURKB	chr17	−0.55	−1.04
STK11	chr19	−0.64	−1.05
CRLF2	chrX	−1.38	−1.41

The number in column of tissue and FDOV1 represent the log2 (sample/germline), consequently, the number more than 0 suggests amplified in copy number, less than 0 suggests decreased in copy number

Methods

Medical history

A 67-year-old woman was admitted into Fudan University Shanghai Cancer Center with the chief complaint of palpable abdominal mass in May 2016. Ultrasound revealed a large pelvic mass (14 × 10 cm) with mixed components and a hyperechoic mural nodule (4 × 3 cm). Serum tumor markers including carbohydrate antigen (CA) 125 and CA199 were not elevated. Intraoperative findings were only significant for a cystic-and-solid mass (15 cm in diameter) in the left adnexa. Frozen pathology was highly suspicious of ovarian clear cell carcinoma. The patient underwent comprehensive staging surgery and the final stage was FIGO (International Federation of Gynecology and Obstetrics) Ia. She gave written informed consent before surgery according to institutional guideline (FUSCC 050432–4-1212B). Six cycles of TC regimen (paclitaxel + carboplatin) chemotherapy were administered. She was followed up every 3 months after treatment. The patient was admitted into outside hospital with chief complain of

Table 3 Cell lines of ovary clear cell carcinoma

	Cell line	Country	Age	Material	DT	Chromosome number	Transplantability	Gene characteristics
1	HUOCA-II (1987)	Japan	51	Ovary	24,28	46	Yes	
2	RMG-I (1988)	Japan	34	Ascites	60	47	Yes	
3	OCC1 (1990)	Hong Kong	47	Ascites	36,38	70–77	Yes	
4	RMG-II (1991)	Japan	53	Ascites	58	hypertetraploid	No	
5	TOV-21G(1991)[a]	French-Canadian descent	62	Ovary	36	47	Yes	ARID1A p.Q758fs[a]75, ARID1A p.Y551fs[a]72, KRAS p.G13C, PIK3CA p.H1047Y
6	ES-2(1991)[a]	Black	47	Ovary	24	66- 88	Yes	BRAF p.V600E, MAP2K1 p.D67N
7	OVISE (1995)	Japan	40	Metastatic tumor	60–70	59–65	Yes	
8	OVTOKO (1995)	Japan	78	Metastatic tumor	60–70	76–83	Yes	
9	JHOC-5 (1999)	Japan	47	Ovary	52	74–85	No	
10	JHOC-6 (1999)	Japan	43	Recurrent tumor	70	46–49	Yes	
11	SMOV-2 (1999)	Japan	46	Ovary	48.2	85–92	Yes	P53 mutation (–)
12	TAYA (2002)	Japan	43	Ascites	50	69–74	No	P53 mutation (codon 132 in exon 5), PTEN mutation(–)
13	RMG-V (2005)	Japan	52	Ascites	15.5	77–85	No	
14	TU-OC-1 (2013)	Japan	65	Ovary	38.4	64–90	Yes	PIK3CA E542K mutation
15	TU-OC-2(2016)	Japan	68	Ovary	37.5	41–96	No	PIK3CA mutation (–), TP53 mutation (–) ARID1A loss
16	HCH-1 (2016)	Japan	67	Ovary	48.7, 66.4	39–44	Yes	PIK3CA mutation (–), P53 mutation(–), PTEN mutation(–), KRAS mutation(–)
17	NOCC(2016)	Japan	48	Ascites	29	60–83	Yes	
18	HCH-3 (2017)	Japan	41	Ovary	82	78–87	Yes	KRAS mutation (+), TP53 mutation(+)
19	FDOV1(2017)	China mainland	67	Ovary	37.4	45–90	Yes	PIK3CA p.H1047R, ARID1A p.L2106 fs, ARID1A p.N201 fs, SPOP p.D82H ARID1B p.E1681X

[a]The biological characteristics of TOV-21G and ES-2 were obtained from ATCC database (http://www.atcc.org), and the genetic variants of TOV-21G and ES-2 were obtained from COSMIC database (https://cancer.sanger.ac.uk/cell_lines), which provide more detailed and complete genetic features of cell lines

intestinal obstruction in May 2017. She developed multiple sites of venous thromboembolism and cerebral infarction. Unfortunately, she died 1 month later with no chance of anti-cancer treatment.

Establishment of cell line

The fresh tissue (1 cm^3) from primary ovarian tumor was obtained during comprehensive staging surgery, and suspended in phosphate buffer solution (PBS) to get rid of necrotic and connective tissue. The material was then finely minced into 1-mm^3 tissue blocks and placed in 10-cm cell culture dishes (Corning, NY, USA) containing Medium 199 medium (HyClone, Thermo Scientific, USA) with 10% fetal bovine serum (Gibco, Life technologies, USA), 100 IU/ml penicillin (HyClone, Thermo Scientific, USA) and 50 μg/ml streptomycin (HyClone, Thermo Scientific, USA). The cells were then incubated in a humidified atmosphere containing 5% CO2 at 37 °C. After repeated passage, a new cell line of FDOV1 was successfully established with more than 80 generations. FDOV1 cells have been sent to China General Microbiological Culture Collection Center for preservation (No. 13812) in March 2017.

Growth characteristics

Cell proliferation and growth curve was determined by Cell Counting Kit-8 (CCK-8) test. FDOV1 cells (2×10^3 cells/100 μl) were seeded in 96-well plates in sextuplicate. Ten days later, 100 μl mixture (CCK-8/medium 1:9) were added into the wells for incubation by 2 hours. We then measured the Optical Density (OD) at 450 nm (OD_{450}) by a microplate reader (Synergy H4, Bio-Tek).

Cell cycle analysis by flow cytometry

Resuspended FDOV1 cells (1×10^6 cell) were kept overnight in 3 ml 75% ethanol at − 20 °C. After treatment, the cells were collected and stained with propidium iodide solution for 20 min at 4 °C in darkness. We then assessed the cell cycle by flow cytometer (BD Biosciences, San Jose, CA, USA).

Chromosome analysis

The cells in exponential phase were treated with 0.25 μg/ml colchicine for 6 hours and kept overnight at 37 °C. We then treated the cells with 0.1% trypsin solution for 15 s at room temperature and stained them with 3% Giemsa for G-band karyotyping. After examing 45 metaphases, the histograms of the chromosomal distribution were determined.

Tumor markers

A total of 2×10^6 cells were cultured for 4 days in total. The medium was changed and collected every 2 days, then were sent for tumor marker detection by chemiluminescence immunoassay. Detected markers included CA 125, CA 199, CA 153, CA 724, AFP, CEA and HE4.

Heterotransplantation

All the procedures were approved by the Department of Laboratory Animal Science in Fudan University. For in vivo studies, 4–6 weeks old NOD/SCID mice (Shanghai SLAC Laboratory Animal, Shanghai, China) were maintained under sterile conditions. FDOV1 cells (1×10^7 cells, passage 18) were injected subcutaneously into the dorsal flanks of two mice. Visible tumors were noted in both mice 20 days after transplantation.

Histological analysis and immunohistochemistry

Transplant tumors were fixed in 10% buffered formalin for 24 h and embedded in paraffin. Hematoxylin and eosin (HE) were used to stain 4-μm sections. The markers used for immunohistochemistry were listed as follows: HNF-1β (Sigma, CA, USA), Napsin A (Abcam, Cambridge, UK), Pax-8 (Cellmarque, CA, USA), ER (Roche, Basel, Swiss) and PR (Roche, Basel, Swiss). Microscopic slides were reviewed by a senior gynecology-dedicated pathologist (Prof. Yang).

Whole-exome sequencing (WES) of FDOV1 cell and patient's tumor tissue

The WES was performed by 3D Medicines Corporation and the specific method was the same as a previous publication [48].

Sanger sequencing

Mutations of the specific genes in FDOV1 cells were validated by Sanger Sequencing. The RNA was extracted by Trizol Methods, then reverse transcription polymerase chain reaction (RT-PCR) was performed as our previous study [49]. The primers were showed in Additional file 1: Table S1. PCR amplification was performed as follows: denaturation at 98 °C for 5 min, 30 cycle of 98 °C for 10s, 58 °C for 30s, and 72 °C for 1 min, then holding at 72 °C for 1 min, finally incubation at 4 °C. Sequencing was performed at Boshang Biotechnology Co.Ltd. (Shanghai, China).

Abbreviations

AFP: Alpha fetoprotein; ARID1A: AT-Rich Interactive Domain-containing protein 1A; CA125: Carbohydrate antigen125; CA199: Carbohydrate antigen 199; CEA: Carcinoembryonic antigen; HE4: Human epididymis protein 4; OCCC: Ovarian clear cell carcinoma; PIK3CA: Phosphoinositide-3-kinase Catalytic Alpha; FIGO: International Federation of Gynecology and Obstetrics; TC: Paclitaxel & Carboplatin; PBS: Phosphate buffer solution; CCK8: Cell counting kit-8; OD450: Optical density (OD) at 450 nm; HE: Hematoxylin and eosin; MRI: Magnetic resonance imaging; WES: Whole-exome sequence; SNV: Single nucleotide variant; CNV: Copy number variation; indel: Insertion and deletion; ER: Estrogen receptor; AR: Androgen receptor; PR: Progesterone receptor; ZNF217: Zinc Finger Protein 217; PFS: Progression-Free Survival; OS: Overall survival

Acknowledgements

We thank Dr. David Chan for his advice in manuscript preparation. We thank 3D Medicines Corporation for WES analysis.

Funding

The study was supported by grants from National Natural Science Foundation of China (81572803 and 81702558).

Authors' contributions

HY and LX treated the patient and collected clinicopathological data. WJ and LX were involved in sample collection, processing and cell culture. WJ, TH and XP studied the biological and molecular characteristics of the cell lines as well as its tumorigenicity. WY performed the histological examination and immunohistological staining of the surgical tissues, cell cultures and tumors from transplants. LG measured tumor markers. HY and WJ analyzed and interpreted the data of the patients, cell line and the transplant. SY was a major contributor in writing the manuscript and HY finalized the paper. All authors read and approved the final manuscript.

Competing interests

The authors declare that they have no competing interests.

Author details

[1]Department of Gynecologic Oncology, Fudan University Shanghai Cancer Center, Shanghai 200032, China. [2]Department of Pathology, Fudan University Shanghai Cancer Center, Shanghai 200032, China. [3]Department of Oncology, Shanghai Medical College, Fudan University, Shanghai 200032, China. [4]Department of Clinical Laboratory, Fudan University Shanghai Cancer Center, Shanghai 200032, China.

References

1. Anglesio MS, Carey MS, Kobel M, Mackay H, Huntsman DG. Clear cell carcinoma of the ovary: a report from the first ovarian clear cell symposium, June 24th, 2010. Gynecol Oncol. 2011;121(2):407–15.
2. del Carmen MG, Birrer M, Schorge JO. Clear cell carcinoma of the ovary: a review of the literature. Gynecol Oncol. 2012;126(3):481–90.
3. Okamoto A, Glasspool RM, Mabuchi S, Matsumura N, Nomura H, Itamochi H, et al. Gynecologic Cancer InterGroup (GCIG) consensus review for clear cell carcinoma of the ovary. Int J Gynecol Cancer. 2014;24(9 Suppl 3):S20–5.
4. Sung PL, Chang YH, Chao KC, Chuang CM. Global distribution pattern of histological subtypes of epithelial ovarian cancer: a database analysis and systematic review. Gynecol Oncol. 2014;133(2):147–54.
5. Jones S, Wang TL, Shih le M, Mao TL, Nakayama K, Roden R, et al. Frequent mutations of chromatin remodeling gene ARID1A in ovarian clear cell carcinoma. Science. 2010;330(6001):228–31.
6. Wiegand KC, Shah SP, Al-Agha OM, Zhao Y, Tse K, Zeng T, et al. ARID1A mutations in endometriosis-associated ovarian carcinomas. N Engl J Med. 2010;363(16):1532–43.
7. Campbell IG, Russell SE, Choong DY, Montgomery KG, Ciavarella ML, Hooi CS, et al. Mutation of the PIK3CA gene in ovarian and breast cancer. Cancer Res. 2004;64(21):7678–81.
8. Kuo KT, Mao TL, Jones S, Veras E, Ayhan A, Wang TL, et al. Frequent activating mutations of PIK3CA in ovarian clear cell carcinoma. Am J Pathol. 2009;174(5):1597–601.
9. Yamamoto S, Tsuda H, Takano M, Tamai S, Matsubara O. Loss of ARID1A protein expression occurs as an early event in ovarian clear-cell carcinoma development and frequently coexists with PIK3CA mutations. Mod Pathol. 2012;25(4):615–24.
10. Huang HN, Lin MC, Huang WC, Chiang YC, Kuo KT. Loss of ARID1A expression and its relationship with PI3K-Akt pathway alterations and ZNF217 amplification in ovarian clear cell carcinoma. Mod Pathol. 2014; 27(7):983–90.
11. Chandler RL, Damrauer JS, Raab JR, Schisler JC, Wilkerson MD, Didion JP, et al. Coexistent ARID1A-PIK3CA mutations promote ovarian clear-cell tumorigenesis through pro-tumorigenic inflammatory cytokine signalling. Nat Commun. 2015;6:6118.
12. Yamada T, Hattori K, Satomi H, Okazaki T, Mori H, Hirose Y. Establishment and characterization of a cell line (HCH-1) originating from a human clear cell carcinoma of the ovary. J Ovarian Res. 2016;9(1):32.
13. Ishiwata I, Ishiwata C, Soma M, Ishikawa H. Establishment of HUOCA-II, a human ovarian clear cell adenocarcinoma cell line, and its angiogenic activity. J Natl Cancer Inst. 1987;78(4):667–73.
14. Nozawa S, Tsukazaki K, Sakayori M, Jeng CH, Iizuka R. Establishment of a human ovarian clear cell carcinoma cell line (RMG-I) and its single cell cloning–with special reference to the stem cell of the tumor. Hum Cell. 1988;1(4):426–35.
15. Nozawa S, Yajima M, Sasaki H, Tsukazaki K, Aoki D, Sakayori M, et al. A new CA125-like antigen (CA602) recognized by two monoclonal antibodies against a newly established ovarian clear cell carcinoma cell line (RMG-II). Jpn J Cancer Res. 1991;82(7):854–61.
16. Gorai I, Nakazawa T, Miyagi E, Hirahara F, Nagashima Y, Minaguchi H. Establishment and characterization of two human ovarian clear cell adenocarcinoma lines from metastatic lesions with different properties. Gynecol Oncol. 1995;57(1):33–46.
17. Yamada K, Tachibana T, Hashimoto H, Suzuki K, Yanagida S, Endoh H, et al. Establishment and characterization of cell lines derived from serous adenocarcinoma (JHOS-2) and clear cell adenocarcinoma (JHOC-5, JHOC-6) of human ovary. Hum Cell. 1999;12(3):131–8.
18. Yonamine K, Hayashi K, Iida T. Establishment and characterization of human ovarian clear cell adenocarcinoma cell line (SMOV-2), and its cytotoxity by anticancer agents. Hum Cell. 1999;12(3):139–48.
19. Saga Y, Suzuki M, Machida S, Ohwada M, Sato I. Establishment of a new cell line (TAYA) of clear cell adenocarcinoma of the ovary and its radiosensitivity. Oncology. 2002;62(2):180–4.
20. Aoki D, Suzuki N, Susumu N, Noda T, Suzuki A, Tamada Y, et al. Establishment and characterization of the RMG-V cell line from human ovarian clear cell adenocarcinoma. Hum Cell. 2005;18(3):143–6.
21. Itamochi H, Kato M, Nishimura M, Oumi N, Oishi T, Shimada M, et al. Establishment and characterization of a novel ovarian clear cell adenocarcinoma cell line, TU-OC-1, with a mutation in the PIK3CA gene. Hum Cell. 2013;26(3):121–7.
22. Sato S, Itamochi H, Oumi N, Chiba Y, Oishi T, Shimada M, et al. Establishment and characterization of a novel ovarian clear cell carcinoma cell line, TU-OC-2, with loss of ARID1A expression. Hum Cell. 2016;29(4):181–7.
23. Wong WS, Wong YF, Ng YT, Huang PD, Chew EC, Ho TH, et al. Establishment and characterization of a new human cell line derived from ovarian clear cell carcinoma. Gynecol Oncol. 1990;38(1):37–45.
24. Ohyama A, Toyomura J, Tachibana T, Isonishi S, Takahashi H, Ishikawa H. Establishment and characterization of a clear cell carcinoma cell line, designated NOCC, derived from human ovary. Hum Cell. 2016;29(4):188–96.
25. Yamada T, Hattori K, Satomi H, Okazaki T, Moriand H, Hirose Y. Characterization of a novel cell line (HCH-3) derived from a human ovarian clear cell carcinoma. J Carcinog Mutagen. 2017;8(3):292.
26. Murakami R, Matsumura N, Brown JB, Higasa K, Tsutsumi T, Kamada M, et al. Exome sequencing landscape analysis in ovarian clear cell carcinoma shed light on key chromosomal regions and mutation gene networks. Am J Pathol. 2017;187(10):2246–58.
27. Kim SI, Lee JW, Lee M, Kim HS, Chung HH, Kim JW, et al. Genomic landscape of ovarian clear cell carcinoma via whole exome sequencing. Gynecol Oncol. 2018;148(2):375–82.
28. Sugiyama T, Okamoto A, Enomoto T, Hamano T, Aotani E, Terao Y, et al. Randomized phase III trial of irinotecan plus cisplatin compared with paclitaxel plus carboplatin as first-line chemotherapy for ovarian clear cell carcinoma: JGOG3017/GCIG trial. J Clin Oncol Off J Am Soc Clin Oncol. 2016;34(24):2881–7.
29. Lai Y, Wang C, Civan JM, Palazzo JP, Ye Z, Hyslop T, et al. Effects of Cancer stage and treatment differences on racial disparities in survival from Colon Cancer: a United States population-based study. Gastroenterology. 2016; 150(5):1135–46.
30. Goutte N, Sogni P, Bendersky N, Barbare JC, Falissard B, Farges O. Geographical variations in incidence, management and survival of hepatocellular carcinoma in a western country. J Hepatol. 2017;66(3):537–44.
31. Keenan T, Moy B, Mroz EA, Ross K, Niemierko A, Rocco JW, et al. Comparison of the genomic landscape between primary breast Cancer in African American versus white women and the Association of Racial Differences with Tumor Recurrence. J Clin Oncol Off J Am Soc Clin Oncol. 2015;33(31):3621–7.
32. Abeshouse A, Ahn J, Akbani R, Ally A, Amin S, Andry CD, et al. The molecular taxonomy of primary prostate cancer. Cell. 2015;163(4):1011–25.
33. Barbieri CE, Baca SC, Lawrence MS, Demichelis F, Blattner M, Theurillat JP, et al. Exome sequencing identifies recurrent SPOP, FOXA1 and MED12 mutations in prostate cancer. Nat Genet. 2012;44(6):685–9.
34. Blattner M, Liu D, Robinson BD, Huang D, Poliakov A, Gao D, et al. SPOP mutation drives prostate tumorigenesis in vivo through coordinate regulation of PI3K/mTOR and AR signaling. Cancer Cell. 2017;31(3):436–51.
35. Boysen G, Barbieri CE, Prandi D, Blattner M, Chae SS, Dahija A, et al. SPOP mutation leads to genomic instability in prostate cancer. Elife. 2015;4:e09207.
36. Yoo SK, Lee S, Kim SJ, Jee HG, Kim BA, Cho H, et al. Comprehensive analysis of the transcriptional and mutational landscape of follicular and papillary thyroid cancers. PLoS Genet. 2016;12(8):e1006239.
37. Ye L, Zhou X, Huang F, Wang W, Qi Y, Xu H, et al. The genetic landscape of benign thyroid nodules revealed by whole exome and transcriptome sequencing. Nat Commun. 2017;8:15533.
38. Le Gallo M, Rudd ML, Urick ME, Hansen NF, Zhang S, Lozy F, et al. Somatic mutation profiles of clear cell endometrial tumors revealed by whole exome and targeted gene sequencing. Cancer. 2017;123(17):3261–8.
39. DeLair DF, Burke KA, Selenica P, Lim RS, Scott SN, Middha S, et al. The genetic landscape of endometrial clear cell carcinomas. J Pathol. 2017; 243(2):230–41.
40. Jones S, Stransky N, McCord CL, Cerami E, Lagowski J, Kelly D, et al. Genomic analyses of gynaecologic carcinosarcomas reveal frequent mutations in chromatin remodelling genes. Nat Commun. 2014;5:5006.
41. Kan Z, Jaiswal BS, Stinson J, Janakiraman V, Bhatt D, Stern HM, et al. Diverse somatic mutation patterns and pathway alterations in human cancers. Nature. 2010;466(7308):869–73.
42. Kim MS, Je EM, Oh JE, Yoo NJ, Lee SH. Mutational and expressional analyses of SPOP, a candidate tumor suppressor gene, in prostate, gastric and colorectal cancers. APMIS. 2013;121(7):626–33.
43. Rahman MT, Nakayama K, Rahman M, Nakayama N, Ishikawa M, Katagiri A, et al. Prognostic and therapeutic impact of the chromosome 20q13.2 ZNF217 locus amplification in ovarian clear cell carcinoma. Cancer. 2012; 118(11):2846–57.

44. Huang HN, Huang WC, Lin CH, Chiang YC, Huang HY, Kuo KT. Chromosome 20q13.2 ZNF217 locus amplification correlates with decreased E-cadherin expression in ovarian clear cell carcinoma with PI3K-Akt pathway alterations. Hum Pathol. 2014;45(11):2318–25.
45. Littlepage LE, Adler AS, Kouros-Mehr H, Huang G, Chou J, Krig SR, et al. The transcription factor ZNF217 is a prognostic biomarker and therapeutic target during breast cancer progression. Cancer Discov. 2012;2(7):638–51.
46. Bellanger A, Donini CF, Vendrell JA, Lavaud J, Machuca-Gayet I, Ruel M, et al. The critical role of the ZNF217 oncogene in promoting breast cancer metastasis to the bone. J Pathol. 2017;242(1):73–89.
47. Shida A, Fujioka S, Kurihara H, Ishibashi Y, Mitsumori N, Omura N, et al. Prognostic significance of ZNF217 expression in gastric carcinoma. Anticancer Res. 2014;34(9):4813–7.
48. Feng F, Cheng Q, Yang L, Zhang D, Ji S, Zhang Q, et al. Guidance to rational use of pharmaceuticals in gallbladder sarcomatoid carcinoma using patient-derived cancer cells and whole exome sequencing. Oncotarget. 2017;8(3): 5349–60.
49. Xiang L, Li J, Jiang W, Shen X, Yang W, Wu X, et al. Comprehensive analysis of targetable oncogenic mutations in chinese cervical cancers. Oncotarget. 2015;6(7):4968–75.

6

Comparison of benign peritoneal fluid- and ovarian cancer ascites-derived extracellular vesicle RNA biomarkers

Cindy M. Yamamoto[1*], Melanie L. Oakes[1], Taku Murakami[1], Michael G. Muto[2], Ross S. Berkowitz[2] and Shu-Wing Ng[2,3]

Abstract

Background: Extracellular vesicles (EVs) are considered as a new class of resources for potential biomarkers. We analyzed expression of specific mRNA and miRNA in EVs derived from ovarian cancer ascites and the ideal controls, peritoneal fluids from benign patients for potential early detection and prognostic biomarkers.

Methods: Fluids were collected from subjects with benign cysts or endometrioma ($n = 10$), or low/high grade serous ovarian carcinoma ($n = 8$). EV particles were captured using primarily ExoComplete filterplate or ultracentrifugation and analyzed by nanoparticle tracking analysis, ELISA, and scanning electron microscopy. EV RNAs extracted from two ascites and three peritoneal fluids were submitted for next-generation sequencing. The expression of 34 mRNA and 18 miRNAs in the EVs isolated from patient fluids and cell line media was determined using qPCR.

Results: EVs isolated from patient samples had concentrations greater than 10^{10} EV particles/mL and 30% were EpCAM-positive based on ELISA. EV particle sizes averaged 113 ± 11.5 nm. The qPCR studies identified five mRNA (*CA11, MEDAG, LAMA4, SPINT2, NANOG*) and six miRNA (*let-7b, miR23b, miR29a, miR30d, miR205, miR720*) that were significantly differentially expressed between cancer ascites and peritoneal fluids. In addition, *CA11* mRNA was decreased to 0.5-fold and *SPINT2* and *NANOG* mRNA were significantly increased up to 100-fold in conditioned media of cancer cells compared to immortalized ovarian surface and fallopian tube epithelial cell lines, the hypothesized cells of origin for ovarian cancer development.

Conclusions: This study indicates that EV mRNA profiles can reflect the disease stage and may provide a potentially novel source for discovery of biomarkers in ovarian cancer.

Keywords: Extracellular vesicles, Ovarian cancer, Biomarkers, Ascites, Peritoneal fluids

Background

Ovarian cancer is the fifth-leading cause of cancer deaths in women [1]. With a lack of early obvious symptoms, women are frequently diagnosed with advanced stage disease. Approximately 60% of women are diagnosed at stage 3 or higher where the 5-year survival rate is below 30% [2]. In contrast, only 15% of cases are diagnosed at stage 1, when the tumor is localized to the primary site and patients have a 5-year survival rate of about 92%. In addition, patients with metastatic ovarian cancer frequently experience high recurrence rates within 16–22 months after conventional platinum-based combination chemotherapy. Identification of novel, specific and sensitive biomarkers for screening, monitoring or prediction may improve clinical outcomes and survival.

Screening tests currently used for ovarian cancer detection include pelvic examination, transvaginal ultrasound, and cancer antigen 125 (CA125). If an adnexal mass is detected by physical examination and/or ultrasound, surgery is ultimately needed for the confirmed ovarian cancer diagnosis and staging. CA125 is more routinely used as a marker for disease recurrence and treatment response [3]. It has been shown to be elevated in 80% of epithelial ovarian carcinomas, but its increase

* Correspondence: cyamamoto@hitachi-chemical.com
[1]Hitachi Chemical Co. America, Ltd. R and D Center, 1003 Health Sciences Rd, Irvine, CA 92617, USA
Full list of author information is available at the end of the article

in other conditions such as endometrial, pancreatic and breast cancer and certain benign conditions have limited its use as an early screening marker [4, 5]. In addition, annual screening with both CA125 and transvaginal ultrasound has not reduced ovarian cancer mortality compared with usual care [6]. Further research is necessary to discover and identify biomarkers that would be effective in early ovarian cancer screening.

Recently, extracellular vesicles (EVs) have been analyzed for their potential as ovarian cancer disease biomarkers [7]. EVs comprise of exosomes (30–100 nm) and microvesicles (100–1000 nm) which are either actively released from cells by fusion of multivesicular bodies to plasma membrane or formed by direct budding of the cell membrane into the extracellular space, respectively. Exosomes and microvesicles contain proteins, lipids and nucleic acids such as mRNA and miRNA from their cell of origin. The increasing evidence of their roles in cell-to-cell communication [8, 9], their high abundance in plasma (10^{12} per mL), and highly stable nature, are several of the reasons for the increased interest to identify EV-based biomarkers. In ovarian cancer, EVs have been explored in ascites and urine for miRNA and protein surface markers [10, 11]. Because of the demonstrated roles of EVs in communication and tumor progression, we initiated a study to examine the expression of EV mRNA and miRNA in ovarian cancer ascites and compared the expression with an ideal but difficult to obtain control source, peritoneal fluids from females inflicted with benign gynecologic diseases. These studies indicate that malignant ascites EVs package quantifiable mRNA and miRNA that can potentially provide insights into diagnostic biomarkers and therapeutic targets.

Methods

Study design

The experimental design is separated into two parts: 1) preliminary characterization of clinical samples and 2) evaluations of the biomarkers in cultured cell line. For the characterization of clinical samples, four main studies were performed: 1) size and concentration of EVs, 2) preliminary qPCR screening of mRNA biomarkers identified through previous literature, 3) pilot RNA-sequencing of EV mRNA, and 4) RT-qPCR validation of mRNA and screening of miRNA. The mRNA biomarkers identified through the RNA-seq qPCR validation were evaluated in several appropriate cell lines.

Biofluid collection

Ascites from advanced stage ovarian cancer patients were collected from the peritoneal cavity using Yankauer suction connected to a drainage bag, or bulb suction from volumes smaller than 500 mL. Bulb suction was also used to collect small volumes (1–5 mL) of peritoneal fluids from patients with non-malignant conditions. Samples were collected at the Brigham and Women's hospital under informed consent and Internal Review Board approval. Fluids were transferred into 50 cm^3 tubes and centrifuged at 2000 x g for 15 min at 4 °C to remove cell debris. The supernatant was then stored at − 80 °C until further use.

Cell culture

Immortalized human fallopian tube secretory epithelial cell line (FTSEC) was kindly provided by Dr. Ronny Drapkin [12]. Ovarian surface epithelial (OSE7, HOSE1–15) and high-grade serous ovarian cancer (SKOV3, OVCA3) cell lines have been previously described [13]. FTSEC cells were cultured in DMEM/Ham's F-12 1:1 (Cellgro, Mediatech, Inc. Manassas, VA) supplemented with 2% Ultroser G serum substitute (Pall Corp., Port Washington, NY). Ovarian epithelial cell lines were cultured in a mixture of medium 199 and MCDB105 medium (1:1) (Sigma, St. Louis, MO) supplemented with 10% fetal bovine serum (FBS, Invitrogen, Carlsbad, CA).

Standard media was replaced with exosome-free fetal bovine serum (System Biosciences, SBI, Palo Alto, CA) containing media 24 h prior to conditioned media collection. Cell counts were determined at the time of conditioned media collection and ranged from 2 to 9×10^5 cells/mL. Conditioned media were transferred to 50 cm^3 tubes and centrifuged at 2000×g for 15 min at 4 °C to remove cells and cell debris. The supernatant was then stored at − 80 °C until further use.

Differential ultracentrifugation and EV characterization

Ascites and peritoneal fluid samples were initially centrifuged at 2000 x g for 10 min to remove large debris. The supernatant was collected and further centrifuged at 10,000 x g for 30 min. EVs in the supernatant were then collected by ultracentrifugation at 100,000 x g for 1 h, washed with PBS, then collected again at 100,000 x g for 1 h in a Ti90 rotor. EV pellet was resuspended in PBS and stored at − 80 °C until further use. Nanoparticle tracking analysis of the EVs was conducted by Nanosight LM10 (Particle Characterization Laboratories, Inc., Novato, CA). Samples were diluted from 1:5 to 1:50 and applied to ELISA assay for EpCAM detection (Thermo Scientific, Frederick, MD) at 450 nm.

Scanning electron microscopy (SEM)

Ascites samples were pre-centrifuged at 3000 x g for 15 min at 4 °C before applying to the ExoComplete filterplate (Hitachi Chemical Diagnostics, Inc., (HCD), Mountain View, CA). EVs were captured on the filter membrane after centrifugation at 2000 x g for 5 min. Filters were fixed with 4% paraformaldehyde, and blocked with casein before incubation with 1:200 anti-human CD63 (Clone H5C6, BioLegend, Dedham, MA) for 1 h with gentle shaking. Samples were washed 3 times with casein PBS followed by incubation with 1:40 goat anti-mouse IgG gold colloid 9.0–11.0 nm (Sigma-Aldrich, St. Louis, MO) for 2 h. EVs were washed 3 times with casein PBS and PBS. Samples were fixed again with 4% paraformaldehyde for 5 min. Samples were washed once with PBS and 2 times with distilled water before incubation with 100 μL Silver Enhancement solution (BBI Solutions) for 10 min. Filters were washed with distilled water and air-dried overnight before analysis with SEM using Hitachi S-4800.

Next generation RNA sequencing

Ascites ($n = 2$) and peritoneal fluid ($n = 3$) samples were centrifuged at 2000 x g for 10 min at 4 °C after thawing as described above. The ExoComplete filterplate (HCD) captured EVs from 400 μL of centrifuged ascites and peritoneal fluid supernatant. Total RNA from EVs attached to the filter membrane was isolated using miRNeasy kit (Qiagen, Valencia, CA). Total RNA was monitored for quality control using the Agilent Bioanalyzer Nano RNA chip and Nanodrop absorbance ratios for 260/280 nm and 260/230 nm. Library construction was performed according to the Illumina TruSeq mRNA stranded protocol. The input quantity for total RNA was within the recommended range and mRNAs and noncoding RNAs with poly(A) tails was enriched using oligo dT magnetic beads. The enriched poly(A)$^+$ RNA was chemically fragmented. First strand synthesis used random primers and reverse transcriptase to make cDNA. After second strand synthesis, the ds cDNA was cleaned using AMPure XP beads, cDNA was end repaired and then the 3′ ends were adenylated. Illumina barcoded adapters were ligated on the ends and the adapter ligated fragments were enriched by nine cycles of PCR. The resulting libraries were validated by qPCR and sized by Agilent Bioanalyzer DNA high sensitivity chip. Concentrations for the libraries were normalized and then multiplexed together. Multiplexed libraries were sequenced using paired end 100 cycles chemistry for the HiSeq 2500. The version of HiSeq control software was HCS 2.2.58 with real time analysis software, RTA 1.18.64. FASTQ files were input into Maverix Biomics platform mRNA-seq for differential expression in eukaryotes version 2.5. Additionally, Ingenuity Pathway Analysis (IPA) (Qiagen) was employed to identify biological pathway modulation.

Extracellular vesicle mRNA analysis

Ascites ($n = 8$), peritoneal fluid ($n = 10$), and cell culture conditioned media (2 mL) were processed by first thawing for 10 min at 37 °C and then placed on ice. For preliminary qPCR screening of mRNA in clinical samples, ascites ($n = 8$) and peritoneal fluid ($n = 2$) were used. Thawed samples were centrifuged at 2000 x g for 10 min at 4 °C. Three hundred fifty μL of supernatant was applied to ExoComplete filterplate (HCD) and centrifuged. For cell culture conditioned media, samples were centrifuged as above and supernatants were applied to EV collection tubes (HCD). EVs were then captured onto the filter membrane after repeated centrifugation. From this step, procedures for mRNA analysis for ascites, peritoneal fluid, and cell culture conditioned media are identical. Exocomplete lysis buffer is applied to the EVs captured on the filter and incubated at 37 °C for 10 min. Centrifugation of the filterplate or filter tips from the collection tube was performed at 2000 x g for 5 min at 4 °C to transfer lysate to the mRNA Capture Plate for hybridization of mRNA to the oligo(dT)-covalently linked wells. After wash steps, on-plate random-primed cDNA synthesis using MMLV was performed at 37 °C for 2 h. For qPCR analysis, 2 μL of cDNA was used with Sso Advanced SYBR mix (Bio-Rad, Hercules, CA) and gene-specific primers (Additional file 1). Real-time PCR was performed on a ViiA7 (Thermo Fisher Scientific, Inc., Waltham, MA) instrument using the following profile: initial denaturation at 95 °C for 10 min, 40 cycles of 95 °C for 30 s and 65 °C for 1 min, melting curve analysis. Ct values greater than 36 were set to 36 cycles for data analysis. Real-time PCR data was processed by Data Assist v3.01 (Thermo Fisher Scientific, Inc.) and analyzed by Excel.

Extracellular vesicle miRNA analysis

Ascites ($n = 8$) and peritoneal fluid ($n = 10$) were thawed for 10 min at 37 °C and then placed on ice. Four hundred μL ascites and peritoneal fluid were centrifuged at 2000 x g for 10 min at 4 °C. Supernatant was applied to ExoComplete filterplate and centrifuged at 2000 x g for 5 min at 4 °C. Lysis buffer from miRNeasy (Qiagen), was applied to the wells in the filterplate. Total RNA was isolated per manufacturer's protocol. Synthesis of cDNA was performed using miScript RT kit (Qiagen). The cDNA was diluted 1:4 and 1 μL was used with the miScript PCR assay (Qiagen) for qPCR screening. For miRNA analysis, Excel and DataAssist v3.01 was used with the following parameters: cut-off value of Ct = 36, *SNORD61* selected as endogenous reference RNA.

Statistical analysis

The statistical analysis was performed using Microsoft Excel software. The statistical significance of the differences was determined by applying the Student's *t*-test.

Results

Patient characteristics and samples

The patient characteristics and clinical information were obtained for ovarian cancer ascites samples (Additional file 2). All samples were collected at the time of diagnosis. Eight patients were diagnosed with serous type ovarian cancer: seven with high grade, and a single patient was diagnosed with low grade serous type. The ages ranged from 48 to 80 years with an average age at diagnosis of 64 ± 12 years old. Using the available data, CA125 levels were elevated with average values at 1289 ± 541 U/mL at diagnosis and average progression-free and overall survival were 19 ± 8 and 33 ± 22 months, respectively. For peritoneal fluid samples, no malignant cells were identified in peritoneal washings or from ovary, fallopian tube, uterus and cervix pathology report (Additional file 3).

Ascites and peritoneal fluid EV characterization

Ascites and peritoneal fluid extracellular vesicles were isolated using differential ultracentrifugation and characterized for size and concentration using nanoparticle tracking analysis (Table 1). This preliminary characterization indicated average sizes of ascites and peritoneal fluid EVs were not statistically different and averaged 113 ± 11.5 nm. CD63-positive particles < 200 nm in diameter were observed in scanning electron micrographs of ovarian cancer ascites samples applied to the ExoComplete EV capture filterplate and correlate to size estimates from nanoparticle tracking analysis (Fig. 1). EV concentrations ranged from 10^{10} to 10^{12}particles/mL and were also not statistically significant between the two sample types. EVs from both ascites and peritoneal fluids were also evaluated for EpCAM surface marker expression by ELISA. EpCAM is a proposed surface marker of ovarian cancer-derived exosomes. Only one of each sample type was found to be positive for EpCAM. The single ascites and peritoneal fluid-derived EV samples had an EpCAM concentration of 670 pg/mL and 1.44 ng/mL, respectively. The other samples were below the limit of detection (50 pg/mL) for the ELISA assay.

Next generation RNA sequencing and qPCR validation

A literature search for potential ovarian cancer biomarkers identified 50 mRNA candidates (Additional file 4) which were then evaluated in a preliminary qPCR screening of ovarian cancer ascites ($n = 8$) and peritoneal fluid EVs ($n = 2$). Three mRNAs, *NANOG, SPINT2, ZEB2*, were found to be significantly elevated (> 2-fold, *p*-value < 0.05) in ascites in the preliminary screening (Additional file 5). To further identify differentially expressed genes and additional mRNA markers, next generation poly(A)$^+$ RNA sequencing was performed on selected samples of ascites ($n = 2$) and peritoneal fluid ($n = 3$). RNA sequencing mapping percentages to hg19 assembly ranged from 50% to 87%, and greater than 70% of the reads were kept after quality assessment (Additional file 6). The read distributions indicate that both samples have a higher percentage of reads mapping to exons and 3' UTR compared to introns and 5' UTR as expected based on sequencing preparation methodology (Additional file 7). Intergenic regions ranged from 2.5–15.9% for peritoneal fluid EVs and 24–47% for ovarian cancer ascites EVs.

Pathway analysis of RNA-seq differential gene expression data from ovarian cancer ascites and peritoneal fluid EVs identified organismal injury, cancer and reproductive system diseases as the main categories of diseases and disorders (Additional file 8). In terms of function, results were consistent with the biological environment of an advanced stage disease. Signaling pathways within growth, malignant tumor and advanced malignancy categories were predicted to be up-regulated whereas tumor cell death pathways were predicted to decline.

RNA-seq differential gene expression analysis identified 114 genes with statistical significance ($p < 0.05$) (Additional file 9). From this list, 30 genes selected for qPCR validation based on fold change, *p*-value, abundance and function were measured in eight ovarian cancer ascites and ten peritoneal fluid samples (Additional file 10). *SPINT2*, one of the three mRNA found to be differentially expressed in the initial screen based on literature-identified biomarkers was identified in the RNA-seq analysis. The remaining two genes, *NANOG* and *ZEB2*, were added to the list of 30 genes in the final RNA-seq qPCR validation assays. *ACTB* was selected as a reference gene for mRNA normalization. Of the selected mRNA for qPCR validation, five were found to be significantly ($p < 0.05$) differentially expressed in ovarian cancer ascites and peritoneal fluid (Fig. 2). Three

Table 1 Ascites ($n = 3$) and peritoneal fluid ($n = 3$) EV characteristics

EV Sample Source[a]	ID	EpCAM ELISA[a]	Concentration (particles/mL)	Size (nm)
Ascites	A2	positive	2.17E + 10	105
Ascites	A3	negative	3.20E + 12	106
Ascites	A10	negative	5.43E + 10	128
Peritoneal Fluid	B7	negative	1.20E + 10	106
Peritoneal Fluid	B11	positive	8.47E + 11	106
Peritoneal Fluid	B13	negative	1.55E + 10	128

[a]EV isolated by differential centrifugation
[b]10E9 – 10E11 EVs applied

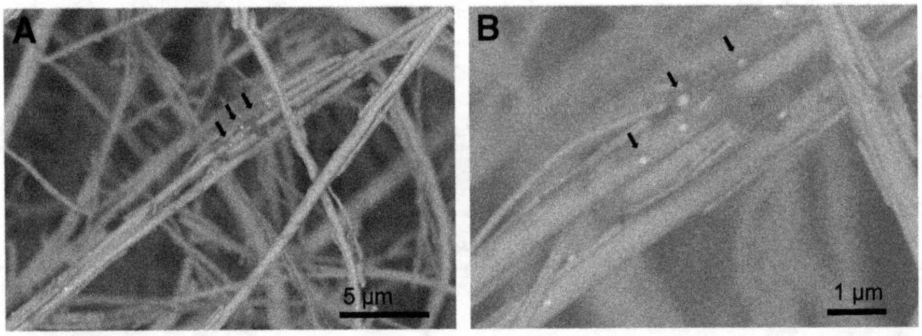

Fig. 1 a,b Scanning electron microscopy of ovarian cancer ascites EVs captured on the membrane of the ExoComplete filterplate. Ovarian cancer ascites was applied to the filterplate, fixed, labeled with anti-CD63 primary monoclonal antibody and anti-mouse IgG colloidal gold with silver enhancement. Black arrows indicate selected extracellular vesicles with diameters < 200 nm captured on the membrane. Images were obtained with accelerating voltages of 2.0 kV in detection mode

mRNAs, *CA11, LAMA4, MEDAG,* were .01–.28-fold lower expressed and two mRNA, *SPINT2* and *NANOG,* were 3.2–5.8-fold higher expressed in ovarian cancer ascites versus peritoneal fluid EVs.

Ascites and peritoneal fluid EV miRNA analysis

Small RNAs are abundant within extracellular vesicles. Here, we quantitate specific miRNA previously identified to be involved in ovarian cancer progression or invasiveness [14–18]. There were six miRNAs, *let-7b, miR23b, miR29a, miR30d, miR205, miR720,* which were found to be significantly ($p < 0.05$) decreased .01–.21-fold in ovarian cancer ascites compared to benign peritoneal fluid when normalized to *SNORD61* (Fig. 3).

Multivariate discriminate analysis

The combined mRNA and miRNA raw qPCR data were used in multivariate discriminate analysis (Additional file 11). The predictors, *LAMA4, CA11, MEDAG, NANOG, SPINT2, let-7b, miR23b, and miR29a* were found to be sufficient to classify 87.5% and 100% of ovarian cancer ($n = 8$) and disease control ($n = 10$) groups, respectively.

Specific EV mRNA from normal and cancer cell lines

The EVs released from normal human fallopian tube epithelial (FTSEC194), ovarian surface epithelial (OSE7, HOSE1–15), and high grade serous ovarian cancer (SKOV3, OVCA3) cell lines were analyzed for specific mRNA that were differentially expressed in ovarian

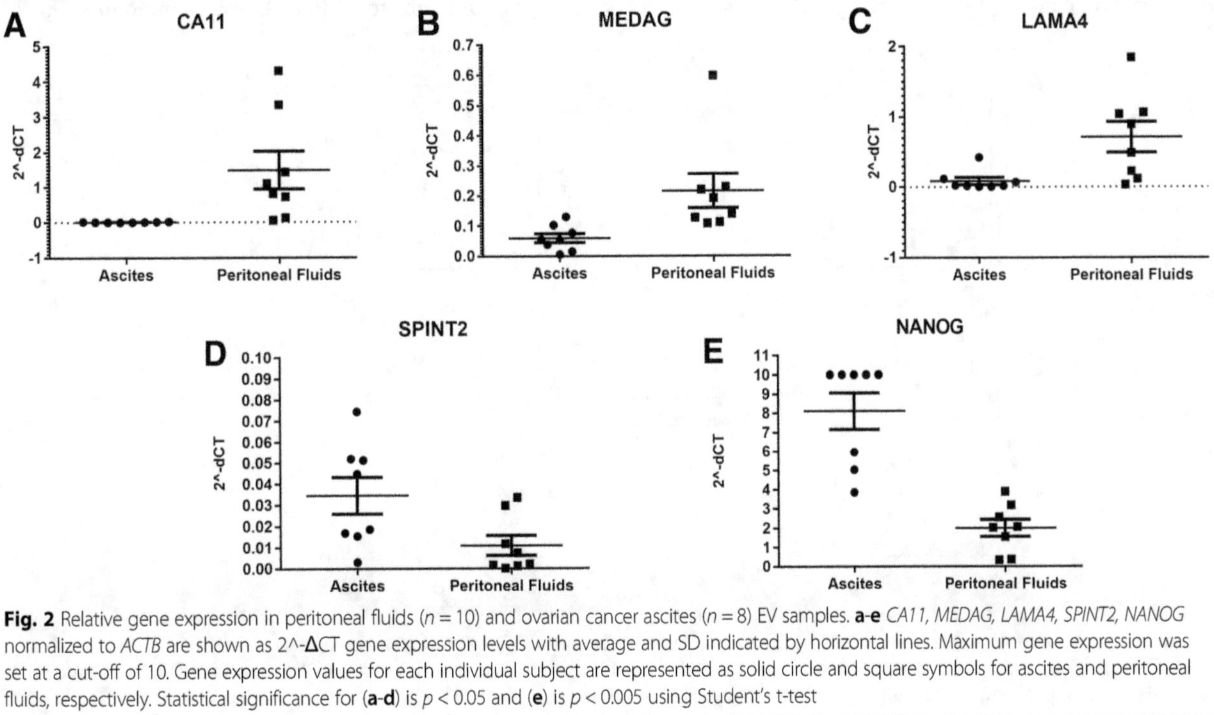

Fig. 2 Relative gene expression in peritoneal fluids ($n = 10$) and ovarian cancer ascites ($n = 8$) EV samples. **a-e** *CA11, MEDAG, LAMA4, SPINT2, NANOG* normalized to *ACTB* are shown as 2^-ΔCT gene expression levels with average and SD indicated by horizontal lines. Maximum gene expression was set at a cut-off of 10. Gene expression values for each individual subject are represented as solid circle and square symbols for ascites and peritoneal fluids, respectively. Statistical significance for (**a-d**) is $p < 0.05$ and (**e**) is $p < 0.005$ using Student's t-test

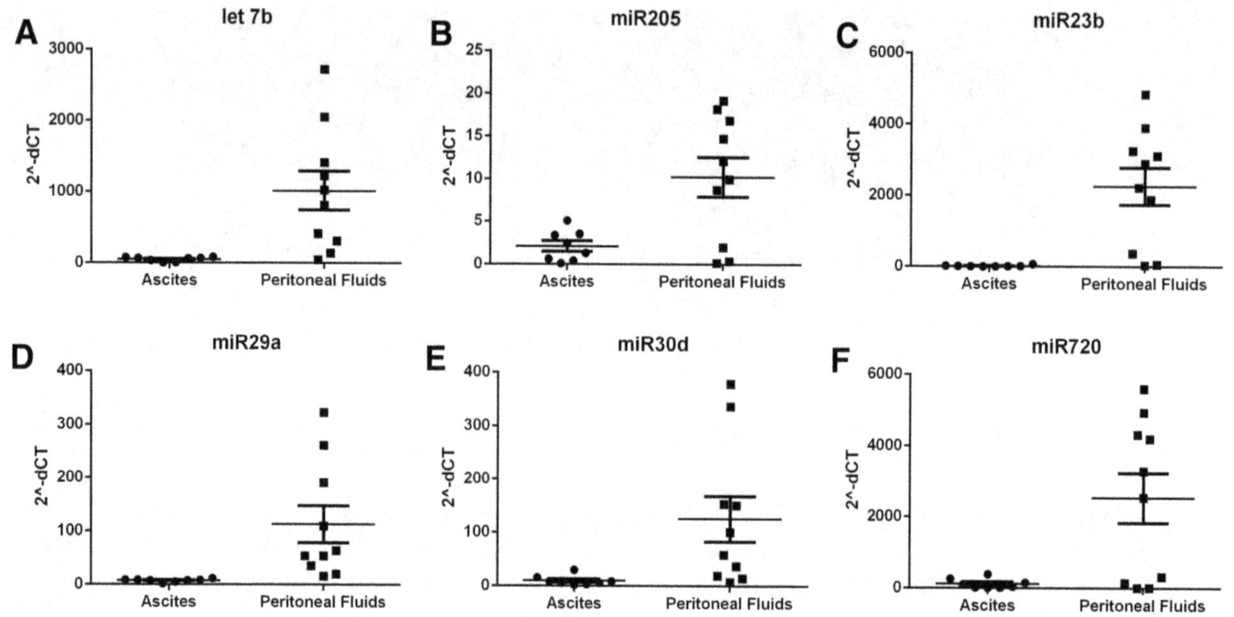

Fig. 3 Relative miRNA expression levels in peritoneal fluids ($n = 10$) and ovarian cancer ascites ($n = 8$) EV samples. **a-f** *Let7b, miR205, miR23b, miR29a, miR30d, miR720* normalized to *SNORD61* are shown as 2^-ΔCT expression levels with average and SD indicated by horizontal lines. Gene expression values for each individual subject are represented as solid circle and square symbols for ascites and peritoneal fluids, respectively. Statistical significance for (**a-d**) is $p < 0.05$ and (**e**) is $p < 0.005$ using Student's t-test

cancer ascites and peritoneal fluids (Fig. 4). The immortalized normal fallopian and ovarian surface epithelial cells were used as controls. Using 3 mL of conditioned media from each cell line, we confirm that *CA11* mRNA is 0.1–0.5-fold lower abundance and *NANOG* is 50-fold higher abundance in EVs released from high-grade serous ovarian cancer cells, OVCA3. Although *CA11* expression appeared to be elevated in SKOV3 cells, mRNA levels for *CA11* as well as *NANOG* were not statistically significant compared to normal cells. *SPINT2*, however, was found to be significantly elevated in both SKOV3 and OVCA 3 cells compared to normal cells. *LAMA4* was expressed in 0.1-fold lower abundance in OVCA3, but up to 2-fold higher abundance in EVs

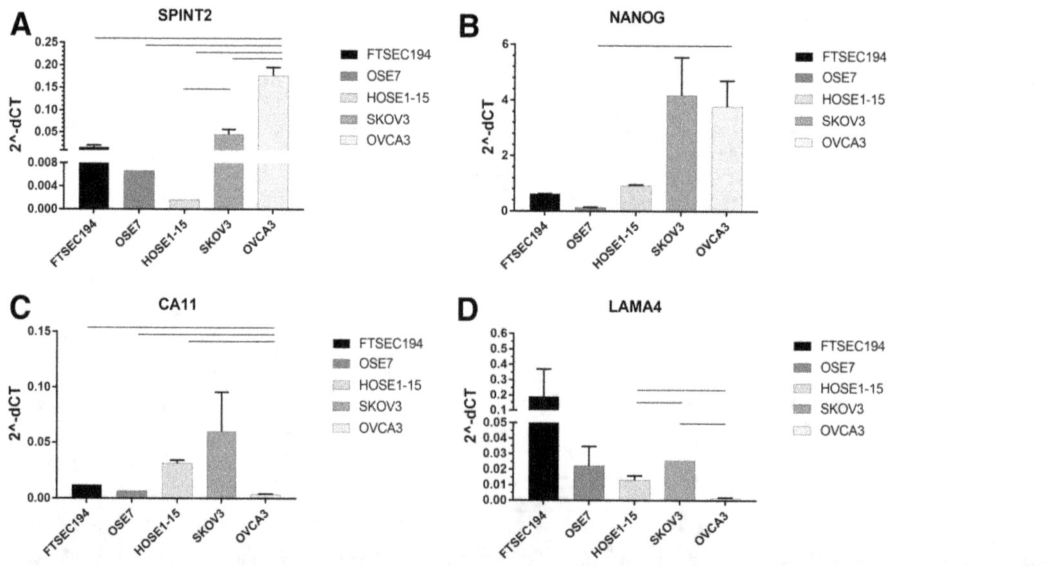

Fig. 4 Specific mRNA expression normalized to *ACTB* from immortalized fallopian (FTSEC194), ovarian surface epithelial (OSE7, HOSE1–15) and ovarian cancer cell lines (SKOV3, OVCA3) EVs released in conditioned media. **a** *SPINT2*, (**b**) *NANOG*, (**c**) *CA11*, (**d**) *LAMA4* mRNA quantitation (2^-ΔCT) is shown as column graph with average and SD ($n = 2$) and statistical significance indicated by a bar representing $p < 0.05$ by Student's t-test

originating from SKOV3 cells compared to ovarian surface epithelial cell-derived EVs (HOSE1–15). The two high grade serous ovarian cancer cell lines, SKOV3 and OVCA3, demonstrated similar expression patterns for *SPINT2* and *NANOG*, but distinct relative expression for *CA11* and *LAMA4*. *MEDAG* mRNA was present in very low levels and was not reproducibly detected in all cell lines.

Discussion

Extracellular vesicles (EVs), including exosomes and microvesicles, are small membranous particles released from all cells and found in many biofluids. These vesicles are thought to provide a mode of cellular communication and deliver their cargo of protein, DNA and RNA, to target cells [10, 11]. As a result, EVs have been a novel source of biomarkers in a wide range of diseases. In this study, we analyzed EV mRNA and miRNA from ovarian cancer ascites and benign peritoneal fluids to determine if they can provide biological insight into metastasis and be a potential source of novel diagnostic biomarkers.

The average size and concentrations of EVs isolated from ovarian cancer ascites and peritoneal fluids were < 120 nm and at least 10^{10} particles/mL and are within range of EVs isolated from other biofluids such as plasma and urine. The variability in particle concentration observed between samples is consistent with what has been observed in previous literature [11]. In addition, EpCAM has been proposed as a marker for ovarian cancer-derived exosomes [11], but only 1 out of 3 of the ovarian cancer and peritoneal fluid EV samples were positive for EpCAM. This may be reflective of the typically low presence of adenocarcinoma cells (< 0.1%) within ovarian cancer ascites and the presence of endometrial epithelial cells in peritoneal fluids [19, 20]. The ovarian cancer ascites EV sample did not demonstrate a higher EpCAM concentration compared to the peritoneal fluid EV sample.

The ovarian cancer ascites and peritoneal fluid EVs were analyzed for differential mRNA expression. The mRNAs in this study were selected based on a combination of next generation sequencing (NGS) results and previous literature. The EV characterization and RNA sequencing were pilot analyses of the EVs and identification of new targets. IPA results confirmed RNA-seq is a methodology which may identify relevant biomarkers for diagnosis. The qPCR validation of the RNA-seq results employed more samples to confirm the gene expression pattern. Based on these qPCR analyses, the mRNAs confirmed to be decreased in ovarian cancer ascites compared to peritoneal fluid EVs included *LAMA4*, *CA11*, and *MEDAG*. EVs from a high grade serous ovarian adenocarcinoma cell line OVCA3 also contained less abundance of *CA11* compared to controls from immortalized epithelial fallopian and ovarian cells. Recently, fallopian tube secretory epithelial cells have been proposed to be the precursor tissue for high grade serous ovarian cancer, and immortalized human fallopian tube secretory epithelial cells are being used for studying early-stage development of high grade serous ovarian cancer [21]. Based on the publicly available genotype-tissue expression (GTEx) database, *CA11* mRNA has high baseline expression in brain and medium expression in tissues such as ovary. Although no previous studies were found to link *CA11* with gynecological cancers, this mRNA was down-regulated in human gastric cancer [22]. CA11 is a member of carbonic anhydrase family known to participate in biological processes such as formation of aqueous humor, CSF and saliva. Similar to *CA11*, *MEDAG* was in lower abundance in ovarian cancer ascites EVs. *MEDAG* expression, however, was either at the limit of detection or undetectable in the fallopian and ovarian cell lines used in this study suggesting low baseline expression of *MEDAG* in these tissues. The GTEx database confirms this observation and shows MEDAG expressed at higher levels in visceral adipose and arterial tissues. *MEDAG* is a gene involved in processes that promote adipocyte differentiation, lipid accumulation, and glucose uptake in mature adipocytes. Because ovarian cancer cells bind preferentially to omental fat and use human omental adipocytes as an energy source, the decrease observed in ovarian cancer ascites *MEDAG* EV mRNA may reflect changes in the ascites microenvironment [23]. A previous study using microarray has also shown a lower *MEDAG* and *LAMA4* expression in ovarian cancer compared to normal epithelial cells [24]. *LAMA4* is a member of the major family of non-collagenous constituents of basement membranes. The decrease in *LAMA4* observed in malignant ascites EV and OVCA3 EV, in contrast to the increase in SKOV3 EV, are interesting and warrants further experimental studies to evaluate the relationship. Ascites EVs could be providing cell-to-cell communication through unique molecular profiles promoting cancer cell survival within the ascites milieu.

In contrast to *LAMA4*, *CA11*, and *MEDAG*, the 2 mRNAs, *SPINT2* and *NANOG*, were found to be increased in ovarian cancer ascites compared to peritoneal fluid EVs. *SPINT2* was also in higher abundance in OVCA3 and SKOV3 EVs compared to controls. Interestingly, although SPINT2 is a putative suppressor, we demonstrate an increase in cancer ascites [25]. Müller-Pillasch et al. also reports that *SPINT2* expression was elevated in pancreatic cancer [26]. NANOG, on the other hand, is a DNA binding homeobox transcription factor involved in embryonic stem cell proliferation, renewal and pluripotency. *NANOG* is increased in expression from normal tissue, benign, borderline, and malignant tumors of ovarian serous cystadenocarcinomas and protein is found selectively associated with high-grade ovarian serous carcinoma [27, 28]. *NANOG* mRNA was found to be significantly increased in OVCA3 EVs compared to OSE7 control. Based on previous studies relating to these mRNA, *CA11* and *MEDAG* may be involved in maintaining malignant ascites microenvironment, while *LAMA4, NANOG* and *SPINT2* activities could regulate ovarian cancer progression and metastasis.

There were six miRNA biomarkers, *let7b, miR205, miR23b, miR29a, miR30d,* and *miR720,* significantly down-regulated in ovarian cancer ascites EVs compared to peritoneal fluids. These miRNAs have previously been shown to be involved in ovarian cancer progression, invasion or metastasis. The *let-7* family regulates downstream gene targets involved in self-renewal of mesenchymal stem cells derived from human embryonic stem cells. *Let-7b* is often dysregulated in ovarian cancer and is associated with poor prognosis [29]. Recently, *miR205* was shown to be elevated in ovarian cancer tissue and associated with tumor growth and metastasis in ovarian cancer [30]. In pre-surgical plasma, *miR720* was elevated in women who had short overall survival (< 2 years) when compared to women with long overall survival (> 4 years) after their diagnosis [31]. In contrast, *miR23b* expression is lower in epithelial ovarian carcinoma and borderline tumors than in normal ovarian tissues and benign tumors consistent with the lower abundance observed in ovarian cancer ascites in this study. *MiR23b* was shown to target cyclin G1 and suppress ovarian cancer tumorigenesis and progression [14]. *MiR29a* was also shown to have tumor suppressive effects and may contribute to cisplatin resistance of ovarian cancer cells [32, 33]. *MiR30d* also functions as a suppressor of ovarian cancer progression notably by decreasing Snail expression and blocking TGF-b1-induced EMT process [34].

Malignant ascites presents in approximately 30% of women with ovarian cancer and is frequently tapped to relieve symptoms. This fluid is composed of lymphocytes, epithelial cells, and EVs, and provides clues into ascites formation and metastatic progression. Functional analysis of each specific mRNA and miRNA will be needed to determine the biological significance of their differential expression in ovarian cancer.

Conclusions

Here, we demonstrate that EVs from ovarian cancer ascites contain distinct RNA expression signatures from benign peritoneal fluids, control samples that are rarely available to research. The two mRNA markers *SPINT2* and *NANOG* that are upregulated in cancer ascites relative to peritoneal fluids may have potential as diagnostic biomarkers. Through continued liquid biopsy investigations, an understanding of the mechanisms involved in advanced stage disease and development of chemo-resistant disease may lead to alternative therapeutic targets and improved palliative care.

Additional files

Additional File 1: Primer sequences (5′ to 3′) for qPCR validation. (DOCX 13 kb)

Additional File 2: Clinical information from patient ascites samples. (DOCX 13 kb)

Additional File 3: Clinical information from benign peritoneal fluid (PF) sample pathology reports. (DOCX 12 kb)

Additional File 4: Preliminary set of genes with primer sequences for screening based on literature search. Additional genes (*MET, EGFR, EPCAM, CLDN3*) were quantitated using Qiagen Quantitect Primer Assays. (DOCX 13 kb)

Additional File 5: Volcano plot displays *p*-values vs. fold change of ovarian cancer ascites ($n = 8$) and peritoneal ($n = 2$) EVs. Three mRNA (*NANOG, SPINT2, ZEB2*) show values above the fold change boundary of 2 (2-fold change) and a p-value of 0.05. Plot generated using. Data Assist v3.01 software. (PPTX 58 kb)

Additional File 6: mRNA sequencing reads and percentage aligned to hg19 assembly. (DOCX 12 kb)

Additional File 7: The distribution of EV mRNA sequencing reads mapping to human genome annotations. The percentage of reads (ave. ± SD) overlapping genomic features including exons, introns, UTR, and intergenic regions are shown for peritoneal fluids ($n = 3$) and ovarian cancer ascites samples ($n = 2$). (PPTX 115 kb)

Additional File 8: Ingenuity Pathway Analysis summary of top diseases and disorders, top canonical pathways, and top molecular and cellular functions. *P*-values are calculated using the right-tailed Fisher Exact Test and number of molecules are based on Ingenuity Knowledge Base with information contained in Canonical Pathways coming from specific journal articles, review articles, textbooks and HumanCyc. (DOCX 22 kb)

Additional File 9: Differentially expressed genes from RNA sequencing analysis. Significantly increased RNA ($p < 0.05$) from ovarian cancer ascites (n = 2) compared to benign peritoneal fluid (n = 3) are listed below as either up-regulated or down-regulated in ascites compared to peritoneal fluids. (DOCX 22 kb)

Additional File10: Next generation RNA sequencing data were plotted for each sample of ovarian cancer ascites (OC) and benign peritoneal fluids (DC). RPKM values for each corresponding gene are indicated in blue and the 30 selected genes for qPCR validation are labeled in red. Solid blue lines indicate linear regression. Both over- and under-expressed genes were selected for validation. (PPTX 318 kb)

Additional File 11: Multivariate discriminant analysis of mRNA and miRNA qPCR data. Linear discriminant functions are listed for ovarian cancer and disease control groups. (DOCX 12 kb)

Abbreviations

CA125: Cancer antigen 125; EOC: Epithelial ovarian cancer; EV: Extracellular vesicles; FTSEC: Fallopian tube secretory epithelial cell

Acknowledgements

N/A

Funding

No external source of funding was used for this study.

Authors' contributions

CMY and SWN designed the study and contributed to writing the manuscript. CMY, MO, and TM collected, analyzed and/or interpreted data. MM and RB collected peritoneal and ascites samples. All authors read and approved final manuscript.

Competing interests

CMY, MO, and TM are employees of Hitachi Chemical Co. America, Ltd. R&D Center and the two authors, CMY and SWN have submitted a provisional patent (Appl. No. 62/507,091) entitled, "Methods for detecting ovarian cancer using extracellular vesicles for molecular analysis".

Author details

[1]Hitachi Chemical Co. America, Ltd. R and D Center, 1003 Health Sciences Rd, Irvine, CA 92617, USA. [2]Department of Obstetrics, Gynecology and Reproductive Biology, Gynecologic Oncology Division, Brigham and Women's Hospital, Harvard Medical School, 75 Francis Street, Boston, MA 02115, USA. [3]Department of Obstetrics and Gynecology, Tuft Medical Center, 800 Washington Street, Boston, MA 02111, USA.

References

1. U.S. Cancer Statistics Working Group. United States cancer statistics: 1999–2013 incidence and mortality web-based report. https://www.cdc.gov/cancer/ovarian/statistics/index.htm (accessed 17 Aug 2017).
2. National Cancer Institute: Surveillance, Epidemiology, and End Results Program. https://seer.cancer.gov/statfacts/html/ovary.html (accessed 17 Aug 2017).
3. Skates SJ, Xu FJ, Yu YH, Sjovall K, Einhorn N, Chang Y, et al. Toward an optimal algorithm for ovarian cancer screening with longitudinal tumor markers. Cancer. 1995;76(Suppl 10):2004–10.
4. Streppel MM, Vincent A, Mukherjee R, Campbell NR, Chen SH, Konstantopoulos K, et al. Mucin 16 (cancer antigen 125) expression in human tissues and cell lines and correlation with clinical outcome in adenocarcinomas of the pancreas, esophagus, stomach, and colon. Hum Pathol. 2012;43:10.
5. Jelovac D, Armstrong DK. Recent progress in the diagnosis and treatment of ovarian cancer. CA Cancer J Clin. 2011;61:3.
6. Buys SS, Partridge E, Black A, et al. Effect of screening on ovarian cancer mortality: the prostate, lung, colorectal and ovarian (PLCO) cancer screening randomized controlled trial. JAMA. 2011;305:22.
7. Dorayappan KDP, Wallbillich JJ, Cohn DE, Selvendiran K. The biological significance and clinical applications of exosomes in ovarian cancer. Gynecol Oncol. 2016;142:1.
8. Crow J, Atay S, Banskota S, Artale B, Schmitt S, Godwin AK. Exosomes as mediators of platinum resistance in ovarian cancer, Oncotarget. 201; doi: https://doi.org/10.18632/oncotarget.14440.
9. Nakamura K, Sawada K, Kinose Y, Yoshimura A, Toda A, Nakatsuka E, et al. Exosomes promote ovarian cancer cell invasion through transfer of CD44 to peritoneal mesothelial cells. Mol Cancer Res. 2017;15:1.
10. Zhou J, Gong G, Tan H, Dai F, Zhu X, Chen Y, et al. Urinary microRNA-30a-5p is a potential biomarker for ovarian serous adenocarcinoma. Onc Rep. 2015;33:6.
11. Im H, Shao H, Park YI, Peterson VM, Castro CM, Weissleder R, et al. Label-free detection and molecular profiling of exosomes with a nano-plasmonic sensor. Nat Biotechnol. 2014;32:5.
12. Karst AM, Levanon K, Drapkin R. Modeling high-grade serous ovarian carcinogenesis from the fallopian tube. PNAS. 2011;108:18.
13. Zhang Y, Kwok JS-L, Choi P-W, Liu M, Yang J, Singh M, et al. Pinin interacts with C-terminal binding proteins for RNA alternative splicing and epithelial cell identity of human ovarian cancer cells. Oncotarget. 2016;7:10.
14. Yan J, Jiang J-Y, Meng X-N, Xiu Y-L, Zong Z-H. MiR-23b targets cyclin G1 and suppresses ovarian cancer tumorigenesis and progression. J Exp Clin Ca Res. 2016;35:31.
15. Li J, Hu K, Gong G, Zhu D, Wang Y, Liu H, et al. Upregulation of miR-205 transcriptionally suppresses SMAD4 and PTEN and contributes to human ovarian cancer progression. Sci Reports. 2016;1:7.
16. Meng X, Muller V, Milde-Langosch K, Trillsch F, Pantel K, Schwrzenbach H. Diagnostic and prognostic relevance of circulating exosomal miR-373, miR-200a, miR-200b and miR-200c in patients with epithelial ovarian cancer. Oncotarget. 2016;7:13.
17. Yeung CLA, Co N-N, Tsuruga T, Yeung T-L, Kwan S-Y, Leung CS, et al. Exosomal transfer of stroma-derived miR21 confers paclitaxel resistance in ovarian cancer cells through targeting APAF1. Nat Commun. 2016;29:7.
18. Wu RL, Ali S, Bandyopadhyay S, Alosh B, Hayek K, Daaboul MHD, et al. Comparative analysis of differentially expressed miRNAs and their downstream mRNAs in ovarian cancer and its associated endometriosis. J cancer Sci Ther. 2105;7:7.
19. Kipps E, DSP T, Kaye SB. Meeting the challenge of ascites in ovarian cancer: new avenues for therapy and research. Nat Rev Ca. 2103;13:4.
20. O DF, Roskams T, Van den Eynde K, Vanhie A, Peterse DP, et al. The presence of endometrial cells in peritoneal fluid of women with and without endometriosis. Reprod Sci. 2017;24:2.
21. Perets R, Wyant GA, Muto KW, Bijron JG, Poole BB, et al. Transformation of the fallopian tube secretory epithelium leads to high-grade serous ovarian cancer in Brca;Tp53;Pten models. Cancer Cell. 2013;24:6.
22. Yoshikawa Y, Mukai H, Hino F, Asada K, Kato I. Isolation of two novel genes, down-regulated in gastric cancer. Jpn J Cancer Res. 2000;91:5.
23. Nieman KM, Kenny HA, Penicka CV, Ladanyi A, Buell-Gutbrod R, Zillhardt MR, et al. Adipocytes promote ovarian cancer metastasis and provide energy for rapid tumor growth. Nat Med. 2011;17:11.
24. Yeung TL, Leung CS, Wong KK, Samimi G, Thompson MS, Liu J, et al. TGF-b modulates ovarian cancer invasion by upregulating CAF-derived versican in the tumor microenvironment. Ca Research. 2013;73:16.
25. Kongkham PN, Northcott PA, Ra YS, Nakahara Y, Mainprize TG, Croul SE, et al. An epigenetic genome-wide screen identifies SPINT2 as a novel tumor suppressor gene in pediatric medulloblastoma. Cancer Res. 2008; https://doi.org/10.1158/0008-5472.CAN-08-2169.
26. Muller-Pillasch F, Wallrapp C, Bartels K, Varga G, Friess H, Buchler M, et al. Cloning of a new Kunitz-type protease inhibitor with a putative transmembrane domain overexpressed in pancreatic cancer. Biochim Biophys Acta. 1998;1395:1.
27. Pan Y, Jiao J, Zhou C, Cheng Q, Hu Y, Chen H. Nanog is highly expressed in ovarian serous cystadenocarcinoma and correlated with clinical stage and pathological grade. Pathobiology. 2011;77:6.
28. Kenda Suster N, Frkovic Grazio S, Virant-Klun I, Verdenik I, Smrkolj S. Cancer stem cell-related marker NANOG expression in ovarian serous tumors: a clinicopathological study of 159 cases. Int J Gynecol Cancer. 2017;9:2006.
29. Zaman MS, Maher DM, Khan S, Jaggi M, Chauhan SC. Current status and implications of microRNAs in ovarian cancer diagnosis and therapy. J Ovarian Research. 2012;5:44.
30. Li J, Hu K, Gong G, Zhu D, Wang Y, Liu H, et al. Upregulation of miR-205 transcriptionally suppresses SMAD4 and PTEN and contributes to human ovarian cancer progression. Sci Rep. 2017; https://doi.org/10.1038/srep41330.
31. Shapira I, Oswald M, Lovecchio J, Khalili H, Menzin A, Whyte J, et al. Circulating biomarkers for detection of ovarian cancer and predicting cancer outcomes. Br J Cancer. 2014; https://doi.org/10.1038/bjc.2013.795.
32. Yu PN, Yan MD, Lai HC, Huang RL, Chou YC, Lin WC, et al. Downregulation of miR-29 contributes to cisplatin resistance of ovarian cancer cells. Int J Cancer. 2014; https://doi.org/10.1002/ijc.28399.
33. Creighton CJ, Hernandez-Herrera A, Jacobsen A, Levine DA, Mankoo P, Schultz N, et al. Integrated analyses of microRNAs demonstrate their widespread influence on gene expression in high-grade serous ovarian carcinoma. PLoS One. 2012; https://doi.org/10.1371/journal.pone.0034546.
34. Ye Z, Zhao L, Li J, Chen W, Li X. MiR-30d blocked transforming growth factor β1-induced epithelial-mesenchymal transition by targeting snail in ovarian cancer cells. Int J Gyn Ca. 2015; https://doi.org/10.1097/IGC.0000000000000546.

7

Is the ovarian reserve influenced by vitamin D deficiency and the dress code in an infertile Iranian population?

Soheila Arefi[1,2,3], Gholamreza Khalili[4], Homa Iranmanesh[5], Fattaneh Farifteh[6], Ahmad Hosseini[6], Human M. Fatemi[7] and Barbara Lawrenz[7,8*]

Abstract

Background: In the recent years, vitamin D has become a topical subject and a focus of research not only in reproductive medicine but across many medical disciplines. In reproductive medicine, studies have identified an association between vitamin D status in women and ovarian reserve. In humans, exposure of the skin to sunlight is the main important source of vitamin D. A dress code of wearing concealing clothing is a risk factor for vitamin D deficiency. The objective of this prospective observational study was to evaluate the correlation between vitamin D deficiency and ovarian reserve in a population of infertile women in Iran. As part of the basic fertility assessment of study participants, blood tests were taken to measure vitamin D concentration and transvaginal ultrasound scans were performed on day 2–5 of the cycle to determine antral follicle count (AFC). All study participants were assessed by a reproductive medicine specialist and consultant dermatologist to classify their skin types according to the Fitzpatrick classification. In addition, the dress code of each study participant was recorded noting the percentage of exposed skin not covered by concealing clothing.

Results: 189 infertility patients were included in this study. The mean concentration of vitamin D in this study population was 15.46 ng/ml, indicating severe vitamin D deficiency. A statistically significant negative correlation between age and vitamin D ($p = 0.008$) and age and AFC ($p = 0.001$) was identified. This study revealed a highly significant correlation between vitamin D concentrations and AFC ($p < 0.001$).

Conclusions: A concealing dress code is an independent risk factor for vitamin D deficiency due to a lack of skin exposure to sunlight. Our study suggests that the so caused severe vitamin D deficiency may play a crucial role in reduced ovarian reserve in the herein described group of an infertile female Iranian population.

Keywords: Dress code, Vitamin D deficiency, Ovarian reserve, Skin-type

Background

In recent years, vitamin D has become a topical subject and a focus of research in several medical disciplines.

Vitamin D is widely recognized to facilitate absorption of calcium and promote bone growth. Vitamin D deficiency in children may result in a condition known as rickets incurring an increased risk of fractures and deformity. In adults, vitamin D deficiency may result in osteomalacia carrying the same risks of fracture and deformity. In addition to its role in bone health, it appears that vitamin D deficiency is also involved in the pathogenesis of many chronic diseases such as autoimmune diseases, inflammatory bowel disease, infections, immune deficiency, cardiovascular diseases, cancer and neurocognitive disorders [1].

As vitamin D receptors are widely found in reproductive tissues, including the ovaries and the endometrium, an important role of vitamin D in human reproduction has been suggested. Vitamin D status has been suggested to be associated with ovarian reserve and with the

* Correspondence: barbara.lawrenz@ivirma.com
[7]IVF department, IVI RMA Middle-East Fertility Clinic, Abu Dhabi, UAE
[8]Women's university hospital Tuebingen, Tuebingen, Germany
Full list of author information is available at the end of the article

outcome of in vitro fertilization (IVF) treatments as well as with features of polycystic ovarian syndrome (PCOS) and endometriosis. In men, associations with semen quality and sperm count, motility and morphology had been described [2].

Vitamin D belongs to a group of fat-soluble vitamins and is responsible for the intestinal absorption of calcium, magnesium, phosphate, zinc and iron. The most important forms of Vitamin D are vitamin D3 (cholecalciferol) and vitamin D2 (ergocalciferol) [3]. According to recent studies, vitamin D deficiency is defined as serum-levels of 25(OH)D below 20 ng/ml. The importance of vitamin D deficiency is underlined by the fact, that an estimated 1 billion people worldwide are vitamin D deficient and deficiencies can be found in all ethnicities and age groups [4]. Therefore vitamin D deficiency is the most common vitamin deficiency worldwide in both, children and adults [5].

Dietary sources of vitamin D alone are not sufficient to maintain normal vitamin D levels.

The most important source of vitamin D for humans is exposure to sunlight, particularly ultraviolet B rays. Several factors influence vitamin D production following sun exposure. These factors include age, skin color, degree of exposed skin, length of time exposed to sunlight, geographic location, time of year, time of day, cloud cover, smog, dust or haze.

The countries of the Middle East have the highest vitamin D deficiency rates in the world, ranging from 67% in Iran, 55–83% in Jordan, 84% in Lebanon up to 90% in Saudi Arabia [6].

Recently, several studies evaluated the influence of vitamin D on the ovarian reserve [7–9]. In contrast to the herein presented study, the participants consisted mainly of women of Caucasian ethnicity and were not subjected to imposed female dress codes. Our study is unique in that our participants are of Iranian ethnicity and wear concealing clothing, a dress code imposed by both, religious and social values.

The aim of this study was to evaluate the vitamin D status in an infertile population in Iran and to correlate vitamin D concentrations with parameters such as female age, skin type, degree of skin concealment and antral follicle count (AFC) as parameter of the ovarian reserve.

Methods

This observational prospective study was performed in 2 independent private infertility centers in Iran. Patients, referred to the fertility centers with both, primary and secondary infertility, were considered eligible for inclusion in the study. Exclusion criteria included any factors which may adversely affect ovarian reserve such as a history of endometriosis, history of previous pelvic surgery, smokers and recreational drug users, history of chemotherapy or pelvic radiation and a history of hormonal treatment in the previous 6 months. Polycystic ovarian syndrome as defined by the Rotterdam-criteria [10] was also included as an indication for exclusion from the study. The intake of calcium, vitamin D or multivitamin supplements in the previous 3 months or a history of poor ovarian response according to the Bologna criteria [11] in a previous ART-treatment were also exclusion factors.

All study participants signed an informed consent agreement. Blood for vitamin D concentrations were measured via venipuncture and was taken together with other blood tests, deemed necessary for evaluation of the existing infertility and further treatment planning. Due to the additional costs which would have been created by performing AMH-testing and which would have to be covered by the patients, no routine AMH-test was performed. Transvaginal 2D ultrasound of the pelvis was performed on day 2–5 of the cycle to exclude pelvic pathology and to determine AFC.

Ultrasound for antral follicle count measurement

All patients were scanned by transvaginal 2D ultrasound on day 2–5 of the cycle. The ultrasound-scans were performed by one designated reproductive medicine specialist in each center in order to reduce the inter-observer variability. The two involved investigators established a common ultrasound technique for the AFC measurement prior of commencing the study in order to avoid any bias through different techniques.

All study participants had a transvaginal scan performed by the same investigator for intra-observer or inter-observer reliability, using a vaginal probe (Honda 5–9 MHZ, HS-2600, Japan). The optimal probe program, providing the best ultrasound image, was used in both fertility centers and the settings were maintained throughout the duration of the ultrasound evaluation. Each patient was asked to empty the bladder and was scanned in a Lloyd Davies position to ensure free manipulation of the transvaginal transducer. Ultrasound assessment of the pelvis excluded pelvic pathology. The ovaries were visualized in the longitudinal plane and the number of antral follicles measuring 2–10 mm in diameter within each ovary was counted as the transducer was moved from one side of the ovary to the other. Two scans were obtained for each ovary and in case of any discrepancy between these two values, a third measurement was done to confirm the final value.

Skin-type

The skin-types of all study participants was evaluated and classified according to the different skin type groups described by the Fitzpatrick classification [12] by a reproductive specialist and a consultant dermatologist.

Type I-II Fitzpatrick classification – abbreviated in this study as F1:

- Type I (scores 0–6) always burns, never tans (pale white; blond or red hair; blue eyes; freckles)
- Type II (scores 7–13) usually burns, tans minimally (white; fair; blond or red hair; blue, green, or hazel eyes)

Type III – IV 3–4 Fitzpatrick classification – abbreviated in this study as F2:

- Type III (scores 14–20) sometimes mild burn, tans uniformly (cream white; fair with any hair or eye color)
- Type IV (scores 21–27) burns minimally, always tans well (moderate brown)

Type V - Fitzpatrick classification – abbreviated in this study as F3:

- Type V (scores 28–34) very rarely burns, tans very easily (dark brown)

Dress-code

According to the Iranian regulations, in any public place women must cover their heads with a headscarf, wear trousers (or a floor length skirt), and a long-sleeved tunic or coat that reaches to mid-thigh or knee. Depending on the amount of skin not covered by concealing cloths, patients were stratified into the dress code (DR) 1, 2 and 3. Patients with DR 1 had an amount of uncovered skin of 10 to 15%, patients in DR 2 between 5 and 10% and patients in group DR 3 below 5% of skin exposed to sunlight.

Measurement of vitamin D-levels

Blood samples were taken to measure vitamin D concentrations within the first week following the initial consultation with a reproductive medicine specialist and at the same time of ultrasonographic assessment of the antral follicle count (AFC). Once the blood sample was taken for vitamin D concentration, the sample was centrifuged and frozen at – 20° Celsius. All blood samples for vitamin D concentrations were measured by the ELISA assay at one time to avoid inter-assay variability, using electrochemiluminescence binding assay (Roche's test) and Cobas e immunoassay analyzers.

Vitamin D deficiency was defined as serum level of $<$ 20 ng /ml 25hydroxy vitamin D [3].

Statistical analysis

Data were analyzed by SPSS v.18 software (IBM, Chicago, IL, USA). The quantitative measurements were described by using the mean and the standard deviation (SD). For nominal variables the relative frequency, using percentages, were reported. For comparison of means among groups, analysis of variance and LSD post hoc test was used.

Results

A total of 189 patients have been included in this prospective observational study. 87.7% ($n = 166$) of the patients attended the clinics due to primary infertility. The mean BMI of the patients was 26.70 kg/m^2 with a range of 17.9–35.5 kg/m^2.

According to the Fitzpatrick classifications, 50 patients (26.4%) were categorized as Fitzpatrick I-II (F1), 89 (47.1%) as Fitzpatrick III-IV (F2) and 50 (26.4%) as Fitzpatrick V (F3).

The patients were also classified according to dress code DR1, DR2 and DR 3 as previously described with the following distribution, 110 (58.2%), 30 (15.9%) and 49 (25.9%) respectively.

The mean age of the study group was 32.21 years and for the groups F1, F2 and F3 31.76 years, 32.40 years and 32.32 years respectively. The mean age of the patients in the different groups classified according to dress-code groups were as follows: DR1: 31.97 years, DR2: 33.07 years and DR3: 32.22 years.

The mean vitamin D level for the total study group was 15.46 ng/ml. In group F1 mean vitamin D level was 16.39 ng/ml, in group F2 14.50 ng/ml and in group F3 16.23 ng/ml. The mean Vitamin D level for groups DR1, DR2 and DR3 were 16.15 ng/ml, 13.66 ng/ml and 14.21 ng/ml, respectively.

The mean AFC count in all patients was 10.84. Patients in group F1 had a mean AFC of 10.14, group F2 a mean AFC of 11.20 and group F3 a mean AFC of 10.90. In the dress-code groups the results were: DR1: 10.59, DR2: 9.87 and DR3: 12.00, respectively. Table 1 provides the summary of the results.

The correlation of the data of all study patients between the parameters age, vitamin D concentrations and AFC showed a significant negative correlation between age and vitamin D ($p = 0.008$), age and AFC ($p = 0.001$) and importantly, a highly statistically significant correlation between vitamin D and AFC ($p < 0.001$).

No significant differences were found between and within the different skin-type groups for age ($p = 0.59$), vitamin D ($p = 0.56$) and AFC ($p = 0.66$). The groups of different dress-codes were also found to have no significant differences between and within the group for the parameters age ($p = 0.34$), Vitamin D ($p = 0.32$) and AFC ($p = 0.31$). Also no correlations were found between vitamin

Table 1 Summary of the results for the means, ranges and standard deviations for the following parameters: age, vitamin D concentrations and AFC in the different skin-type- and dress-code-groups

Groups		Total group	F1	F2	F3	DR1	DR2	DR3	Significance
Number of patients and %		189 (100%)	50 (26.4%)	89 (47.1%)	50 (26.4%)	110 (58.2%)	30 (15.9%)	49 (25.9%)	n.a.
Age (years)	Mean	32.21	31.76	32.4	32.32	31.97	33.07	32.22	n.s.
	Range	21–42	21–38	23–43	21–38	21–39	27–42	26–40	
	SD	3.64	3.63	3.69	3.58	3.67	3.83	3.44	
Vitamin D level (ng/ml)	Mean Vit. D level (ng/ml)	15.46	16.39	14.50	16.23	16.15	13.66	14.21	n.s.
	Range	2.5–73	2.5–43.8	2.5–73	4–48	2.5–73	2.5–48	4.0–44	
	SD	11.5	11.01	11.32	11.05	11.91	10.54	11.08	
AFC	Mean AFC	10.84	10.14	11.20	10.90	10.59	9.87	12.00	n.s.
	Range	1–31	2–29	2–31	1–30	1–31	2–29	2–29	
	SD	6.63	6.45	7.06	6.06	6.43	7.54	6.37	

n.a. not applicable, *n.s.* not significan, *SD* Standard deviation

D and BMI ($p = 0.968$) and vitamin D and the type of infertility ($p = 0.451$). The performance of multiple comparisons in the groups age, vitamin D and AFC within the different skin types as well as within the different dress codes did not show any significant differences.

Discussion

The presence of vitamin D receptors in reproductive tissues [13, 14] and the fact that in animal studies impaired folliculogenesis [15] was found in rats with compromised expression of vitamin D receptors suggests, that vitamin D deficiency may play an important role in determining the ovarian reserve. It was previously described that 1.25-dihydroxyvitamin D3 alters Anti-Mullerian-Hormone (AMH) sensitivity in human granulosa cells by inhibiting the expression of the AMH receptor (AMHR-II). Due to a reduced AMH sensitivity, more follicle might reach terminal maturation and ovulation, thereby influencing the ovarian reserve [16]. This possible interaction between the ovarian reserve and vitamin D is underlined by a correlation of seasonal fluctuations in serum AMH with seasonal changes in the vitamin D levels [17]. Due to this correlation, Irani et al. [7] even considered vitamin D to be a clinically useful marker of the ovarian reserve and suggested to include vitamin D into the routine workup in patients with infertility.

The herein presented study findings result from a prospective observational study in 189 female infertility patients in Iran, who are obliged to wear a specific dress code. The results demonstrate clearly a highly significant correlation ($p < 0.001$) between vitamin D deficiency and a reduced ovarian reserve. In this setting of self-payer patients, ovarian reserve was assessed by the antral follicle count (AFC), which is an established parameter to evaluate the ovarian reserve [18].

The most commonly used parameters for ovarian reserve testing are FSH (Follicle-stimulating-hormone), AMH (Anti-Muellerian-Hormone) and the antral follicle count. Nowadays, FSH is regarded as a parameter with poor sensitivity towards the detection of a diminished ovarian reserve and FSH testing has several major limitations including significant inter-cycle and intra-cycle variability and elevated FSH levels are almost only found in patients with an existing diminished ovarian reserve [19]. AMH is produced by the granulosa cells of small and large preantral and small antral follicles, therefore reflecting the primordial follicle pool. Whereas it was suggested that AMH is relatively stable throughout the cycle [20, 21], recent publications demonstrated significant fluctuations within a menstrual cycle [22, 23]. The antral follicle count (AFC) is calculated as the sum of follicles in both ovaries in the early follicular phase (day 2–4) of the menstrual cycle. The assessment can be performed in the context of the primary ultrasound evaluation of the internal genital organs and it provides an immediate result, has a good inter-cycle reliability and, if performed by experienced and a limited number of investigators, a good inter-observer reliability [24]. Several studies have shown that AFC and AMH are both good predictors of the ovarian response in the context of hormonal stimulation for ART (assisted reproductive techniques) treatment [25, 26], with each method having special advantages, disadvantages and limitations.

Studies to date, investigating the role of vitamin D on the ovarian reserve are conflicting and our results are in contrast to the findings from the recently published studies of Fabris et al. [8] and Drakopoulos et al. [9] who could not find a correlation between the ovarian reserve parameters AFC / AMH and vitamin D deficiency.

The contradictory finding between the studies may be attributed to the different ethnicities of the study population, having different socio-cultural religious habits and different dress-codes. Drakopoulos et al. [9] evaluated women with Caucasian ethnicity, who have been treated in an infertility center due to primary / secondary infertility in Belgium. The study of Fabris et al. [8] included only oocyte donors, who are usually young and healthy and don't have any infertility problems. The ethnicity of the study population is not revealed. However, their data are derived from an oocyte-donation-program based at a Spanish IVF-clinic. Therefore it can be assumed that their study patients had Caucasian ethnicity as well. In contrast to those mentioned studies, the herein described study population presents firstly a completely different ethnicity and secondly around 40% of the study population is dressed in a dress-code, which leaves less than 90% of the skin uncovered, thereby limiting the skin-exposure to the sun dramatically.

The Middle East countries have the highest vitamin D deficiency rates in the world and different factors contribute to low sun exposure and low vitamin D levels in women of reproductive age in these countries [27]. One of the most important factors leading to a high rate of vitamin D deficiency is the dress code of wearing concealing clothing due to social and religious habits [28]. The concealing dress code has been found to be an independent prognostic factor of vitamin D deficiency in Lebanese women, confirming the significance of sunlight exposure in vitamin D synthesis [28] and differences observed in vitamin D deficiency rates between Christian and Muslim women in Middle East highlight the importance of the dress code [29].

Skin-type is an important factor in determining the time needed for sufficient vitamin D synthesis via sunlight exposure. Persons with a skin-type classification I or II achieve maximal vitamin D photosynthesis rapidly after approximately 2–8 min of midday spring or summer sun exposure in New York or Boston and only slightly longer in Alaska or Scandinavia. Persons with phototype III skin produce vitamin D at similar rates to persons with phototype I or II skin after a first UV exposure. Persons with skin-type IV have high epidermal melanin content and therefore photosynthesize relatively limited amounts of vitamin D because of UV absorption by melanin [30]. Other authors deem the exposure of arms and legs for 5 to 30 min between 10 a.m. and 3 p.m. twice a week for sufficient to achieve adequate vitamin D levels [31].

However, in most Middle-East Islamic populations, girls start to wear concealing clothing with the onset of puberty or even earlier, leading to long-lasting non-exposure of the skin to the sun and therefore to long-lasting Vitamin D deficiencies.

Evaluation of the influence of the skin-type and dress-code on the Vitamin D deficiency was performed in a subgroup-analysis and no significant correlations between the different skin-types / dress-codes and vitamin D deficiency were found. Due to wearing concealing clothing with coverage of most of the body surface, the skin-type is of negligible importance. Absence of a correlation between the different dress-codes and vitamin D deficiency is explained by the fact, that even the group with the least skin coverage (10–15% at most of body skin surface which could be exposed to the sun) is still far below the required 20%.

Our study population is characterized by a severe vitamin D deficiency with 71.4% (135 patients) of the patients being vitamin D deficient and a mean vitamin D level in the study group of 15.48 ng/ml. In contrast, the mean vitamin D levels are not mentioned in the studies of Drakopoulos and Fabris [8, 9]. In addition, less than 50% of their study populations were vitamin D deficient (30 and 18% respectively). Therefore the severity of vitamin D deficiency in their studies, when compared to our study, was less and may be the reason why no correlation between vitamin D deficiency and the ovarian reserve parameters was identified.

Conclusions

The herein presented data may indicate, that severe and long-lasting vitamin D deficiency, caused by inadequate sun-exposure to the skin, could be a cause of the reduced ovarian reserve in the herein investigated group of infertile female Iranian patients. Future studies are required to investigate further the interaction between dress-code, vitamin D and fertility.

Acknowledgements

We thank Dr. Carol Coughlan for the linguistic revision and correction of the manuscript.

Authors' contributions

SA Conceptualization: Lead; Supervision: Lead; Investigation: Lead; Methodology: Lead; Writing – review & editing: Supporting. GK Conceptualization: Supporting; Formal analysis: Lead; Investigation: Equal; Writing – review & editing: Supporting. HI Conceptualization: Supporting; Investigation: equal. FF Conceptualization: Supporting; Investigation: equal. AH Conceptualization: Supporting; Formal analysis: lead; Investigation: equal. HMF Conceptualization: Supporting; Supervision: equal; Writing – review editing: equal. BL formal analysis: Supporting; writing- original draft: Lead. All authors read and approved the final manuscript.

Competing interests

Soheila Arefi, Gholamreza Khalili, Homa Iranmanesh, Fattaneh Farifheh, Ahmad Hosseini, Human M. Fatemi and Barbara Lawrenz have no competing interests.

Author details
[1]Avicenna Research Institute, ACECR, Tehran, Iran. [2]Bahman Hospital Infertility Center, North Iran Zamin St, Shahrak Gharb, Tehran, Iran. [3]Givar Infertility Center, Tehran, Iran. [4]Department of Epidemiology and Reproductive Health, Reproductive Research Center, Royan Institute for Reproductive Biomedicine, ACECR, Tehran, Iran. [5]Sarem Infertility Center, Sarem Women's Hospital, Shahrak Ekbatan, Tehran, Iran. [6]Cellular and Molecular Biology Research Center, Shahid Beheshti University of Medical science, Arabi Ave, Daneshjoo Blvd, Velenjak, Tehran, Iran. [7]IVF department, IVI RMA Middle-East Fertility Clinic, Abu Dhabi, UAE. [8]Women's university hospital Tuebingen, Tuebingen, Germany.

References

1. Groeber U, Spitz J, Reichrath J, Kisters K, Holick MF. Vitamin D update 2013: from rickets prophylaxis to general preventive healthcare. Dermatoendocrinol. 2013;5(3):331–47.
2. Anagnostis P, Karras S, Goulis DG. Vitamin D in human reproduction: a narrative review. Int J Clin Pract. 2013;67(3):225–35.
3. Holick MF. Vitamin D deficiency. N Engl J Med. 2007;357(3):266–81.
4. Lips P. Worldwide status of vitamin D nutrition. J Steroid Biochem Mol Biol. 2010;121:297–300.
5. Hossein-Nezhad A, Holick MF. Vitamin D for health: a global perspective. Mayo Clin Proc. 2013;88(7):720–55.
6. Lips P. Vitamin D status and nutrition in Europe and Asia. J Steroid Biochem Mol Biol. 2007;103(3–5):620–5.
7. Irani M, Merhi Z. Role of vitamin D in ovarian physiology and its implication in reproduction: a systematic review. Fertil Steril. 2014;102:460–8.
8. Fabris AM, Cruz M, Iglesias C, Pacheco A, Patel A, Patel J, et al. Impact of vitamin D levels on ovarian reserve and ovarian response to ovarian stimulation in oocyte donors. Reprod BioMed Online. 2017;35(2):139–44.
9. Drakopoulos P, van de Vijver A, Schutyser V, Milatovic S, Anckaert E, Schiettecatte J, et al. The effect of serum vitamin D levels on ovarian reserve markers: a prospective cross-sectional study. Hum Reprod. 2017;32(1):208–14.
10. The Rotterdam ESHRE/ASRM-Sponsored PCOS Consensus Workshop Group. Revised 2003 consensus on diagnostic criteria and long-term health risks related to polycystic ovary syndrome (PCOS). Hum Reprod. 2004;19:41–7.
11. Ferraretti AP, La Marca A, Fauser BC, Tarlatzis B, Nargund G, Gianaroli L. ESHRE working group on poor ovarian response definition. ESHRE consensus on the definition of 'poor response' to ovarian stimulation for in vitro fertilization: the bologna criteria. Hum Reprod. 2011;26(7):1616–24.
12. Fitzpatrick TB. The validity and practicality of sun-reactive skin types I through VI. Arch Dermatol. 1988 Jun;124(6):869–71.
13. Shahbazi M, Jeddi-Tehrani M, Zareie M, Salek-Moghaddam A, Akhondi MM, Bahmanpoor M, et al. Expression profiling of vitamin D receptor in placenta, decidua and ovary of pregnant mice. Placenta. 2011;32:657–64.
14. Zarnani AH, Shahbazi M, Salek-Moghaddam A, Zareie M, Tavakoli M, Ghasemi J, et al. Vitamin D3 receptor expressed in the endometrium of cycling mice throughout the estrous cycle. Fertil Steril. 2010;93:2738–43.
15. Halloran BP, DeLuca HF. Effect of vitamin D deficiency on fertility and reproductive capacity in the female rat. J Nutr. 1980;110:1573–80.
16. Merhi Z, Doswell AD, Krebs K, Cipolla MJ. Vitamin D alters genes involved in follicular development and steroidogenesis in human cumulus granulosa cells. J Clin Endocrinol Metab. 2014;14:jc20134161.
17. Dennis NA, Houghton LA, Jones GT, van RijAM MK, McLennan IS. The level of serum anti-mullerian hormone correlates with vitamin D status in men and women but not in boys. J Clin Endocrinol Metab. 2012;97:2450–5.
18. Fleming R, Seifer DB, Frattarelli JL, Ruman J. Assessing ovarian response: antral follicle count versus anti-Müllerian hormone. Reprod BioMed Online. 2015;31(4):486–96.
19. Broekmans FJ, Kwee J, Hendriks DJ, Mol BW, Lambalk CB. A systematic review of tests predicting ovarian reserve and IVF outcome. Hum Reprod Update. 2006;12(6):685–718.
20. Hehenkamp WJ, Looman CW, Themmen AP, de Jong FH, Te Velde ER, Broekmans FJ. Anti-Mullerian hormone levels in the spontaneous menstrual cycle do not show substantial fluctuation. J Clin Endocrinol Metab. 2006; 91(10):4057–63.
21. La Marca A, Stabile G, Artenisio AC, Volpe A. Serum anti-Mullerian hormone throughout the human menstrual cycle. Hum Reprod. 2006;21(12):3103–7.
22. Kissell KA, Danaher MR, Schisterman EF, Wactawski-Wende J, Ahrens KA, Schliep K, et al. Biological variability in serum anti-Mullerian hormone throughout the menstrual cycle in ovulatory and sporadic anovulatory cycles in eumenorrheic women. Hum Reprod. 2014;29(8):1764–72.
23. Hadlow N, Longhurst K, McClements A, Natalwala J, Brown SJ, Matson PL. Variation in antimullerian hormone concentration during the menstrual cycle may change the clinical classification of the ovarian response. Fertil Steril. 2013;99(6):1791–7.
24. Tal R, Seifer DB. Ovarian reserve testing: a user's guide. Am J Obstet Gynecol. 2017;217(2):129–40.
25. La Marca A, Sighinolfi G, Radi D, Argento C, Baraldi E, Artenisio AC, Stabile G, Volpe A. Anti-Mullerian hormone (AMH) as a predictive marker in assisted reproductive technology (ART). Hum Reprod Update. 2010;16(2):113–30.
26. Lukaszuk K, Kunicki M, Liss J, Lukaszuk M, Jakiel G. Use of ovarian reserve parameters for predicting live births in women undergoing in vitro fertilization. Eur J Obstet Gynecol Reprod Biol. 2013;168(2):173–7.
27. Mishal AA. Effects of different dress styles on vitamin D levels in healthy young Jordanian women. Osteoporos Int. 2001;12(11):931–5.
28. Hatun S, Islam O, Cizmecioglu F, Kara B, Babaoglu K, Berk F, et al. Subclinical vitamin D deficiency is increased in adolescent girls who wear concealing clothing. J Nutr. 2005;135(2):218–22.
29. Gannagé-Yared MH, Maalouf G, Khalife S, Challita S, Yaghi Y, Ziade N, et al. Prevalence and predictors of vitamin D inadequacy amongst Lebanese osteoporotic women. Br J Nutr. 2009;101(4):487–91.
30. Gilchrest BA. Sun exposure and vitamin D sufficiency. Am J Clin Nutr. 2008; 88(2):570S–7S.
31. Holick MF. Vitamin D: the underappreciated D-lightful hormone that is important for skeletal and cellular health. Curr Opin Endocrinol Diabetes. 2002;9:87–98.

8

DNA damage repair in ovarian cancer: unlocking the heterogeneity

Mary Ellen Gee[1,2], Zahra Faraahi[1], Aiste McCormick[3] and Richard J. Edmondson[1,2*]

Abstract

Treatment for advanced ovarian cancer is rarely curative; three quarters of patients with advanced disease relapse and ultimately die with resistant disease. Improving patient outcomes will require the introduction of new treatments and better patient selection. Abrogations in the DNA damage response (DDR) may allow such stratifications.
A defective DNA-damage response (DDR) is a defining hallmark of high grade serous ovarian cancer (HGSOC). Indeed, current evidence indicates that all HGSOCs harbour a defect in at least one major DDR pathway. However, defective DDR is not mediated through a single mechanism but rather results from a variety of (epi)genetic lesions affecting one or more of the five major DNA repair pathways. Understanding the relationship between these pathways and how these are abrogated will be necessary in order to facilitate appropriate selection of both existing and novel agents. Here we review the current understanding of the DDR with regard to ovarian, and particularly high grade serous, cancer, with reference to existing and emerging treatments as appropriate.

Keywords: Non-homologous end joining, Homologous recombination, Nucleotide excision repair, Base excision repair, Mismatch repair, Ovarian cancer

Background

Epithelial ovarian cancer is not one homogenous disease, but a collection of disparate cancers arising from different tissues, including the fallopian tube and the ovary, each of which represents a very different biological entity. Current evidence suggests five major subtypes of epithelial ovarian cancer, namely, high grade serous, low grade serous, endometrioid, clear cell and mucinous cancers, of which high grade serous is the commonest.

Teasing out the heterogeneity between these types is of major importance but remains a challenge. Understanding is hampered by the relative lack of driver mutations and the massive genetic instability that characterises many forms of the disease and makes molecular profiling difficult.

Genomic and transcriptomic studies have managed to identify a limited number of driver mutations, restricted at present largely to p53 and BRCA1/2, but have grossly failed to identify predictive patterns that can be used to determine therapy. A notable exception is the identification of defective homologous recombination as a predictor of response to both platinum [1] and PARP inhibitor therapy [2].Building upon this, and using defects in other DNA damage repair (DDR) mechanisms as a stratification tool, has enormous potential. The inability to repair DNA damage is one of the hallmarks of the cancer cell, however rendering a cell defective in DNA damage repair is not mediated through a single process, rather it is conferred by a wide variety of genomic defects and this can result in differing sensitivities to conventional and novel chemotherapeutic agents.

In general, DNA damage results in either single strand or double strand breaks. Current understanding suggests that there are five mechanisms used by mammalian cells to identify and repair DNA damage. These are mismatch repair (MMR), base excision repair (BER), and nucleotide excision repair (NER) for single strand breaks and homologous recombination (HR) and non homologous end joining (NHEJ) for double strand breaks (see Fig. 1). Single strand breaks may be repaired directly but if left unrepaired will result in a stalled replication fork. Replication stress is the term coined to describe the effects on the cell

* Correspondence: richard.edmondson@manchester.ac.uk
[1]Division of Cancer Sciences, Faculty of Biology, Medicine and Health, University of Manchester, St Mary's Hospital, Manchester, UK
[2]Department of Obstetrics and Gynaecology, Manchester Academic Health Science Centre, St Mary's Hospital, Central Manchester NHS Foundation Trust, Manchester Academic Health Science Centre, Level 5, Research, Oxford Road, Manchester, UK
Full list of author information is available at the end of the article

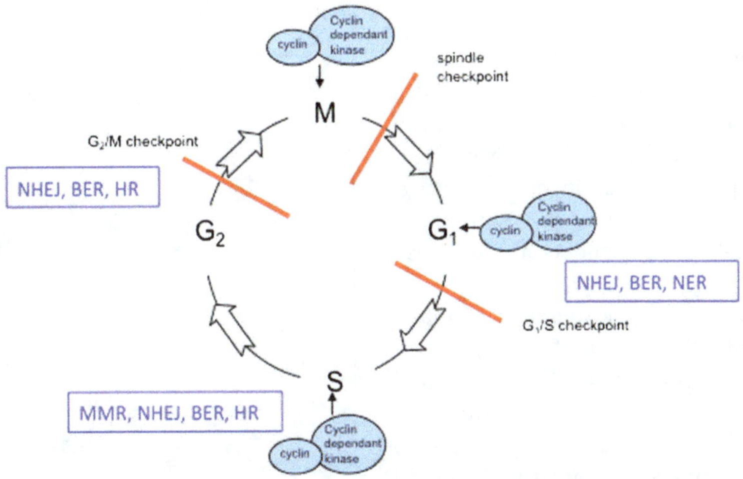

Fig. 1 The phases of the cell cycle and DNA repair mechanisms active during the four stages. Both classical and alternative non homologous end joining (C-NHEJ and A-NHEJ) repair double strand breaks and are active throughout the cell cycle, they are especially active in G1 [25]. Base excision repair (BER) removes damaged nucleotides and repairs single strand breaks throughout the cell cycle [60]. Nucleotide excision repair is concerned with the removal of bulky damaged DNA lesions and single strand breaks during G1. Mismatch repair corrects DNA mismatches and repairs single strand breaks during S phase [91]. Homologous recombination repairs double strand breaks during S phase and G2 [4]

of a stalled replication fork. Replication stress should activate functional DNA checkpoint proteins to trigger the commencement of the double strand DNA repair pathways. However, in cancer cells the combination of a high replication rate and defective DNA repair mechanisms can lead instead to genomic instability. This is particularly the case in high grade serous ovarian cancer which is characterised by genomic instability. Given the high levels of genomic instability and subsequent chromosomal rearrangements which are tolerated by high grade serous cancer cells in particular, it is highly likely that at least one of these five pathways is dysfunctional in each cell (Table 1).

Through the understanding of these DNA repair mechanisms, their interaction and how they may be defective in women with different subtypes of EOC, it may be possible to target chemotherapy to the molecular mechanisms underlying a cancer. Synthetic lethality is the term coined to describe the effect of the combination of two genetic alterations that are lethal to cells, but alone do not have a negative effect (reviewed by Kaelin [3]). Discovery of novel drugs which exploit synthetic lethality is one such way that the understanding of defective DNA repair mechanisms can advance the management of ovarian cancer.

Treatments exploit the exquisite balance of DNA damage in a cancer cell by either inducing further DNA damage, with which the cell's already impaired DNA capacity cannot cope, or by impairing the capacity of the DDR even further. Either strategy leads to catastrophic DNA damage causing cell death. The benefit of the latter approach in which DDR pathways are inhibited in the cell, is that it has little effect on normal cells which include many overlapping pathways that can cope with loss of a single pathway. Thus the toxicity of these targeted treatments is often more acceptable than conventional cytotoxic chemotherapy.

Here we review the current state of knowledge regarding the role of the various DNA repair pathways in ovarian cancer; using high grade serous cancer as the exemplar, but referring to the other subtypes where appropriate.

Table 1 The known contribution of defective DNA repair pathways to ovarian cancer

DNA repair pathway	Type of repair	Contribution to serous ovarian cancer	Contribution to all histological subtypes of ovarian cancer
Homologous Recombination	Double Strand Breaks	50% [4]	50%
Non Homologous Enjoining	Double Strand Breaks		
Base Excision Repair	Nucleotide Excision and Single Strand Breaks		Polymorphisms and altered expression of BER components in 63–67% ovarian cancers [60, 91]
Mismatch Repair	Single Strand Breaks, Nucleotide Mismatches	0.18% [94]	0.76% [94], mostly clear cell
Nucleotide Excision Repair	Single Strand Breaks, Bulky Lesions	8%	

Homologous recombination

Mechanism

Homologous recombination (HR) is a high fidelity mechanism for repairing double strand breaks or stalled replication forks that occur during S and G2 phases of the cell cycle [4]. DSBs can be caused by ionising radiation, reactive oxygen species and antineoplastic drugs, such as anthracyclines and bleomycin. Inability to repair DSB causes chromosomal rearrangements and can lead to cell death [4].

HR uses the sister chromatid as a template to repair the DSB. The damaged DNA ends of the DSB are resected by the RAD50, MRE11 and NBS1 complex (mediated by BRCA1). The complex, using a 3′-5′ exonuclease exposes the 3′ strand ends on either side of the DSB [5]. Single strand DNA is unwound and the 3′ strand from the damaged chromosome invades into the sister chromosome, at the complementary sequence, using BRCA2 and the single strand binding protein RAD51. DNA polymerase then reads off the complimentary sequence to extend the previously damaged 3′ end. The replication continues past the original DSB and continues to the end of the chromosome (see Fig. 2) [6].

It has been estimated that there are at least 40 proteins participating in this pathway, but it was the recognition that this included BRCA1 and BRCA2 that provided the stimulus to study this pathway in breast and ovarian cancer.

The role of homologous recombination in high grade serous ovarian Cancer

Overall, defects in HR, whether through mutation or epigenetic silencing of key proteins, have been found in up to 50% EOC [1, 7].

BRCA1 and 2

Mutations in BRCA1 and BRCA2 are well documented in hereditary ovarian cancer syndromes. As a result of carrying mutations in BRCA1 and BRCA2 women carry a 40% lifetime risk of epithelial ovarian cancer [8].

BRCA1 and 2 dysfunction is also prevalent in sporadic epithelial ovarian cancer [9]. The term "BRCAness", which is synonymous with defective homologous recombination (HRD), has been coined to describe the phenotype of dysfunctional BRCA1 and 2, brought about by epigenetic silencing. Mechanisms contributing to HRD in sporadic EOC include BRCA1 hypermethylation, occurring in 5–31% of sporadic ovarian cancer [10, 11]. Estimates of the prevalence of BRCA1 and 2 mutations in the general population range from 1 in 400 to 1 in 800 [12].

Of the histological subtypes of EOC, high grade serous EOC is associated with a BRCA1/2 mutations of 10.9 and 5.6% respectively, whilst endometrioid EOC is associated with a 2.1% mutation rate [13]. BRCA1 and 2 do not appear to play a role in mucinous EOC.

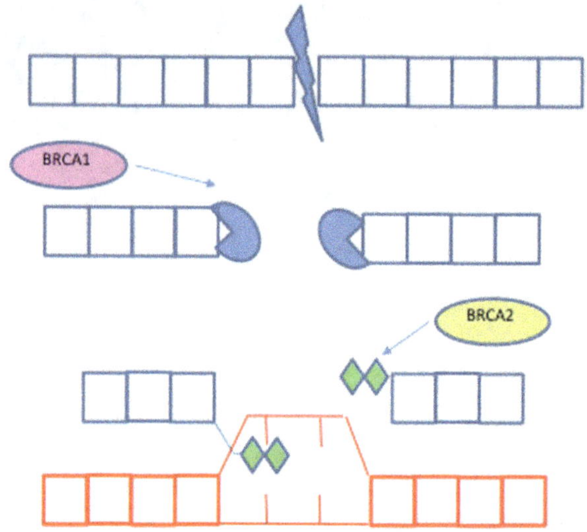

Fig. 2 Double Strand Break (DSB) repair by Homologous Recombination. When a DSB is recognised, BRCA1 mediates the recruitment of the MRN complex, which comprises MRE11, RAD50 and NBS1 [3]. The MRN complex recruits ataxia-telangiectasia mutated (ATM) which, in turn, activates MRN components by phosphorylating them. The MRN complex work with CtIP and EXO1 to resect 3′ ends of the DS. Replication protein A (RPA) covers the DNA overhang to prevent it from being degraded. This stage of HR, nucleolytic processing, can be defunct in hereditary ovarian cancer; a single base mutation in exon 10 of MRE11 is reported in hereditary ovarian cancers [92] and RAD50 protein truncation is reported in hereditary breast and ovarian cancer families. As well as activating nucleolytic processing machinery, ATM phosphorylates and activates BRCA1 and RAD51. ATM is mutated in 2% of high grade EOC [7] and is significantly associated with platinum resistance [41]. Single strand DNA is unwound and the damaged chromosome invades the sister chromosome to form a Holliday junction. This occurs when RPA is replaced by RAD51, facilitated by BRCA2, allowing for strand invasion [93]. RAD51 is hypermethylated in 3% of high grade serous EOC, resulting in ineffective strand invasion [7]. MSY (not shown) is an oncogene that can silence the activation domain of BRCA2 it is overexpressed in 17% sporadic high grade serous ovarian cancer [15]

Implications for therapy

Defective HR allows accumulation of mutations thereby promoting oncogenesis, but appears to also confer a prognostic advantage, possibly through improved sensitivity to chemotherapeutic agents and ionising radiation [14, 15].

This effect is not limited just to BRCA related cancers and it is now clear that all HR defective tumours, identified using a RAD51 immunoflourescence assay, are associated with improved survival compared to HR competent tumours when managed with platinum based chemotherapy [1].

Therefore, disruption of functional HR is a potential therapeutic target to prevent chemotherapy resistance. A clinical example, although with little current clinical to support it, is the use of the BCR-ABL inhibitor, Imatinib. RAD51 requires phosphorylation in order to become active during the process of homologous recombination and phosphorylation is dependent on the proto-oncogene ABL1. Thereby using Imatinib, HR is inhibited and cells are sensitised to crosslinking chemotherapy agents and ionising radiation [16].

PARP inhibitors

Since the landmark papers of Bryant and Farmer [17, 18], the therapeutic effect of PARP inhibition has been presumed to be mediated via the inhibition of the base excision repair pathway in cells already defective in homologous recombination. The concept of HR/BER synthetic lethality is based upon the idea that most single strand breaks would be repaired by BER, if this is inhibited by PARPi then they persist to become stalled replication forks during replication which then cannot be repaired by the defective HR in the cell.

PARP inhibitors have shown clinical efficacy in tumours with defective HR. The PARPi, olaparib, has shown efficacy in both the relapsed setting, in women with BRCA1/2 mutations and ovarian cancer [19], and when used as maintenance therapy in women with sporadic high grade serous ovarian cancer, improving progression-free survival time, when compared to placebo [20]. However the remaining challenge is to identify HR defective tumours; in a recent phase III study of niraparib, which demonstrated efficacy in women with platinum sensitive relapse, the greatest effect was, not surprisingly, seen in tumours with a germline BRCA mutation but the test used to determine HR status in the non BRCA related tumours failed to provide a clinically useful stratification [21].

Other HR related targets

Whilst PARP inhibitors have clear clinical utility and serve as a great example of synthetic lethality, there are other opportunities to target HR related proteins including ATR.

ATR is a potential target as it works upstream in the HR process and is influential over the whole pathway. ATR initiates HR in response to radiation or platinum induced stalled replication forks and ATR inhibition should render the cell defective for HR [22]. NU6027 has been shown to inhibit ATR in preclinical studies and has been found to enhance hydroxyurea and cisplatin cytotoxicity, inhibit RAD51 focus formation, and lead to cell cycle arrest at G2/M. Further, when used with PARPi or cells with defective XRCC1, NU6027 demonstrates synthetic lethality [23].Two ATR inhibitors, VX-970 (similar to VE-821) and AZD-6738, are currently undergoing clinical evaluation. VX-970 is being evaluated both as a single agent and in combination with platinum-based chemotherapy (clinicaltrials.gov identifier: NCT02157792) and AZD-6738 in haematological malignancies with 11q deletions (ATM defective) (clinicaltrials.gov identifier: NCT01955668).

A further way to block HR is to inhibit CDK1, which activates BRCA1. Preclinical studies showed that CDK1 inhibitor AG024322 is synthetically lethal with PARPi [24].

Non homologous End Joining

Mechanism

Non homologous end joining (NHEJ), the other pathway in the repair of DNA DSBs, has received less attention than HR as a determinant of response to therapy. Emerging evidence suggests that this may be a serious oversight and that NHEJ may have a major role in determining outcome to treatment. NHEJ occurs during G0 and G1 of the cell cycle, with some activity in late S and G2 [25] and is considered to be responsible for the majority of DSB repairs caused by ionising radiation [26].

NHEJ has always been considered to be an error prone process relying on modification of DNA breaks to allow joining (or synapsis), rather than directly replicating the sister chromatid [27]. Whilst it is not entirely clear why cells choose one pathway over the other it has been hypothesised that higher eukaryotes use the error prone NHEJ more than HR because NHEJ allows for faster DNA repair during a dynamic cell cycle and does not have the same steric constraints as HR, where the sister chromatid needs to be in close proximity [25, 28]. The NHEJ process comprises two pathways, a classical and an alternative pathway [29].

The classical NHEJ pathway

The classical, canonical, or DNA-PK dependent pathway, is active in normally functioning cells and occurs in the absence of a DNA template or extended regions of microhomology. The classical pathway is inherently accurate but is adaptable and therefore infidelity can creep into the process as a result of the nature of the damage that requires repair [30].

Classical NHEJ involves the actions of 6 key proteins: DNA-PKcs, the Ku70/Ku80 heterodimer, Artemis, DNA ligase IV, XRCC4 and XLF [29].

Ku (Ku70/Ku80 heterodimer), a ring like structure, binds to the DNA DSB with high affinity and recruits the serine-threonine protein kinase DNA-PK. Ku is able to stabilise DNA-PK's affinity for the DNA terminus [31] and may act as a docking site for other proteins in NHEJ. If the ends of the DNA DSB are not compatible then 'overhangs' of DNA need to be removed, trimmed back to a microhomology and resynthesized by nucleases and DNA polymerases such as Artemis. Artemis can form both a 3′ and a 5′ endonuclease when complexed with DNA-PK [32]. Once the ends are compatible they can be ligated. DNA ligase IV and XRCC4 co-factor, along with XLF appear to be responsible in humans for this ligation in NHEJ [33, 34].

The alternative NHEJ (A-EJ) pathway

The alternative, (also known as the back up or microhomology mediated end joining) pathway is less well characterised than the classical pathway. As the name suggests, it has been found to be active when other mechanisms, (classical NHEJ and HR) are inhibited or absent. It can be activated throughout the cell cycle and is slower than the classical pathway [35]. A-EJ pathway is independent of Ku and frequently uses microhomologies distant from the DSB. A-EJ is typically associated with deletions at the repair junction and therefore is highly mutagenic. The key proteins proposed to be active in the alternative pathway are PARP1, DNA ligase III and XRCC1 and thought to be promoted by DNA polymerase Θ [36]. PARP1 recognises and binds to DNA at DSB in competition with Ku to fulfil a similar role [37]. XRCC1 and LIG III form a complex to ligate the broken DSB strands [38].

Ku is biochemically more competitive than PARP1, however in cells that are Ku80 deficient, inhibiting PARP results in both arms of NHEJ being defective, resulting in the cell being sensitive to the effects of ionising radiation [39].

Role in high grade serous epithelial ovarian Cancer

Errors in NHEJ are associated with therapeutic resistance. Defective NHEJ has been found in up to 50% of ovarian cancers, is independent of HR function and appears to confer resistance to PARP inhibitor therapy, at least in the ex vivo setting [40]. Defective NHEJ may be conferred by a wide range of molecular aberrations affecting either the classical or the alternative pathways. In general, molecular events can either be in the germline, conferring an altered risk of developing the disease, or somatic, implying that the genomic event is affecting cell survival and subsequent sensitivity to therapy.

Classical pathway components

DNA-PK complex DNA-PK is the complex made up of DNA-PKcs, Ku70/Ku80. Molecular study of platinum resistant ovarian cancer has shown that DNA-PK is responsible for phosphorylating AKT at S743 and relocating it to the nucleus. High expression of DNA-PKCS is a common finding in high grade serous cancer and associates with advanced stage, higher grade and poorer survival due to reduced platinum sensitivity [41]. PARP-1 has been shown to interact with Ku protein [42]. Genetic ablation of KU70 and LIG IV has been shown to restore survival of PARP-1 deficient cells exposed to DSBs inducing agents [43]. Also, DNA-PK inhibition and depletion has been shown to result in HR function recovery and PARPi resistance in vitro [44].

DNA LIG iv

Single nucleotide polymorphisms have been associated with an increased risk of developing ovarian cancer [45] although this remains controversial [46]. It is possible that LIG IV variants result in dysfunctional NHEJ with an associated hypersensitivity to DNA damage [33].

Alternative pathway components

Pol Θ Pol Θ is thought to promote A-EJ. Pol Θ expression has been found to be inversely proportional to HR competency in epithelial ovarian cells in vitro and increased expression has been found in serous ovarian cancer [47].

XRCC1 Although often thought of as a protein whose role is limited to NER, XRCC1 is relatively promiscuous and appears to have functional roles in both the base excision repair (BER) and non homologous end joining pathways. Deficiency in XRCC1 can result in cell death due to genomic stress, but can also allow for accumulation of mutations, as SSBs remain unrepaired. In ovarian cancer patients XRCC1 polymorphisms are associated with poorer prognosis and higher levels of platinum resistance [48].

Pre-clinical studies of cells deficient in XRCC1 show that these cells have higher sensitivity to platinum chemotherapy than controls [49]. This is supported by clinical data suggesting that EOC tumours overexpressing XRCC1 and were more likely to be high grade serous cancer, demonstrate platinum resistance, increased risk of death and increased risk of tumour progression [49].

Implications for therapy

PARP inhibitors

Knowledge of NHEJ status may allow further enrichment of a population that is likely to have a high response rate to PARPi therapy.

DSB are repaired by the dominant, but more error prone NHEJ pathway. Only if cells are NHEJ defective (classical pathway) will DSB will be repaired by HR. Recent data suggest that cells which are NHEJ defective develop upregulated HR, as evidenced by increased RAD51 foci formation and are resistant to rucaparib [40]. However cells which are HR defective are still sensitive to PARPi, as the alternative, PARP dependent pathway is also inhibited.

DNA-PK

It is now becoming clear that platinum resistant clones may be present in the primary tumour and can be selected for, inadvertently, through the use of platinum based chemotherapy [50]. Platinum resistant high grade serous EOC are associated with phosphorylated AKT, relocated to the nucleus. By inhibiting DNA-PK or inhibiting AKT, platinum sensitivity can be restored in cells rendered previously resistant [51].

Preclinical studies have found that treatment of malignant ovarian cell lines with the combination of an EGFR inhibitor, Gefitinib, plus cisplatin is able to reduce DNA-PK expression, even in cisplatin resistant cells [52]. Cisplatin has also been reported to inhibit NHEJ in vitro [53]. Unravelling intracellular signalling properties of already established drugs may be a rewarding avenue in the future management of high grade serous ovarian cancer.

The finding that Wortmannin, a member of the DNA-PK family which inhibits PIKK, and is a radiosensitiser in preclinical models, [54] led to the investigation of other DNA-PK inhibitors as potential targets such as Nu7441, a small molecule DNA-PK inhibitor found to sensitise HeLa cells to ionising radiation and etoposide [55, 56]in colon cancer. There are other small molecular DNA-PK inhibitors, however none are yet reported to have shown activity to high grade serous ovarian cancer.

XRCC1

XRCC1 expression has been suggested as a predictive biomarker in human ovarian cancer with expression being associated with platinum resistance, suggesting that XRCC1 positive tumours should be considered for non platinum based chemotherapy [49].

Furthermore, XRCC1 may be a target for synthetic lethality, it is active in multiple DNA repair pathways, with important activity in single strand repair pathways, meaning that cells deficient in XRCC1 have higher reliance on DSB repair pathways to maintain genomic integrity. Pre-clinical data, albeit regarding breast cancer, has examined the synthetic lethality of inhibiting pathways for DSB in cells deficient in XRCC1 and found that potent ATM and DNA-PKc inhibitors are synthetically lethal in XRCC1 deficient cells [57].

Base excision repair

Mechanism of base excision repair

Base excision repair (BER) is responsible for both removing small base lesions from DNA and also effecting SSB repair (via a subpathway of BER called single strand break repair (SSBR)). Bases may become damaged due to reactive oxygen species (ROS), spontaneous deamination or due to alkylation [58]. Single strand breaks (SSBs) are the commonest endogenous DNA lesion. They arise from DNA damage due to reactive oxygen species (ROS) or via BER when damaged bases are excised [59].

BER repairs lesions generated endogenously by aerobic respiration, but also therapeutically by ionising radiation, topoisomerase I agents and DNA methylating agents.

BER can work by repairing one nucleotide in the predominant, short patch BER (SP-BER)pathway or by replacing 2–12 nucleotides as a long patch BER (LP-BER) [58] (Fig. 3).

Role in high grade serous epithelial ovarian Cancer

The extent to which defective BER plays a role in high grade serous epithelial ovarian cancer is not well identified, probably because of the difficulty of studying this pathway independently of other DNA repair pathways. However, there are some studies identifying how the components of BER may contribute to ovarian cancer.

Polymorphisms of other BER components, notably the glycosidase OGG1, result in an increased risk of ovarian cancer, especially in women who are BRCA1 deficient [60], and are a common finding with up to 63% of women with ovarian cancer carrying these germline variants [61].

DNA polymerase activity upregulates the error prone BER pathway, via pol β overexpression, in up to 67% of ovarian cancers. Subsequent silencing of pol β induces sensitivity to platinum chemotherapy, thus implicating pol β in the low fidelity DNA repair mechanism which allows cells to escape apoptosis by bypassing DNA lesions [62].

High nuclear expression of APE1 is associated with high grade serous epithelial ovarian cancer and correlates with poor surgical outcome, a poor overall survival and possibly higher rates of platinum resistance when compared to APE1 negative patients [63].

Implications for therapy

BER has the capacity to repair DNA which has been intentionally damaged by therapy such as IR and alkylating agents. Therefore, by undermining BER whilst managing patients with IR and chemotherapy, the effects can be potentiated.

PARP inhibitors

PARP recruits and activates DNA repair proteins by causing the post translational modification, poly ADP-ribosylation. PARP1 has a key role in SSBR, as it binds at single strand breaks, stabilising the DNA ends and recruiting downstream proteins such as XRCC1. Inhibition of PARP has been found to sensitize ovarian cancer cells to chemotherapy because when PARP is inhibited, BER cannot proceed and the SSB causes replication fork collapse when it is met in S phase, resulting in DSB [64, 65], If the DSB cannot be repaired, then the cell dies. As previously mentioned, PARP inhibition is synthetically lethal in women with known defective homologous recombination. Olaparib is being investigated in clinical trials, not only as a monotherapy

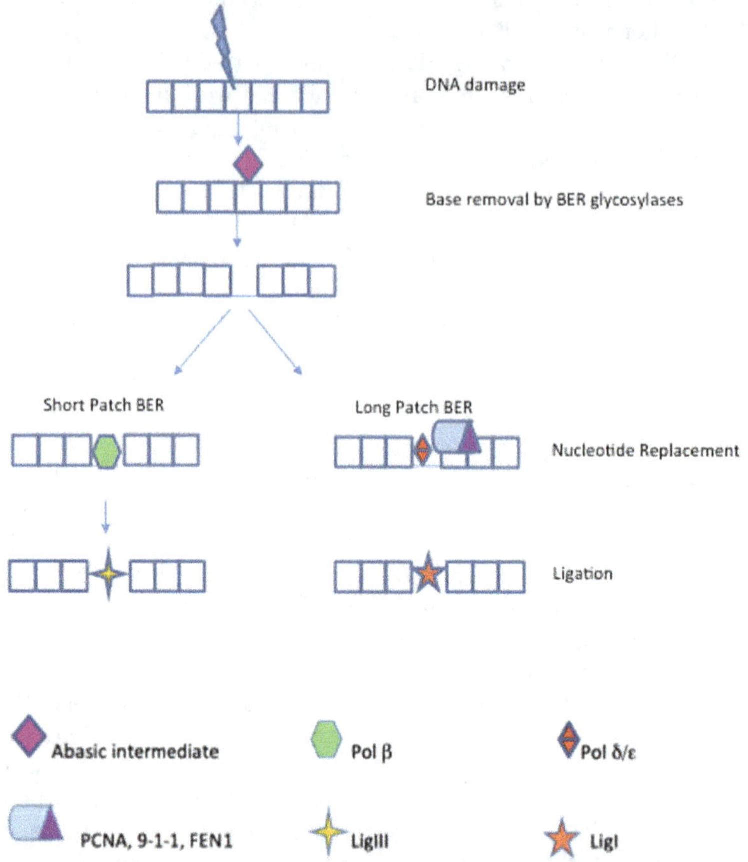

Fig. 3 The Base Excision Repair Pathway. BER consists of 5 stages: Damaged bases are recognised and removed by BER glycolases to produce an abasic intermediate. BER endonucleases (commonly APE1) make a site incision, generating a SSB. The sugar backbone is modified by phosphodiesterase. The newly formed nucleotide gap is filled by DNA polymerase. DNA ligase seals the nucleotide patch together. In SP-BER DNA polymerase B (Pol β) replaces the damaged nucleotide and the ends are ligated by DNA Lig III [58]. In LP-BER the patch is processed by proliferating cell nuclear antigen (PCNA), 9–1-1 complex and flap endonuclease 1 (FEN1), the nucleotides replaced by Pol δ and Pol ε with ligation by Lig I. in the single strand break repair (SSBR) pathway, PARP1 senses nicks in DNA, recruits XRCC1which acts as a scaffold for the other BER components to stabilise the SSB

(clinicaltrials.gov identifier: NCT01844986) but also in combination with AZD1775, a cell cycle checkpoint inhibitor (clinicaltrial.gov identifier NCT02511795), [66].

Pol β

Pol β has been identified as a potential target for inhibition which would result in abrogation of BER and prevent the tumour cell from withstanding oncogenic stress. One inhibitor, masticadienomic acid (MA) has been identified as a potent and selective Pol β inhibitor, which competes for the active site of Pol β in ovarian cancer cell lines and sensitises the cells to cis-platin [67]. Additional in vitro studies have found Pol β inhibitors able to cause sensitisation to bleomycin and ionising radiation [68, 69].

APE1 inhibitors (APEX1)

In vitro studies of silencing APE1 using siRNA rendered ovarian cancer cell lines sensitive to cisplatin and resulted in cell apoptosis [70].Methoxyamine has been found to inhibit APE1 in other cancers and studies of methoxyamine in ovarian cancer cell lines have found it to increase sensitivity to alkylatortemozolmide [71, 72]. There are multiple ongoing clinical trials of methoxyamine in various advanced or relapsed solid tumours, including ovarian cancer (clinicaltrials.gov identifiers NCT02535312, NCT01851369).

Mismatch repair

Mechanism of mismatch repair

Mismatch repair (MMR) is a mechanism for repairing incorrect base matches and insertion/deletion errors generated during replication. Defects in MMR are associated with genome instability due to higher rates of spontaneous mutation and thus high levels of microsatellite instability (MSI). MMR plays an instrumental role in DNA repair but is also required for effective cell cycle arrest and apoptosis in severely damaged cells [73]. Hence, defective MMR results in a predisposition to certain cancers and a loss of sensitivity to chemotherapeutic agents.

MMR has been extensively studied in E.coli, but is incompletely defined in eukaryotic cells. MMR comprises 3 general stages, initiation, excision and resynthesis (Fig. 4).

MutS homologs (MSK2, MSH3, MSH6) recognise and bind to mismatches and loops caused by the insertion/deletion of up to 4 bases to form the hMutα or hMutβ heterodimer complex. This occurs as hMutLα stabilises the bind and distinguishes the newly formed, mutated, DNA by scanning DNA for SSB or 'nicks'. Nicks are present transiently in newly synthesised lagging strand DNA, before DNA ligase seals them, so nicks are the eukaryotic method for distinguishing new DNA from template DNA. The next stages are incompletely understood in eukaryotes, but overall, DNA is then unwound by a helicase and excised by exonuclease I (Exo I), this is followed by resynthesis by polymeraseδ and ligation by DNA ligase I, with the aid of the DNA sliding clamp, proliferating cell nuclear antigen (PCNA).

Induction of cell apoptosis using MMR machinery is hypothesised to happen by one of two possible mechanisms (futile repair mechanism or the direct signalling model), which both result in the recruitment of AMT/ATR by hMutSα and hMutLα.

Role of mismatch repair in high grade serous epithelial ovarian cancer

Microsatellite instability occurs when there are variable lengths of unrepaired nucleotide repeats, MSI is used as a marker for defective MMR in studies to determine the frequency and contribution of defective MMR to cancer development.

Defective MMR is understood to be a driver in Lynch Syndrome, an autosomal dominant syndrome where individuals are predisposed to colorectal, endometrial and ovarian cancers. The study of Lynch Syndrome, like other hereditary cancer syndromes, has allowed a better understanding of the role of MMR proteins in cancer (Table 2). Lynch Syndrome confers a 10–15% lifetime ovarian cancer risk, with ovarian cancer occurring at a younger age. In contrast to BRCA1 and 2 mutations, the Lynch Syndrome phenotype predisposes to low grade [74] or clear cell histology [75]. A large study of 2222 ovarian cancer cases found that defective MMR contributed to only 0.18% cases of high grade serous ovarian cancer [76].

MMR is defective in sporadic ovarian cancer also, where promotor methylation results in epigenetic silencing of key genes (Table 2). The main proteins defective in Lynch Syndrome are MHLH1 and MSH6.

Implications for therapy

In vitro studies have found an association between MMR deficiency and resistance to platinum agents and DNA methylating agents such as 6-thioguanine, due to an inactivation of MMR driven apoptosis in ovarian cancer cell lines [77, 78]. The extent to which defective MMR contributes to therapy resistance in vivo, however, is inconclusive [79] for high grade serous ovarian cancer, but is better defined in ovarian clear cell carcinoma where defective MMR plays a larger role in oncogenesis [80]. Nonetheless, reactivation of MMR by demethylation of epigenetically silenced MMR genes is an interesting area of study. In vitro and mice studies, 5-azacytidine and 2′-deoxy-5-azacytidine (DAC or decitabine) have been found to reactivate MMR by demethylating the mMLH1 promoter, resulting in the return of sensitivity to platinum therapies, temozolomide and epirubicin [81, 82]. However, phase II clinical trials using decitabine with carboplatin in ovarian

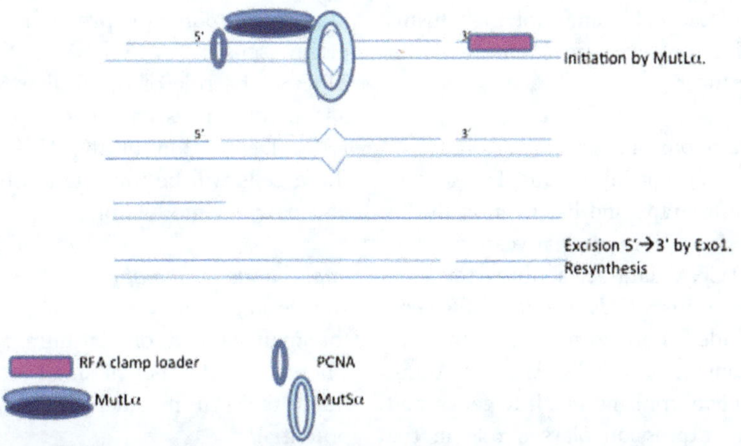

Fig. 4 Eukaryotic mismatch repair mechanism. DNA mismatches are recognised by the mismatch recognition factor MutSα, which then prompts binding and DNA stabilisation by the MLH1-PMS2 heterodimer (MutLα). The PCNA and RFA clamp loader are able to load on at a nearby 'nick'. MutSα activated exonuclease 1 (Exo1) excise the mismatch in a 5′ to 3′ direction and the excised fragment of DNA is removed by the DNA polymerase δ holoenzyme. DNA polymerase δ refills the DNA gap and it is ligated by DNA ligase I

Table 2 Defective MMR proteins in ovarian cancer

Gene/Protein	Role	Defect	Clinical Effect	Evidence of mutation in cases of HGS
MLH1	Forms MutLα with PMS2 [95] which has endonuclease activity.	Promoter methylation	Spontaneous tumours	0.1%
		Exon deletion	Lynch Syndrome	
MSH6	Forms hMutSβ with MSH2 to recognise and initiate repair [95]	Exon deletion	Lynch Syndrome	0.45%
MSH2	Forms hMutSβ			0.18%
PMS2	Forms MutLα	Loss		0.05%
MutLα and MutSβ	Recruit ATM/ATR	Loss	Resistance to DNA methylating agents [77]	

cancer were abandoned due to a lack of efficacy and the development of adverse reactions (DACROC study).

Nucleotide excision repair

Mechanism of nucleotide excision repair

Nucleotide excision repair (NER) is a highly conserved and versatile pathway used to remove 'bulky lesions' caused by UV light and carcinogens such as benzopyrene, which would otherwise distort the DNA double helix. Large protein complexes scan the DNA and identify distortions at the bulky lesion. Lesions that stall transcription use the 'transcription coupled NER pathway' using RNA Pol II. The 'global NER pathway' manages lesions elsewhere affecting the genome. The transcription factor, TF11H, has helicase activity and is recruited to unwind the DNA duplex. XPG and ERCC1-XPF then cleave the abnormal strand either side of the lesion and DNA polymeraseδ or ε and ligase 3(LIG III) repair the gap with PCNA and replication factors C [59].

Defective NER is implicated in various cancers, notably the syndrome xerodermapigmentosa which is characterised by UV sensitivity, where global NER is defective. Epigenetic alterations, gene polymorphisms and SNP's of global NER proteins are associated with lung, skin and bladder cancer.

Role of NER in high grade serous ovarian cancer

NER is responsible for repairing intrastrand DNA cross links caused by platinum therapy and has been found to determine platinum resistance in ovarian cancer cells in vitro [83, 84]. The TCGA data set analysis revealed that 8% of high-grade serous EOCs have an NER gene alternation which included homozygous deletions of NER genes and nonsynonymous or splice site mutations. The extent to which polymorphisms of NER genes and their subsequent protein expression plays a role in the platinum resistance of ovarian cancer is controversial, with some studies finding direct correlation between protein levels to platinum resistance and other studies finding no correlation, (see Table 3) [85, 86]. However, Ceccaldi et al.'s extensive TCGA study demonstrated that NER gene alterations in high grade serous EOCs were associated improved overall and progression-free survival compared to tumours that did not have NER alterations. Specifically, two NER mutations; ERCC6-Q524 and ERCC4-A583T were functionally associated with platinum sensitivity in vitro.

In the same study the survival of patients with tumours harbouring NER alterations was similar to patients with *BRCA1/2*-altered tumours suggesting that NER pathway alterations may contribute to EOC platinum sensitivity to a similar extend as that of the effect of *BRCA1/2* loss. Ceccaldi's data reported that NER pathway alterations, unlike *BRCA1/2* alterations, were not associated with sensitivity to PARP inhibitors. Importantly, their findings identified a subset of NER-deficient, HR-competent EOCs with distinct platinum and PARP-inhibitor profiles [87].

An interesting study by Wang et al. looked at the roles of both NER and HRR in platinum resistance. They found that the importance of NER's contribution to platinum resistance varies between in vitro cell lines. Additionally, overall there was no correlation between NER protein component expression and NER activity, nor cisplatin sensitivity [88]. Yet, they did highlight that ERCC1, the role of which is extensively studied in NER and platinum resistance, also plays an influential role in HRR. Delineation of the NER and HRR pathways in these cells will be important when developing DNA repair pathway modulators.

Implications for therapy

Development of NER inhibitors is a potential target for the management of platinum resistant ovarian cancer. There are a number of small molecular inhibitors, identified through in silico screens, with variable clinical potential.

One promising agent is Trabectedin, which is thought to disrupt the NER pathway by binding NER machinery and DNA at the damaged DNA site, sequestering NER proteins and resulting in cytotoxic complexes [83, 89].

Table 3 NER components and response to platinum therapy in ovarian cancer

Protein	Role	Relevant to Ovarian Cancer
ERCC1	Forms heterodimer with ERCC4 to form XPF, which binds DNA with nuclease activity	SNP C8092A, which affects mRNA stability associated with reduced tumour size and more differentiation [96].
		In vitro cell line experiments found high ERCC1 expression correlated to platinum resistance due to upregulated NER [97]
XPA	Binds and stabilises damaged DNA	Paradoxically XPA expression associated with better overall survival in women with metastatic ovarian cancer and chemotherapy response [98]
XPB	A transcription factor that can also aid unwinding of DNA at sites of damage	Five fold higher mRNA expression in platinum resistant ovarian cancer cell lines than non resistant cells [89].
XPG	Endonuclease that catalyses 3′ incision	No statistically significant effect of XPG polymorphisms [94]
CSB	ATP dependent helicase that enables DNA repair	Six times higher mRNA expression in platinum resistant ovarian cancer cells [98]

The INOVATYON study is a phase III trial investigating Trabectedin and pegylated liposomal doxorubicin (PLD) vs carboplatin and PLD in women with platinum resistant ovarian cancer(clinicaltrials.gov identifier NCT01379989).

The importance of developing a DDR stratification system

Targeting functional and dysfunctional DNA repair pathways in ovarian cancer, to overcome therapeutic resistance is a frontier for improving the prognosis of ovarian cancer. However multiple challenges exist. Firstly, clinicians require a way of identifying which DNA pathways are important in a particular tumour. Secondly, an understanding of the interactions and overlap between the pathways will be key to accurately targeting therapy. Thirdly, although there are numerous small molecular DNA repair pathway modulators which appear promising at a pre-clinical stage these need to be rapidly translated through clinical development.

The first two issues may be overcome through the development and use of functional assays to either identify key DNA repair pathways or identify key DNA repair proteins ('key drivers'), which may interact across numerous pathways.

Importantly however, determining the DDR status of any given HGSOC cancer is not trivial. Despite multiple attempts to an assay for HR an ideal test remains elusive. While BRCA-mutated cancers display a distinctive gene expression signature, this in itself is not necessarily predictive. In a recent study, 11 out of 12 tumours with dominant BRCA signatures were refractory to primary treatment, consistent with intact HR [84]. Furthermore, attempts to use indirect methods such as genomic scarring have been equally ineffective within the context of clinical trials [21].

Studies to identify HR proficiency using the identification of Rad51 focus formation in primary cultures, gathered from ascitic fluid in women with ovarian cancer have shown a promising way of identifying women with HR deficiency who are susceptible to PARP inhibition [85]. Similar functional assays have been developed for the assessment of NHEJ and NER status [86]. Development of these assays further, for clinical use, may prove useful in selecting women for targeted therapy via identification of their DNA repair status.

If we know that a drug targets a specific protein in a specific DNA repair pathway, then assessing function of that protein represents an important biomarker. This can be carried out by assessing the DNA, RNA or protein directly. Immunohistochemistry of tissue samples can be used to screen for key proteins and stratify patients into groups likely to respond to the drug. Early work using immunohistochemistry and RT-PCR to identify DNA-PK/mRNA in solid tissue as a predictor for NHEJ and correlation with sensitivity to PARPi and cisplatin sensitivity is one such promising example of this [90].

Conclusions

With the increasing realisation that ovarian cancer is not one disease, the increased use of molecular diagnostics, and the development of new targeted agents the ability to deliver personalised medicine for patients with ovarian cancer is perhaps finally on the horizon.

An understanding of the DNA damage repair pathways and how they are abrogated will allow the development of personalised treatment algorithms but as we have outlined here this is likely to be complex given the high degree of interaction, overlap and perhaps redundancy that is shown between the various pathways.

Authors' contributions

MEG and RJE devised the review and carried out the literature search. ZF and AM provided comments and review. All authors approved the final manuscript.

Competing interests

The authors declare that they have no competing interests.

Author details
[1]Division of Cancer Sciences, Faculty of Biology, Medicine and Health, University of Manchester, St Mary's Hospital, Manchester, UK. [2]Department of Obstetrics and Gynaecology, Manchester Academic Health Science Centre, St Mary's Hospital, Central Manchester NHS Foundation Trust, Manchester Academic Health Science Centre, Level 5, Research, Oxford Road, Manchester, UK. [3]Northern Institute for Cancer Research, Newcastle University, Framlington Place, Newcastle upon Tyne NE2 4AD, UK.

References

1. Mukhopadhyay A, et al. Clinicopathological features of homologous recombination deficient epithelial ovarian cancers: sensitivity to PARP inhibitors, platinum and survival. Cancer Res. 2012;72(22):5675–82.
2. Ledermann J, et al. Olaparib maintenance therapy in patients with platinum-sensitive relapsed serous ovarian cancer: a preplanned retrospective analysis of outcomes by BRCA status in a randomised phase 2 trial. Lancet Oncol. 2014;15(8):852–61.
3. Kaelin WG Jr. The concept of synthetic lethality in the context of anticancer therapy. Nat Rev Cancer. 2005;5(9):689–98.
4. Kennedy R, AD D'A. DNA Repair Pathways in Clinical Practice: Lessons From Pediatric Cancer Susceptibility Syndromes. J Clin Oncol. 2006;24(23):3799–808.
5. Zhong Q, Chen CF, Li S, et al. Association of BRCA1 with the hRad50-hMre11-p95 complex and the DNA damage response. Science. 1999;285:747–50.
6. Khanna KK, Jackson SP. DNA double-strand breaks: signaling, repair and the cancer connection. Nat Genet. 2001;27:247–54.
7. TCGA. Integrated genomic analyses of ovarian carcinoma. Nature. 2011; 474(7353):609–15.
8. King MC, Marks JH, Mandell JB. Breast and ovarian Cancer risks due to inherited mutations in BRCA1 and BRCA2. Science. 2003;302(5645):643–6.
9. Hilton J, Geisler JP, Rathe J, Hattermann-Zogg M, DeYoung B, Buller R, Inactivation of BRCA1 and BRCA2 in ovarian Cancer. J Natl Cancer Inst. 2002; 94(18):1396–406.
10. Catteau A, Harris WH, Xu CF, Solomon E. Methylation of the BRCA1 promoter region in sporadic breast and ovarian cancer: correlation with disease characteristics. Oncogene. 1999;18(11):1957–65.
11. Baldwin RL, Nemeth E, Tran H, Shvartsman H, Cass I, Nardod S, Karlan BY. BRCA1 promoter region hypermethylation in ovarian carcinoma: a population-based study. Cancer Res. 2000;60(19):5329–33.
12. Petrucelli N, Daly MB, Feldman GL. Hereditary breast and ovarian cancer due to mutations in BRCA1 and BRCA2. Genet Med. 2010;12(5):245–59.
13. Risch HA, McLaughlin JR, Cole D, Rosen B, et al. Prevalence and penetrance of Germline BRCA1 and BRCA2 mutations in a population series of 649 women with ovarian Cancer. Am J Human Genet. 2001;68(3):700–10.
14. Boyd J, Sonoda Y, Federici MG. Clinicopathologic features of BRCA-linked and sporadic Ovarioan Cancer. JAMA. 2000;283:2260–5.
15. Cass I, Baldwin RL, Varkey T. Improved Survival in Women with BRCA-Associated Ovarian Carcinoma. Cancer. 2003;97(9):2187–95.
16. Choudhury A, Zhao H, Jalali F, Al Rashid S, Ran J, Supiot S, Kiltie AE, Bristow RG. Targeting homologous recombination using imatinib results in enhanced tumor cell chemosensitivity and radiosensitivity. Mol Can Ther. 2009;8(1):203–13.
17. Bryant HE, et al. Specific killing of BRCA2-deficient tumours with inhibitors of poly(ADP-ribose) polymerase. Nature. 2005;434(7035):913–7.
18. Farmer H, et al. Targeting the DNA repair defect in BRCA mutant cells as a therapeutic strategy. Nature. 2005;434(7035):917–21.
19. Fong PC, Yap TA, Boss DS, et al. Poly(ADP) - Ribose Polymerase Inhibition: Frequent Durable Responses in BRCA Ovarian Cancer Correlating with Platinum-Free Interval. J Clin Oncol. 2010;28(15):2512–9.
20. Ledermann J, Harter P, Gourley C, et al. Olaparib maintenance therapy in platinum-sensitive relapsed ovarian Cancer. N Engl J Med. 2012;366:1382–92.
21. Mirza MR, et al. Niraparib maintenance therapy in platinum-sensitive, recurrent ovarian cancer. N Engl J Med. 2016;375:2154–64.
22. Wang H, Wang H, Powell SN, Iliakis G, Wang Y. ATR affecting cell radiosensitivity is dependent on homologous recombination repair but independent of nonhomologous end joining. Cancer Res. 2004;64(19):7139–43.
23. Peasland A, Wang LZ, Rowling E, Kyle S, Chen T, et al. Identification and evaluation of a potent novel ATR inhibitor, NU6027, in breast and ovarian cancer cell line. Br J Cancer. 2011;105:372–81.
24. Johnson N, Li YC, Walton ZE, et al. Compromised CDK1 acticity sensitizes BRCA profecient cancers to PARP inhibition. Nat Med. 2011;17:875–82.
25. Lieber MR, Ma Y, Pannicke U, Schwarz K. Mechanism and regulation of human non-homologous DNA end-joining. Nat Rev Mol Cell Biol. 2003;4: 712–20.
26. Beucher A, Birraux J, Tchouandong L, Barton O, et al. ATM and Artemis promote homologous recombination of radiation-induced DNA double-strand breaks in G2. EMBO J. 2009;28:3413–27.
27. Burma S, Chen BP, Chen DJ. Role of non-homologous end joining (NHEJ) in maintaining genomic integrity. DNA Repair. 2006;5(9–10):1042–8.
28. Valerie K, Povirk LF. Regulation and mechanisms of mammalian double-strand break repair. Oncogene. 2003;22:5792–812.
29. McCormick A, S.N., Curtin NJ, Edmondson RJ, (n.d.) Non Homologous End Joining pathways defects in human cancers.
30. Betermier M, Bertrand P, Lopez BS. Is non-homologous end-joining really an inherently error-prone process? PLoS Genet. 2014;10(1):e1004086.
31. West RB, Yaneva M, Lieber MR. Productive and Nonproductive complexes of Ku and DNA-dependent protein kinase at DNA termini. Mol Cell Biol. 1998; 18:5908–20.
32. Ma Y, Pannicke U, Schwarz K, Leiber MR. Hairpin Opening and Overhang processing by an Artemis/DNA-dependent protein kinase complex in nonhomologous end joining and V(D)J recombination. Cell. 2002;108:781–94.
33. Assis J, Pereira D, Medeiros R. Ovarian Cancer and DNA repair: DNA ligase IV as a potential key. World J Clin Oncol. 2013;4:14–24.
34. Ahnesorg P, Smith P, Jackson SP. XLF Interacts with the XRCC4-DNA Ligase IV Complex to Promote DNA Nonhomologous End-Joining. Cell. 2005; 124(2):287–99.
35. Dueva R, Iliakis G. Alternative pathways of non-homologous end joining (NHEJ) in genomic instability and cancer. Transl Cancer Res. 2013;2(3):163–77.
36. Kent T, Chandramouly G, McDevitt SM, et al. Mechanism of microhomology-mediated end-joining promoted by human DNA polymerase Θ. Nat Struct Mol Biol. 2015;22(3):230–9.
37. Wang M, Wu W, Wu W, Rosidi B, Zhang L, Wang H, Iliakis G. PARP-1 and Ku compete for repair of DNA double strand breaks by distinct NHEJ pathways. Nucleic Acids Res. 2006;34(21):6170–82.
38. Audebert M, Salles B, Calsou P. Involvement of poly(ADP-ribose) polymerase 1 and XRCC1/DNA ligase III in an alternative route for DNA double-strand breaks rejoining. J Biol Chem. 2004;279(53):55117–26.
39. Mansour WY, Rhein T, Dahm-Daphi J. The alternative end-joining pathway for repair of DNA double-strand breaks requires PARP1 but is not dependent upon microhomologies. Nucleic Acids Res. 2010;38(18):6065–77.
40. McCormick, A., et al., Ovarian Cancers Harbour Defects in Non-Homologous End Joining Resulting in Resistance to Rucaparib. Clin Canc res, 2016. Published OnlineFirst October 4, 2016.
41. Abdel-Fatah T, Arora A, Moseley P, Coveney C, Perry C, Johnson K, Kent C, Ball G, Chan S, Madhusudan S. AMT, ART and DNA-PKcs expressions correlate to adverse clinical outcomes in epithelial ovarian cancers. BBA Clinical. 2014;2:10–7.
42. Couto CA, Wang HY, Green JC, et al. PARP regulates nonhomologous end joining through retention of Ku at double strand breaks. J Cell Biol. 2011; 194(3):367–75.
43. Hochegger H, Dejsuphong D, et al. PARP 1 protects homolgous recombination from interference by Ku and Ligase IV in vertebrate cells. EMBO J. 2006;**25**(6):1305–14.
44. Patel AG, Sarkaria JN, Kaufmann SH. Nonhomologous end joining drives poly (ADP-ribose) polymerase (PARP) inhibitor lethality in homologous recombination-deficient cells. Proc Natl Acad Sci U S A. 2011;108(8):3406–11.
45. Schildkraut JM, Iversen ES, Wilson MA, Clyde MA, et al. Association between DNA damage response and repair genes and risk of invasive serous ovarian Cancer. PLoS One. 2010;5(4):e10061.
46. Pearce CL, Near AM, Van Den Berg DJ, et al. Validating genetic risk associations for ovarian cancer through the international ovarian Cancer association consortium. Br J Cancer. 2009;100:412–20.
47. Ceccaldi R, Liu JC, Amunugama R et al, Homologous recombination deficient tumours are dependent on PolΘ mediated repair. Nature. 2015;518:258–62.
48. Miao J, Zhang X, Tang QL, Wang XY, Kai L. Prediction value of XRCC1 gene polymorphisms on the survival of ovarian cancer treated by adjuvant chemotherapy. Asian Pac J Cancer Prev. 2012;13:5007–10.
49. Adel-Fatah T, Sultana R, Abbotts R, Hawkes C, Seedhouse C, Chan S, Madhasudan S. Clinicopathological and functional significance of XRCC1 expression in ovarian cancer. Int J Cancer. 2012;132:2778–86.

50. Cooke SL, Ng CK, Melnyk N, Garcia MJ, Hardcastle T, Temple J, Langdon S, Huntsman D, Brenton JD. Genomic analysis of genetic heterogeneity and evolution in high-grade serous ovarian carcinoma. Oncogene. 2010;29(35): 4905–13.
51. Stronach EA, Chen M, Maginn EN, Agarwal R, Mills GB, Wasan H, Gabra H. DNA-PK mediates AKT activation and apoptosis inhibition in clinically acquired platinum resistance. Neoplasia. 2011;13(11):1069–80.
52. Ohtaa T, Ohmichi M, et al. Gefitinib (ZD1839) increases the efficacy of cisplatin in ovarian cancer cells. Cancer Biol Ther. 2012;13(6):408–16.
53. Diggle CP, Bentley J, et al. Inhibition of double strand break non-homologous end-joining by cisplatin adducts in human cell extracts. Nucleic Acids Res. 2005;33(8):2531–9.
54. Wipf P, Halter RJ. Chemistry and Biology of Wortmannin. Org Biomol Chem. 2005;3:2053–61.
55. Leahy JJ, Golding BT, Griffin RJ, et al. Identification of a highly potent and selective DNA-dependent protein kinase (DNA-PK) inhibitor (NU 7441) by screening of chromosome libraries. Bioorg Med Chem Lett. 2004;14:6083–7.
56. Zhao Y, Thomas HD, Batey MA, et al. Preclinical evaluation of a potent novel DNA-dependent protein kinase inhibitor NU7441. Cancer Res. 2006;66:5354–62.
57. Sultana R, Abdel-Fatah T, Abbotts R, Hawkes C, Albarakati N, Seedhouse C, Ball G, Chan S, Rakha EA, Ellis IO, Madhusudan S. Targeting XRCC1 Deficiency in Breats Cancer for Personalised Therapy. Cancer Res. 2012;73(5):1621–34.
58. Kim YJ, Wilson DM. Overview of Base Excision Repair Biochemistry. Curr Mol Pharmacol. 2012;5(1):3–13.
59. Curtin NJ. DNA repair dysregulation from cancer driver to therapeutic target. Nat Rev Cancer. 2012;12:801–17.
60. Osorio A, Milne RL, et al. DNA glycosylases involved in base excision repair may be associated with cancer risk in BRCA1 and BRCA2 mutation carriers. PLoS Genet. 2014;10(4):e1004256.
61. Pieretti M, Khattar NH, Smith SA. Common polymorphisms and somatic mutations in human base excision repair genes in ovarian and endometrial cancers. Mut Res Gen. 2001;432:53–9.
62. Albertella MR, Lau A, O'Connor MJ. The overexpression of specialized DNA polymerases in cancer. DNA Repair. 2005;4(5):583–93.
63. Al-Attar A, Gossage L, Fareed KR, et al. Human apurinic/apyrimidinic endonuclease (APE1) is a prognostic factor in ovarian, gastro-oesophageal and pancreatico-biliary cancers. Br J Cancer. 2010;102:704–9.
64. Huehls AM, Wagner JM, Huntoon CJ, Karnitz LM. Identification of DNA repair pathways that affect the survival of ovarian Cancer cells treated with a poly(ADP-ribose) polymerase inhibitor in a novel drug combination. Mol Pharmacol. 2012;82:767–76.
65. Rouleau M, Patel A, Hendzel MJ, Kaufmann SH, Poirier GG. PARP inhibition: PARP1 and beyond. Nat Rev Cancer. 2010;10(4):293–301.
66. MJ OC. Targeting the DNA damage response in Cancer. Mol Cell. 2015;60:547–60.
67. Boudsocq F, Benaim P, et al. Modulation of Cellular Response to Cisplatin by a Novel Inhibitor of DNA Polymerase. Mol Pharmacol. 2005;67(5):1485–97.
68. Gao Z, Maloney DJ, Dedkova LM, Hecht SM. Inhibitors of DNA polymerase β: activity and mechanism. Bioorg Med Chem. 2008;16:4331–40.
69. Kumamoto-Yonezawa Y, et al. Enhancement of human cancer cell radiosensitivity by conjugated eicosapentaenoic acid - a mammalian DNA polymerase inhibitor. Int J Oncol. 2010;36:577–84.
70. Zhang Y, Wang J, Xiang D, Wang D, Xin X. Alterations in the expression of the apurinic/apyrimidinic endonuclease-1/redox factor-1 (APE1/Ref-1) in human ovarian cancer and indentification of the therapeutic potential of APE1/Ref-1 inhibitor. Int J Oncol. 2009;35:1069–79.
71. Taverna P, Liu L, Hwang HS, et al. Methoxyamine potentiates DNA single strand breaks and double strand breaks induces by temozolomide in colon cancer cells. Mutat Res. 2001;485(4):269–81.
72. Fishel ML, He Y, Smith ML, Kelley MR. Manipulation of base excision repair to sensitize ovarian cancer cells to alkylating agent temozolomide. Clin Cancer Res. 2007;13(1):260–7.
73. G-M L. Mechanisms and functions of DNA mismatch repair. Cell Res. 2008; 18:85–98.
74. Watson P, Bützow R, Lynch HT, et al. The clinical features of ovarian cancer in hereditary nonpolyposis colorectal cancer. Gynaecol Oncol. 2001;82:223–8.
75. Jensen KC, Mariappan MR, Putcha GV, Husain A, Chun N, Ford JM, et al. Microsatellite instability and mismatch repair protein defects in ovarian epithelial neoplams in patients 50 years of age and younger. Am J Surg Pathol. 2008;32(7):1029–37.
76. Song H, Cicek MS, Dicks E, et al. The contibution of deleterious germline mutations in BRCA1, BRCA2 and the mismatch repair genes to ovarian cancer in the population. Hum Mol Genet. 2014;23(17):4703–9.
77. P, K. Mechanisms of tolerance to DNA damaging therapeutic drugs. Carcinogenesis. 2001;22(12):1931–7.
78. Martin LP, Hamilton TC, Schilder RJ. Platinum Resistance: The Role of DNA Repair Pathways. Clin Cancer Res. 2008;14(5):1291–5.
79. Helleman J, van Staveren IL et al. Mismatch repair and treatment resistance in ovarian cancer. BMC Cancer. 2006;6(201):201.
80. Tan DSP, Miller RE, Kaye SB. New perspectives on olecula targeted therapy in ovarian clear cell carcinoma. Br J Cancer. 2013;108:1553–9.
81. Branch P, Masson M, Aquilina G, et al. Spontaneous development of drug resistance: mismatch repair defects in resistance to cisplatin in human tumor cells. Oncogene. 2000;19:3138–45.
82. Plumb JA, Strathdee G, Sludden J, Kaye SB, Brown R. Reversal of drug resistance in human tumor xenografts by 2'-deoxy-5-azacytidine-induced demethylation of the hMLH1 gene promoter. Cancer Res. 2000;60:6039–44.
83. Herrero AB, Martín-Castellanos C, Marco E, et al. Cross-Talk between Nucleotide Excision and Homologous Recombination DNA Repair Pathways in the Mechanism of Action of Antitumor Trabectedin. Cancer Res. 2006;66(16):8155–62.
84. Patch AM, et al. Whole-genome characterization of chemoresistant ovarian cancer. Nature. 2015;521(7553):489–94.
85. Mukhopadhyay A, Elattar A, Cerbinskaite A, Wilkinson S, Drew Y, Kyle S, Los G, Hostomsky Z, Edmondson R, Curtin N. Development of a Functional Assay for Homolgous Recombination Status in Primary Culture of Epithelial Ovarian Tumor and Correlation with Sensitivity to Poly(ADP-Ribose) Polymerase Inhibitors. Clinical Cancer Research. 2010;16(8):2344–51.
86. Woodhouse L, Mcormick A, O'Donnell R, Kauffmann A, Edmondson R. Development of a functional assay to determine the nucleotide excision repair status of epithelial ovarian cancer. Liverpool: NCRI Cancer Conference; 2014.
87. Ceccaldi R, et al. A unique subset of epithelial ovarian cancers with platinum sensitivity and PARP inhibitor resistance. Cancer Res. 2015;75(4):628–34.
88. Wang Q-E, Milum K, Han C, Huang Y-W et al Differential contributory roles of nucleotide excision and homologous recombination repair for enhancing cisplatin sensitivity in human ovarian cancer cells Mol Cancer. 2011;10(24):24.
89. Buterin T, Hess MT, Gunz D, et al. Trapping of DNA Nucleotide Excision Repair Factors by Nonrepairable Carcinogen Adducts. Cancer Res. 2002; 62(15):4229–35.
90. O'Sullivan R, D P, Curtin N, Kaufmann A, McCormick A, Edmondson RJ. DNA-PK as a biomarker of non-homologous end joining in ovarian cancer. Liverpool: NCRI Cancer Conference; 2014.
91. Tomkinson AE, Vijayakumar S, Pascal JM, Ellenberger T. DNA ligases: structure, reaction mechanism, and function. Chem Rev. 2006;106:687–99.
92. Heikkinen K, Karppinen SM, Soini Y, Makinen M, Wingvist R, Mutation screening of Mre11 complex genes: indication of RAD50 involvement in breast and ovarian cancer susceptibility. J Med Genet. 2003;40(12):e131.
93. Jensen RB, Carreira A, Kowalczykowski SC. Purified human BRCA1 stimulates RAD51-mediated recombination. Nature. 2010;467(7316):678–83.
94. Caiola E, Porcu L, Fruscio R, et al. DNA-damage response gene polymorphisms and therapeutic outcomes in ovarian cancer. Pharmacogenomics J. 2013;13:159–72.
95. Kunkel TA, Erie DA. DNA mismatch repair. Annu Rev Biochem. 2005;74:681–710.
96. Ferry KV, Hamilton TC, Johnson SW. Increased nucleotide excision repair in Cisplatin-resistant ovarian Cancer cells. Biochem Pharmacol. 2000;60:1305–13.
97. Stevens EV, Raffeld M, Espina V, et al. Expression of xeroderma pigmentosum A protein predicts improved outcome in metastatic ovarian carcinoma. Cancer. 2005;103(11):2313–9.
98. Dabholkar M, Thornton K, Vionnet J, Bostick-Bruton F, et al. Increased mRNA levels of Xeroderma Pigmentosum complementation group B (XPB) and Cockayne's syndrome complementation group B (CSB) without increased mRNA levels of multidrug-resistance gene (MDR1) or Methallothionein-II (MT-II) in platinum resistant human ovarina cancer tissues. Biochem Pharmacol. 2000;60:1611–9.

9

Use of a Small Animal Radiation Research Platform (SARRP) facilitates analysis of systemic versus targeted radiation effects in the mouse ovary

Allison R. Grover[1], Bruce F. Kimler[2] and Francesca E. Duncan[1,3*]

Abstract

Background: Radiation exposure is known to cause accelerated aging and damage to the ovary, but the contribution of indirect versus direct effects is not well understood. We used the Small Animal Radiation Research Platform (SARRP) (Xstrahl) to deliver radiation to precise fields equivalent to clinical practice, allowing us to investigate systemic versus targeted damage in a structure as small as the mouse ovary. The X-ray dose was kept constant at 1 Gy, but the field varied. Mice either received total body irradiation (TBI), radiation targeted to both ovaries (T2), or radiation targeted to one ovary (left) while the contralateral ovary (right) was spared (T1). Sham mice, handled similarly to the other cohorts but not exposed to radiation, served as controls. Two weeks post-exposure, ovaries were harvested and analyzed histologically to identify and count follicles within each ovary.

Results: Radiation significantly reduced primordial follicles in the TBI and T2 cohorts compared to the Sham cohort. There were no significant differences between these two irradiated groups. These findings suggest that at 1 Gy, the extent of damage to the ovary caused by radiation is similar despite the different delivery methods. When investigating the T1 cohort, targeted ovaries showed a significant decrease in primordial and growing follicles compared to non-targeted contralateral ovaries.

Conclusions: These findings demonstrate that the SARRP is an effective strategy for delivering precise ionizing radiation to small organs such as mouse ovaries. Such tools will facilitate identifying the relative risks to ovarian function associated with different radiation fields as well as screening the efficacy of emerging fertoprotective agents.

Keywords: Ovary, Follicle, Radiation, Total body irradiation, Fertility preservation, Iatrogenic

Background

Within the United States, more than 120,000 women under the age of 45 are diagnosed with cancer every year [1]. The three-pronged approach of surgical resection, chemotherapy, and radiation therapy has been a mainstay of cancer treatment [2, 3]. Although these approaches are lifesaving, they can have unintended off target health consequences. For example, exposure to radiation can accelerate reproductive aging and entry into menopause [4, 5]. This accelerated reproductive aging in turn can lead to subfertility, infertility, or increased complications during pregnancies that are achieved [6, 7]. As cancer treatments improve, survivorship is projected to increase to 20.3 million people in the United States by 2026, representing a 4 million increase in survivors in the span of a decade [2, 3, 8]. Thus, off target effects of treatment that may have detrimental consequences on these survivors' overall health and quality of life must be addressed.

Radiation therapy is a delicate balance between destruction of malignant cells and minimizing damage to healthy tissue, but it can unintentionally damage key organs of the reproductive system. For example,

* Correspondence: f-duncan@northwestern.edu
[1]Center for Reproductive Science, Northwestern University, Chicago, IL 60611, USA
[3]Department of Obstetrics and Gynecology, Feinberg School of Medicine, Northwestern University, 303 E. Superior Street, Lurie 7-117, Chicago, IL 60611, USA
Full list of author information is available at the end of the article

in treatment of acute myeloid leukemia and conditioning therapy for bone marrow transplantation in Hodgkins and non-Hodgkins lymphoma, total body irradiation exposes the whole body to radiation, including the hypothalamus-pituitary-gonad axis (HPG axis) [2, 3, 9]. When the HPG axis is targeted, hormone secretion such as gonadotropin pulses can be perturbed leading to amenorrhea, hypogonadism, precocious puberty, and other endocrine disruptions [10–13]. The uterus may be exposed to radiation in cases where there is a uterine tumor or a solid abdominal tumor, and in both scenarios, the uterus would be in the radiation field [5, 14]. Radiation exposure can result in uterine vascular insufficiency and decreased uterine volume [9, 11, 14]. When the ovary is exposed to radiation through total body or abdominal radiation, oocytes are lost through cell death pathways; granulosa cell damage results in impaired gonadal hormone production; and the ovarian vasculature and stroma are compromised. These changes may ultimately lead to premature ovarian failure, subfertility, or infertility [5, 6, 9, 11, 12, 14].

From a mechanistic perspective, radiation primarily affects cells via direct induction of DNA damage, including base damage, base losses, single-strand breaks, double-strand breaks, and DNA-protein crosslinks [15, 16]. Such damage leads to activation of DNA damage repair pathways that if not repaired properly can result in cell death, cell transformation, or heritable genetic mutations [15, 17]. Irradiated cells may also initiate damage signals that affect nearby non-irradiated cells, and this phenomenon is referred to as the radiation-induced bystander effect (RIBE) [18, 19]. The RIBE then induces several cellular responses in the non-irradiated cells including oxidative DNA damage and inflammatory networks [20, 21]. Importantly, the RIBE appears to dominate at low dose radiation exposures (< 1 Gy) and thus may be a significant contributor to ovarian damage [22, 23]. Finally, there are abscopal effects where radiation induces damage to non-irradiated tissues and organs that are remote from the site of exposure [15]. For example, radiation restricted to the hypothalamus or pituitary may result in effects observable in the ovaries [9].

Of all reproductive organs, the ovary – including both its somatic and germ cell compartments – is particularly susceptible to radiation damage. In fact, the radiation dose required for 50% loss of function (LD_{50} value) in the human oocyte is estimated at < 2 Gy, but oocyte radiosensitivity is also highly dependent on species, developmental stage, and animal age [6, 24, 25]. In some mouse strains, the LD_{50} value has been reported to be as low as 0.15 Gy, and in both mouse and rat, oocytes within primordial follicles appear to be much more radiosensitive relative to the larger follicle stages [6, 26]. The DNA damage checkpoints and cell death pathways that are elicited in response to radiation exposure have been extensively investigated in the oocyte [6, 27]. However, whether or not radiation damage in the ovary is due solely to direct and targeted effects or to systemic effects has been difficult to distinguish, especially in animal model systems such as the rodent, because of the technical limitations in the ability to administer precise radiation doses to small fields [28–30]. The mouse ovary represents a significant challenge for targeted irradiation methods because, compared to the human ovary, it is substantially smaller and has a different anatomy [31]. The mouse ovary is surrounded by a bursa, a layer of epithelial cells that isolates the ovary from the abdominal cavity, it is located caudal to the kidneys instead of in the pelvic cavity, and it is connected to a uterine horn via the oviduct [31–33].

Recently, innovative microirradiators that mimic the treatment conditions used in modern clinical radiation oncology facilities and veterinary practices have been developed for use in small animals [34, 35]. These platforms can achieve targeting and imaging accuracy to 0.1 mm resolution, thus enabling radiation-based preclinical and basic science studies [35, 36]. In this study, we used the Xstrahl Small Animal Radiation Research Platform (SARRP) to compare ovarian damage due to a single low dose of ionizing radiation in three cohorts of reproductively adult mice: one that received total body irradiation (TBI), one that received targeted radiation to both ovaries, and one that received targeted radiation to one ovary while sparing the contralateral ovary. We found that both low dose TBI and targeted radiation caused a similar significant reduction in follicle numbers and that off target effects were negligible. These findings provide proof-of-concept that the SARRP is an effective means of delivering precise radiation to organs as small as a mouse ovary and an innovative tool to explore and decipher mechanisms of targeted versus systemic radiation-induced damage to reproductive organs.

Results

Use of the SAARP to examine systemic versus targeted effects of ionizing radiation on ovarian tissue

We have previously demonstrated that a single dose of 1 Gy TBI is sufficient to cause a significant reduction in ovarian follicles 2 weeks post-exposure in adult female CD1 mice, whereas a lower dose of 0.1 Gy is not [37]. Consequently, we exposed mice to a single dose of 1 Gy radiation but varied the field (Fig. 1a-c). We used the SAARP to generate three experimental cohorts of mice: one that received TBI, one that received targeted

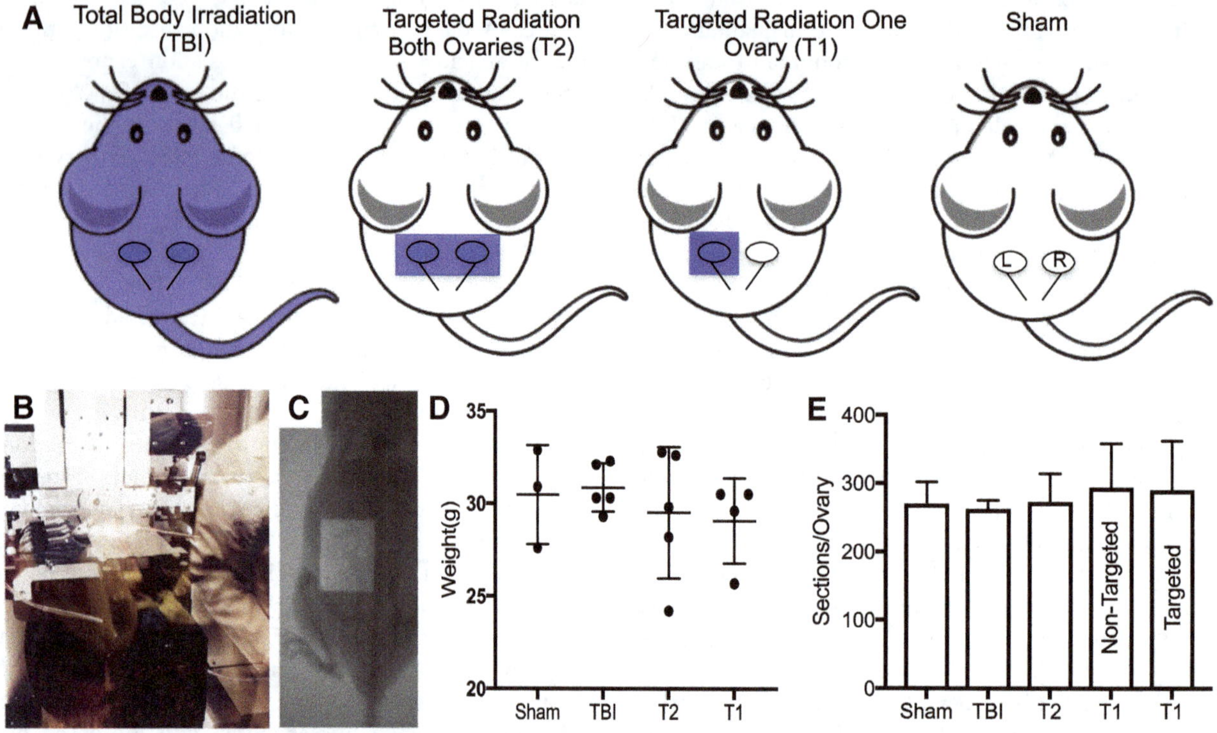

Fig. 1 Use of the SAARP to examine the effect of differences in radiation field on ovarian damage. a A schematic of the experimental paradigm. Adult female mice received a single X-ray dose of 1 Gy and ovaries were harvested 2 weeks post-exposure. The Total Body Irradiation (TBI) cohort received the dose to the entire organism ($n = 5$). The targeted radiation cohort to both ovaries (T2) received the radiation dose to a 20 mm × 10 mm field encompassing both ovaries ($n = 5$). The targeted radiation cohort to one ovary (T1) received the radiation to a 10 mm × 10 mm field focused on the left ovary ($n = 4$). The Sham cohort underwent the same procedures as the experimental cohorts but was not irradiated ($n = 3$). **b** A representative image of how a mouse was anesthetized for immobilization in the beam field of the SARRP to target the ovaries. **c** A representative image that highlights the specified area of the collimating X-ray beam that was used to target the field of a single ovary. **d** Mouse weights were monitored 2 weeks post-exposure prior to euthanasia to examine whether there were acute health effects due to radiation. A one-way ANOVA test was performed and no differences were observed in weight between the groups ($p = 0.73$). **e** The total number of 5 μm serial sections generated per ovary was averaged and used as a proxy for ovarian size. A one-way ANOVA test was performed and no differences were observed between the groups ($p = 0.68$)

ionizing radiation to both ovaries, and one that received targeted radiation to a single ovary while the contralateral ovary was spared (Fig. 1a). Comparison of ovaries from mice that received TBI to those that were exposed to a targeted radiation field containing both ovaries allowed us to investigate systemic damage relative to targeted damage. In addition, by comparing targeted ovaries to contralateral non-targeted ovaries within individual animals, we were able to assess off-target effects in a paired organ system. For all cohorts, ovaries were harvested 2 weeks post-exposure. Importantly, we did not observe significant differences in animal weight among the cohorts at the time of tissue harvest (Fig. 1d). This consistency in weight in addition to the absence of animal lethality, suggests that the exposures to 1 Gy did not cause acute toxicity at this time point. We also did not observe any difference in the total number of serial sections obtained per ovary, suggesting that radiation exposure did not cause dramatic changes in ovarian size (Fig. 1e).

Comparison of ovarian damage following total body irradiation versus targeted radiation to both ovaries

To examine the ovarian effects of systemic versus targeted radiation, we compared the ovaries from the animals that received TBI and targeted radiation to both ovaries (T2) to each other and to the Sham controls (Fig. 1). Ovarian histological sections were used to evaluate tissue appearance and to perform quantitative analysis of healthy follicles. Analysis of histological sections revealed that ovaries from all cohorts, irrespective of radiation exposure, had morphologically normal antral follicles and corpora lutea providing evidence of both follicle growth and estrous cyclicity (Fig. 2a-c). Whereas primordial and primary follicles were clearly

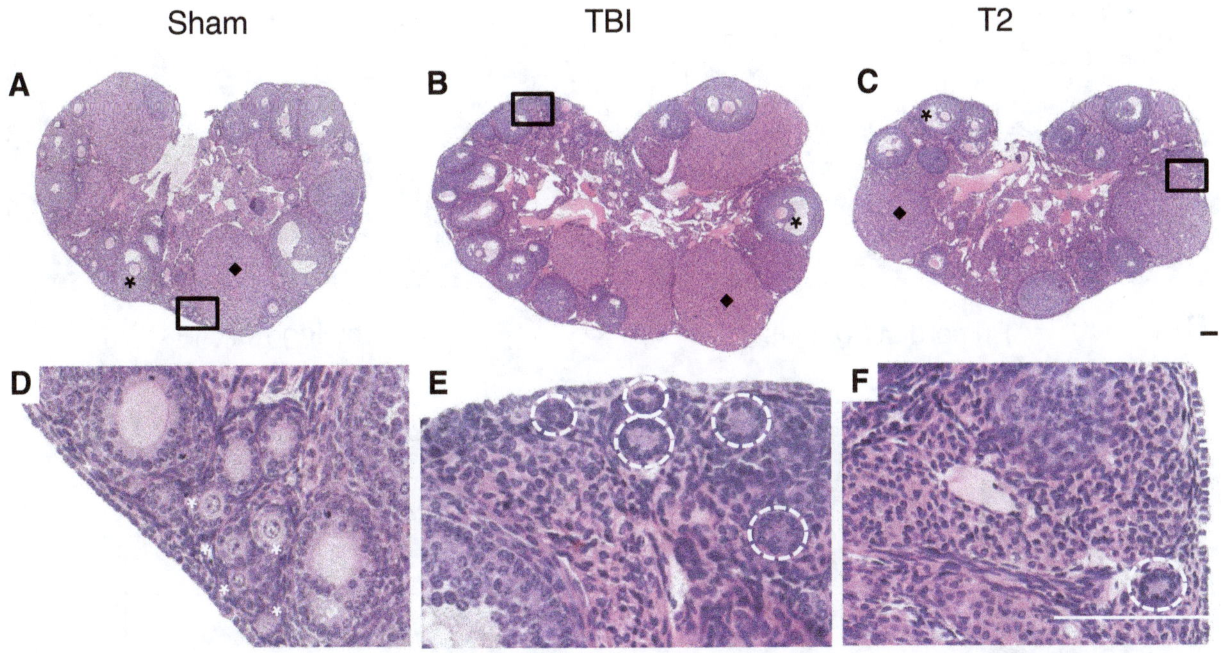

Fig. 2 TBI and targeted radiation to the ovary with X-rays at a dose of 1 Gy cause ovarian damage that is evident by histology. Representative images of whole histological sections of ovaries from the following cohorts are shown: (**a**) Sham, (**b**) TBI, and (**c**) targeted radiation to both ovaries (T2). Examples of healthy antral follicles are highlighted with black asterisks and corpora lutea are highlighted with black diamonds. Corresponding higher magnification images of the boxed regions are shown in (**d-f**) to visualize primordial and primary follicles at the ovarian cortex. White asterisks in (**d**) highlight specific primordial and primary follicles that are absent in (**e**) and (**f**). Remnants of primordial and primary follicles that lack oocytes are shown with dashed circles in (**e**) and (**f**) in the TBI and T2 cohorts. The scale bars are 125 μm

visible in ovarian sections from the Sham cohort, they were not visible in the irradiated cohorts (Fig. 2d-f). In fact, in ovarian sections from both the TBI and T2 cohorts, only remnants of small follicles were visible, and these were not included in the follicle counts (Fig. 2e and f). To quantify these differences between the experimental groups and the Sham control, we classified and counted healthy follicles according to previously established morphological criteria (Fig. 3a) [38]. When examining all follicle classes together, both TBI and T2 cohorts showed a significant decrease in total counts relative to the Sham cohort (343.5 ± 92.0 follicles, 1761.0 ± 2620.3 follicles, and 6689.2 ± 2289.6 follicles, respectively; Additional file 1). We were particularly interested in primordial follicles, since they dictate the ovarian reserve and reproductive lifespan of an individual. Thus, we examined the number of primordial follicles in each experimental cohort separately from growing follicles. Within the Sham cohort, there was an average of 17.8 ± 2.0 primordial follicles per section (Fig. 3b) and 9.9 ± 1.4 growing follicles per section (Fig. 3c). Exposure to radiation significantly reduced the amount of average primordial follicles to 0.1 ± 0.1 follicles per section in the TBI cohort and 3.6 ± 6.6 follicles per section in the T2 cohort (Fig. 3b). Exposure to radiation also reduced the number of growing follicles to an average of 1.3 ± 0.3 growing follicles per section in the TBI cohort and an average of 4.7 ± 7.5 follicles per section in the T2 cohort (Fig. 3c). However, this reduction was only significant when comparing the TBI to the Sham cohort (Fig. 3c). If we further examined growing follicles on a class-specific basis, we observed that there were significantly fewer primary and secondary follicles in both the TBI and T2 cohorts relative to the Sham controls, but there were no differences in the number of antral follicles across cohorts, suggesting that the largest follicles are not sensitive to radiation-induced damage (Additional file 2).

Because we kept the ovaries from each individual animal separate for processing, we were able to further analyze the data to see if there were any differences in follicle counts depending on the animal or the respective ovary (Fig. 4, Additional file 3). In the Sham cohort, both primordial and growing follicle counts were similar across mice (Fig. 4a and b). The follicle counts between left and right ovaries were similar in two of the three mice, but in one mouse, the right ovary had significantly more follicles per section than the left (18.6 ± 6.9 and 14.5 ± 9.4 primordial follicles per section, respectively, and 12.5 ± 5.0 and 9.6 ± 6.7 growing follicles per section, respectively). In the TBI cohort, follicle counts were similarly

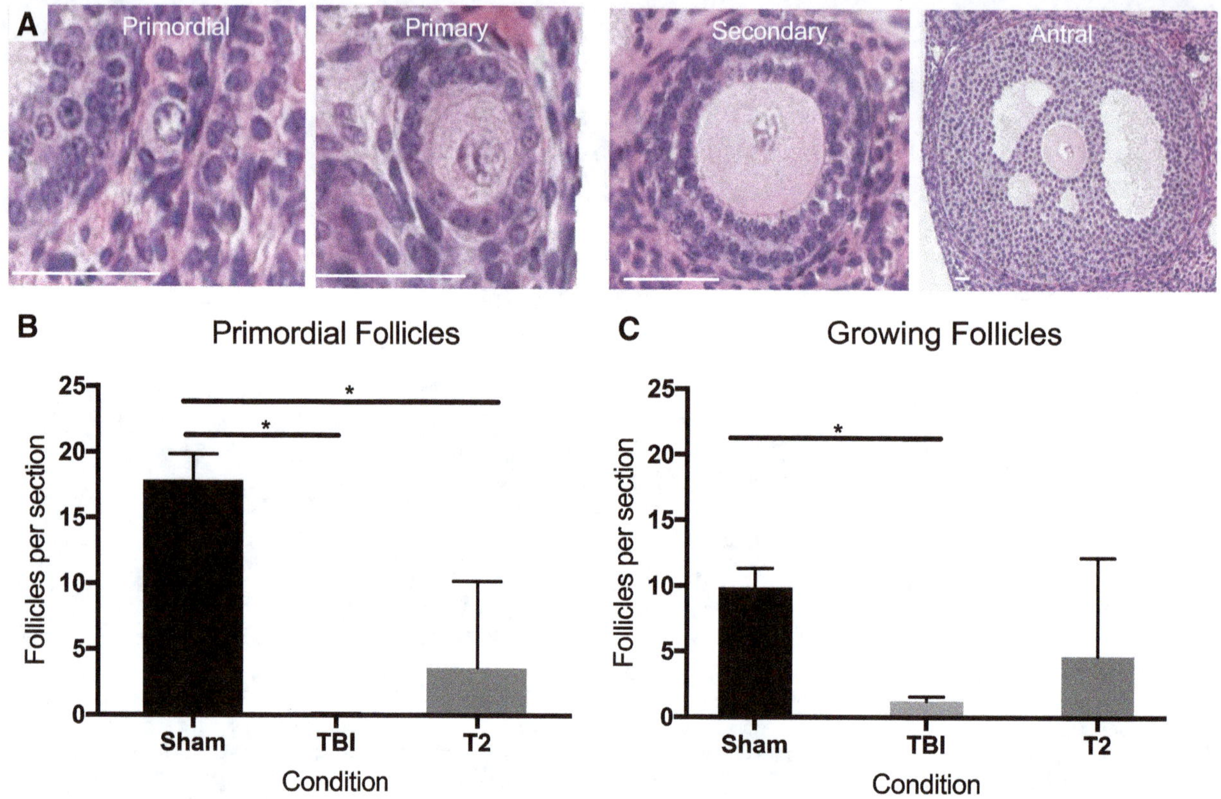

Fig. 3 TBI and targeted radiation to the ovary with X-rays at a dose of 1 Gy cause significant follicle loss. a Follicle classes were defined according to morphological criteria. Primordial follicles were identified as an oocyte surrounded by squamous granulosa cells. Primary follicles were defined as an oocyte surrounded by one layer of cuboidal granulosa cells. Secondary follicles were defined as an oocyte surrounded by two or more layers of cuboidal granulosa cells. Antral follicles were defined as an oocyte surrounded by multiple layers of cuboidal cells with an antral space filled with follicular fluid forming in the middle of the follicle. Growing follicles were considered to be follicles at the primary stage or beyond. The average number of (**b**) primordial follicles per section and (**c**) growing follicles per section were quantified in ovaries from each cohort (Sham, TBI, and T2). A one-way ANOVA was performed between cohorts, and statistical significance was defined as $*p < 0.05$. The scale bar is 50 μm

low across all mice, and no differences were seen between the left and right ovaries in both primordial and growing follicle counts (Fig. 4c and d). In the T2 cohort, three of the five mice exhibited a near loss of all primordial and growing follicles in response to radiation, but two mice still had follicles present (Fig. 4e and f). In fact, one of the animals (mouse C) had follicle counts that were similar to those in the Sham cohort (Fig. 4a and c). Thus, the observation that mice in the T2 cohort had a less pronounced reduction in follicle numbers compared to the TBI cohort was primarily due to the response of two animals rather than a global phenomenon across the cohort (Fig. 3b-c and Fig. 4c-f). Specifically, mouse C and E still had primordial follicles present (Fig. 4e). Also in mice from the T2 cohort, all the right and left ovaries had similar numbers of follicles except for one mouse in which the right ovary had more follicles than the left ($4.3 \pm 2.$ and 0.0 ± 0.3 primordial follicles per section, respectively; Fig. 4e and 3.5 ± 2.7 and 1.1 ± 1.1 growing follicles per section, respectively, Fig. 4f).

Comparison of ovarian damage following targeted radiation to a single ovary relative to the non-targeted contralateral ovary

To examine potential off-target effects of radiation damage to the ovary, we used the SAARP to deliver precise radiation to one ovary while sparing the contralateral ovary for each mouse (Fig. 1a; T1 cohort). In this case, the non-targted ovary served as an internal control or a within-animal comparison, which is typically not possible, i.e., when only TBI is used. Based on gross assessment of ovarian histological sections, both non-targeted and targeted ovaries still had antral follicles and corpora lutea present in the tissue similar to what we observed in the TBI and T2 cohorts; providing evidence of follicle growth and estrous cyclicity (Fig. 5a and b). However, there was a visible difference in the primordial and primary follicles between the targeted and non-targeted ovaries. Whereas the non-targeted ovaries had clearly visible primordial and primary follicles at the cortex, the targeted ovaries did not (Fig. 5c and d). These observations were confirmed with follicle counting. When

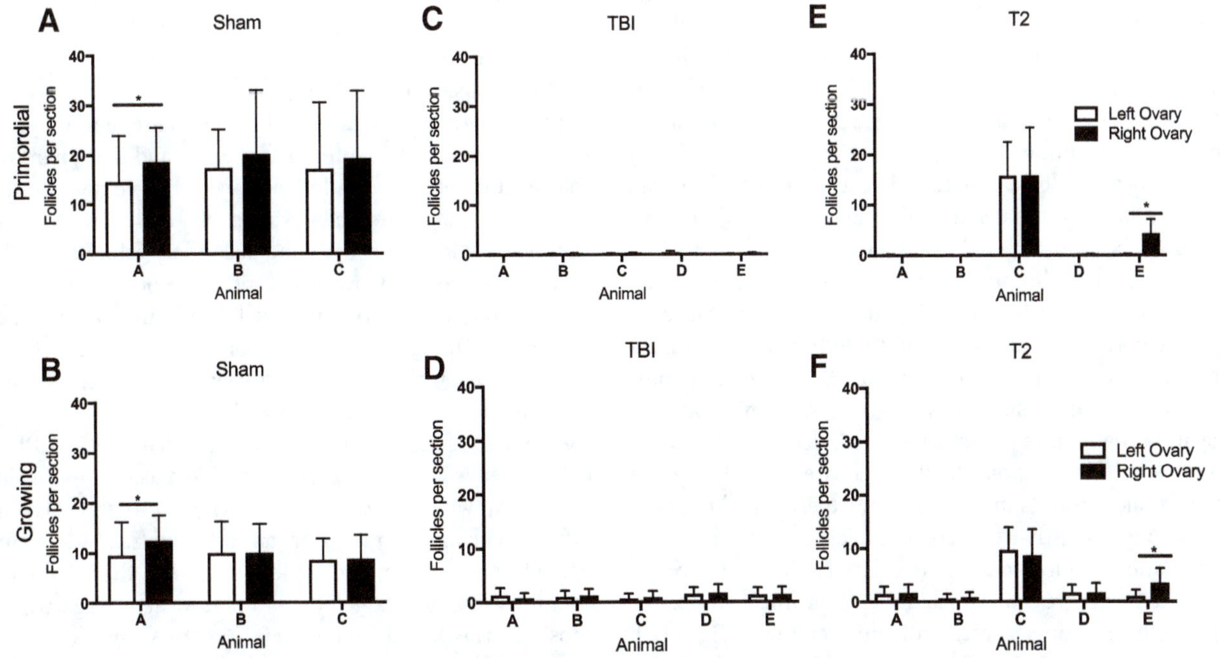

Fig. 4 Individual animal variation in ovarian follicle numbers in response to radiation damage. The follicle data shown in Fig. 3 was further broken down by individual animal (letter) and by right (black) and left (white) ovaries for the (**a-b**) Sham (**c-d**) TBI, and (**e-f**) T2 cohorts. Data for primordial follicles are shown in (**a**, **c**, **e**) and data for growing follicles are shown in (**b**, **d**, **f**). Unpaired t-tests were performed with statistical significance defined as $^*p < 0.05$

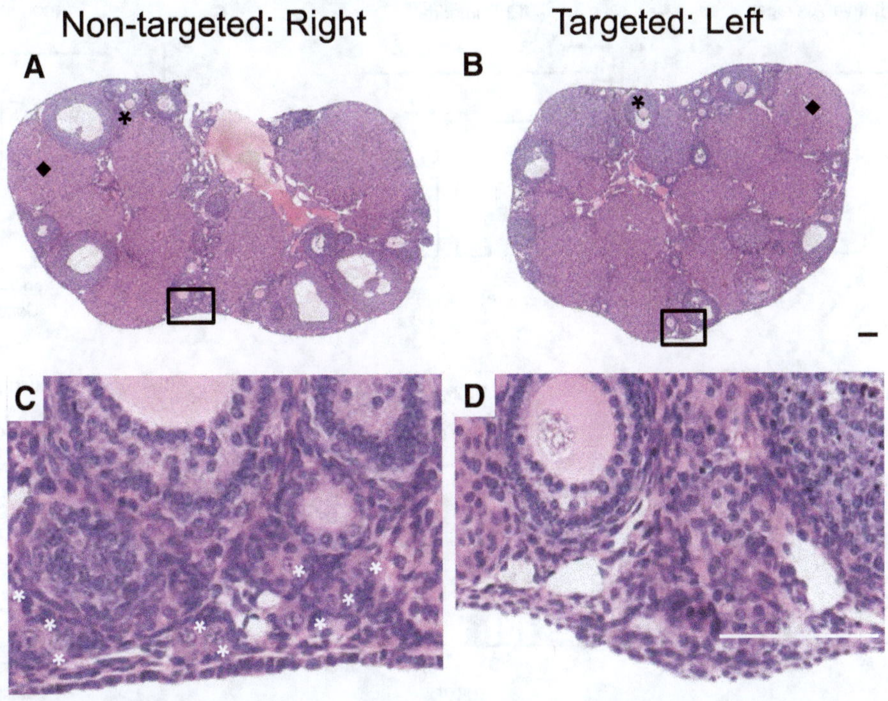

Fig. 5 Histological evidence supports that the SAARP can effectively target and damage a single ovary at a dose of 1 Gy. Representative images of whole histological sections of ovaries from the (**a**) non-targeted (right) and (**b**) targeted (left) ovary of the same mouse. Examples of healthy antral follicles are highlighted with black asterisks and corpora lutea are highlighted with black diamonds. Corresponding higher magnification images in the boxed regions are shown in (**c-d**) to visualize primordial and primary follicles at the ovarian cortex. White asterisks in (**c**) highlight specific primordial follicles in the cortex that are absent in (**d**). The scale bar is 125 μm

examining all follicle classes together, we observed that the targeted ovaries had significantly fewer total follicles relative to the non-targeted ovaries, which were similar to the total in Sham controls (1356.3 ± 2222.5 follicles, 6508.8 ± 2723.4 follicles, and 6689.2 ± 2289.6 follicles, respectively; Additional file 1). When focusing specifically on primordial follicles, we found that the targeted ovaries had significantly less primordial follicles per section compared to the non-targeted ovaries (2.3 ± 4.7 vs. 18.0 ± 11.7 primordial follicle per section, respectively, Fig. 6a). There were also fewer growing follicles in the targeted ovaries compared to the non-targeted ovaries (2.2 ± 2.4 growing follicles per section vs. 6.9 ± 1.5 growing follicles per section, respectively, Fig. 6b), and this was primarily attributable to changes in secondary follicles (Additional file 4). Interestingly, there were no changes in antral follicle counts in the different experimental cohorts, again suggesting that the largest follicles are not sensitive to radiation-induced damage (Additional file 4). To examine whether there was variability among mice, we examined follicle counts across individual animals (Fig. 6c-d, Additional file 4). While the number of primordial follicles in the non-targeted ovaries was similar in three of the four mice, mouse A had significantly more follicles than mouse D (34.1 ± 18.3 primordial follicles per section vs. 6.1 ± 4.7 follicles per section, respectively, Fig. 6c). There were no animal-specific differences in the number of growing follicles (Fig. 6d). Nevertheless, across animals, the targeted ovaries consistently exhibited a significant decrease in both primordial and growing follicle counts compared to their non-targeted counterparts (Fig. 6c and d). When further examining growing follicles according to specific follicle class, the targeted ovaries in each animal had significantly fewer primary and secondary follicles relative to the non-targeted ovary except for mouse B that had similar numbers of primary follicles in both ovaries (Additional file 4). Again across animals, there were no differences in antral follicles between the targeted and non-targeted ovaries (Additional file 4).

Although these results demonstrate that the SARRP is able to deliver precise radiation to a field as small as a single ovary, we wanted to assess whether there was any off-target damage to the non-targeted contralateral ovary. Therefore, we compared follicle counts in the T1 cohort (right ovary: non-targeted; and left ovary: targeted) to those in the Sham cohort (Fig. 6e-f). As expected, we found that when comparing the average primordial follicle counts in Sham controls to the targeted ovary in the T1 cohort, there was a marked decrease in primordial follicle counts: 17.8 ± 2.0 and 2.3 ± 4.7 primordial follicles per

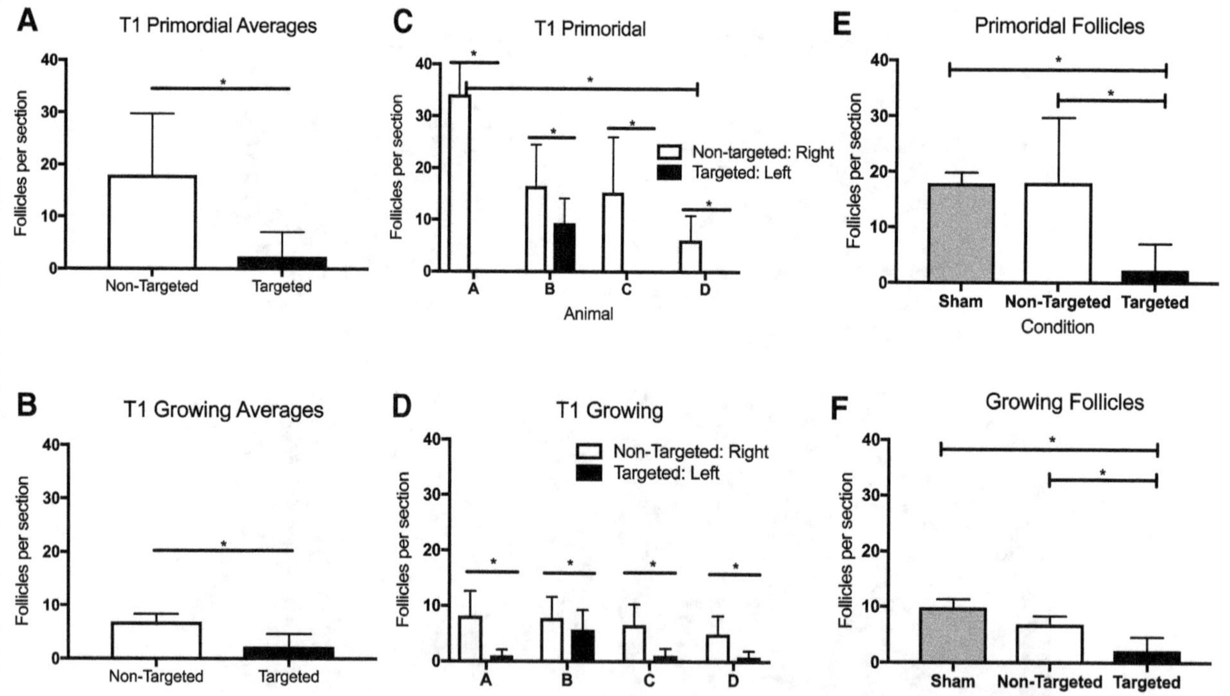

Fig. 6 Targeted radiation to a single ovary causes significant damage to the targeted ovary without having off target effects on the contralateral ovary. The average number of (**a**) primordial follicles per section and (**b**) growing follicles per section were quantified in both the non-targeted and targeted ovaries. These data were delineated by individual animal (letter) (**c-d**). In (**e-f**), the same data that are shown in (**a-b**) were plotted alongside the average follicle counts for the Sham cohort shown in Fig. 3b-c. The data were analyzed either by unpaired t-tests or one-way ANOVAS. Statistical significance was defined as $*p < 0.05$

section, respectively (Fig. 6e). This decrease was also true for growing follicles where there were 9.9 ± 1.4 growing follicles per section in the Sham cohort but only 2.2 ± 2.4 growing follicles per section in the targeted ovaries from the T1 cohort (Fig. 6f). In contrast, there was no difference when comparing the average follicle counts in the Sham ovaries relative to the counts in non-targeted ovaries from the T1 cohort for either primordial or growing follicles, indicating negligible off target effects (Fig. 6e-f). Interestingly, when examining the growing follicles according to class, there did appear to be a decrease in primary follicles between the Sham and non-targeted cohorts, suggesting that primary follicles may be sensitive to off-target radiation effects (Additional file 4).

Discussion

In this study, we used the SARRP to examine the effect of a single dose of ionizing radiation delivered to precise fields on ovarian damage in an adult whole animal mouse model. Although a limitation of our study is the small sample size in each experimental cohort, we nevertheless were able to draw important conclusions based on several robust findings. Overall, consistent with previous studies, we found that 1 Gy was sufficient to decrease follicle counts within the mouse ovary [28, 37, 39]. In fact, 1 Gy caused significant depletion of the ovarian reserve – or the number of primordial follicles – when delivered either as TBI or as targeted radiation to a field containing both ovaries (T2). This dose is much lower compared to humans where the effective sterilizing dose at which premature ovarian failure occurs immediately after treatment in 97.5% of patients is 16.5 Gy at 20 years and 14.3 Gy at 30 years [24]. Similarly, in nonhuman primates, a single dose of 15 Gy targeted radiation to the ovary resulted in a rapid decline in reproductive function [40]. Although we observed a significant reduction in the number of primordial follicles within the ovaries in the TBI and T2 cohorts, some follicles do remain. However, it is difficult to extrapolate whether this reduction would lead to partial or complete infertility in these mice because we do not know how the rate of follicle loss is affected when the ovarian reserve experiences such a significant depletion nor how residual follicles are recruited to contribute to fertility. In a recent study, cyclophosphamide-treated mice that showed a 90% reduction in follicle counts remarkably still maintained fertility [41]. However, previously we have shown that while follicles are still present following a single dose exposure of 1 Gy TBI at 2 weeks post-exposure, they are virtually all eliminated at 5 weeks post-exposure [37]. Thus, we anticipate that our treatment paradigm would likely affect fertility quite rapidly. Interestingly, we still observed the presence of antral follicles and corpora lutea in all the tissues we examined, and in fact, the number of antral follicles did not change across experimental cohorts. It takes approximately 18–24 days for a primordial follicle to reach the antral follicle stage in mouse [42]. Thus, any antral follicles or corpora lutea observed at the 2 week time point would be derived from a growing follicle that was present at the time of radiation and escaped damage to continue growth into a morphologically normal antral follicle.

Although the difference did not reach statistical significance, the TBI cohort tended to exhibit a more severe follicle loss phenotype compared to the cohort that received targeted radiation to both ovaries when considering both primordial and growing follicles. TBI could be more damaging to the ovary relative to targeted radiation due to compounding systemic effects. Radiation can induce systemic effects in which complex tissue responses are observed in non-irradiated regions due to signaling from irradiated cells. These systemic effects include inflammatory responses that may indirectly contribute to ovarian damage and follicle loss [15, 20, 22, 23, 43]. Ultimately, distinguishing the relative contribution of systemic damage compared to targeted damage in the ovary will require additional dose response studies with a larger sample size. Our findings parallel clinical data which demonstrated that female cancer survivors with spontaneous menstrual cycles who had been exposed to TBI and alkylating chemotherapy had a lower ovarian volume and follicle numbers compared to those who had received radiotherapy below the diaphragm with or without alkylating chemotherapy [5]. These findings suggest that TBI has a compounding effect on ovarian damage relative to targeted radiation. However, controlled human studies are nearly impossible due to variability in factors such as treatment regimen and radiation dose, further warranting animal studies and technologies such as the SARRP.

While systemic effects may account for the potential differences between the TBI and targeted radiation cohorts, it is also possible that individual animal variability contributes the extent of ovarian damage. For example, we observed that the larger number of remaining follicles in the cohort receiving targeted radiation to both ovaries compared to the TBI cohort was not a global phenomenon but rather due to the follicle numbers of two mice. This animal-specific response could be due to genetic variations in outbred CD-1 mice that confer differential radiosensitivity.

We also can not rule out the possibility that there could be technical inconsistencies with the targeting especially due to the challenging in vivo anatomy and small size of the mouse ovary. However, we do not think mis-targeting was a major limitation in our study. Geographic misalignment of the radiation field with respect to the ovary would be reflected in one of several possibilities. First, a portion of the ovary could have been outside the radiation field and, therefore, received less than the prescribed dose. Given the mm size of the ovary and the 1 cm field size, the probability is low that this would occur and result in a difference in dose (and therefore, damage and thus sequelae) within the ovary. However, if it did, this would be visible at the macroscopic level when individual ovaries (from either T1 or T2 protocols) were examined, and we did not observe evidence of a portion of the ovary being under-dosed. The second possibility is that ovary was completely outside the radiation field. If this were to happen in the T1 protocol, we would expect no reduction in follicles in the targeted ovary compared to the non-targeted ovary – since neither would have received radiation. This reduction was not observed. Rather, follicle number was substantially reduced in targeted ovaries relative to paired non-targeted ovaries. Conceivably, a misalignment of the 2 cm wide field could occur under the T2 protocol such that only one ovary received the full dose and the other received no dose (in the extreme situation). Misalignment would then result in a difference in follicle count between the two ovaries where there should not be such an effect. This difference was observed in one animal even though the follicle counts were obviously reduced from the shams, indicating a radiation effect. However, a difference between ovaries was also detected in one Sham animal. While inherent differences between ovaries within the same animal may make it more difficult to use a paired ovary as an internal control (T1 protocol), this variability was the exception rather than the rule and does not support the existence of dose inhomogeneity. Finally, the least likely scenario is that there was complete misalignment of the field during the T2 protocol such that both ovaries were completely excluded from the large radiation field. Although it is difficult to imagine how such a severe positioning error could have been made (and not noticed), there is one animal where the data would be consistent with this possibility. Because of this one potentially spurious result, we acknowledge the possibility of field misalignment as an unavoidable limitation of our experimental set-up.

Another key finding in our study was that significant follicle loss was often only observed in the targeted ovary when 1 Gy was delivered to a single ovary and not the contralateral ovary. This finding provides important proof-of-concept that the SAARP is a powerful method to target even the smallest structures within the mouse such as the ovary. In our experimental paradigm, we noted that the average primordial and growing follicle counts in the non-targeted ovaries were nearly identical to the Sham controls suggesting that the near complete loss of follicles in one ovary does not cause a dramatic change in the overall follicle profile of the remaining ovary despite individual animal variability in follicle numbers. In addition, the bystander effect appears to be negligible in our model. Although doses of 1 Gy can elicit bystander effects, this cell-signaling typically occurs through gap junction communication and paracrine signaling mechanisms which act over distances of a few millimeters. Thus, it is possible that paired mouse ovaries are too physically separated from each other to produce a biological effect. Another possibility is that 2 weeks post-radiation exposure is not sufficient to observe off target effects or compensatory effects in the non-targeted ovary that may take place over a longer time scale. In fact, we recently showed that a single dose exposure to 1 Gy TBI elicited significant germ cell damage without any overt stromal damage even up to 5 weeks post-exposure [44]. Thus, additional impacts of radiation damage that have been observed in human ovaries, such as stromal fibrosis and impaired vasculature, are late effects [4, 9, 14].

Conclusion

Taken together our findings demonstrate the SARRP is an innovative tool to examine the impact and underlying mechanisms of targeted radiation damage as well as systemic effects. This system can be applied to modeling specific scenarios relevant to the field of fertility preservation. For example, it can be used to screen and determine the efficacy of fertoprotective agents against radiation damage in whole animal models [40, 45–47]. Furthermore, implementation of the SARRP will allow accurate modeling of clinical radiation therapies to better understand how they impact the ovary and reproductive function, thereby ultimately improving personalized medicine.

Methods

Animals

Female CD-1 mice (6 weeks old) from Envigo (Indianapolis, IN) were used in this study. Mice were housed in a controlled barrier facility at the University of Kansas Medical Center (KUMC) under constant temperature, humidity, and a 12 h light/dark cycle. Food and water were provided ad libitum. All animal experiments were approved by the Institutional Animal Care and Use Committee and were performed in accordance with the National Institutes of Health Guidelines.

Irradiation procedure

Mice were randomized into experimental cohorts 1) those that were exposed to total body irradiation (TBI), 2) those that received radiation targeted to both ovaries (T2), and 3) those that received radiation targeted to one ovary (T1) (Fig. 1a). Sham mice served as controls.

Between 3 and 5 mice were used in each experimental cohort. The Xstrahl Small Animal Radiation Research Platform (SARRP, Xstrahl Inc., Suwanee, GA) was used to deliver a conformal dose of 1 Gy at a dose rate of 0.037 Gy/sec with an exposure time of 27 s to a designated field (Fig. 1b-c). Mice were anesthetized using a subcutaneous injection of buprenorphine (0.05–0.1 mg/kg) and then placed on the irradiator platform (Fig. 1b). The mice in the TBI group were irradiated in a field containing the whole mouse with the collimator removed. Mice in the T2 cohort were irradiated in a 20 mm × 10 mm collimated field containing both ovaries, whereas mice in the T1 cohort had only the left ovary exposed to radiation in a 10 mm × 10 mm collimated field (Fig 1c). The spine and the knee served as landmarks for defining the exposure field. Sham mice were handled the same way as those that were irradiated (i.e. handled, anesthetized, placed in the microirradiator) but were not exposed to radiation. Mice in all cohorts were monitored post-exposure to ensure that there were no visible acute effects of radiation and were weighed and euthanized 2 weeks post-procedure.

Ovarian tissue fixation and histological processing

Ovaries were harvested from all mice, and the bursa was removed by careful dissection under a light microscope. The right and left ovaries for each mouse were processed separately. Ovaries were fixed in Modified Davidson's fixative which is a prepared combination of 14% ethyl alcohol, 37.5% formalin, 37–39% glacial acetic acid, in 1 L of deionized water (Electron Microscopy Sciences, Hatfield, PA). Ovaries were rocked gently in fixative for 6 h at room temperature and then transferred to 4 °C overnight (~ 15 h). Samples were washed in 70% ethanol and processed and dehydrated using an automated tissue processor (Leica Biosystems, Buffalo Grove, IL). Ovaries were placed in molds and embedded in paraffin wax (Leica EG1160, Leica Biosystems, Buffalo Grove, IL). Paraffin embedded ovarian blocks were serial sectioned at a thickness of 5 μm using a Leica RM2335 microtome (Leica Biosystems, Buffalo Grove, IL). Every fifth section was placed on a separate slide designated for hematoxylin and eosin (H&E) staining to facilitate follicle counting. Stained sections were counted as a proxy for ovarian size to determine any differences between experimental groups (Fig. 1e). Slides were H&E stained using the AutostainerXL (Leica Biosystems, Buffalo Grove, IL). Whole slides were digitally imaged at the University of Washington Histology and Imaging Core using the Hamamatsu-HT imaging system (Hamamatsu Photonics, Hamamatsu City, Japan). NanoZoomer Digital Pathology Software (Hamamatsu Photonics) was used to analyze the images for follicle counting.

Follicle classification and counting

We used established morphological criteria to classify and count healthy follicles [38]. Atretic follicles with pyknotic granulosa cells or abnormal oocytes were excluded. In brief, a primordial follicle was defined as an oocyte surrounded by a complete or incomplete layer of squamous granulosa cells; a primary follicle was defined as an oocyte surrounded by a single complete layer of cuboidal granulosa cells; a secondary follicle was defined as an oocyte surrounded by two or more layers of granulosa cells; finally, antral follicles were defined as an oocyte surrounded by multiple layers of granulosa cells and containing a clear fluid filled cavity. Secondary and antral follicles were only counted if the oocyte nucleus was visible to avoid double counting. Follicles were grouped into two classes: primordial and growing. Growing follicles were defined as any follicle that was primary, secondary, or antral. Follicles were counted on every 5th section and either reported as total counts per experimental cohort or the number of follicles per total number of sections counted for each respective ovary.

Statistics

Follicle counts were analyzed based on cohort, animal, and ovary. Data represented in all graphs represent the mean ± standard deviation. Comparisons of two independent groups were done using unpaired t-test, and comparisons of more than two independent groups were done using a one-way ANOVA test followed by a post-hoc test. Statistical significance was defined as $p < 0.05$. All analyses were completed using GraphPad PRISM software (GraphPad Software Inc., La Jolla, CA).

Additional files

Additional file 1: Total follicle counts. The total number of follicles (primordial, primary, secondary, and antral) were quantified, and the average total number per each experimental cohort (Sham, TBI, T2, and T1) are plotted. A one-way ANOVA was performed between cohorts, and statistical significance was defined as $*p < 0.05$. (PDF 480 kb)

Additional file 2: The effect of TBI and targeted radiation on growing follicles analyzed by specific class. The average number of (A) primary follicles per section, (B) secondary follicles per section, and (C) antral follicles per section were quantified in ovaries from each cohort (Sham, TBI, and T2). A one-way ANOVA was performed between cohorts, and statistical significance was defined as $*p < 0.05$. (PDF 480 kb)

Additional file 3: Individual animal variation in growing follicle numbers in response to radiation damage. The growing follicle data shown in Fig. 4 was further broken down into follicle classes, including (A-C) primary follicles, (D-F) secondary follicles, and (G-I) antral follicles. Data for the Sham cohort are shown in A, D, G, for the TBI cohort in B, E, H, and for the T2 cohort in C, F, and I. Data for individual animals are denoted by letters and for the right and left ovaries by black and white bars, respectively. Unpaired t-tests were performed to compare follicle counts between the right and left ovaries with statistical significance defined as $*p < 0.05$. (PDF 480 kb)

Additional file 4: Stage-specific effects on growing follicles of targeted radiation to a single ovary relative to its non-targeted contralateral counterpart. The average number of (A) primary follicles per section, (B) secondary follicles per section, and (C) antral follicles per section were quantified in both the non-targeted and targeted ovaries and compared to the Sham cohort. These data were also delineated by individual animal (letter) (D-F). The data were analyzed either by unpaired t-tests or one-way ANOVAS. Statistical significance was defined as *$p < 0.05$. (PDF 480 kb)

Abbreviations

H&E: Hematoxylin and eosin; HPG axis: Hypothalamus-pituitary-gonad axis; RIBE: Radiation-induced bystander effect; SARRP: Small Animal Radiation Research Platform; T1: Radiation targeted to one ovary; T2: Radiation targeted to both ovaries; TBI: Total body irradiation

Acknowledgements

The authors would like to thank Drs. Subhrajit Saha and Payel Bhanja for assistance with the irradiations; Mr. Shawn Briley, Mr. Austin Armstrong, and Dr. Susmita Jasti for assistance with sample collection and processing; Ms. Keisha Barreto for histology training; and the University of Washington Histology and Imaging Core for assistance with slide scanning. We also acknowledge Dr. Teresa Woodruff and Dr. Mary Ellen Pavone for insightful discussions.

Funding

This work was supported by the Center for Reproductive Health After Disease (P50 HD076188) from the National Centers for Translational Research in Reproduction and Infertility (NCTRI) and the Master of Science in Reproductive Science and Medicine as part of Feinberg School of Medicine at Northwestern University.

Authors' contributions

All authors contributed significantly to this work and were involved in experimental design, data collection and analysis, and manuscript writing. ARG was involved with the sectioning and staining of tissue, data collection and analysis, and wrote the manuscript. BFK was involved in the experimental design and irradiation of the animals, as well as manuscript writing. FED was involved in the experimental design, manuscript writing, and oversaw the project. All authors read and approved the final manuscript.

Competing interests

The authors declare that they have no competing interests.

Author details

[1]Center for Reproductive Science, Northwestern University, Chicago, IL 60611, USA. [2]Department of Radiation Oncology, Kansas University Medical Center, Kansas City, KS 66160, USA. [3]Department of Obstetrics and Gynecology, Feinberg School of Medicine, Northwestern University, 303 E. Superior Street, Lurie 7-117, Chicago, IL 60611, USA.

References

1. ACS. Cancer Facts and Figures 2017. Atlanta: American Cancer Society; 2017.
2. DeSantis CE, Lin CC, Mariotto AB, Siegel RL, Stein KD, Kramer JL, Alteri R, Robbins AS, Jemal A. Cancer treatment and survivorship statistics, 2014. CA Cancer J Clin. 2014;64:252–71.
3. Siegel R, DeSantis C, Virgo K, Stein K, Mariotto A, Smith T, Cooper D, Gansler T, Lerro C, Fedewa S, et al. Cancer treatment and survivorship statistics, 2012. CA Cancer J Clin. 2012;62:220–41.
4. Duncan FE, Kimler BF, Briley SM. Combating radiation therapy-induced damage to the ovarian environment. Future Oncol. 2016;12(14):1687–90.
5. Larsen EC, Müller J, Schmiegelow K, Rechnitzer C, Andersen AN. Reduced ovarian function in long-term survivors of radiation- and chemotherapy-treated childhood Cancer. J Clin Endocrinol Metab. 2003;88:5307–14.
6. Adriaens I, Smitz J, Jacquet P. The current knowledge on radiosensitivity of ovarian follicle development stages. Hum Reprod Update. 2009;15:359–77.
7. Reulen RC, Bright CJ, Winter DL, Fidler MM, Wong K, Guha J, Kelly JS, Frobisher C, Edgar AB, Skinner R, et al. Pregnancy and Labor Complications in Female Survivors of Childhood Cancer: The British Childhood Cancer Survivor Study. J Natl Cancer Inst. 2017;109:djx056.
8. Bluethmann SM, Mariotto AB, Rowland JH. Anticipating the "silver tsunami": prevalence trajectories and comorbidity burden among older cancer survivors in the United States. Cancer Epidemiol Biomarkers Prev. 2016;25(7):1029–36.
9. Meirow D, Biederman H, Anderson RA, Wallace WHB. Toxicity of chemotherapy and radiation on female reproduction. Clin Obstet Gynecol. 2010;53:727–39.
10. Metzger ML, Meacham LR, Patterson B, Casillas JS, Constine LS, Hijiya N, Kenney LB, Leonard M, Lockart BA, Likes W. Female reproductive health after childhood, adolescent, and young adult cancers: guidelines for the assessment and management of female reproductive complications. J Clin Oncol. 2013;31:1239–47.
11. Ogilvy-Stuart AL, Shalet SM. Effect of radiation on the human reproductive system. Environ Health Perspect. 1993;101:109.
12. Bath LE, Critchley HO, Chambers SE, Anderson RA, Kelnar CJ, Wallace WHB. Ovarian and uterine characteristics after total body irradiation in childhood and adolescence: response to sex steroid replacement. BJOG Int J Obstet Gynaecol. 1999;106:1265–72.
13. Filicori M, Santoro N, Merriam GR, Crowley WR Jr. Characterization of the physiological pattern of episodic gonadotropin secretion throughout the human menstrual cycle. J Clin Endocrinol Metab. 1986;62:1136–44.
14. Grigsby PW, Russell A, Bruner D, Eifel P, Koh W-J, Spanos W, Stetz J, Stitt JA, Sullivan J. Late injury of cancer therapy on the female reproductive tract. Int J Radiat Oncol Biol Phys. 1995;31:1281–99.
15. Sologuren I, Rodríguez-Gallego C, Lara PC. Immune effects of high dose radiation treatment: implications of ionizing radiation on the development of bystander and abscopal effects. Transl Cancer Res. 2014;3:18–31.
16. Klammer H, Mladenov E, Li F, Iliakis G. Bystander effects as manifestation of intercellular communication of DNA damage and of the cellular oxidative status. Cancer Lett. 2015;356:58–71.
17. Desouky O, Ding N, Zhou G. Targeted and non-targeted effects of ionizing radiation. J Radiat Res Appl Sci. 2015;8:247–54.
18. Rzeszowska-Wolny J, Przybyszewski WM, Widel M. Ionizing radiation-induced bystander effects, potential targets for modulation of radiotherapy. Eur J Pharmacol. 2009;625:156–64.
19. Kadhim M, Salomaa S, Wright E, Hildebrandt G, Belyakov OV, Prise KM, Little MP. Non-targeted effects of ionizing radiation–implications for low dose risk. Mutat Res. 2013;752:84–98.
20. Lorimore S, Wright E. Radiation-induced genomic instability and bystander effects: related inflammatory-type responses to radiation-induced stress and injury? A review. Int J Radiat Biol. 2003;79:15–25.
21. Mothersill C, Rusin A, Seymour C. Low doses and non-targeted effects in environmental radiation protection; where are we now and where should we go? Environ Res. 2017;159:484–90.
22. Rödel F, Frey B, Multhoff G, Gaipl U. Contribution of the immune system to bystander and non-targeted effects of ionizing radiation. Cancer Lett. 2015; 356:105–13.
23. Frey B, Hehlgans S, Rödel F, Gaipl US. Modulation of inflammation by low and high doses of ionizing radiation: implications for benign and malign diseases. Cancer Lett. 2015;368:230–7.
24. Wallace WHB, Thomson AB, Saran F, Kelsey TW. Predicting age of ovarian failure after radiation to a field that includes the ovaries. Int J Radiat Oncol Biol Phys. 2005;62:738–44.

25. Shah D, Sachs R, Wilson D. Radiation-induced cancer: a modern view. Br J Radiol. 2012;85:e1166–73.
26. Baker T. Effects of ionizing radiations on mammalian oogenesis: a model for chemical effects. Environ Health Perspect. 1978;24:31.
27. Winship AL, Stringer JM, Liew SH, Hutt KJ. The importance of DNA repair for maintaining oocyte quality in response to anti-cancer treatments, environmental toxins and maternal ageing. Hum Reprod Update. 2018;24(2): 119–34.
28. Pesty A, Doussau M, Lahaye J-B, Lefèvre B. Whole-body or isolated ovary 60Co irradiation: effects on in vivo and in vitro folliculogenesis and oocyte maturation. Reprod Toxicol. 2010;29:93–8.
29. Lee CJ, Park HH, Do BR, Yoon Y-D, Kim JK. Natural and radiation-induced degeneration of primordial and primary follicles in mouse ovary. Anim Reprod Sci. 2000;59:109–17.
30. Lee CJ, Yoon Y-D. γ-Radiation-induced follicular degeneration in the prepubertal mouse ovary. Mutat Res Fundam Mol Mech Mutagen. 2005;578: 247–55.
31. Kaufman M, Nikitin AY, Sundberg JP. Histologic basis of mouse endocrine system development: a comparative analysis. CRC Press Taylor & Francis Group;Boca Raton, FL. 2016.
32. Clement PB. Anatomy and histology of the ovary. In: Blaustein's pathology of the female genital tract: Springer;New York, NY. 1987. p. 438–70.
33. Treuting PM, Dintzis SM, Liggitt D, Frevert CW. Comparative anatomy and histology: a mouse and human atlas (expert consult): Academic Press;New York, NY. 2011.
34. Bazalova M, Nelson G, Noll JM, Graves EE. Modality comparison for small animal radiotherapy: a simulation study. Med Phys. 2014;41:011710.
35. Brodin NP, Velcich A, Guha C, Tomé WA. A model for precise and uniform pelvic-and limb-sparing abdominal irradiation to study the radiation-induced gastrointestinal syndrome in mice using small animal irradiation systems. Dose-Response. 2017;15:1559325816685798.
36. Tillner F, Thute P, Löck S, Dietrich A, Fursov A, Haase R, Lukas M, Rimarzig B, Sobiella M, Krause M. Precise image-guided irradiation of small animals: a flexible non-profit platform. Phys Med Biol. 2016;61:3084.
37. Kimler BF, Briley SM, Johnson BW, Armstrong AG, Jasti S, Duncan FE. Radiation-induced ovarian follicle loss occurs without overt stromal changes. Reproduction. 2018;155:553–62.
38. Duncan FE, Jasti S, Paulson A, Kelsh JM, Fegley B, Gerton JL. Age-associated dysregulation of protein metabolism in the mammalian oocyte. Aging Cell. 2017;16:1381–93.
39. Zhang H, Zhang X, Yuan Z, Li X, Li W, Zhou Q, Min F, Xie Y, Liu B, Duan X. Germ cell loss induced by 12C6+ ion irradiation in young female mice. J Radiat Res. 2006;47:131–4.
40. Zelinski MB, Murphy MK, Lawson MS, Jurisicova A, Pau KF, Toscano NP, Jacob DS, Fanton JK, Casper RF, Dertinger SD. In vivo delivery of FTY720 prevents radiation-induced ovarian failure and infertility in adult female nonhuman primates. Fertil Steril. 2011;95:1440–5.
41. Nguyen QN, Zerafa N, Liew SH, Morgan FH, Strasser A, Scott CL, Findlay JK, Hickey M, Hutt KJ. Loss of PUMA protects the ovarian reserve during DNA-damaging chemotherapy and preserves fertility. Cell Death Dis. 2018;9:618.
42. Eppig JJ, Wigglesworth K, Pendola FL. The mammalian oocyte orchestrates the rate of ovarian follicular development. Proc Natl Acad Sci U S A. 2002; 99:2890–4.
43. Wright EG, Coates PJ. Untargeted effects of ionizing radiation: implications for radiation pathology. Mutat Res Fundam Mol Mech Mutagen. 2006;597: 119–32.
44. Briley SM, Jasti S, McCracken JM, Hornick JE, Fegley B, Pritchard MT, Duncan FE. Reproductive age-associated fibrosis in the stroma of the mammalian ovary. Reproduction. 2016;152:245–60.
45. Myers M, Morgan FH, Liew SH, Zerafa N, Gamage TU, Sarraj M, Cook M, Kapic I, Sutherland A, Scott CL. PUMA regulates germ cell loss and primordial follicle endowment in mice. Reproduction. 2014;148:211–9.
46. Kim S-Y, Kim SK, Lee JR, Woodruff TK. Toward precision medicine for preserving fertility in cancer patients: existing and emerging fertility preservation options for women. J Gynecol Oncol. 2015;27:e22.
47. Bolcun-Filas E, Rinaldi VD, White ME, Schimenti JC. Reversal of female infertility by Chk2 ablation reveals the oocyte DNA damage checkpoint pathway. Science. 2014;343:533–6.

10

KLK10 exon 3 unmethylated PCR product concentration: a new potential early diagnostic marker in ovarian cancer?

Mustafa A. El Sherbini[1*], Amal A. Mansour[1], Maha M. Sallam[1], Emtiaz A. Shaban[1], Zeinab A. Shehab ElDin[2] and Amr H. El-Shalakany[2]

Abstract

Background: *KLK10* exon 3 hypermethylation correlated to tumor-specific lack of *KLK10* expression in cancer cell lines and primary tumors. In the present study we investigate the possible role of *KLK10* exon 3 methylation in ovarian tumor diagnosis and prognosis.

Results: Qualitative methylation-specific PCR (MSP) results did not show statistically significant differences in patient group samples (normal and tumor) where all samples were positive only for the unmethylated-specific PCR except for two malignant samples that were either doubly positive (serous carcinoma) or doubly negative (Sertoli-Leydig cell tumor) for the two MSP tests. However, *KLK10* exon 3 unmethylated PCR product concentration (ng/μl) showed statistically significant differences in benign and malignant patient group samples; mean ± SD (n): tumor: 0.077 ± 0.035 (14) and 0.047 ± 0.021 (15), respectively, *p*-value = 0.011; and normal: 0.094 ± 0.039 (7) and 0.046 ± 0.027 (6), respectively, *p*-value = 0.031. Moreover, ROC curve analysis of *KLK10* exon 3 unmethylated PCR product concentration in overall patient group samples showed good diagnostic ability (AUC = 0.778; *p*-value = 0.002). Patient survival (living and died) showed statistically significant difference according to preoperative serum CA125 concentration (U/ml); median (n): 101.25 (10) and 1252 (5), respectively, *p*-value = 0.037, but not *KLK10* exon 3 unmethylated PCR product concentration (ng/μl) in overall malignant patient samples; mean ± SD (n): 0.042 ± 0.015 (14) and 0.055 ± 0.032 (7), *p*-value = 0.228.

Conclusion: To the best of our knowledge, this is the first report on *KLK10* exon 3 unmethylated PCR product concentration as potential early epigenetic diagnostic marker in primary ovarian tumors. Taken into account the limitations in our study (small sample size and semi-quantitative PCR product analysis) further studies are strongly recommended.

Keywords: Ovarian cancer, CA125, KLK10, KLK6, *KLK10* exon 3 methylation

Background

DNA methylation is one of the well-studied epigenetic modifications in DNA/chromatin metabolism. It is a dynamic process and involves the reversible and heritable methylation of the 5′ carbon of cytosine residues to yield 5-methylcytosine (5-MC) [1]. The reaction belongs to one carbon metabolism where DNA methyltransferases (DNMT1, DNMT3a and DNMT3b) are the biocatalysts and S-adenosylmethionine (SAM) is the methyl-donor [2]. Besides having important physiological roles in cell differentiation, development and gene regulation [3], DNA methylation can provide clues to other physiological processes, e.g. cell and tissue aging [4] and establishment of memory [5].

In DNA the cytosine residues occur either in frequencies that are far less than expected or in CpG-rich short stretches (0.5–4 kbp) in gene promoters and other regulatory regions known collectively as CpG islands

* Correspondence: me_sherbini@yahoo.com
[1]Medical Biochemistry Department, Faculty of Medicine, Ain Shams University, Cairo, Egypt
Full list of author information is available at the end of the article

[6]. In the CpG context the two cytosines on the opposing DNA strands are usually symmetrical as for their methylation status, i.e. both are either unmethylated or methylated [7]. The effect of DNA methylation on gene regulation may differ according to the context in which it occurs; however, in CpG-rich gene promoters it is well known to share in gene silencing [8]. Deregulated gene methylation was implicated in several diseases including cancer [9]. Nonetheless, aberrant gene methylation in cancer can be a promising diagnostic and prognostic target in tumor and naked DNA samples; e.g. in lung cancer [10].

The kallikrein-related peptidase 10 gene (*KLK10*) is one of 15 members in a serine protease gene subfamily located in tandem on chromosome 19q13.3–13.4 [11]. The gene product (KLK10) is a secreted protein found in normal human mammary epithelial cells (MECs) but downregulated or absent in the majority of human breast cancer cell lines [12]. *KLK10* has a wide tissue expression [13] and is regulated by mechanisms that include steroid hormones [14] and micRNA [15]. The gene was reported as candidate tumor suppressor in some cancer types, e.g. in prostate cancer cells [16]; however, it showed contrasting expression profiles in different cancers, e.g. underexpressed in breast [17], testis [18] and prostate [19], and overexpressed in ovary [20], colon [21], and pancreas [22].

Liu and colleagues did not find mutation in *KLK10* gene in different cancer types [12]. Indeed, tumor-specific lack of *KLK10* expression correlated to *KLK10* exon 3 hypermethylation in a majority of cell lines and in primary breast cancer [23]. The rationale behind such correlation may be understood as *KLK10* exon 3 methylation was shown to perfectly follow that of *KLK10* gene promoter [24]. Results of previous works were consistent about the confinement of *KLK10* exon 3 hypermethylation in malignant samples; but not normal ones, in cell lines [23–25] and in primary tumors [23–26]. However, in some sample sets *KLK10* expression did not show simple correlation with *KLK10* exon 3 methylation [23–26]. In the present study, *KLK10* exon 3 methylation is assessed for its possible role in the biology, diagnosis and/or prognosis of ovarian tumors.

Methods

Patients and samples

This is a further study for our previous work on serum KLK6 and 10 in ovarian cancer patients [27]. The protocol of the present study was approved by the Ethics and Research Committee of Ain Shams University.

Patients' demographic data and preoperative serum marker levels (CA125, KLK10 and KLK6) were taken from our previous data as mentioned above. Patients or their relatives were contacted from October 2012 to January 2013 to collect patient follow-up data and have their written informed consent.

The studied samples were archival FFPE-ovarian tissue samples that are available at the Gynecologic Oncology Unit, Ain Shams University Maternity Hospital. The included samples were tumors and their contralateral normal ovarian samples (for some cases), while non-neoplastic ovarian masses, i.e. inflammation and endometriosis, were excluded.

Experimental protocol

Using histopathology microtome (microTec® *cut 4050*, UK) 10 to 15 tissue sections, each of ~ 2 × 2 cm in diameter and 1–2 µm thickness were cut and put in clean and autoclaved 1.5 ml microcentrifuge tube, one day before DNA extraction. An H&E stained tissue section was prepared and examined microscopically for each sample.

DNA extraction

Commercially available QIAamp DNA FFPE Tissue Kit (Qiagen) was used. The steps of the experiment were done according to the product insert provided by the manufacturer. Xylol (Sigma-Aldrich, Germany) was used to dissolve the paraffin and 98–100% ethanol (Sigma-Aldrich, Germany) was used to remove the xylol and to reconstitute the buffers. The concentration of the extracted pure DNA was measured spectrophotometrically (Ultraspec® 1000, Amersham Pharmacia Biotech, Cambridge, England) at 260 nm and the DNA samples were stored at – 80 °C until the time of DNA sodium bisulfite treatment.

Sodium bisulfite treatment of DNA

One µg of extracted DNA was treated by sodium bisulfite using commercially available EpiTect Bisulfite Kit (Qiagen). The steps of the experiment and the thermal cycler program were done according to the product insert given by the manufacturer for FFPE-samples. The sodium bisulfite converted DNA samples were kept at – 80 °C until the time of MSP experiment.

MSP for *KLK10* exon 3

Commercially available HotStarTaq Master Mix kit (Qiagen) was used. Methylated- and unmethylated-specific PCRs were run in parallel in separate PCR tubes where each tube contained either methylated- or unmethylated-specific primer pair, respectively. The two primer pairs were provided by Invitrogen (USA), as described elsewhere [23]. Each PCR reaction contained ~ 0.5 µg sodium bisulfite-treated DNA sample. The concentrations of the PCR reaction components were made according to the manufacturer's instructions in the product insert. A methylation positive control MSP was done using 2 µg (1 µg for each MSP test type) fully methylated DNA (EpiTect® Control DNA (human), methylated and bisulfite converted (100), Qiagen). The thermal cycler program was as follows: 1 cycle of 95 °C for 15 min; 35 cycles of

94 °C for 1 min, 55 °C for 1 min, and 72 °C for 1 min; and 1 cycle of 72 °C for 10 min.

Capillary gel electrophoresis

PCR products were assessed by capillary gel electrophoresis using QIAxcel system (Qiagen). A QIAxcel kit (QIAxcel DNA High Resolution Kit (1200)) was used and the experiment steps were done according to the manufacturer's instructions in the product insert. Determination of DNA fragment size and concentration was done using the BioCalculator software provided with the QIAxcel (Qiagen).

Statistical analysis

Statistical analysis of data was done using SPSS (version 15.0 for Windows). $p < 0.05$ was considered the cutoff value for significance. Chi-square test (χ^2) was used to test the association of categorical data. Parametric or non-parametric tests were used to compare mean ± SD (Student *t*-test or ANOVA test) or median and interquartile range (Mann-Whitney test or Kruskal Wallis test) in two or more populations, respectively, involving independent samples. Spearman's test was used to evaluate correlations between continuous variables. A receiver operating characteristic (ROC) curve was used to illustrate the diagnostic properties of a test on a numerical scale. Marker's diagnostic parameters were calculated as follows: sensitivity = true positive tests/ all positive samples by gold standard test; specificity = true negative tests/ all negative samples by gold standard test; positive predictive value (PPV) = true positive tests/ all positive tests; negative predictive value (NPV) = true negative tests/ all negative tests; and accuracy = true positive and true negative tests/all positive and all negative tests.

Results

Patients and samples

This study included 14 benign and 16 malignant ovarian tumor patients. Patient clinicopthological data are shown in Table 1. There were no statistically significant differences of patient age mean ± SD according to disease grade (1, 2 and 3): mean ± SD (n): 36.8 ± 11.2 (5), 48.0 ± 19.6 (5) and 46.5 ± 11.0 (6), respectively; *p*-value = 0.422, or disease stage (I/II and III/IV): mean ± SD (n): 42.5 ± 16.4 (9) and 45.7 ± 11.7 (7), respectively; *p*-value = 0.675.

Each patient participated by one tumor sample. In addition, samples from contralateral normal ovaries of some patients in benign and malignant patient groups were included as normal controls (n = 7 and 6, respectively). Table 2 shows the pathological characteristics of tumor samples in the two patient groups. Histopathological H&E examination of all samples showed good quality of the tissue samples and confirmed the previously known diagnoses.

Table 1 Clinicopathological parameters of patient groups

	Patient group		*p*-value
	Benign (*N* = 14)	Malignant (*N* = 16)	
Age (mean ± SD)	45.2 ± 12.7	43.9 ± 14.2	0.788[c]
Menstrual cycle			
Premenopausal	7	11	0.296[a]
Postmenopausal	7	5	
Ascites			
Absent	13	8	0.011[a]
Present	1	8	
Serum marker (median)			
CA125 (U/ml)	11.6	186.0	0.001[b]
KLK10 (ng/ml)	1.41	1.99	0.236[b]
KLK6 (ng/ml)	3.05	3.17	0.678[b]

SD standard deviation
[a]χ^2 test
[b]Mann-Whitney test
[c]Student *t*-test

MSP

In the overall there were 42 unmethylated-specific positive PCR tests and only one methylated-specific positive PCR test. The unmethylated PCR band size was as follows: min.-max.: 101.30–274.00 bp; median: 123.45 bp and mean ± SD: 126.25 ± 23.61 bp, whereas the methylated band was 134.5 bp. The methylation positive control sample was positive for the methylated-specific PCR (band size: 129.0 bp) but negative for unmethylated-specific PCR.

Qualitative results of MSP did not show statistically significant difference in the two patient groups for both tumor and normal samples (Table 3). However, comparison of *KLK10* exon 3 unmethylated PCR product concentration mean ± SD (ng/μl) showed statistically significant differences in benign (n = 14), malignant (n = 15) and overall normal (n = 13) samples; mean ± SD: 0.077 ± 0.035, 0.047 ± 0.021, and 0.072 ± 0.041, respectively; *p*-value = 0.046. Moreover, *KLK10* exon 3 unmethylated PCR product concentration mean ± SD (ng/μl) showed statistically significant differences in tumor and normal samples in the two patient groups (Fig. 1).

Spearman's correlation of *KLK10* exon 3 unmethylated PCR product concentration (ng/μl) showed statistically significant positive correlation with patient age (ρ = 0.398; *p*-value = 0.009) and statistically significant negative correlation with serum KLK10 (ρ = − 0.300; *p*-value = 0.054) but not KLK6 (ρ = − 0.114; *p*-value = 0.471) or CA125 (ρ = − 0.214; p-value = 0.197). Comparisons of *KLK10* exon 3 unmethylated PCR product concentration mean ± SD (ng/μl) in overall samples and in sample pathology types in the two patient groups according to patient age and serum KLK10 are shown in Tables 4 and 5, respectively.

Table 2 Pathological characteristics of tumor samples

		Benign tumors (*N*, %)	Malignant tumors (*N*, %)
Pathology subgroup/subtype		Neoplastic (14, 100%)	Epithelial (11, 68.75%)
		Serous cystadenoma (3)	Serous (4)
		Serous cystadenofibroma (1)	Mucinous (2)
		Simple serous cyst (2)	Endometrioid (4)
		Granulosa cell tumor (3)	Clear cell (1)
		Mature cystic teratoma (3)	Non-epithelial (3, 18.75%)
		Mucinous cystadenoma (1)	Yolk sac tumor (1)
		Brenner tumor (1)	Liposarcoma (1)
			Sretoli-leydig cell tumor (1)
			Metastatic (2, 12.5%)
			Colon cancer (2)
Grade			
	1	–	5 (31.3%)
	2	–	5 (31.3%)
	3	–	6 (37.5%)
Stage			
	I/II	–	9 (56.3%)
	III/IV	–	7 (43.8%)

ROC curves

ROC curves for *KLK10* exon 3 unmethylated PCR product concentration (ng/μl) and preoperative serum markers in the two patient groups are shown in Figs. 2a and b, respectively.

Combination of *KLK10* exon 3 unmethylated PCR product concentration and serum marker showed enhanced combined marker sensitivity with all 3 markers and better specificity with CA125 but not KLK10 or KLK6. Combined marker profile of *KLK10* exon 3 unmethylated PCR product concentration with serum marker was as follows; CA125: sensitivity: 100%, specificity: 94.4%, PPV: 68.9%, NPV: 73.9% and accuracy: 71.1%; KLK10: sensitivity: 90.4%, specificity: 85.7%, PPV: 67.8%, NPV: 62% and accuracy: 64.9%; and KLK6: sensitivity: 85.7%, specificity: 71.4%, PPV: 60%, NPV: 60% and accuracy: 60%.

Table 3 MSP qualitative results in patient group samples

MSP	Normal samples		Tumor samples	
	Benign patient	Malignant patient	Benign patient	Malignant patient
Methylated-specific PCR				
Positive	0	0	0	1[b]
Negative	7	6	14	15
p-value	–		0.341[a]	
Unmethylated-specific PCR				
Positive	7	6	14	15
Negative	0	0	0	1[b]
p-value	–		0.341[a]	

- not applicable
[a]χ^2 test
[b]The two odd results in the malignant samples belonged to two samples; one was doubly positive (ovarian serous adenocarcinoma) and the other was doubly negative (Sertoli-Leydig cell tumor) for the two MSP test types

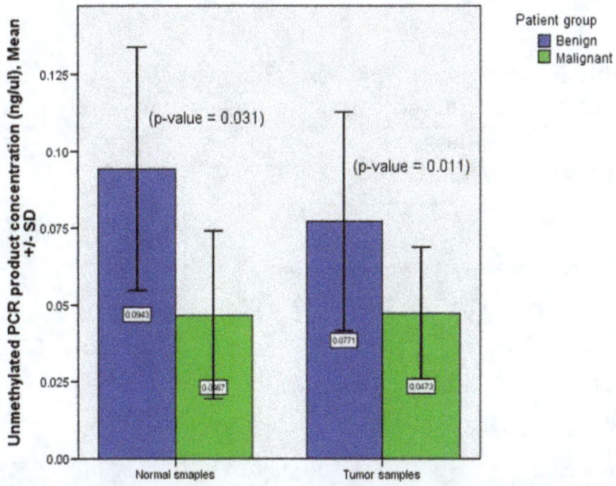

Fig. 1 *KLK10* exon 3 unmethylated PCR product concentration (ng/μl) mean ± SD in patient group samples. Number of samples in benign and malignant patient groups were: normal sample: 7 and 6, respectively, and tumor sample: 14 and 15, respectively

Table 4 Comparison of *KLK10* exon 3 unmethylated PCR product concentration (ng/μl) according to patient age

KLK10 exon 3 unmethylated PCR product; ng/μl, mean ± SD	Age group			*p*-value
	16–32 years	33–55 years	> 55 years	
Overall samples (*n* = 6–27)	0.032 ± 0.029	0.064 ± 0.029	0.090 ± 0.037	0.004[b]
Benign patients:				
Normal ovary (*n* = 0–5)	-	0.078 ± 0.034	0.135 ± 0.007	0.078[b]
Benign ovary (*n* = 2–10)	0.060 ± 0.042	0.078 ± 0.034	0.090 ± 0.056	0.728[b]
p-value	-	1.00[a]	0.380[a]	
Malignant patients:				
Normal ovary (*n* = 1–3)	0.020 ± –	0.040 ± 0.000	0.070 ± 0.042	0.335[b]
Malignant ovary (*n* = 3–9)	0.017 ± 0.011	0.049 ± 0.010	0.073 ± 0.015	0.000[b]
p-value	0.826[a]	0.188[a]	0.903[a]	

- no samples or statistical test not applicable, *SD* standard deviation
[a]Student *t*-test
[b]ANOVA test

Patients' survival

Five-year patient follow-up data were available between 2007 and 2012. Five patients died within the first two years of the follow-up period. In the living 11 patients there were 9 disease-free and 2 relapsed. Comparisons of patient clinicopathological parameters according to patient survival (living and died) showed statistically significant differences in preoperative serum CA125 concentration (U/ml); median (n): 101.25 (10) and 1252 (5), respectively; *p*-value = 0.037, and disease stage (I/II and III/IV): late stage was more frequent in died patients compared to the living (4 vs. 1, respectively); *p*-value = 0.049. The *p*-values for other clinicopathological parameters were as follows: patient age mean ± SD: 0.355; serum KLK10 (ng/ml) mean ± SD: 0.798; serum KLK6 (ng/ml) mean ± SD: 0.278; ascites (absent and present): 0.106; disease grade (1, 2, and 3): 0.622; pathology subgroup (epithelial, nonepithelial and metastatic): 0.402; and epithelial pathology subtype (serous, mucinous, endometrioid and clear cell carcinoma): 0.735.

Comparison of *KLK10* exon 3 unmethylated PCR product concentration (ng/μl) mean ± SD according to patient survival (living and died) did not show statistically significant differences in overall malignant patient samples: mean ± SD (n): 0.042 ± 0.015 (14) and 0.055 ± 0.032 (7), respectively; *p*-value = 0.228, normal samples: mean ± SD (n): 0.035 ± 0.010 (4) and 0.070 ± 0.042 (2), respectively; *p*-value = 0.153, or malignant samples: mean ± SD (n): 0.046 ± 0.017 (10) and 0.050 ± 0.030 (5), respectively; *p* = 0.748. However, the oddly methylated-specific PCR positive sample in our results was serous carcinoma of grade 3, stage III/IV and its unmethylated PCR product concentration was 0.06 ng/μl; the patient of which died one year after diagnosis and start of treatment.

Table 5 Comparison of *KLK10* exon 3 unmethylated PCR product concentration (ng/μl) according to preoperative serum KLK10

KLK10 exon 3 unmethylated PCR product; ng/μl, mean ± SD	Serum KLK10		*p*-value
	< 2 ng/ml	≥ 2 ng/ml	
Overall samples (*n* = 15–27)	0.075 ± 0.038	0.046 ± 0.018	0.007[a]
Benign patients:			
Normal ovary (*n* = 1–6)	0.100 ± 0.040	0.060 ± –	0.397[a]
Benign ovary (*n* = 3–11)	0.086 ± 0.033	0.043 ± 0.023	0.060[a]
p-value	0.463[a]	0.596[a]	
Malignant patients:			
Normal ovary (*n* = 2–4)	0.070 ± 0.042	0.035 ± 0.010	0.153[a]
Malignant ovary (*n* = 7–8)	0.044 ± 0.023	0.051 ± 0.019	0.511[a]
p-value	0.252[a]	0.156[a]	

- not applicable, *SD* standard deviation
[a]Student *t*-test

Discussion

In the literature we could find only one study on *KLK10* exon 3 methyaltion in primary ovarian tumors that was reported by Sidiropoulos and colleagues [25]. Our results agree with those in the previous work with some logic approximation due to differences in the used technique for gene methylation assessment (MSP vs. direct DNA sequencing, respectively) and the examined *KLK10* expression parameter (serum KLK10 vs. cytosolic KLK10, respectively). The two studies showed *KLK10* exon 3 methylation only in malignant samples (methylated-specific PCR positive samples: 1/16 and samples with partially methylated *KLK10* exon 3: 6/7, respectively) but not in normal samples (methylated-specific PCR negative samples: 13/13 and samples with fully unmethylated *KLK10* exon 3: 2/2, respectively). Additionally, we studied *KLK10* exon 3 methylation in benign ovarian tumors – not included in the previous work – and they all were unmethylated (Table 3). Differences in the internal working of MSP and direct DNA

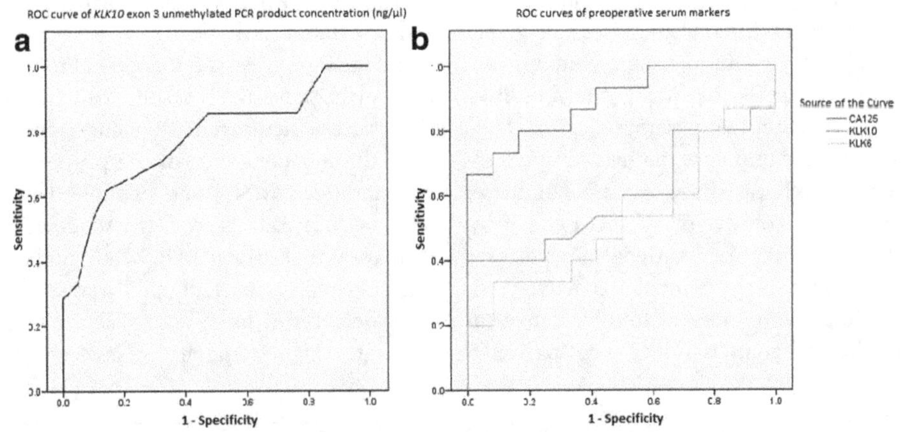

Fig. 2 ROC curve analysis of *KLK10* exon 3 unmethylated PCR product concentration (ng/µl) in overall patient group samples (**a**) and ROC curves of preoperative serum markers CA125, KLK10 and KLK6 in patient groups (**b**). Markers' diagnostic profiles were as follows:

	Best cutoff	Area under the curve	p-value	Sensitivity	Specificity	PPV	NPV	Accuracy
KLK10 exon 3 unmethylated PCR product (ng/µl)	0.065	0.778	0.002	61.9%	85.7%	69.2%	81.2%	73.8%
CA125 (U/ml)	26.85	0.894	0.001	80%	83.3%	85.7%	76.9%	81.4%
KLK10 (ng/ml)	2	0.627	0.236	50%	78.6%	72.7%	57.8%	62.06%
KLK6 (ng/ml)	3.11	0.545	0.678	56.3%	57.1%	60%	53.3%	56.6%

sequencing would make comparison of frequencies of methylated samples in the two studies practically unfeasible (see later).

Moreover, as for the correlation between *KLK10* gene expression and *KLK10* exon 3 methylation the two studies showed similar results. In the previous work there was fair *KLK10* expression in normal samples (fully unmethylated) and high expression in the partially methylated malignant samples (3 out of 6). In concordance to those results our samples showed negative correlation between serum KLK10 level (ng/ml) and *KLK10* exon 3 unmethylated PCR product concentration (ng/µl) by Spearman's correlation and by comparing the unmethylated PCR product concentration mean ± SD in overall samples according to KLK10 level (Table 5).

While our qualitative MSP results did not show statistically significant differences in patient group samples (Table 3), *KLK10* exon 3 unmethylated PCR product concentration (ng/µl) mean ± SD showed statistically significant differences in normal and tumor samples in the two patient groups (Fig. 1). Because our MSP experiment conditions were almost constant for all PCR tests (including the operator, instruments and machines, kits and reagents, DNA template concentration, PCR program, simultaneous unmethylated- and methylated-specific PCRs, and random sample sets in 4 PCR runs done in 4 different days) those statistically significant differences of *KLK10* exon 3 unmethylated PCR product concentration should be due to differences in the methylation patterns of samples rather than due to unfounded chance (see later).

Individual cells in the same tissue may show heterogeneity as regard their DNA methylation patterns [28]. Indeed, understanding that methylation pattern heterogeneity is fundamental in interpreting qualitative and quantitative DNA methyaltion data and also for appreciating and understanding several aspects of gene functions. Each cell contains two copies of each CpG site; one on each of the two homologous chromosomes, and, therefore, can have on its own 3 different methylation patterns for that particular CpG site: fully unmethylated, fully methylated or partially methylated. The possible methylation patterns of a number (n) of CpG sites are given mathematically as 2^n. For example, when studying an average number of 12 CpGs by MSP, the possible methylation patterns in the DNA sample are 2^{12} = 4096, which reflects possible immense methylation pattern heterogeneity when the cell can have any two of these patterns. However, in the context of *KLK10* exon 3 in ovarian cancer the property of methylation pattern heterogeneity would be present almost exclusively in malignant samples but not in normal ones because in the previous work the malignant samples were partially methylated, whereas the normal samples were fully unmethylated [25].

In Fig. 3 we present a theoretical rationale for qualitative and quantitative MSP results based on possible methylation pattern heterogeneity in individual cells of a sample [28], the independency of the primer pairs in MSP from one another [23, 29] and previous DNA methylation results by MSP and direct DNA sequencing in cell lines and primary breast cancer [23]. We hypothesize that the existence of different partially methylated patterns in the sample would result in the stratification of the starting DNA template into template classes with varying MSP-

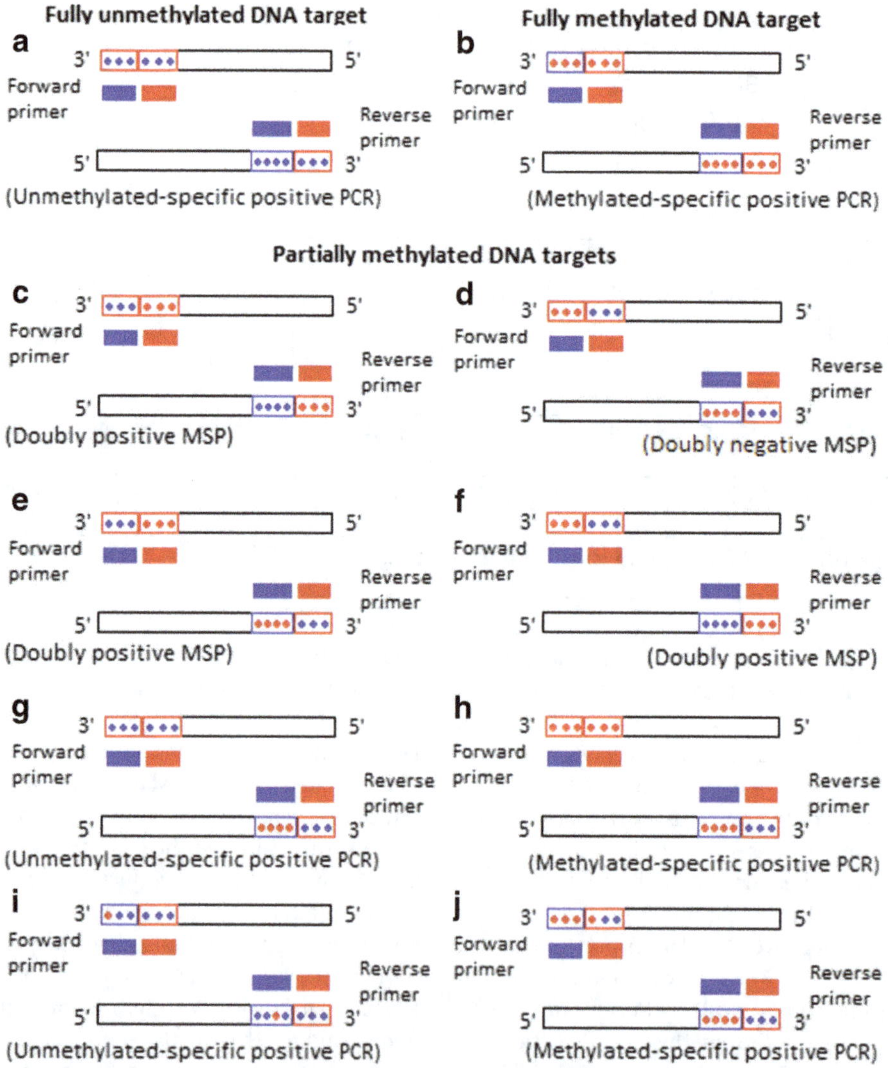

Fig. 3 The Figure shows a schematic representation of a theoretical rationale for MSP results based on previous works [23, 28, 29]. The DNA templates (long bars with 3'- > 5' directionality designation) show blue and red dots representing unmethylated and methylated CpGs, respectively. The short blue and red bars represent unmethylated- and methylated-specific primer pairs, respectively. For simplicity, we show methylation patterns with uniform methylation status at the primer's annealing site on DNA template (**a-h**) and only two with non-uniform methylation status (**i** and **j**). While fully unmethylated (**a**) and fully methylated (**b**) patterns provide unmethylated- and methylated-specific positive PCRs, respectively, partially methylated patterns (**c-j**) can have any of the four possible qualitative MSP results. MSP-inexpressible partially methylated pattern (**d**) may rationalize our doubly negative malignant sample (Sertoli-Leydig cell tumor), in addition to possible mutation as methylated CpGs are known hotspot for mutations [39, 40]

expressivities according to the number of methylation-wise matching CpG sites with their corresponding nucleotides in the respective PCR primer. While some patterns would be more or less favorable for primer annealing (Fig. 3: elements C, and E-J), other patterns may not be at all (Fig. 3: element D). Differences of the proportions of those differentially MSP-expressible partially methylated patterns in the samples may be effected practically as differences in the unmethylated PCR product concentration. Given that those partially methylated patterns would occur only in malignant samples but not in normal – and probably also benign – samples (see above), such proportionate decreases in the unmethylated PCR product concentration would happen in malignant samples only.

Our results showed statistically significant positive correlation between *KLK10* exon 3 unmethylated PCR product concentration (ng/μl) and patient age by Spearman's correlation and on comparing its mean ± SD in overall samples and in malignant samples according to age groups (Table 4). However, because there was no statistically significant difference of patient age in the two patient groups (Table 1), comparison of *KLK10* exon 3 unmethylated PCR product concentration in patient group samples should be valid and justifiable.

KLK10 exon 3 methylation correlated to high disease grade (breast cancer [30]), late stage (lung cancer [26]) and bad patient prognosis (acute lymphoblastic leukemia [24]). Similarly, the only methylated-specific PCR positive sample in our results was serous carcinoma of high grade (3) and late stage (III/IV) whose patient died within one year after starting the treatment. However, in our results comparison of *KLK10* exon 3 unmethylated PCR product concentration (ng/μl) according to disease grade, stage or patient survival did not show statistically significant differences that may be attributable to early implication of deregulated *KLK10* exon 3 methylation in the disease or lack of significant information about site-specific CpG methylation in MSP data (see later).

The notion that information about the exact location of DNA methylation maybe crucial for correct clues about disease diagnosis, prognosis and gene function [31] would greatly restrain the translational impact of DNA methylation data by MSP. For example, lack of site-specific CpG methylation data (in MSP) and/or data about their pattern distribution in the sample (in MSP and direct DNA sequencing, respectively) may explain – at least in part – the inconsistent results, in sample subsets or sample types, about the downregulation of *KLK10* through *KLK10* exon 3 hypermethylation in previous works [23–26]. At the functional aspect, the reported antitumor role of *KLK10* was demonstrated in vector-mediated transfection experiments in vitro and/or in tumor xenograft in mice using different cancer cell lines; e.g. breast [32], prostate [16] and gastric cell [33], including ovarian cell line [34]. Noteworthy is that overexpression of *KLK10* was found in malignant sample subsets (tissues or sera) in cancer types in which *KLK10* was shown experimentally as tumor suppressor; breast [35], prostate [19], gastric [36] and ovary [20, 27]. Taken together, the antitumor role of *KLK10* may be understood only in relation to the context of the given study as regard type of tissue and the underlying pathophysiologic processes [37].

Indeed, the translational impact of DNA methylation data can vary greatly with the pros and cons of the used tools. While MSP studies only a few of CpGs without regard to their exact location, direct DNA sequencing can give site-specific CpG methylation data for all CpGs of interest as percent methylation in the sample. Unfortunately, both tools fall short of providing information about site-specific CpG methylation pattern distribution in sample. The more recently discovered next generation sequencing have the advantage of presenting site-specific DNA methylation data in absolute numbers and may tackle the problem of methylation pattern distribution in hand of sophisticated computational methods [38]. Nonetheless, considering possible dynamicity of DNA methylation as a mechanism for gene regulation [1] another dimension for DNA methylation pattern resolution may be necessary in order to spot and trace such spatiotemporal DNA methylation events rather than making statements based merely on single static snapshot image.

Conclusions

In summary, our results agreed with those in the previous work as for the exclusive occurrence of *KLK10* exon 3 methylation in malignant but not in normal ovarian samples. Additionally, we assessed *KLK10* exon 3 methylation in benign ovarian tumors (not included in the previous work) and found that they were unmethylated. Although our qualitative MSP results did not show statistically significant differences in patient group samples, semi-quantitative *KLK10* exon 3 unmethylated PCR product concentration (ng/μl) showed statistically significant differences not only in tumor samples but also in otherwise histologically normal samples in benign and malignant patients. These findings would suggest, for the first time, *KLK10* exon 3 unmethylated PCR product concentration as potential early epigenetic diagnostic marker in ovarian cancer. The diagnostic potential of *KLK10* exon 3 unmethylated PCR product concentration in overall patient group samples was also evident in ROC curve analysis, and it could enhance the sensitivity of preoperative serum markers CA125, KLK10 and KLK6. Taking into account the limitations in the present study (small sample size and semi-quantitative assessment of PCR product concentration) further studies are needed before making a statement about the validity and reproducibility of these results. Moreover, we highlighted the translational limitations of DNA methylation data in MSP and direct DNA sequencing and addressed future challenges of the more recent next generation sequencing (NGS) to further enhance the translational impact of DNA methylation data.

Abbreviations

5-MC: 5-methylcytosine; bp: Base pair; CA125: Cancer antigen 125; DNA: Deoxyribonucleic acid; DNMT1: DNA methyltransferase 1; DNMT3a: DNA methyltransferase 3a; DNMT3b: DNA methyltransferase 3b; FFPE: Formalin-fixed paraffin-embedded; H&E: Hematoxylin and eosin; KLK10: Kallikrein-related peptidase 10; *KLK10*: Kallikrein-related peptidase10 gene; KLK6: Kallikrein-related peptidase 6; MECs: Human mammary epithelial cells; micRNA: micro RNA; MSP: Methylation-specific PCR; NEC: Human normal epithelial cell line; NGS: Next generation sequencing; NPV: Negative predictive value; PCR: Polymerase chain reaction; PPV: Positive predictive value; SAM: S-adenosylmethionine

Acknowledgments

We thank Dr. Mohamed Badr (PhD) from the Medical Research Center, Ain Shams Faculty of Medicine for helping in DNA extraction. We thank also Drs. Nashwa Khazragy (PhD, MD), Manar Mahmoud (PhD), Fatma Shehata (PhD) and Aisha Hussein (PhD) from the Oncology Diagnostic Unit, Biochemistry Department, Ain Shams Faculty of Medicine for helping in MSP experiments. Our thanks are due to Colors for Research laboratory in Cairo for conducting the capillary gel electrophoresis experiments. We are also much indebted to Drs. Hala El Sallaly (PhD, MD) and Sahar Ezz Elarab (PhD, MD) for helping in histopathology grading and in the statistical analysis of data, respectively.

Funding

This work was supported in part by cash money grant given once to PhD students (MAE) by The Academy of Scientific Research and Technology in Cairo. The funding body had no role in the design of the study and collection, analysis, and interpretation of data and in writing the manuscript.

Authors' contributions

MAE and AAM contributed equally to the conception and design of this work. MAE collected patient data and tissue samples and performed the experiments. ZAS performed and examined H&E sections of tissue samples. MAE interpreted the data and wrote the manuscript. AAM, MMS, EAS, ZAS and AHE revised the manuscript critically for important intellectual content. All authors read and approved the final manuscript.

Competing interests

The authors declare that they have no competing interests.

Author details

[1]Medical Biochemistry Department, Faculty of Medicine, Ain Shams University, Cairo, Egypt. [2]Gynecologic Oncology Unit, Ain Shams University Maternity Hospital, Cairo, Egypt.

References

1. Wallace K, Grau MV, Levine AJ, Shen LL, Hamdan R, Chen XL, Gui JA, Haile RW, Barry EL, Ahnen D, McKeown-Eyssen G, Baron JA, Issa JPJ. Association between folate levels and CpG Island Hypermethylation in normal colorectal mucosa. Cancer Prev Res (Phila). 2010;3:1552–64.
2. Bird A, Tate P, Nan X, Campory J, Meehan R, Cross S, Tweedie S, Charlton J, Macleod D. Studies of DNA methyaltion in animals. J Cell Sci. 1995;Suppl 19:37–9.
3. Bird AP. Functions of DNA methylation in vertebrates. Cold Spring Harb Symp Quant Biol. 1993;58:281–5.
4. Horvath S. DNA methylation age of human tissues and cell types. Genome Biol. 2013; https://doi.org/10.1186/gb-2013-14-10-r115.
5. Miller C, Sweatt J. Covalent modification of DNA regulates memory formation. Neuron. 2007;53(6):857–69. https://doi.org/10.1016/j.neuron.2007.02.022.
6. Gardiner-Garden M, Frommer M. CpG islands in vertebrate genomes. Mol Biol. 1987;196:261–82.
7. Jones PA, Liang G. Rethinking how DNA methylation patterns are maintained. Nat Rev Genet. 2009;10(11):805–11.
8. Miranda TB, Jones PA. DNA methylation: the nuts and bolts of repression. J Cell Physiol. 2007;213:384–90.
9. Costello JF, Plass C. Methylation matters. J Med Genet. 2001;38(5):285–303.
10. Balgkouranidou I, Triantafyllou P, Theodoropoulos C, Tsaroucha EG, Kaklamanis L, Lianidou E. Prognsotic significance of DNA methylation markers in tissue and corresponding cell-free circulating DNA in plasma of NSCLC patients, vol. 2009. Denver: AACR 2009. 100st Annual Meeting of American Association of Cancer Research (AACR).
11. Yousef GM, Chang A, Scorilas A, Diamandis EP. Genomic organization of the human kallikrein gene family on chromosome 19q13.3-q13.4. Biochem Biophys Res Commun. 2000;276(1):125–33.
12. Liu XL, Wazer DE, Watanabe K, Band V. Identification of a novel serine protease-like gene, the expression of which is down-regulated during breast cancer progression. Cancer Res. 1996;56(14):3371–9.
13. Shaw JL, Diamandis EP. Distribution of 15 human kallikreins in tissues and biological fluids. Clin Chem. 2007;53(8):1423–32.
14. Luo LY, Grass L, Diamandis EP. Steroid hormone regulation of the human kallikrein 10 (*KLK10*) gene in cancer cell lines and functional characterization of the *KLK10* gene promoter. Clin Chim Acta. 2003;337(1–2):115–26.
15. Chow TF, Crow M, Earle T, El-Said H, Diamandis EP, Yousef GM. Kallikreins as microRNA targets: an in silico and experimental-based analysis. Biol Chem. 2008;389(6):731–8.
16. Hu J, Lei H, Fei X, Liang S, Xu H, Qin D, Wang Y, Wu Y, Li B. NES1/KLK10 gene represses proliferation, enhances apoptosis and downregulates glucose metabolism of PC3 prostate cancer cells. Sci Rep. 2015; https://doi.org/10.1038/serp17426.
17. Dhar S, Bhargava R, Yunes M, Li B, Goyal J, Naber SP, Wazer DE, Band V. Analysis of normal epithelial cell specific-1 (NES1)/kallikrein 10 mRNA expression by in situ hybridization, a novel marker for breast cancer. Clin Cancer Res. 2001;7(11):3393–8.
18. Luo LY, Rajpert-De Meyts ER, Jung K, Diamandis EP. Expression of the normal epithelial cell-specific 1 (NES1; KLK10) candidate tumor suppressor gene in normal and malignant testicular tissue. Br J Cancer. 2001;85(2):220–4.
19. Petraki CD, Gregorakis AK, Papanastasiou PA, Karavana V, Luo LY, Diamandis EP. Immunohistochemical localization of human kalikreins 6, 10 and 13 in benign and malignant prostatic tissues. Prostate Cancer Prostatic Dis. 2003; 6(3):223–7.
20. Shvartsman HS, Lu KH, Lee J, Lillie J, Deavers MT, Clifford S, Wolf JK, Mills GB, Bast RC Jr, Gershenson DM, Schmandt R. Overexpression of kallikrein 10 in epithelial ovarian carcinoma. Gynecol Oncol. 2003;90(1):44–50.
21. Talieri M, Alexopoulou DK, Scorilas A, Kypraios D, Arnogiannaki N, Devetzi M, Patsavela M, Xynopoulos D. Expression analysis and clinical evaluation of kallikrein-related peptidase 10 (KLK10) in colorectal cancer. Tumour Biol. 2011;32(4):737–44.
22. Rückert F, Hennig M, Petraki CD, Wehrum D, Distler M, Denz A, Schröder M, Dawelbait G, Kalthhoff H, Saeger HD, Diamandis EP, Pilarsky C, Grützmann R. Co-expression of KLK6 and KLK10 as prognostic factors for survival in pancreatic ductal adenocarcinoma. Br J Cancer. 2008;99(9):1484–92.
23. Li B, Goyal J, Dhar S, Dimri G, Evron E, Sukumar S, Wazer DE, Band V. CpG methylation as a basis for breast tumor-specific loss of NES1/KLK10 expression. Cancer Res. 2001;61(21):8014–21.
24. Roman-Gomez J, Jimenez-Velasco A, Agirre X, Castillejo JA, Barrios M, Andreu EJ, Prosper F, Heiniger A, Torres A. The normal epithelial cell-specific 1 (NES1) gene, a candidate tumor suppressor gene on chromosome 19q13. 3-4, is downregulated by hypermethylation in acute lymphoblastic leukemia. Leukemia. 2004;18(2):362–5.

25. Sidiropoulos M, Pampalakis G, Sotiropoulo G, Katsaros D, Diamandis EP. Downregulation of human kallikrein 10 (KLK10/NES1) by CpG hypermethylation in breast, ovarian and prostate cancers. Tumour Biol. 2005;26(6):324–36.
26. Zhang Y, Song H, Miao Y, Wang R, Chen L. Frequent transcriptional inactivation of Kallikrein 10 gene by CpG island hypermethylation in non-small cell lung cancer. Cancer Sci. 2010;101(4):934–40.
27. El Sherbini MA, Sallam MM, Shaban EA, El-Shalakany AH. Diagnostic value of serum kallikrein-related peptidases 6 and 10 versus CA125 in ovarian cancer. Int J Gynecol Cancer. 2011;21(4):625–32.
28. Crider KS, Yang TP, Berry RJ, Bailey LB. Folate and DNA methylation: a review of molecular mechanisms and the evidence for Folate's role. Adv Nutr. 2012;3:21–38. https://doi.org/10.3945/an.111.000992.
29. Herman JG, Graff JR, Myöhänen S, Nelkin BD, Baylin SB. Methylation-specific PCR: a novel PCR assay for methylation status of CpG islands. Proc Natl Acad Sci U S A. 1996;93(18):9821–6.
30. Kioulafa M, Kaklamanis L, Stathopoulos E, Mavroudis D, Georgoulias V, Lianidou ES. Kallikrein 10 (KLK10) methylation as a novel prognostic biomarker in early breast cancer. Ann Oncol. 2009;20(6):1020–5.
31. van Vlodrop IJH, Niessen HE, Derks S, Baldewijns MM, van Criekinge W, Herman JG, van Engeland M. Analysis of promoter CpgG island hypermethylation in cancer: location, location, location! Clin Cancer Res. 2011;17(13):4225–31.
32. Goyal J, Smith KM, Cowan JM, Wazer DE, Lee SW, Band V. The role for NES1 serine protease as a novel tumor suppressor. Cancer Res. 1998;58(21):4782–6.
33. Huang W, Tian X-L, Wu Y-L, Zhong J, Yu L-F, Hu SP, Li B. Suppression of gastric cancer growth by baculovirus vector-mediated transfer of normal epithelial cell specific-1 gene. World J Gastroenterol. 2008;14:5810–5.
34. Pépin D, Shao ZQ, Huppé G, Wakefield A, Chu CW, Sharif Z, Vanderhyden BC. Kallikreins 5, 6 and 10 differentially alter pathophysiology and overall survival in an ovarian cancer xenograft model. PLoS One. 2011;6(11):e26075. https://doi.org/10.1371/journal.pone.0026075.
35. Ewan King L, Li X, Cheikh Saad Bouh K, Pedneault M, Chu CW. Human kallikrein 10 ELISA development and validation in breast cancer sera. Clin Biochem. 2007;40(13–14):1057–62.
36. Jiao X, Lu H-J, Zhai M-M, Zhang D-P. Overexpression of kallikrein gene 10 is a biomarker for predicting poor prognosis in gastric cancer. World J Gastroenterol. 2013;19(48):9425–31.
37. Borgoño CA, Diamandis EP. The emerging roles of human tissue kallikreins in cancer. Nat Rev Cancer. 2004;4:876–90. https://doi.org/10.1038/nrc1474.
38. Xu H, Podolsky RH, Ryu D, Wang X, Su S, Shi H, George V. A method to detect differentially methylated loci with next-generation sequencing. Genet Epidemiol. 2012;37(4):377–82.
39. Cooper DN, Youssoufian H. The CpG dinucleotide and human genetic disease. Hum Genet. 1988;78:151–5.
40. Rideout WM, Coetzee GA, Olumi AF, Jones PA. 5-Methylcytosine as an endogenous mutagen in the human LDL receptor and p53 genes. Science. 1990;249(4974):1288–90.

11

Differential cyclooxygenase expression levels and survival associations in type I and type II ovarian tumors

Alicia Beeghly-Fadiel[1,2], Andrew J. Wilson[3], Spencer Keene[1], Meral El Ramahi[3], Shu Xu[4], Lawrence J. Marnett[4,5], Oluwole Fadare[6], Marta A. Crispens[2,3] and Dineo Khabele[7*]

Abstract

Background: High cyclooxygenase (COX)-2 expression in ovarian tumors has been associated with poor prognosis, but the role of COX-1 expression and its relation to survival is less clear. Here, we evaluated COX expression and associations with survival outcomes between type I (clear cell, mucinous, low grade endometrioid and low grade serous) and type II (high grade serous and high grade endometrioid) ovarian tumors.

Methods: We developed and validated a new COX-1 antibody, and conducted immunohistochemical (IHC) staining for COX-1 and COX-2 on a tissue microarray (TMA) of 190 primary ovarian tumors. In addition to standard IHC scoring and H-scores to combine the percentage of positive cells and staining intensity, we also measured COX-1 and COX-2 mRNA expression by QPCR. High expression was defined as greater than or equal to median values. Clinical characteristics and disease outcomes were ascertained from medical records. Associations with disease-free survival (DFS) and overall survival (OS) were quantified by hazard ratios (HRs) and confidence intervals (CIs) from proportional hazards regression.

Results: Type I tumors had high COX-2 expression, while type II tumors had high COX-1 expression. In multivariable adjusted regression models, higher COX-1 mRNA expression was associated with shorter DFS (HR: 6.37, 95% CI: 1.84–22.01) and OS (HR: 2.26, 95% CI: 1.04–4.91), while higher H-scores for COX-2 expression were associated with shorter DFS (HR: 1.92, 95% CI: 1.06–3.49). Stratified analysis indicated that COX-2 was significantly associated with DFS among cases with Type II tumors (HR: 1.93, 95% CI: 1.06–3.53).

Conclusions: These findings suggest that ovarian tumor type contributes to differences in COX expression levels and associations with survival.

Keywords: Cyclooxygenase, Ovarian cancer, Tumor subtype, Survival analysis

Background

Ovarian cancer is the 5th leading cause of cancer deaths among women in the United States (US), and has an overall five year survival rate of only 46% [1]. Surgical tumor debulking and a combination of platinum and taxane chemotherapy are standard treatment for ovarian cancer [2]. While survival rates have modestly improved over time, the mortality rate of ovarian cancer has not substantially changed for nearly 50 years, remaining at approximately 10 women per 100,000 [2–4]. Identifying additional ways to improve treatment, extend survival, and decrease mortality are critical research priorities for ovarian cancer [2, 3].

Ovarian cancer is classified into two distinct types with different etiologies based on histology and grade: indolent type I and aggressive type II tumors [2, 5, 6]. Clear cell, mucinous, low grade endometrioid and low grade serous cancers are type I, whereas high grade serous, high grade endometrioid, carcinosarcomas, and undifferentiated cancers are type II tumors [2, 5]. Type I tumors typically arise from benign precursor lesions and are

* Correspondence: dkhabele@kumc.edu
[7]Department of Obstetrics and Gynecology, Division of Gynecologic Oncology, The University of Kansas Medical Center, MS 2028, 3901 Rainbow Boulevard, Kansas City, KS 66160, USA
Full list of author information is available at the end of the article

generally slow-growing, low grade, and chromosomally stable. In contrast, type II tumors are fast-growing, high grade, and genetically unstable [2, 5]. In addition to differences in etiology, prognosis differs, as women with type I tumors generally fare much better than those with type II tumors [2, 7].

Two cyclooxygenase (COX) isoforms, also known as prostaglandin H_2 synthases (PTGS or PGHS), are rate-limiting enzymes that produce prostaglandins by catalyzing the oxidation of arachidonic acid to tissue-specific lipid prostanoids [8, 9]. Effects downstream of COX include inflammation, platelet activation, cellular proliferation, angiogenesis, invasion, and metastasis [9, 10]. COX-2 is strongly implicated in ovarian cancer progression; meta-analysis of 15 studies found 35% significantly worse survival for cases with COX-2 positive tumors [11]. Despite this evidence, questions remain, as studies included in the meta-analysis were small (average $N =$ 104), included predominantly non-US study populations, and had significant heterogeneity across findings [11]. COX-1 may also be relevant to ovarian cancer progression. Unlike most other solid malignancies where COX-2 expression is high, our group and others have found higher COX-1 than COX-2 levels in high grade serous ovarian cancer [12–14]. Despite this unique expression, only a few small studies have evaluated COX-1 in ovarian cancer survival, and evidence of an association has been limited [15–17]. In one small study, semi-quantitative PCR indicated that serous and entrometrioid had higher, while clear cell carcinomas had lower COX-2 levels [18]. Other studies that used immunohistochemistry (IHC) found that both COX-1 and COX-2 were higher in non-mucinous than mucinous tumors [16, 19]. Our prior report showed higher COX-1 than COX-2 in serous tumors [12]. One study of 65 cases found no difference in COX-2 expression by tumor type [20], but both COX isozymes were significantly associated with tumor type in another studyof 82 type I and 131 type II tumors [21]. Analyses stratified by tumor type are limited with regard to survival, and no prior reports have evaluated the significance of an interaction term between COX expression and tumor type in multivariable regression models.

The purpose of this study was to determine if COX expression and associations with survival outcomes differ between type I and type II ovarian tumors. Since possible cross-reactivity between IHC antibodies for COX-1 and COX-2 may have influenced prior findings, we generated and validated a new COX-1 antibody. We then measured COX-1 and COX-2 expression in type and type II ovarian tumors and tested associations with disease-free survival (DFS) and overall survival (OS) from ovarian cancer. These findings may have important implications for disease prognosis and for COX targeted therapeutic interventions for women with ovarian cancer.

Methods

Antibody generation

Generation of a new rabbit polyclonal anti-COX-1 antibody was conducted at the Vanderbilt Antibody and Protein Resource. The protein sequence of human COX-1 and COX-2 were compared to identify unique COX-1 sequences [22]. Anti–human COX-1 antibodies were generated by immunization of two New Zealand white rabbits with three KLH-conjugated human COX-1 specific peptides (peptide sequences: CQDDGPAVERPS, ADPGAPTPVC, and LMHYPRGIPPQSQMAC) which have no overlap with the corresponding COX-2 protein sequence (Additional file 1). Bleeds from sequential boosts were collected from both rabbits and tested by Western blot and ELISA. Antisera from both animals were mixed for affinity purification. Polyclonal antibodies were purified using affinity against immunizing peptides and then the elution was sequentially cleared by a mouse COX-2 immobilized affinity column. Final antibodies were further validated by Western blot, and demonstrated to have no cross-reactivity with COX-2 (Additional file 1). Antibodies used for Western blot included the newly generated Vanderbilt rabbit polyclonal anti-COX-1 (1:2000 overnight), rabbit polyclonal anti-COX-2 (1:1000 overnight; Cayman Chemicals, Ann Arbor, MI), and mouse monoclonal anti-actin (1:10000 for 15 mins; Sigma Chemical Co, St Louis, MO); positive controls included recombinant ovine COX-1 and human COX-2 (both from Cayman Chemicals).

Laboratory analysis

A tissue microarray (TMA) was created from primary ovarian cancer samples from the Vanderbilt Tissue Repository for Ovarian Cancer (TROC), as previously described [12]. We conducted immunostaining with the newly generated rabbit polyclonal COX-1 antibody (designated Vanderbilt), the well-characterized commercially available mouse monoclonal COX-1 antibody (Cat#sc-19,998; Santa Cruz Biotechnology, Dallas, TX), and a widely-used mouse monoclonal COX-2 antibody l (Cat# 18–7379; Thermo Fisher Scientific, Inc., Waltham, MA), as previously described [12]. Immunohistochemistry (IHC) was performed in the Vanderbilt Translational Pathology Shared Resource. Whole-slide imaging and semi-quantitative measurement of the percentage of tumor cells showing positive cytoplasmic expression was performed using the automated Ariol® SL-50 Platform in the Digital Histology Shared Resource (DHSR) of the Vanderbilt University Medical Center (VUMC). For comparability with existing literature, IHC staining was first categorized as weak (< 10% positive), moderate (10–50% positive), or strong (> 50% positive). In addition to this standard IHC scoring, we also multiplied the the percentage of cells staining positive (0–100) by staining intensity (weak: 1, moderate: 2, strong: 3), which resulted in an H-score ranging from 0 to 300 [23]. Steady-state expression levels of COX-1 and COX-2 were also measured at the mRNA level by quantitative real-time PCR (QPCR), as previously described [12].

Statistical analysis

Correlations between continuous variables were evaluated with Pearson's correlation coefficient. Standard IHC scoring was dichotomized as weak or moderate/strong; expression measured by H-scores and QPCR was dichotomized, with high defined as greater than or equal to median values. Associations with COX expression were assessed with Student's t-tests for continuous or x^2 tests for categorical variables. Overall survival (OS) was defined as the interval between cancer diagnosis and death, or else censored at the date of last contact in medical records. Disease-free survival (DFS) was defined as the interval between cancer diagnosis and evidence of disease recurrence, or else censored at the date of death or last contact; women that died without a disease-free interval were excluded from these analyses. Associations with survival were evaluated using Cox proportional hazards regression to calculate hazard ratios (HR) and corresponding 95% confidence intervals (CI). Clinical covariates of interest included age, stage of disease, histologic subtype, grade, residual disease, and platinum sensitivity. High grade serous and high grade endometrioid tumors were classified as type II tumors; all others were classified as type I tumors [24]. Differences in associations by tumor type were evaluated in stratified models; to formally test statistical interactions, multiplicative terms were created and included in regression models. Kaplan-Meier functions were employed to visually evaluate survival outcomes; differences in curves were evaluated with Log Rank tests. A P-value ≤ 0.05 was interpreted as statistically significant. All analyses were conducted with SAS v 9.4.

Results

A total of 190 epithelial ovarian cancer cases from the Vanderbilt TROC were evaluated for COX expression by IHC; representative staining images in a high-grade serous tumor are shown in Fig. 1. The majority of cases evaluated were Caucasian (88.4%), and had high grade (82.6%), late stage (III or IV = 69.0%), and serous histology (60.0%; Table 1). COX-1 H-scores for the new Vanderbilt and Santa Cruz commercial antibody were 97.6% correlated, and were not related to COX-2 expression levels by IHC (Fig. 2a & Additional file 2). Unless otherwise stated, COX-1 IHC expression data was hereafter from the new Vanderbilt developed antibody.

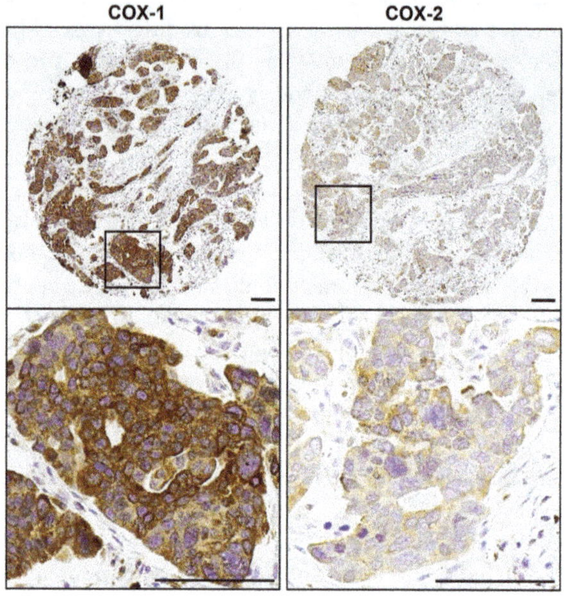

Fig. 1 Representative IHC Images for COX-1 and COX-2, the Vanderbilt TROC. Representative immunohistochemical staining for COX-1 and COX-2 in a high-grade serous (VOC-A-155) section from a TMA of 190 ovarian tumors. Higher power images of the boxed areas are shown in the corresponding right panels. Scale bars represent 100 μM

Expression of both COX isozymes, as measured by H-score, significantly differed in high grade serous, mucinous, and endometrioid ovarian cancers (Fig. 2b). High COX-1 levels were observed in both low and high grade serous tumors, and were significantly lower in tumors of non-serous histology. Biologically aggressive Type II tumors (high grade serous and high grade endometrioid) had significantly higher COX-1 expression than Type I tumors. A similar pattern of COX-1 expression was observed with the commercial antibody (Additional file 2). In contrast, COX-2 levels were significantly higher in non-serous and type I tumors (Fig. 2b and c). To further validate the specificity of our antibodies, we also measured COX gene expression by QPCR. Among 49 serous cases with both COX-1 measures available, protein and mRNA levels were highly correlated for both the newly developed Vanderbilt COX-1 antibody ($r = 0.764$, $P < 0.0001$) and the commercial COX-1 antibody ($r = 0.763$, $P < 0.0001$); similarly, for 36 serous cases with both COX-2 measures available, H-scores and mRNA measures were highly correlated ($r = 0.738$, $P < 0.0001$) (Additional file 3).

Associations between COX IHC and clinical covariates are shown in Table 2. Regardless of whether standard IHC or H-Scores were evaluated, cases with high COX-1 expression levels were more likely to have late stage disease, serous histology, and to be type II tumors (all P-values < 0.05). For COX-2, cases with high expression

Table 1 Clinical characteristics of 190 epithelial ovarian cancer cases from the Vanderbilt TROC

Characteristic	N or mean	% or std. dev
Age at Diagnosis, years	57.9	(13.7)
Overall Survival, years	4.3	(3.4)
Disease-Free Survival, years	3.9	(3.4)
Race		
White	168	(88.4)
African American	11	(5.8)
Other/Unknown	11	(5.8)
Histologic Subtype		
Serous	131	(69.0)
Endometrioid	25	(13.2)
Mucinous	14	(7.4)
Clear Cell	9	(4.7)
Mixed	6	(3.2)
Other	5	(2.6)
Stage		
I	50	(26.3)
II	7	(3.7)
III	110	(57.9)
IV	21	(11.1)
Unstaged	2	(1.1)
Grade		
Low Grade	33	(17.4)
High Grade	157	(82.6)
Tumor Type		
Type I	65	(34.2)
Type II	125	(65.8)
Residual Disease		
Optimal Debulking	47	(24.7)
Suboptimal Debulking	89	(46.8)
Unknown or Not Applicable	54	(28.4)
Platinum Sensitive Disease		
Resistant	39	(20.5)
Sensitive	81	(42.6)
Unknown or Not Applicable	70	(36.8)

Percentages may not sum to 100 due to rounding error

levels were more likely to have early stage disease, non-serous histology, less differentiation, optimal debulking, platinum sensitivity, and be type I tumors (all *P*-values < 0.05). High COX-2 was also associated with younger age at diagnosis, but only when measured by H-score.

Next, we evaluated COX expression in relation to ovarian cancer survival (Table 3). By standard IHC scoring, high COX-1 was associated with significantly worse DFS in unadjusted analysis (HR: 2.34, 95% CI: 1.30–4.24), but this association was attenuated after multivariable adjustment. On the contrary, COX-1 expression by QPCR was associated with a significantly shorter disease-free interval after both minimal (HR: 4.12, 95% CI: 1.51–11.26) and full multivariable adjustment (HR: 6.37, 95% CI: 1.84–22.01), and significantly shorter OS after multivariable adjustment (HR: 2.26, 95% CI: 1.04–4.91). In crude analyses, high COX-2 was associated with significantly better DFS (HR: 0.51, 95% CI: 0.30–0.87) and OS (HR: 0.52, 95% CI: 0.36–0.77) by standard IHC, and significantly better OS by H-score (HR: 0.57, 95% CI: 0.39–0.82). However, these associations did not withstand adjustment for clinical covariates, and instead high COX-2 by H-score was associated with significantly shorter DFS in both minimally (HR: 1.93, 95% CI: 1.08–3.46) and fully adjusted models (HR: 1.92, 95% CI: 1.06–3.49).

To further clarify the role of COX expression in ovarian cancer survival, we also evaluated data for 489 high grade serous ovarian cancer cases from The Cancer Genome Atlas (TCGA). We downloaded normalized RNA-seq mRNA data and survival times from the Broad Institute Firehose (https://gdac.broadinstitute.org) and found that cases with median or higher COX-1 levels tended to have shorter DFS (HR: 1.25, 95% CI: 0.93–1.68), but no association with OS (HR: 1.07, 95% CI: 0.80–1.44). When we applied this approach to COX-2, no association was found for DFS (HR: 0.91, 95% CI: 0.68–1.27), but high COX-2 was significantly associated with worse OS (HR: 1.36, 95% CI: 1.02–1.82). As expected, Kaplan-Meier survival functions (Fig. 3) were found to be in agreement with unadjusted analyses, with a suggestive association for high COX-1 and DFS (*P*-value = 0.142) and significantly worse OS for high COX-2 (*P*-value = 0.035).

Because TCGA includes only high grade serous ovarian cancers, interactions with tumor type could not be evaluated in this data. Similarly, nearly all cases for which we conducted QPCR were type II tumors. Thus, to determine if associations differed between type I and type II tumors, we evalutated dichotomized COX H-scores in stratified analyses (Table 4). High COX-2 was associated with better OS in unadjusted analysis among type I cases (HR: 0.38, 95% CI: 0.16–0.88), and worse DFS in multivariable adjusted analyses among type II cases (HR: 1.93, 95% HR: 1.06–3.53). While these associations were significant within strata, they did not significantly differ across strata, as statistical interaction terms between COX-2 and tumor type were only suggestive for DFS (P-interaction = 0.181) and OS (P-interaction = 0.051).

Discussion

To test our hypothesis that COX expression levels differ across type I and type II ovarian tumors, we measured

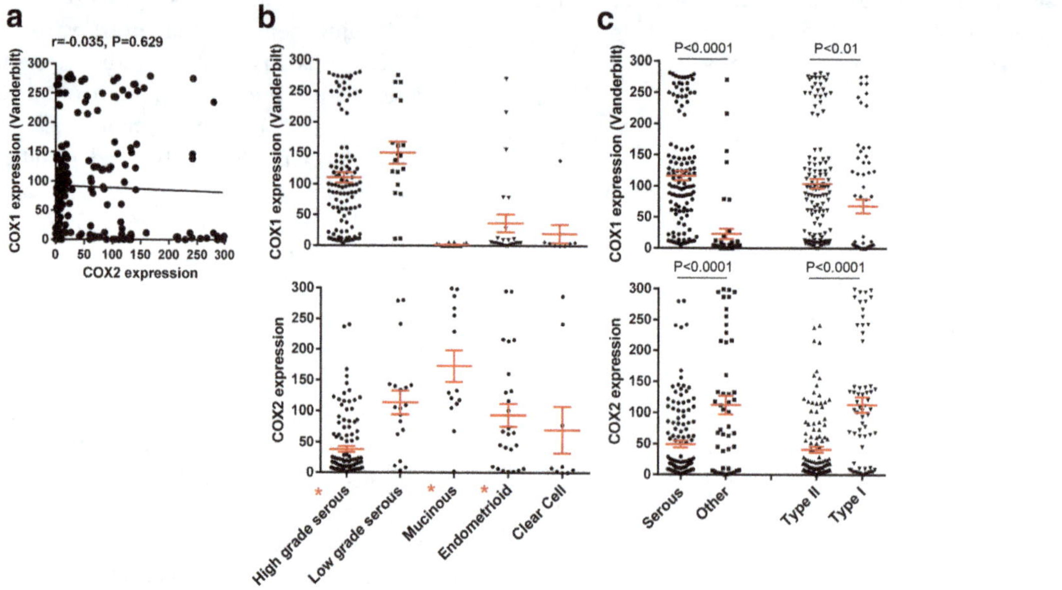

Fig. 2 COX-1 and COX-2 protein expression in ovarian cancer. The percentage of tumor cells positive for COX-1 and COX-2 was determined by automated image analysis and then scaled by intensity for H-scores, ranging from 0 to 300. **a** Pearson correlation between expression levels of COX-1 and COX-2. H-scores for COX-1 and COX-2 expression in (**b**) serous, endometrioid, mucinous and clear cell tumors, and in (**c**) serous tumors versus all other epithelial tumors and type II tumors (high grade serous and high grade endometrioid) versus type I tumors (all other types). *P*-values from Student's t-tests

both COX-1 and COX-2 isozymes in samples from 190 primary ovarian cancer cases from the Vanderbilt TROC. Because cross-reactivity between COX-1 and COX-2 may have influenced prior findings, we developed and validated a new rabbit COX-1 polyclonal antibody. Our new COX-1 antibody had no cross-reactivity with COX-2 and excellent correlation with the commercial COX-1 antibody that we previously evaluated [12]. Our assays were both sensitive and specific as indicated by significant correlations between protein and mRNA expression for both COX-1 and COX-2, and no relationship between measures across the two isoforms. For protein expression by IHC, we also compared standard scoring and H-scores that incorporated both the percentage of positive tumor cells and the staining intensity. Regardless of assay, our analysis indicates that COX-1 and COX-2 expression levels differ across ovarian tumor types: high COX-1 expression was found in type II tumors and high COX-2 expression was found in type I tumors.

With regard to patient outcomes, high COX-1 was associated with shorter DFS in unadjusted models when measured by IHC and in models adjusted for clinical covariates when measured by QPCR. On the contrary, COX-2 measured by QPCR was not associated with any outcome, while high COX-2 by IHC was associated with shorter DFS after adjustment for clinical covariates. RNA-seq data from TCGA also suggested an association between high COX-1 and worse DFS, and showed a significant association for high COX-2 and worse OS. Thus, methodological differences, such as measurement of mRNA or protein, adjustment for clinical covariates, and heterogeneity of tumor types contribute to variation in associations between COX expression and ovarian cancer survival.

Numerous prior reports on COX-2 support a relation with ovarian cancer survival [15, 18, 19, 21, 25–28], and meta-analysis of 15 studies yielded a significantassociation with OS (HR: 1.34, 95% CI: 1.05–1.71) [11]. However, results across studies were highly heterogeneous ($I^2 = 56.5\%$) [11]. Based on current findings, possible reasons underlying the wide variation across prior reports includes differences in statistical methods, such as covariates adjusted for in regression models, and laboratory differences, such as assays and thresholds used to define positive expression. With regard to DFS, our findings from standard IHC and H-scores did show some variation, with HRs of 1.54 and 1.92, respectively. These generally agreewith findings from meta-analysis of 5 studies (HR: 1.36, 95% CI: 0.79–2.33) [11]. However, our results also suggest that COX-2 OS associations may vary by tumor type, with increased hazards only among type II tumors. Prior studies that stratified by tumor type are limited. In one analysis of 23 type I and 42 type II ovarian cancers, high COX-2 expression was not significantly associated with survival [20].

Table 2 Associations between COX expression levels and clinical covariates, the Vanderbilt TROC

	COX-1 / PTGS-1					COX-2 / PTGS-2				
	Standard IHC scoring			H-Score		Standard IHC scoring			H-Score	
Characteristic	N (%) weak	Moderate & strong	*P*-value	Mean (std err)	*P*-value	N (%) weak	Moderate & strong	*P*-value	Mean (std err)	*P*-value
Age										
< 57.6	39 (50.7)	56 (49.6)	0.883	91.2 (9.4)	0.889	46 (44.7)	49 (56.3)	0.109	77.6 (8.8)	**0.047**
≥57.6	38 (49.4)	57 (50.4)		93.0 (9.3)		57 (55.3)	38 (43.7)		54.6 (7.3)	
Stage										
I/II	32 (41.6)	25 (22.1)	**0.004**	72.1 (11.9)	**0.047**	17 (16.5)	40 (46.0)	**< 0.001**	111.5 (12.8)	**< 0.001**
III/IV/Unstaged	45 (58.4)	88 (77.9)		100.6 (7.9)		86 (83.5)	47 (54.0)		46.7 (5.4)	
Histologic Subtype										
Serous	47 (61.0)	12 (10.6)	**< 0.001**	116.5 (7.6)	**< 0.001**	82 (79.6)	49 (56.3)	**< 0.001**	49.7 (5.4)	**< 0.001**
Non-Serous	30 (39.0)	101 (89.4)		37.9 (9.7)		21 (20.4)	38 (43.7)		102.7 (13.2)	
Grade										
Low Grade	15 (19.5)	18 (15.9)	0.526	92.4 (16.4)	0.982	5 (4.9)	28 (32.2)	**< 0.001**	134.0 (16.1)	**< 0.001**
High Grade	62 (80.5)	95 (84.1)		92.0 (7.2)		98 (95.2)	59 (67.8)		51.9 (5.5)	
Type										
Type I Tumors	39 (50.7)	26 (23.0)	**< 0.001**	68.4 (11.1)	**0.009**	19 (18.5)	46 (52.9)	**< 0.001**	113.4 (12.2)	**< 0.001**
Type II Tumors	38 (49.4)	87 (77.0)		104.4 (8.0)		84 (81.6)	41 (47.1)		41.5 (4.8)	
Residual Disease[a]										
Optimal	22 (43.1)	25 (29.4)	0.103	78.4 (12.2)	0.177	16 (21.1)	31 (51.7)	**< 0.001**	109.1 (14.0)	**< 0.001**
Suboptimal	29 (56.9)	60 (70.6)		97.3 (9.3)		60 (79.0)	29 (48.3)		42.4 (6.1)	
Platinum Sensitivity[b]										
Resistant	12 (30.0)	27 (33.8)	0.679	93.0 (13.6)	0.884	28 (40.0)	11 (22.0)	**0.038**	37.7 (8.7)	**0.030**
Sensitive	28 (70.0)	53 (66.3)		95.5 (9.7)		42 (60.0)	39 (78.0)		63.8 (8.2)	

Bold values denote signficant associations; column percentages may not sum to 100% due to rounding error
[a]Among cases with known cytoreductive status
[b]Among cases treated with platinum with response to treatment known

Table 3 Associations between COX expression levels and ovarian cancer survival, the Vanderbilt TROC

	Disease-free survival (DFS), hazard ratio (95% CI), *P*-value						Overall survival (OS), hazard ratio (95% CI), *P*-value					
	IHC[1]		H-Score[2]		QPCR[3]		IHC[1]		H-Score[2]		QPCR[3]	
COX-1 / PTGS1												
N cases / events[a]	47 / 15 vs 71 / 42		60 / 26 vs 58 / 31		15 / 12 vs 17 / 13		77 / 43 vs 113 / 77		95 / 57 vs 95 / 63		24 / 19 vs 25 / 18	
Unadjusted	**2.34 (1.30–4.24)**	**0.005**	1.49 (0.88–2.50)	0.138	1.77 (0.79–3.98)	0.168	1.13 (0.78–1.65)	0.515	1.09 (0.76–1.56)	0.647	1.17 (0.61–2.23)	0.641
Adjusted[b]	1.58 (0.85–2.94)	0.148	1.44 (0.85–2.43)	0.180	**4.12 (1.51–11.26)**	**0.006**	0.79 (0.54–1.16)	0.227	0.97 (0.68–1.40)	0.882	2.02 (0.96–4.22)	0.063
Adjusted[c]	1.55 (0.81–2.98)	0.187	1.30 (0.75–2.34)	0.356	**6.37 (1.84–22.01)**	**0.003**	0.87 (0.59–1.30)	0.495	1.14 (0.78–1.65)	0.504	**2.26 (1.04–4.91)**	**0.039**
COX-2 / PTGS2												
N cases / events	50 / 33 vs 68 / 24		46 / 29 vs 72 / 28		10 / 10 vs 14 / 9		103 / 80 vs 87 / 40		95 / 72 vs 95 / 48		18 / 16 vs 18 / 11	
Unadjusted	**0.51 (0.30–0.87)**	**0.013**	0.61 (0.36–1.02)	0.061	0.51 (0.20–1.29)	0.154	**0.52 (0.36–0.77)**	**< 0.001**	**0.57 (0.39–0.82)**	**0.002**	0.59 (0.27–1.27)	0.173
Adjusted[b]	1.53 (0.85–2.76)	0.160	**1.93 (1.08–3.46)**	**0.028**	0.86 (0.30–2.45)	0.772	0.85 (0.57–1.27)	0.420	0.89 (0.61–1.31)	0.559	0.77 (0.35–1.71)	0.519
Adjusted[c]	1.54 (0.84–2.80)	0.161	**1.92 (1.06–3.49)**	**0.033**	0.87 (0.31–2.47)	0.798	1.05 (0.69–1.59)	0.818	1.05 (0.71–1.56)	0.802	1.40 (0.56–3.51)	0.477

[1]COX protein measured by immunohistochemistry: moderate & strong vs weak
[2]COX protein measured by H-Score: dichotomized at median
[3]COX gene expression measured by quantitative real-time PCR: dichotomized at median
[a]N cases / N events, reference vs high COX
[b]Adjusted for age at diagnosis (continuous), stage (early, late), and tumor type (I, II)
[c]Additionally adjusted for debulking (optimal, suboptimal, missing) and platinum sensitivity (sensitive, resistant, missing)
Bold values denote signficant associations; column percentages may not sum to 100% due to rounding error

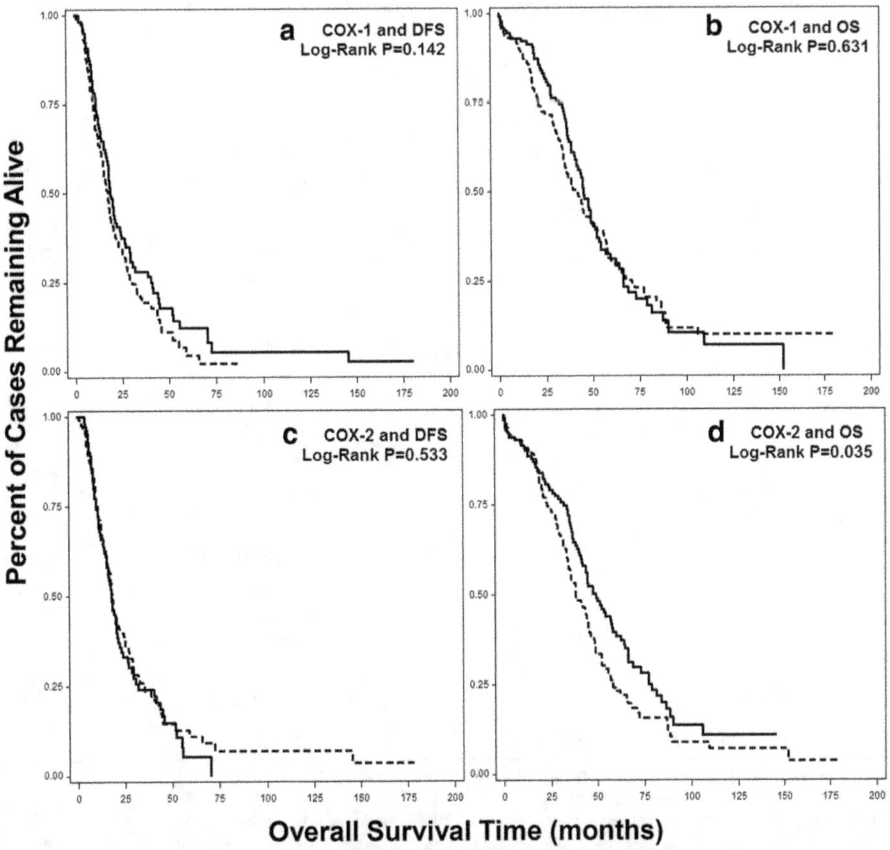

Fig. 3 Kaplan-Meier Survival Functions for COX-1 and COX-2 by RNA-seq from TCGA. Normalized RNA-seq data downloaded from the Broad Firehose for 489 high grade serous (type II) cases, analyzed for (**a**) COX-1 and DFS, (**b**) COX-1 and OS, (**c**) COX-2 and DFS, and (**d**) COX-2 and OS. Solid line = lower than median COX expression; dotted line = median or higher COX expression. X-axis is overall survival time in months, Y-axis is percentage of cases remaining alive, *P*-values from Log-Rank tests

However, in a larger study where COX-2 was not associated with OS among all cases, significantly worse survival was found when analyses were restricted to 131 type II tumors [21]. Thus, studies that include both type I and type II tumors without conducting stratified analysis may also contribute to the high heterogeneity of results in the existing COX-2 literature.

Our group and others have previously shown that COX-1 is highly expressed in ovarian cancer [12–14]. However, prior studies on COX-1 and ovarian cancer survival are limited. Among 30 optimally debulked serous cases, patients whose tumors had high COX-1 tended to have worse OS (HR: 2.5, 95% CI: 0.81–7.95) [17]. Among 70 and 107 cases, Kaplan-Meier plots for COX-1 were not significant, but proportional hazards regression was not conducted [16, 29]. Two more studies also reported no association, but showed no COX-1 results among 75 and 213 cases [15, 21]. In the current study, analysis of TCGA data was suggestive, and COX-1 was significantly associatedwith shorter DFS and OS when measured by QPCR. As our previous findings indicatethat COX-1 is associated with multiple pro-tumorigenic pathways in high grade serous ovarian cancer [12], more research is needed to determine if COX-1 has utility as a prognostic biomarker for type II serous ovarian cancer.

Strengths of the current study include measuring both COX isozymes by QPCR and IHC, and evaluating both standard IHC and H-scores. Our rigorous statistical analysis included multivariable adjusted regression models, stratified analyses, and interactions with tumor type. We found that tumor type and adjustment for clinical covariates markedly influenced many results, so analyses that do not consider these important factors may have inaccurate results. The primary limitation of this study is our small sample size, such that precision, and power to detect associations, especially in stratified analyses, may be low. However, our TMA is larger than what was included in many prior reports on COX expression and ovarian cancer survival.

Table 4 Associations between COX H-score and ovarian cancer survival by tumor type, the Vanderbilt TROC

	Disease-free survival			Overall survival		
	HR (95% CI), *P*-value		P-interaction	HR (95% CI), *P*-value		P-interaction
COX-1 / PTGS1						
Among Type I Cases (*N* = 65)						
N cases / events[a]	28 / 3 vs 21 / 5			39 / 14 vs 26 / 8		
Unadjusted	2.20 (0.52–9.20)	0.282	0.537	0.71 (0.29–1.70)	0.435	0.210
Adjusted[b]	2.88 (0.55–15.04)	0.209		0.56 (0.23–1.38)	0.210	
Among Type II Cases (*N* = 125)						
N cases / events[a]	32 / 23 vs 37 / 26			56 / 43 vs 69 / 55		
Unadjusted	1.32 (0.75–2.31)	0.339		1.10 (0.74–1.64)	0.636	
Adjusted[b]	1.34 (0.76–2.37)	0.313		1.07 (0.72–1.60)	0.740	
COX-2 / PTGS2						
Among Type I Cases (*N* = 65)						
N cases / events[a]	10 / 2 vs 39 / 6			19 / 11 vs 46 / 11		
Unadjusted	0.90 (0.18–4.52)	0.899	0.181	**0.38 (0.16–0.88)**	**0.023**	0.051
Adjusted[b]	0.51 (0.08–3.40)	0.490		0.49 (0.20–1.15)	0.102	
Among Type II Cases (*N* = 125)						
N cases / events[a]	36 / 27 vs 33 / 22			76 / 61 vs 49 / 37		
Unadjusted	1.07 (0.60–1.88)	0.829		0.84 (0.56–1.27)	0.413	
Adjusted[b]	**1.93 (1.06–3.53)**	**0.033**		1.08 (0.71–1.63)	0.723	

[a]N cases / N events, reference vs high COX, measured by H-score, dichotomized at the median
[b]Adjusted for age at diagnosis (continuous) and stage (early, late)
Bold values denote signficant associations; column percentages may not sum to 100% due to rounding error

Conclusions

In conclusion, this study indicates that COX-1 expression is high in type II tumors, COX-2 expression is high in type I tumors, and that both COX-1 and COX-2 may influence ovarian cancer outcomes, with possible variation by tumor type. These findings provide strong rationale for additional research that includes larger study populations and methods to disentangle the roles of the two COX isozymes in type I and type II ovarian tumors, which may impact disease prognosis and COX targeted therapeutic interventions for women with ovarian cancer.

Additional files

Additional file 1: Characterization of new rabbit polyclonal anti-COX-1. **A)** Protein sequences of human COX-1 and COX-2 show that peptides used in anti-COX-1 generation (shaded in yellow) had no overlap with the corresponding COX-2 sequence. **B)** Western blot analysis using the newly generated Vanderbilt anti-COX-1 (1:2000 overnight) show detection of COX-1 at the expected molecular weight (approximately 68 kDa). COX-2 was detected by rabbit polyclonal anti-COX-2. Actin was used as loading control. Samples used were COX-1-expressing OVCAR-3 cell lysate, COX-2-expressing 4 T1 cell lysate, recombinant ovine COX-1 and recombinant human COX-2. (PPTX 71 kb)

Additional file 2: COX-1 expression in ovarian cancer measured by the commercial Santa Cruz antibody (IHC). **A)** Pearson correlation between IHC expression levels of COX-1 and COX-2. H-scores for COX-1 expression in **B)** serous, endometrioid, mucinous and clear cell tumors, and in **C)** serous tumors versus all other epithelial tumors, and type II versus type I tumors. *P* values were determined by Student's t-test. (PPTX 377 kb)

Additional file 3: COX Expression: Correlation between QPCR and IHC. Pearson correlations between COX expression levels measured by quantitative PCR and H-scores from IHC. (PPTX 235 kb)

Abbreviations

CI: Confidence interval; COX: Cyclooxygenase; DFS: Disease-free survival; DHSR: Digital Histology Shared Resource; HR: Hazard ratio; IHC: Immunohistochemistry; OS: Overall survival; PTGS or PGHS: Prostaglandin H_2 synthases; QPCR: Quantitative real-time RT PCR; TCGA: The Cancer Genome Atlas; TMA: Tissue microarray; TROC: Tissue repository for ovarian cancer; VUMC: Vanderbilt University Medical Center

Acknowledgements

Special thanks to members and supporters of the Vanderbilt Ovarian Cancer Alliance (VOCAL).

Funding

Grant Support was 5P30 CA068485, CA091408 5 U54, 1UL1 RR024975, K08CA148887 (DK); the Kay Yow Cancer Fund/V Foundation (DK&LM), and 2R01 CA089450 (LM). The polyclonal anti-COX-1 was generated by the Vanderbilt Antibody and Protein Resource. The Vanderbilt Antibody and Protein Resource is supported by the Vanderbilt Institute of Chemical Biology and the Vanderbilt Ingram Cancer Center (P30 CA68485). Immunohistochemical staining was performed by the Vanderbilt Translational Pathology Shared Resource is supported by NCI/NIH Cancer Center Support Grant 2P30 CA06848.

Authors' contributions

Conceptions and design: ABF, AJW, LJM, DK. Acquisition of data: AJW, SX, MER, MAC, DK. Analysis and interpretation of data: ABF, AJW, SK, LJM, OF, MAC, DK. Writing, review and/or revision of the manuscript: ABF, AJW, LJM, OF, MAC, DK. Administrative, technical or material support: MER, SX. Study supervision: DK. All authors read and approved the final manuscript.

Competing interests

Authors Marnett, Khabele, and Crispens disclose potential conflicts of interest.
Dr. Khabele reports grants from Kay Yow Cancer Fund/V Foundation, during the conduct of the study; other from Astra Zeneca, personal fees from Vertex Pharmaceuticals, personal fees from Genentech, outside the submitted work.
Dr. Marnett reports grants from National Institutes of Health, grants from Kay Yow Cancer Fund/ V Foundation, during the conduct of the study.
Dr. Crispens reports other from Janssen Pharmaceuticals (clinical trial), other from Astra-Zeneca (clinical trial), personal fees from Helomics, outside the submitted work.
Authors Beeghly-Fadiel, Wilson, Keene, El Ramahi, and Xu disclose no competing interests.

Author details

[1]Department of Medicine, Division of Epidemiology, Vanderbilt Epidemiology Center, Institute for Medicine and Public Health, Vanderbilt University Medical Center, Nashville, TN, USA. [2]Vanderbilt-Ingram Cancer Center, Nashville, TN, USA. [3]Department of Obstetrics & Gynecology, Division of Gynecologic Oncology, Vanderbilt University Medical Center, Nashville, TN, USA. [4]Department of Biochemistry, Vanderbilt University Medical Center, Nashville, TN, USA. [5]Vanderbilt Institute of Chemical Biology, Vanderbilt University Medical Center, Nashville, TN, USA. [6]Department of Pathology, School of Medicine, University of California, San Diego, La Jolla, CA, USA. [7]Department of Obstetrics and Gynecology, Division of Gynecologic Oncology, The University of Kansas Medical Center, MS 2028, 3901 Rainbow Boulevard, Kansas City, KS 66160, USA.

References

1. Siegel RL, Miller KD, Jemal A. Cancer statistics, 2017. CA Cancer J Clin. 2017;67:7–30.
2. Jayson GC, Kohn EC, Kitchener HC, Ledermann JA. Ovarian cancer. Lancet. 2014;384:1376–88.
3. Vaughan S, et al. Rethinking ovarian cancer: recommendations for improving outcomes. Nat Rev Cancer. 2011;11:719–25.
4. Siegel R, Naishadham D, Jemal A. Cancer statistics, 2013. CA Cancer J Clin. 2013;63:11–30.
5. Nezhat FR, Apostol R, Nezhat C, Pejovic T. New insights in the pathophysiology of ovarian cancer and implications for screening and prevention. Am J Obstet Gynecol. 2015;213:262–7.
6. Wentzensen N, et al. Ovarian cancer risk factors by histologic subtype: an analysis from the ovarian cancer cohort consortium. J Clin Oncol. 2016; 34: 2888–98.
7. Prahm KP, et al. The prognostic value of dividing epithelial ovarian cancer into type I and type II tumors based on pathologic characteristics. Gynecol Oncol. 2015;136:205–11.
8. Adelizzi RA. COX-1 and COX-2 in health and disease. J Am Osteopath Assoc. 1999;99(11 Suppl):S7–12.
9. Rizzo MT. Cyclooxygenase-2 in oncogenesis. Clin Chim Acta. 2011;412:671–87.
10. Gurpinar E, Grizzle WE, Piazza GA. COX-independent mechanisms of cancer chemoprevention by anti-inflammatory drugs. Front Oncol. 2013;3:181.
11. Lee J-Y, Myung S-K, Song Y-S. Prognostic role of cyclooxygenase-2 in epithelial ovarian cancer: a meta-analysis of observational studies. Gynecol Oncol. 2013;129:613–9.
12. Wilson AJ, et al. Aberrant over-expression of COX-1 intersects multiple pro-tumorigenic pathways in high-grade serous ovarian cancer. Oncotarget. 2015;6:21353–68.
13. Daikoku T, et al. Cyclooxygenase-1 is a potential target for prevention and treatment of ovarian epithelial cancer. Cancer Res. 2005;65:3735–44.
14. Daikoku T, et al. Extracellular signal-regulated kinase is a target of cyclooxygenase-1-peroxisome proliferator-activated receptor-delta signaling in epithelial ovarian cancer. Cancer Res. 2007;67:5285–92.
15. Denkert C, et al. Expression of cyclooxygenase 2 is an independent prognostic factor in human ovarian carcinoma. Am J Pathol. 2002;160:893–903.
16. Khunnarong J, Tangjitgamol S, Manusirivithaya S, Suekwattana P, Leelahakorn S. Expression of cyclooxygenase-1 in epithelial ovarian cancer: a clinicopathological study. Asian Pac J Cancer Prev. 2008;4:757–62.
17. Taşkin S, et al. Roles of E-cadherin and cyclooxygenase enzymes in predicting different survival patterns of optimally cytoreduced serous ovarian cancer patients. Asian Pac J Cancer Prev. 2012;13:5715–9.
18. Shigemasa K, Tian X, Gu L, Shiroyama Y, Nagai N, Ohama K. Expression of cyclooxygenase-2 and its relationship to p53 accumulation in ovarian adenocarcinomas. Int J Oncol. 2003;22:99–105.
19. Seo SS, et al. Expression of cyclooxygenase-2 in association with clinicopathological prognostic factors and molecular markers in epithelial ovarian cancer. Gynecol Oncol. 2004;92:927–35.
20. Magnowska M, Zaborowski M, Surowiak P, Nowak-Markwitz E, Zabel M, Spaczyński M. COX-2 expression pattern is related to ovarian cancer differentiation and prognosis, but is not consistent with new model of pathogenesis. Ginekol Pol. 2014;85:335–41.
21. Ali-Fehmi R, et al. Molecular typing of epithelial ovarian carcinomas using inflammatory markers. Cancer. 2011;117:301–9.
22. Nagini M, Reddy GV, Hemalatha GR, Guruprasad L, Reddanna P. Functional correlation of cyclooxygenases-I, 2 and 3 from amino acid sequences and three dimensional model structures. IJC. 2006;45:A01.
23. Cass JD, et al. Automated quantitative analysis of p53, cyclin D1, Ki67 and pERK expression in breast carcinoma does not differ from expert pathologist scoring and correlates with clinico-pathological characteristics. Cancers. 2012;4:725–42.
24. Kurman RJ, Shih I-M. Molecular pathogenesis and extraovarian origin of epithelial ovarian cancer–shifting the paradigm. Hum Pathol. 2011;42:918–31.
25. Ferrandina G, et al. Increased cyclooxygenase-2 (COX-2) expression is associated with chemotherapy resistance and outcome in ovarian cancer patients. Ann Oncol. 2002;13:1205–11.
26. Erkinheimo T-L, et al. Elevated cyclooxygenase-2 expression is associated with altered expression of p53 and SMAD4, amplification of HER-2/neu, and poor outcome in serous ovarian carcinoma. Clin Cancer Res. 2004;10:538–45.
27. Raspollini MR, et al. Expression of inducible nitric oxide synthase and cyclooxygenase-2 in ovarian cancer: correlation with clinical outcome. Gynecol Oncol. 2004;92:806–12.
28. Steffensen KD, Waldstrøm M, Jeppesen U, Jakobsen E, Brandslund I, Jakobsen A. The prognostic importance of cyclooxygenase 2 and HER2 expression in epithelial ovarian cancer. Int J Gynecol Cancer. 2007;17:798–807.
29. Hamanishi J, et al. The comprehensive assessment of local immune status of ovarian cancer by the clustering of multiple immune factors. Clin Immunol. 2011;141:338–47.

12

The role of vitamin D in ovarian cancer: epidemiology, molecular mechanism and prevention

Hui Guo[1,2], Jing Guo[1,2], Wenli Xie[1,3], Lingqin Yuan[1*] and Xiugui Sheng[1,4*]

Abstract

Vitamin D is a fat-soluble prohormone best known for its role in maintaining calcium homeostasis. Large numbers of epidemiological studies have shown that vitamin D plays an important role in cancer prevention by regulating cellular proliferation and metabolism. Studies of the cellular mechanism of vitamin D in ovarian cancer strongly suggest that it exhibits protective and antitumorigenic activities through genomic and nongenomic signal transduction pathways. These results indicate that vitamin D deficiency results in an increase in the risk of developing ovarian cancer and that vitamin supplements may potentially be an efficient way of preventing cancer. Consequently, this review describes the epidemiology, molecular mechanism and evidence linking vitamin D deficiency to ovarian cancer.

Keywords: Ovarian cancer, $1,25(oh)_2D_3$, Angiogenesis, Metastasis, Inflammatory, Tumor metabolism, Prevention

Background

Ovarian cancer is the fifth leading cause of cancer death, with the highest fatality rate among women [1]. It is often diagnosed at an advanced stage in most patients with a survival rate of less than 40% at 5 years [2]. No significant improvement in ovarian cancer therapies using surgical debulking combined with platinum-based drug therapies has emerged over the past few decades. Consequently, new biomarkers that enable the early detection and prevention before disease onset are required for ovarian cancer.

Vitamin D is a fat-soluble prohormone best known for its role in calcium and bone homeostasis. Nearly 3% of the human genome are regulated by the vitamin D endocrine system [3]. Some epidemiological, preclinical and clinical studies have shown that vitamin D exhibited impressive antioncogenic activity and cancer prevention properties. Vitamin D level are determined by sunlight exposure, diet and supplements. Increasing evidences showed that low vitamin D level was associated with an increased risk of developing ovarian cancer [4–6]. This review aims to highlight the advancements of vitamin D in ovarian cancer that might provide new therapeutic methods and preventative information. The Literature identification and selection were supplied in supplemental methods (Additional file 1).

* Correspondence: ylqsd@aliyun.com; shengxiugui@163.com
[1]Department of Gynecologic Oncology, Shandong Cancer Hospital Affiliated to Shandong University, Shandong Academy of Medical Sciences, Jinan, Shandong, China
Full list of author information is available at the end of the article

Vitamin D and its receptor: Synthesis, sources and metabolism

Synthesis and sources of vitamin D

As shown in Fig. 1, vitamin D is synthesized in skin exposed to sunlight or obtained from dietary sources. Sunlight, specifically ultraviolet-B radiation, is the main pathway for producing adequate levels of vitamin D. It could convert 7-dehydrocholesterol (7-DHC) into vitamin D_3 in the skin. Vitamin D_3 then enters the blood stream as complexes with vitamin D binding protein (DBP) and albumin. Levels of DBP-bound vitamin D and free vitamin D are maintained at equilibrium to ensure adequate levels of circulating hormone. $1,25(OH)_2D_3$ (calcitriol), the active form of vitamin D_3, is synthesized by a series of enzymes that are mainly distributed in the liver and kidney. Firstly, vitamin D_3 is converted to 25-hydroxyvitamin D_3 ($25(OH)D_3$) in the liver, which is the main vitamin D metabolite present in the blood and the most reliable indicator of vitamin D status. $25(OH)D_3$ is then converted into $1,25(OH)_2D_3$ in the kidneys or other target tissues through

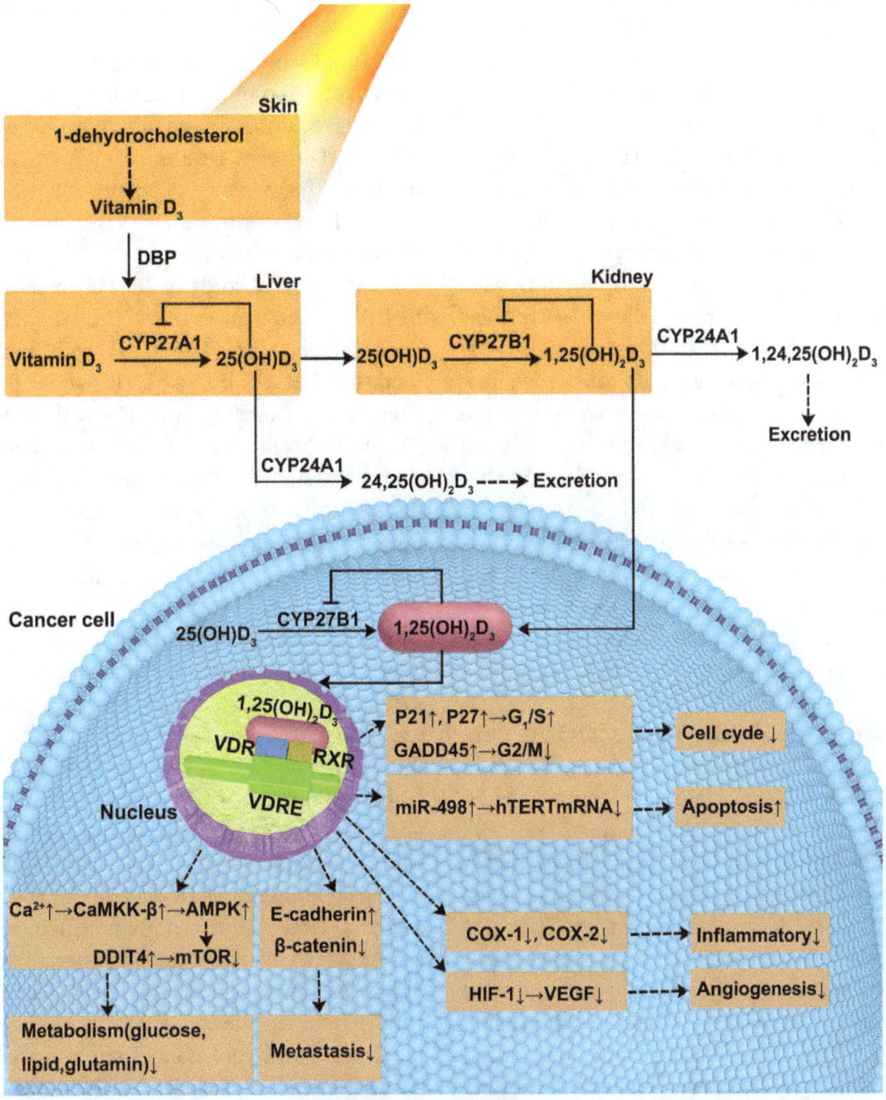

Fig. 1 Synthesis, metabolism and anticancer mechanism of vitamin D. Sunlight, specifically ultraviolet-B radiation, converts 7-dehydrocholesterol (7-DHC) into vitamin D_3 in the skin. Vitamin D_3 then enters the blood stream as complexes with vitamin D binding protein (DBP) and albumin. Liver mitochondrial and microsomal 25-hydroxylases (25-OHases), encoded by the gene CYP27A1, carry out the first hydroxylation of vitamin D to form $25(OH)D_3$. $25(OH)D_3$ is then 1a-hydroxylated by mitochondrial 1a-hydroxylase (1a-OHase) encoded by the CYP27B1 gene to form $1a,25(OH)_2D_3$ in the kidneys and other tissues. The vitamin D receptor (VDR) is a member of the nuclear receptor family that regulates gene transcription by forming a hetero-dimer with RXR, which binds to vitamin D-response elements (VDRE) in the promoter regions of target genes. Several $1,25(OH)_2D_3$ target genes have been reported multiple molecular pathways of anti-tumor actions of $1,25(OH)_2D_3$ in ovarian cancer. These include (1) the up-regulation of cyclin-dependent kinase(CDK) inhibitors P21 and P27 and the subsequent inhibition of G_1/S checkpoint; (2) G_2/M arrest by $1,25(OH)_2D_3$ through the induction of GADD45; (3) the inhibition of tumor angiogenesis due to suppressive effects on the expression of HIF-1/VEGFR pathway; (4) the suppression of invasion and metastasis via the up-regulation of E-cadherin and the down-regulation of β-catenin; (5) the induction of cell apoptosis by the suppression of hTERT mRNA transcription which miR-498 was a primary target gene of $1,25(OH)_2D_3$; (6) the down-regulation of the expression of COX-1 and COX-2 to inhibit the inflammatory process; (7) 1,25(OH)2D3 can induce a slow increase of Ca^{2+} that activates CaMKK-β, a Ca^{2+}-activated kinase that was identified as a direct activator of AMPK. DNA-damage-inducible transcript 4 (DDIT4) played a critical role in the cellular response to cell metabolism by the mTOR pathway

a series of enzymatic reactions. $1,25(OH)_2D_3$ then enters target cells, where it binds to vitamin D receptor (VDR) in the nucleus that regulate cellular function [7].

The vitamin D receptor is a member of the nuclear receptor family that regulates gene transcription by forming a hetero-dimer with RXR, which binds to vitamin D-response elements (VDRE) in the promoter regions of target genes [8]. VDR is weakly expressed in normal ovarian cells, but it is highly expressed in ovarian cancer cell lines and tumor tissues [9]. High levels of VDR expression was associated with improved survival rates in ovarian cancer [9, 10].

Enzyme regulation

Enzymatic reactions play an important role in the biosynthesis and degradation of $1,25(OH)_2D_3$. Liver mitochondrial and microsomal 25-hydroxylases (25-OHases), encoded by the gene CYP27A1, carry out the first hydroxylation of vitamin D to form $25(OH)D_3$. $25(OH)D_3$ is then 1a-hydroxylated by mitochondrial 1a-hydroxylase (1a-OHase) encoded by the CYP27B1 gene to form $1a,25(OH)_2D_3$ in the kidneys and other tissues. These two enzymes represent the rate-limiting steps for $25(OH)D_3$ and $1a,25\ (OH)_2D_3$ biosynthesis, with their activity regulated by high concentrations of $25(OH)D_3$ and $1a,25(OH)_2D_3$ respectively, as part of a negative feedback loop [11, 12]. A 24-hydroxylase encoded by the CYP24A1 gene is primarily responsible for catabolizing $1,25(OH)_2D_3$ which is converted into calcitroic acid that is then excreted. In addition, CYP24A1 expression is strongly induced by high levels of $1,25(OH)_2D_3$, with this feedback mechanism operating to maintain appropriate $1,25(OH)_2D_3$ serum level [12]. However, the amount of $1,25(OH)_2D_3$ present in tumor cells is decreased by this feedback loop [8]. The self-regulation of $1,25(OH)_2D_3$ induces its own inactivation.

It has been reported that CYP27A1 and CYP27B1 were overexpressed in ovarian cancer cells, which can result in an increase in localized $1,25(OH)_2D_3$ concentrations in the tumor and promote anticancer activity [7, 13]. Additionally, CYP24A1 has also been found to be highly expressed in many cancers including ovarian cancer, which is associated with the inverse impact of $25(OH)D_3$ on cancer risk levels [14–16]. Another study showed that decreased CYP27B1 was associated with a more aggressive phonotype for ovarian cancer [17]. Therefore, increasing CYP27A1 and CYP27B1 expression and decreasing CYP24A1 production may be beneficial for inhibiting tumor growth.

The epidemiology of vitamin D and ovarian cancer

Circulating vitamin D and ovarian cancer risk

The hypothesis that levels of vitamin D might be related to cancer rates was first proposed by the Garland brothers in 1980, who reported that people living at higher latitudes with vitamin D deficiency had an increased risk of developing malignant tumors [18]. Their subsequent ecologic study provided further evidence that there is a strong inverse correlation between mean daily solar radiation levels and ovarian cancer mortality [19]. $25(OH)_2D_3$ has a longer half-life than $1,25(OH)_2D_3$, whose serum levels are currently the gold standard for evaluating vitamin D status. Yin et al. provided meta-analysis of 10 cohort studies on the incidence of ovarian cancer, finding an average increase in $25(OH)_2D_3$ of 20 ng/ml, with an RR (95% confidence interval, CI) value of 0.83 (0.63–1.08) [4]. Ong et al. used two-sample MR methodology to demonstrate a causal role relating low levels of circulating vitamin D with high-grade serous ovarian cancer [5]. These studies suggested the possibility of an inverse association, however these associations were not considered statistically significant. Different results may be attributed to racial disparities, the season of diagnosis, different cut-off of 25(OH)D concentration, UVB exposure, obesity and socioeconomic status.

A case-control study of 1631 women diagnosed with epithelial ovarian cancer have shown that higher 25(OH)D concentrations are associated with longer survival rates (adjusted HR: 0.93; 95%CI: 0.88–0.99 per 10 nmol/L) [6]. Colorectal cancer patients with high prediagnostic 25(OH)D levels (>30 ng per mL) have a lower risk of cancer-specific and total mortality [20–22]. Vitamin D status at the time of diagnosis may also be an independent predictor of prognosis, implying that vitamin D supplementation may be an effective treatment for early stage cancer.

UVB and ovarian cancer risk

Several ecological studies have shown that ovarian cancer incidence and mortality are inversely associated with UVB exposure that is responsible for vitamin D production in the skin. [10, 23, 24] A population-based case-control study examined the association between lifetime ambient UVR and ovarian cancer risk, which found that women who spent their lives in areas with high levels of ambient UVR had a lower risk of developing epithelial ovarian cancer [25]. They reported a greater incidence of ovarian cancer in North America and northern Europe than in Asia or Africa. Furthermore, increasing latitude is associated with higher mortality levels in the United States [19]. However, a different cohort study using the TOMS database to estimate ambient UVR found no association between UVB exposure and the risk of ovarian cancer [26].

VDR polymorphisms and ovarian cancer risk

Several VDR gene polymorphisms have been identified that may influence cancer risk. The most frequently studied single nucleotide polymorphisms in ovarian cancer is FokI (rs2228570/ rs10735810), which is located at the 5′ end of the VDR gene. This polymorphism results in the VDR protein sequence being altered, producing a protein that is 3 amino acids longer for carriers of the f allele, than for carriers of the F allele. Lurie et al. were the first to report that the FokI f allele was associated with increased risk of ovarian cancer in Caucasian women [27]. It was subsequently found that the incidence of the f allele was highest amongst younger women (age < 50), which may be due to the promoting effect of estrogen on mRNA expression for VDR [28]. Tworoger et al. also observed that the pooled OR comparing ovarian cancer women with ff versus FF genotype was 1.26 (95% CI, 1.01–1.56) [29]. In Indian population, FokI is also associated with the incidence of ovarian cancer [30]. Meta-analysis has also shown that populations with FokI ff allele were associated with a 10% increased cancer risk (pooled OR = 1.10, 95%CI = 0.99–1.22) [31].

BsmI (rs1544410), ApaI (rs7975232), and TaqI (rs731236) are situated in the 3′ untranslated region of the VDR gene, which does not affect VDR protein structure, so these polymorphisms are likely to regulate VDR mRNA stability [32]. Meta-analysis of 7 case-control studies showed that the BsmI G/A gene variant may be a moderate risk factor for the development of ovarian cancer in European populations when compared to North American or Asian populations [33]. ApaI has been shown to affect VDR mRNA stability. Grant et al. detected a significant association between Apa1 and invasive ovarian cancer in African American women [34]. However, no association of the Taq1 variant with ovarian cancer was found. In addition, another single nucleotide polymorphism Cdx2 A allele was found to improve VDR activity and decrease ovarian cancer risk [27]. Therefore, these genetic differences may be important factors that impact VDR association with ovarian cancer. Other factors including circulating vitamin D levels, sun exposure and disease stage may also modify the effect of VDR variants on ovarian cancer risk [35]. Therefore, more studies in different ethnic populations are required to identify the role of VDR gene polymorphisms in the development of ovarian cancer.

The anticancer mechanism of vitamin D in ovarian cancer

Different studies have described several mechanisms through which VDR can inhibit tumor growth including genomic and non-genomic signal transduction pathways. $1,25(OH)_2D_3$ binds to vitamin D receptor (VDR), translocates to nucleus, where it forms a VDR/retinoid X receptor complex that binds to vitamin D response elements (VDREs) that regulate gene transcription (illustrated in Fig. 1). In addition, vitamin D exerts some non-genomic effects including regulation of calcium and phosphate homeostasis pathways, as well as activating protein kinase C, protein kinase A (PKA), phosphatidylinositol-3 kinase (PI3K) and phospholipase C (PLC) [8, 36].

The VDR variant may also be involved in ovarian cancer carcinogenesis. For example, the FokI f allele resulted in three amino acids longer VDR protein than the F allele. This mutant VDR protein was less responsive to $1,25(OH)_2D_3$ and had lower transcriptional activity [37, 38]. Etten et al. reported that this extended VDR results in lower NF-kB transcriptional activation, leading to reduced IL-12 expression and a weaker immune response [39].

Cell cycle and apoptosis

Expression of VDR is an important factor in tumor cell response to $1,25(OH)_2D_3$, which is known to influence gene expression of p53, Ras, MAPK, PI3, MYC, HIF1a, BRCA1, CDKN1A and GADD45 [8, 12, 40–43]. Jiang et al. have shown that $1,25(OH)_2D_3$ could inhibit cancer growth by arresting cells at the G_2–M transition phase and induce cell death through VDR-mediated, p53-independent induction of GADD45 in ovarian cancer cells [44]. They also demonstrated that the $1,25(OH)_2D_3$ analogue EB1089 inhibited the proliferation of ovarian cancer without inducing hypercalcemia in vivo [45]. VDR-mediated induction of BRCA1 was found to be closely correlated with the anti-proliferative activity of $1,25(OH)_2D_3$ in breast and prostate cancer cells [40]. Studies have also shown that profound cross-talk exists between p53 and VDR, with the VDR gene being a direct target of p53 and its family members [41].

$1,25(OH)_2D_3$ promotes the expression of cyclin-dependent kinase(CDK) inhibitors P21 and P27 with reduced CDK activity. Li et al. demonstrated that $1,25(OH)_2D_3$ arrested ovarian cancer cells at the G_1/S checkpoint and stabilized the p27 protein through downregulation of cyclin E/cyclin-dependent kinase 2 and Skp1-Cullin-F-box protein/Skp2 ubiquitin ligase [46]. Bai et al. identified that $1,25(OH)_2D_3$ suppressed ovarian cancer cells at the G_1/S checkpoint through downregulation of epidermal growth factor receptor (EGFR) transcription [47]. Collectively, these studies confirmed that vitamin D suppressed cell proliferation through inhibitory effects on several regulators of the cell cycle.

Down-regulation of telomerase activity by vitamin D that induce apoptosis and suppress ovarian cancer cell growth may occur via other pathways [48]. Studies by Kasiappan et al. showed that $1,25(OH)_2D_3$ decreased hTERT mRNA transcription to induce cell apoptosis, suggesting that miR-498 was a primary target gene of $1,25(OH)_2D_3$ for ovarian cancer [49]. Microarray analysis has also revealed that $1,25(OH)_2D_3$ regulated the extrinsic apoptotic pathway through tumor necrosis factor such as TRAIL, Fas and caspase-7 in ovarian cancer cells [50].

Angiogenesis

Growing evidence indicates that vitamin D has a potential role for inhibiting tumor angiogenesis [51–54]. Hypoxic regions exist in most solid tumors is a major pathophysiologic condition that regulates angiogenesis. Increased angiogenesis occurs as a cellular adaptation to hypoxia, which is controlled by hypoxia inducible factor-1(HIF-1). HIF1 target genes, such as vascular endothelial growth factor (VEGFR), are inhibited by $1,25(OH)_2D_3$, and this molecular inhibition is mediated via a HIF-dependent pathway [55]. A study by Chung et al. has shown that vitamin D decreased growth inhibition of tumor-derived endothelial cells from VDR knockout mice. Moreover, loss of VDR resulted in an increase in HIF-1α, VEGF, angiopoietin 1 and platelet-derived growth factor levels [56].

Invasion and metastasis

Tumor metastasis is the primary factor for treatment failure in patients with ovarian cancer. The omentum is the most common tissue type affected by ovarian cancer metastasis, because it is comprised of large numbers of adipocytes, immune cells, microvascular cells and fibroblasts, which create a good microenviroment for cancer cell growth. In vivo and vitro experiments suggested that $1,25(OH)_2D_3$ and its analog EB1089 could suppress the spread of cancer cells through the omentum by binding to VDR present in epithelial cancer and stromal cells [57]. Moreover, Liu et al. found that $1,25(OH)_2D_3$ upregulated the expression of E-cadherin and VDR and downregulated the expression of β-catenin in ovarian cancer induced by 7,12-dimethylbenz[a]anthracene (DMBA) [58].

Inflammatory response

Increased inflammation has been recognized as a risk factor for the development of cancer [59]. Mantovani et al. proposed that a continuous inflammatory environment would result in reduced levels of 25(OH)D, which may provide an explanation why cancer is associated with low levels of 25(OH)D [60, 61]. The two isoenzymes cyclooxygenase 1 and 2 (COX-1 and COX-2) are involved in inflammatory process arrised in ovarian cancer. High-expression levels of COX-2 was associated with poor survival rates in ovarian cancer patients [62]. Vitamin D combined with the COX-2 inhibitor celecoxib was shown to obviously decrease ovarian cancer growth rates when compared to celecoxib alone [63].

Tumor metabolism

Dysregulated tumor cell metabolism has recently been identified to play an important role in the development of cancer. Several studies have shown that vitamin D influences regulation of glucose and fatty acid metabolism in cancer cells. Santos et al. have reported that $1,25(OH)_2D_3$ inhibited the expression of glycolytic enzymes including hexokinase II (HKII) and lactate dehydrogenase A (LDHA) in breast cancer [64]. Tomasz et al. described that $1,25(OH)_2D_3$ also inhibited de novo fatty acid synthesis through down-regulation of pyruvate carboxylase, while acetyl-CoA carboxylase (ACC) and fatty acid synthase (FASN) were not altered in breast cancer cell [65]. $1,25(OH)_2D_3$ has also been shown to decrease the expression of genes regulating glucose, fatty acid and glutamine metabolism in prostate cancer cells [66]. Moreover, glutamine metabolism in breast cancer was also decreased by $1,25(OH)_2D_3$ intervention [67]. However, no studies were found about the impact of $1,25(OH)_2D_3$ on ovarian cancer cell metabolism.

Recent studies have demonstrated the effects of $1,25(OH)_2D_3$ on metabolism-related signaling molecules, including AMPK, DDIT4, mTOR and AKT [68–71]. $1,25(OH)_2D_3$ can induce a slow increase in Ca^{2+} concentration that activates CaMKK-β, which is a Ca^{2+}-activated kinase that was identified as a direct activator of AMPK [72]. DNA-damage-inducible transcript 4 (DDIT4), also known as REDD1/Dig2/RTP801, was over-expressed in high-grade ovarian cancer and significantly linked with late stage cancer patients [73]. DDIT4 played a critical role in cellular response to energy stress via the TSC/mTOR pathway [74]. It has been reported that $1,25(OH)_2D_3$ regulates mTOR signaling through inducing DDIT4 expression [75]. In addition, study found that AKT S473 activation was associated with over-expression of DDIT4 in ovarian cancer tissues [73]. These observations implied that the action of $1,25(OH)_2D_3$ on the mTOR signal pathway may have a key role in cancer metabolism. Therefore, it is clear that further understanding of the pathway relating vitamin D to cancer cell metabolism is required.

Obesity has been proposed to lead to low body vitamin D status, because vitamin D is a fat soluble molecule that can be stored in excess adipose tissue [76]. Strong links between vitamin D and obesity have been further established [77]. It was reported that vitamin D deficiency was associated with an increased risk of ovarian cancer in overweight and obese women [78, 79]. Obesity has been a significant risk factor for ovarian cancer [80]. It was meaningful to elucidate the regulatory mechanisms of vitamin D in the metabolic pathway between obesity and cancer. Leptin is an adipocyte-derived adipokine that plays a crucial role in regulating appetite and energy balance, that is strongly elevated in obese ovarian cancer patients [81]. Bai et al. reported evidence that $1,25(OH)_2D_3$ had a suppressive effect on leptin and HFD-induced ovarian cancer through miR498 pathway [82]. This means that appropriate control of $1,25(OH)_2D_3$ levels may offer an effective strategy for reducing ovarian cancer risk in obese women.

Vitamin D for the treatment and prevention of ovarian cancer

Compared with traditional chemotherapy regiments, the use of $1,25(OH)_2D_3$ or its analogs as a treatment for cancer is not an effective therapy. However, increased antitumor effects using $1,25(OH)_2D_3$ combination therapies offer an opportunity for developing clinical treatments for ovarian cancer [12]. Administration of $1,25(OH)_2D_3$ in vitro, has been shown to significantly enhance antitumor efficacy in the presence of chemotherapeutic agents such as cisplatin, carboplatin, docetaxel or paclitaxel [36, 83].

Growing evidence suggests that vitamin D deficiency is correlated to ovarian cancer, $1,25(OH)_2D_3$ and its analogs have been shown to be promising agents for cancer prevention. Excess exposure to sunlight can result in skin diseases, however vitamin D supplementation can be used to improve the vitamin D status of patients. A healthy blood level of 25-hydroxyvitamin D of > 30 ng/mL has been recommended by the Endocrine Society's Practice Guidelines [84]. Vitamin D supplementation alone was found no association with a decreased risk of ovarian cancer in African-American women [85]. Trivedi et al. reported no effects of 4 monthly doses of 100,000 IU vitamin D on cancer incidence or mortality in 2686 people over a 5-year period [86]. However, randomized controlled trials using vitamin D and calcium on post-menopausal women have found more beneficial effect in reducing the incidence of cancer compared with vitamin D supplement alone. Lappe et al. have reported 4-year trials on the RR of patients developing cancer. They compared patients who took an average of 1450 mg/day calcium with those taking 1450 mg/day calcium plus 1000 IU/day vitamin D3, which gave values of 0.532 (95%CI: 0.27 to 1.03; $P = 0.063$) and 0.40 (95%CI, 0.20 to 0.82; $P = 0.013$), respectively [87, 88]. Bolland et al. have reported that women who took 1000 mg/day calcium and 400 IU/day vitamin D for 8 years had a 14–20% reduced risk of developing breast cancer, and a 17% reduced risk of developing colorectal cancer [89]. In addition, Bolland suggested that higher doses of Ca plus vitamin D did not decrease cancer incidence when compared with lower doses of Ca plus vitamin D. Conversely, a case-control study involving supplementation of 2303 healthy postmenopausal women (55 years and older) with vitamin D (2000 IU/day) and calcium (1500 IU/day) did not result in a significant decrease in cancer rates over a 4 year period [90]. Collectively, there exsits a possibility that vitamin D and calcium combination therapy may be benefit for cancer prevention. Further research is needed in order to select the right clinical dose in preventing the occurrence of ovarian cancer.

Conclusion

The role of Vitamin D in human cancers, including ovarian cancer, has been widely investigated, where it was proposed to play a protective and antitumorigenic role by regulating cellular proliferation and metabolism. In this review, we have shown that vitamin D status may be an independent predictor of prognosis in ovarian cancer patients.Vitamin D combination therapy improves antitumor effects allowing for potential clinical application. Supplement of vitamin D and calcium combination may be an efficient method for cancer prevention.

Abbreviations

1a-OHase: 1a-hydroxylase; 25(OH)D3: 25-hydroxyvitamin D3; 25-OHases: 25-hydroxylases; 7-DHC: 7-dehydrocholesterol; ACC: Acetyl-CoA carboxylase; CDK: Cyclin-dependent kinase; COX-1: Cyclooxygenase 1; COX-2: Cyclooxygenase 2; DBP: Vitamin D binding protein; DMBA: 7,12-dimethylbenz[a]anthracene; EGFR: Epidermal growth factor receptor; FASN: Fatty acid synthase; HIF-1: Hypoxia inducible factor-1; HKII: Hexokinase II; LDHA: Lactate dehydrogenase A; PI3K: Phosphatidylinositol-3 kinase; PKA: Protein kinase A; PLC: Phospholipase C; VDR: Vitamin D receptor; VDRE: Vitamin D-response elements; VEGFR: Vascular endothelial growth factor

Funding

This work was supported by the National Natural Science Fundation of China to Dr. Xiugui Sheng(No.81672591).

Authors' contributions

GH and GJ performed literature review and wrote the manuscript. XW contributed critical discussion about the study. YL and SX designed the review. All authors read and approved the final manuscript.

Competing interests

The authors declare that they have no competing interests.

Author details

[1]Department of Gynecologic Oncology, Shandong Cancer Hospital Affiliated to Shandong University, Shandong Academy of Medical Sciences, Jinan, Shandong, China. [2]School of Medicine and Life Sciences, University of Jinan, Shandong Academy of Medical Sciences, Jinan, Shandong, China. [3]Shandong University, Jinan, Shandong, China. [4]Cancer Hospital Chinese Academy of Medical Sciences, Shenzhen Center, Guangdong, China.

References

1. Gloss BS, Samimi G. Epigenetic biomarkers in epithelial ovarian cancer. Cancer Lett. 2014;342(2):257–63.
2. Mirandola L, J Cannon M, Cobos E, Bernardini G, Jenkins MR, Kast WM, et al. Cancer testis antigens: novel biomarkers and targetable proteins for ovarian cancer. Int Rev Immunol. 2011;30(2–3):127–37.
3. Bouillon R, Carmeliet G, Verlinden L, van Etten E, Verstuyf A, Luderer HF, et al. Vitamin D and human health: lessons from vitamin D receptor null mice. Endocr Rev. 2008;29(6):726–76.
4. Yin L, Grandi N, Raum E, Haug U, Arndt V, Brenner H. Meta-analysis: circulating vitamin D and ovarian cancer risk. Gynecol Oncol. 2011;121(2):369–75.
5. Ong J-S, Cuellar-Partida G, Lu Y, Fasching PA, Hein A, Burghaus S, et al. Association of vitamin D levels and risk of ovarian cancer: a Mendelian randomization study. Int J Epidemiol. 2016;45(5):1619–30.
6. Webb PM, de Fazio A, Protani MM, Ibiebele TI, Nagle CM, Brand AH, et al. Circulating 25-hydroxyvitamin D and survival in women with ovarian cancer. Am J Clin Nutr. 2015;102(1):109–14.
7. Feldman D, Krishnan AV, Swami S, Giovannucci E, Feldman BJ. The role of vitamin D in reducing cancer risk and progression. Nat Rev Cancer. 2014;14(5):342–57.
8. King AN, Beer DG, Christensen PJ, Simpson RU, Ramnath N. The vitamin D/CYP24A1 story in cancer. Anti Cancer Agents Med Chem. 2010;10(3):213–24.
9. Silvagno F, Poma CB, Realmuto C, Ravarino N, Ramella A, Santoro N, et al. Analysis of vitamin D receptor expression and clinical correlations in patients with ovarian cancer. Gynecol Oncol. 2010;119(1):121–4.

10. Campbell MJ, Trump DL. Vitamin D Receptor Signaling and Cancer. Endocrinol Metab Clin N Am. 2017;46(4):1009–38.
11. Brenza HL, DeLuca HF. Regulation of 25-hydroxyvitamin D3 1alpha-hydroxylase gene expression by parathyroid hormone and 1,25-dihydroxyvitamin D3. Arch Biochem Biophys. 2000;381(1):143–52.
12. Deeb KK, Trump DL, Johnson CS. Vitamin D signalling pathways in cancer: potential for anticancer therapeutics. Nat Rev Cancer. 2007;7(9): 684–700.
13. Friedrich M, Rafi L, Mitschele T, Tilgen W, Schmidt W, Reichrath J. Analysis of the vitamin D system in cervical carcinomas, breast cancer and ovarian Cancer. Recent Results Cancer Res. 2003;164:239–46.
14. Anderson MG, Nakane M, Ruan X, Kroeger PE, Wu-Wong JR. Expression of VDR and CYP24A1 mRNA in human tumors. Cancer Chemother Pharmacol. 2006;57(2):234–40.
15. Ge N, Chu XM, Xuan YP, Ren DQ, Wang Y, Ma K, et al. Associations between abnormal vitamin D metabolism pathway function and non-small cell lung cancer. Oncol Lett. 2017;14(6):7538–44.
16. Rodriguez GC, Turbov J, Rosales R, Yoo J, Hunn J, Zappia KJ, et al. Progestins inhibit calcitriol-induced CYP24A1 and synergistically inhibit ovarian cancer cell viability: an opportunity for chemoprevention. Gynecol Oncol. 2016; 143(1):159–67.
17. Brozyna AA, Jozwicki W, Jochymski C, Slominski AT. Decreased expression of CYP27B1 correlates with the increased aggressiveness of ovarian carcinomas. Oncol Rep. 2015;33(2):599–606.
18. Holick MF. Vitamin D, sunlight and cancer connection. Anti Cancer Agents Med Chem. 2013;13(1):70–82.
19. Lefkowitz ES, Garland CF. Sunlight, vitamin D, and ovarian cancer mortality rates in US women. Int J Epidemiol. 1994;23(6):1133–6.
20. Fedirko V, Riboli E, Tjonneland A, Ferrari P, Olsen A, Bueno-de-Mesquita HB, et al. Prediagnostic 25-hydroxyvitamin D, VDR and CASR polymorphisms, and survival in patients with colorectal cancer in western European ppulations. Cancer Epidemiol Biomark Prev. 2012;21(4):582–93.
21. Gong C, Long Z, Yu Y, Zhu L, Tian J, Li S, et al. Dietary factors and polymorphisms in vitamin D metabolism genes: the risk and prognosis of colorectal cancer in Northeast China. Sci Rep. 2017;7(1):8827.
22. Zhu Y, Wang PP, Zhai G, Bapat B, Savas S, Woodrow JR, et al. Vitamin D receptor and calcium-sensing receptor polymorphisms and colorectal cancer survival in the Newfoundland population. Br J Cancer. 2017;117(6): 898–906.
23. Garland CF, Mohr SB, Gorham ED, Grant WB, Garland FC. Role of ultraviolet B irradiance and vitamin D in prevention of ovarian cancer. Am J Prev Med. 2006;31(6):512–4.
24. Boscoe FP, Schymura MJ. Solar ultraviolet-B exposure and cancer incidence and mortality in the United States, 1993–2002. BMC Cancer. 2006;6:264.
25. Tran B, Jordan SJ, Lucas R, Webb PM, Neale R. Association between ambient ultraviolet radiation and risk of epithelial ovarian cancer. Cancer Prev Res (Phila). 2012;5(11):1330–6.
26. Lin SW, Wheeler DC, Park Y, Cahoon EK, Hollenbeck AR, Freedman DM, et al. Prospective study of ultraviolet radiation exposure and risk of cancer in the United States. Int J Cancer. 2012;131(6):E1015–23.
27. Lurie G, Wilkens LR, Thompson PJ, McDuffie KE, Carney ME, Terada KY, et al. Vitamin D receptor gene polymorphisms and epithelial ovarian cancer risk. Cancer Epidemiol Biomark Prev. 2007;16(12):2566–71.
28. Lurie G, Wilkens LR, Thompson PJ, Carney ME, Palmieri RT, Pharoah PD, et al. Vitamin D receptor rs2228570 polymorphism and invasive ovarian carcinoma risk: pooled analysis in five studies within the ovarian cancer association consortium. Int J Cancer. 2011;128(4):936–43.
29. Tworoger SS, Gates MA, Lee IM, Buring JE, Titus-Ernstoff L, Cramer D, et al. Polymorphisms in the vitamin D receptor and risk of ovarian cancer in four studies. Cancer Res. 2009;69(5):1885–91.
30. Mohapatra S, Saxena A, Gandhi G, Koner BC, Ray PC. Vitamin D and VDR gene polymorphism (FokI) in epithelial ovarian cancer in Indian population. J Ovarian Res. 2013;6(1):37.
31. Liu Y, Li C, Chen P, Li X, Li M, Guo H, et al. Polymorphisms in the vitamin D receptor (VDR) and the risk of ovarian cancer: a meta-analysis. PLoS One. 2013;8(6):e66716.
32. Jurutka PW, Whitfield GK, Hsieh JC, Hompson PD, Haussler CA, Haussler MR. Molecular nature of the vitamin D receptor and its role in regulation of gene expression. Rev Endocr Metab Disord. 2001;2(2):203–16.
33. Qin X, Lu Y, Qin A, Chen Z, Peng Q, Deng Y, et al. Vitamin D receptor BsmI polymorphism and ovarian cancer risk: a meta-analysis. Int J Gynecol Cancer. 2013;23(7):1178–83.
34. Grant DJ, Hoyo C, Akushevich L, Iversen ES, Whitaker R, Marks J, et al. Vitamin D receptor (VDR) polymorphisms and risk of ovarian cancer in Caucasian and African American women. Gynecol Oncol. 2013;129(1):173–8.
35. Prescott J, Bertrand KA, Reid BM, Permuth-Wey J, De Vivo I, Cramer DW, et al. Evidence of differential effects of vitamin d receptor variants on epithelial ovarian cancer risk by predicted vitamin d status. Front Oncol. 2014;4:286.
36. Trump DL, Hershberger PA, Bernardi RJ, Ahmed S, Muindi J, Fakih M, et al. Anti-tumor activity of calcitriol: pre-clinical and clinical studies. J Steroid Biochem Mol Biol. 2004;89-90(1–5):519–26.
37. Uitterlinden AG, Fang Y, Van Meurs JB, Pols HA, Van Leeuwen JP. Genetics and biology of vitamin D receptor polymorphisms. Gene. 2004;338(2):143–56.
38. Colin EM, Weel AE, Uitterlinden AG, Buurman CJ, Birkenhager JC, Pols HA, et al. Consequences of vitamin D receptor gene polymorphisms for growth inhibition of cultured human peripheral blood mononuclear cells by 1, 25-dihydroxyvitamin D3. Clin Endocrinol. 2000;52(2):211–6.
39. van Etten E, Verlinden L, Giulietti A, Ramos-Lopez E, Branisteanu DD, Ferrira GB, et al. The vitamin D receptor gene FokI polymorphism: functional impact on the immune system. Eur J Immunol. 2007;37(2):395–405.
40. Campbell MJ, Gombart AF, Kwok SH, Park S, Koeffler HP. The anti-proliferative effects of 1a,25(OH)2D3 on breast and prostate cancer cells are associated with induction of BRCA1 gene expression. Oncogene. 2000; 19(44):5091–7.
41. Reichrath J, Reichrath S, Heyne K, Vogt T, Roemer K. Tumor suppression in skin and other tissues via cross-talk between vitamin D- and p53-signaling. Front Physiol. 2014;5:166.
42. Semenza GL. HIF-1: upstream and downstream of cancer metabolism. Curr Opin Genet Dev. 2010;20(1):51–6.
43. Salehi-Tabar R, Nguyen-Yamamoto L, Tavera-Mendoza LE, Quail T, Dimitrov V, An BS, et al. Vitamin D receptor as a master regulator of the c-MYC/MXD1 network. Proc Natl Acad Sci U S A. 2012;109(46):18827–32.
44. Jiang F, Li P, Fornace AJ, Nicosia SV, Bai W. G2/M arrest by 1,25-dihydroxyvitamin D3 in ovarian cancer cells mediated through the induction of GADD45 via an exonic enhancer. J Biol Chem. 2003;278(48):48030–40.
45. Zhang X, Jiang F, Li P, Li C, Ma Q, Nicosia SV, et al. Growth suppression of ovarian cancer xenografts in nude mice by vitamin D analogue EB1089. Clin Cancer Res. 2005;11(1):323–8.
46. Li P, Li C, Zhao X, Zhang X, Nicosia SV, Bai W. p27Kip1 stabilization and G1 arrest by 1,25-dihydroxyvitamin D3 in ovarian cancer cells mediated through down-regulation of cyclin E/cyclin-dependent kinase 2 and Skp1-Cullin-F-box protein/Skp2 ubiquitin ligase. J Biol Chem. 2004;279(24):25260–7.
47. Shen Z, Zhang X, Tang J, Kasiappan R, Jinwal U, Li P, et al. The coupling of epidermal growth factor receptor down regulation by 1alpha,25-dihydroxyvitamin D3 to the hormone-induced cell cycle arrest at the G1-S checkpoint in ovarian cancer cells. Mol Cell Endocrinol. 2011;338(1–2):58–67.
48. Jiang F, Bao J, Li P, Nicosia SV, Bai W. Induction of ovarian cancer cell apoptosis by 1,25-dihydroxyvitamin D3 through the down-regulation of telomerase. J Biol Chem. 2004;279(51):53213–21.
49. Kasiappan R, Shen Z, Tse AK, Jinwal U, Tang J, Lungchukiet P, et al. 1,25-dihydroxyvitamin D3 suppresses telomerase expression and human cancer growth through microRNA-498. J Biol Chem. 2012;287(49):41297–309.
50. Zhang X, Li P, Bao J, Nicosia SV, Wang H, Enkemann SA, et al. Suppression of death receptor-mediated apoptosis by 1,25-dihydroxyvitamin D3 revealed by microarray analysis. J Biol Chem. 2005;280(42):35458–68.
51. Mantell DJ, Owens PE, Bundred NJ, Mawer EB, Canfield AE. 1 ,25-dihydroxyvitamin D3 inhibits angiogenesis in vitro and in vivo. Circ Res. 2000;87(3):214–20.
52. Pendas-Franco N, Garcia JM, Pena C, Valle N, Palmer HG, Heinaniemi M, et al. DICKKOPF-4 is induced by TCF/beta-catenin and upregulated in human colon cancer, promotes tumour cell invasion and angiogenesis and is repressed by 1alpha,25-dihydroxyvitamin D3. Oncogene. 2008;27(32):4467–77.
53. Maj E, Filip-Psurska B, Milczarek M, Psurski M, Kutner A, Wietrzyk J. Vitamin D derivatives potentiate the anticancer and anti-angiogenic activity of tyrosine kinase inhibitors in combination with cytostatic drugs in an A549 non-small cell lung cancer model. Int J Oncol. 2018;52(2):337–66.
54. Bao BY, Yao J, Lee YF. 1alpha, 25-dihydroxyvitamin D3 suppresses interleukin-8-mediated prostate cancer cell angiogenesis. Carcinogenesis. 2006;27(9):1883–93.
55. Ben-Shoshan M, Amir S, Dang DT, Dang LH, Weisman Y, Mabjeesh NJ. 1alpha,25-dihydroxyvitamin D3 (Calcitriol) inhibits hypoxia-inducible factor-1/vascular endothelial growth factor pathway in human cancer cells. Mol Cancer Ther. 2007;6(4):1433–9.

56. Chung I, Han G, Seshadri M, Gillard BM, Yu WD, Foster BA, et al. Role of vitamin D receptor in the antiproliferative effects of calcitriol in tumor-derived endothelial cells and tumor angiogenesis in vivo. Cancer Res. 2009; 69(3):967–75.
57. Lungchukiet P, Sun Y, Kasiappan R, Quarni W, Nicosia SV, Zhang X, et al. Suppression of epithelial ovarian cancer invasion into the omentum by 1alpha,25-dihydroxyvitamin D3 and its receptor. J Steroid Biochem Mol Biol. 2015;148:138–47.
58. Liu L, Hu Z, Zhang H, Hou Y, Zhang Z, Zhou G, et al. Vitamin D postpones the progression of epithelial ovarian cancer induced by 7, 12-dimethylbenz [a] anthracene both in vitro and in vivo. Onco Targets Ther. 2016;9:2365–75.
59. Allavena P, Garlanda C, Borrello MG, Sica A, Mantovani A. Pathways connecting inflammation and cancer. Curr Opin Genet Dev. 2008;18(1):3–10.
60. Mantovani A, Allavena P, Sica A, Balkwill F. Cancer-related inflammation. Nature. 2008;454(7203):436–44.
61. Autier P, Boniol M, Pizot C, Mullie P. Vitamin D status and ill health: a systematic review. Lancet Diabetes Endocrinol. 2014;2(1):76–89.
62. Lee JY, Myung SK, Song YS. Prognostic role of cyclooxygenase-2 in epithelial ovarian cancer: a meta-analysis of observational studies. Gynecol Oncol. 2013;129(3):613–9.
63. Thill M, Woeste A, Reichert K, Fischer D, Rody A, Friedrich M, et al. Vitamin D inhibits ovarian Cancer cell line proliferation in combination with celecoxib and suppresses cyclooxygenase-2 expression. Anticancer Res. 2015;35(2): 1197–203.
64. Santos JM, Khan ZS, Munir MT, Tarafdar K, Rahman SM, Hussain F. Vitamin D3 decreases glycolysis and invasiveness, and increases cellular stiffness in breast cancer cells. J Nutr Biochem. 2017;53:111–20.
65. Wilmanski T, Buhman K, Donkin SS, Burgess JR, Teegarden D. 1alpha,25-dihydroxyvitamin D inhibits de novo fatty acid synthesis and lipid accumulation in metastatic breast cancer cells through down-regulation of pyruvate carboxylase. J Nutr Biochem. 2017;40:194–200.
66. Abu El Maaty MA, Alborzinia H, Khan SJ, Buttner M, Wolfl S. 1,25(OH)2D3 disrupts glucose metabolism in prostate cancer cells leading to a truncation of the TCA cycle and inhibition of TXNIP expression. Biochim Biophys Acta. 2017;1864(10):1618–30.
67. Zhou X, Zheng W, Nagana Gowda GA, Raftery D, Donkin SS, Bequette B, et al. 1,25-Dihydroxyvitamin D inhibits glutamine metabolism in Harvey-ras transformed MCF10A human breast epithelial cell. J Steroid Biochem Mol Biol. 2016;163:147–56.
68. Li HX, Gao JM, Liang JQ, Xi JM, Fu M, Wu YJ. Vitamin D3 potentiates the growth inhibitory effects of metformin in DU145 human prostate cancer cells mediated by AMPK/mTOR signalling pathway. Clin Exp Pharmacol Physiol. 2015;42(6):711–7.
69. Bothwell KD, Shaurova T, Merzianu M, Suresh A, Kuriakose MA, Johnson CS, et al. Impact of short-term 1,25-dihydroxyvitamin D3 on the chemopreventive efficacy of erlotinib against oral cancer. Cancer Prev Res. 2015;8(9):765–76.
70. Bakhshalizadeh S, Amidi F, Shirazi R, Shabani Nashtaei M. Vitamin D3 regulates steroidogenesis in granulosa cells through AMP-activated protein kinase (AMPK) activation in a mouse model of polycystic ovary syndrome. Cell Biochem Funct. 2018;36(4):183–93.
71. Wang H, Wang JM, Qu H, Wei HL, Ji BL, Yang ZS, et al. In vitro and in vivo inhibition of mTOR by 1,25- dihydroxyvitamin D3 to improve early diabetic nephropathy via the DDIT4/TSC2/mTOR pathway. Endocrine. 2016;54(2):348–59.
72. Hoyer-Hansen M, Bastholm L, Szyniarowski P, Campanella M, Szabadkai G, Farkas T, et al. Control of macroautophagy by calcium, calmodulin-dependent kinase kinase-beta, and Bcl-2. Mol Cell. 2007;25(2):193–205.
73. Jia W, Chang B, Sun L, Zhu H, Pang L, Tao L, et al. REDD1 and p-AKT over-expression may predict poor prognosis in ovarian cancer. Int J Clin Exp Pathol. 2014;7(9):5940–9.
74. Sofer A, Lei K, Johannessen CM, Ellisen LW. Regulation of mTOR and cell growth in response to energy stress by REDD1. Mol Cell Biol. 2005;25(14):5834–45.
75. Lisse TS, Liu T, Irmler M, Beckers J, Chen H, Adams JS, et al. Gene targeting by the vitamin D response element binding protein reveals a role for vitamin D in osteoblast mTOR signaling. FASEB J. 2011;25(3):937–47.
76. Jorde R, Sneve M, Emaus N, Figenschau Y, Grimnes G. Cross-sectional and longitudinal relation between serum 25-hydroxyvitamin D and body mass index: the Tromso study. Eur J Nutr. 2010;49(7):401–7.
77. Kim JH, Kang S, Jung YN, Choi HS. Cholecalciferol inhibits lipid accumulation by regulating early adipogenesis in cultured adipocytes and zebrafish. Biochem Biophys Res Commun. 2016;469(3):646–53.
78. Tworoger SS, Lee IM, Buring JE, Rosner B, Hollis BW, Hankinson SE. Plasma 25-hydroxyvitamin D and 1,25-dihydroxyvitamin D and risk of incident ovarian cancer. Cancer Epidemiol Biomark Prev. 2007;16(4):783–8.
79. Zheng W, Danforth KN, Tworoger SS, Goodman MT, Arslan AA, Patel AV, et al. Circulating 25-hydroxyvitamin D and risk of epithelial ovarian cancer: cohort consortium vitamin D pooling project of rarer cancers. Am J Epidemiol. 2010;172(1):70–80.
80. Horowitz NS, Wright AA. Impact of obesity on chemotherapy management and outcomes in women with gynecologic malignancies. Gynecol Oncol. 2015;138(1):201–6.
81. Uddin S, Bu R, Ahmed M, Abubaker J, Al-Dayel F, Bavi P, et al. Overexpression of leptin receptor predicts an unfavorable outcome in middle eastern ovarian cancer. Mol Cancer. 2009;8:74.
82. Kasiappan R, Sun Y, Lungchukiet P, Quarni W, Zhang X, Bai W. Vitamin D suppresses leptin stimulation of cancer growth through microRNA. Cancer Res. 2014;74(21):6194–204.
83. Zhang Z, Zhang H, Hu Z, Wang P, Wan J, Li B. Synergy of 1,25-dihydroxyvitamin D3 and carboplatin in growth suppression of SKOV-3 cells. Oncol Lett. 2014;8(3):1348–54.
84. Holick MF, Binkley NC, Bischoff-Ferrari HA, Gordon CM, Hanley DA, Heaney RP, et al. Evaluation, treatment, and prevention of vitamin D deficiency: an Endocrine Society clinical practice guideline. J Clin Endocrinol Metab. 2011; 96(7):1911–30.
85. Qin B, Moorman PG, Alberg AJ, Barnholtz-Sloan JS, Bondy M, Cote ML, et al. Dairy, calcium, vitamin D and ovarian cancer risk in African-American women. Br J Cancer. 2016;115(9):1122–30.
86. Trivedi DP, Doll R, Khaw KT. Effect of four monthly oral vitamin D3 (cholecalciferol) supplementation on fractures and mortality in men and women living in the community: randomised double blind controlled trial. BMJ. 2003;326(7387):469.
87. Lappe JM, Travers-Gustafson D, Davies KM, Recher RR, Heaney RP. Vitamin D and calcium supplementation reduces cancer risk: results of a randomized trial. Am J Clin Nutr. 2007;85(6):1586–91.
88. Moukayed M, Grant WB. Molecular link between vitamin D and cancer prevention. Nutrients. 2013;5(10):3993–4021.
89. Bolland MJ, Grey A, Gamble GD, Reid IR. Calcium and vitamin D supplements and health outcomes: a reanalysis of the Women's Health Initiative (WHI) limited-access data set. Am J Clin Nutr. 2011;94(4):1144–9.
90. Lappe J, Watson P, Travers-Gustafson D, Recker R, Garland C, Gorham E, et al. Effect of vitamin D and calcium supplementation on cancer incidence in older women: a randomized clinical trial. JAMA. 2017;317(12):1234–43.

13

Clinical analysis of chemo-resistance risk factors in endometriosis associated ovarian cancer

Tong Ren[1†], Ting-Ting Sun[1†], Shu Wang[1*], Jian Sun[2], Yang Xiang[1*], Keng Shen[1] and Jing-He Lang[1*]

Abstract

Background: To analyze the clinical characteristics and chemo-resistance related factors of patients with resistant and non-resistant endometriosis-associated ovarian cancer (ovarian clear cell carcinoma and endometrioid carcinoma) by reviewing the data of epithelial ovarian cancer patients who received initial treatment in our hospital over a 12-year period.

Results: Among the 304 patients, 17.1% were seen with platinum-based drug resistance. The ROC curve of continuous variables was drawn according to resistance situation, then they were grouped by age (< 48 or ≥ 48 years), tumor size (< 7 cm or ≥ 7 cm) and Ca125 (< 90 and ≥ 90 U/ml). In univariate analysis, age ≥ 48 years, initial symptom of abdominal distension or weight loss, abnormal preoperative serum Ca125, Ca125 < 90 U/ml, advanced FIGO stage, absence of endometriosis, bilateral tumors, lack of lymphadenectomy, positive lymph nodes, unsatisfactory initial cytoreduction surgery and history of breast cancer were all related to drug resistance in ovarian cancer. In multivariate analysis, advanced stage, lack of lymphadenectomy, positive lymph nodes and history of breast cancer were independent risk factors related to platinum-based drug resistance ($P < 0.05$).

Conclusion: For patients of endometriosis-related ovarian cancer, platinum-based drug resistance were associated with advanced FIGO stage, lack of lymphadenectomy, positive lymph nodes and history of breast cancer.

Keywords: Chemo-resistance, Risk factors, Endometriosis associated ovarian cancer

Background

At present, many scholars regard endometriosis-associated ovarian cancer(EAOC) as a special pathological type of epithelial ovarian cancer(EOC), including ovarian clear cell carcinoma (OCCC) and endometrioid carcinoma. Studies have reported that the clinical features and prognosis of patients with EAOC were different from those with other EOCs. Compared with ovarian serous carcinoma, the onset age of OCCC was younger (55 vs 64 years; median age) [1]. A study comparing early ovarian cancer and advanced ovarian cancer (I/II vs. III/IV) reported that 57–81% of OCCC were diagnosed in early stage (I/II) [2]. Since most patients of OCCC were with unilateral pelvic mass of early stage, their prognosis was better than other types of EOC. The 5-year survival rate of OCCC patients with early stage was higher than 80% [3]. However, the prognosis of those with advanced stage was poorer than that of other EOCs with the 5-year survival rate about 20%, which might be related to the resistance to platinum-based chemotherapy [4]. The clinical risk factors of chemo-resistance in patients with EAOC have not been reported. By retrospectively analyzing the data of EOC patients who received initial treatment in our hospital over a 12-year period, this study intended to analyze the clinical features and chemo-resistance related factors of patients with resistant and non-resistant EAOC (OCCC and endometrioid carcinoma), expecting to provide references for the guidance of clinical treatments and the prediction of survival outcomes.

* Correspondence: wangshu219@hotmail.com; XiangY@pumch.cn; langjh@hotmail.com
†Tong Ren and Ting-Ting Sun contributed equally to this work.
[1]Department of Obstetrics and Gynecology, Peking Union Medical College Hospital, Chinese Academy of Medical Science and Peking Union Medical College, 1 ShuaiFuYuan, DongCheng District, Beijing 100730, China
Full list of author information is available at the end of the article

Table 1 Clinical and morphological characteristics of patients with or without chemo-resistance

Variable	Category	Number(%)	Chemo-sensitive(%)	Chemoresistance(%)	*P*
		304	252(82.9%)	52(17.1%)	
Age	< 48	129(42.43)	114(45.24)	15(28.85)	0.0294*
	≥48	175(57.57)	138(54.76)	37(71.15)	
Menopausal status	Pre	161(52.96)	139(55.16)	22(42.31)	0.0909
	Post	143(47.04)	113(44.84)	30(57.69)	
Gravidity	< 1	35(11.51)	31(12.3)	4(7.69)	0.3431
	> = 1	269(88.49)	221(87.7)	48(92.31)	
Parity	< 1	51(16.78)	46(18.25)	5(9.62)	0.1290
	> = 1	253(83.22)	206(81.75)	47(90.38)	
Abdominal pain	No	210(69.08)	174(69.05)	36(69.23)	0.9016
	Yes	93(30.59)	77(30.56)	16(30.77)	
Bloating	No	243(79.93)	208(82.54)	35(67.31)	0.0125*
	Yes	61(20.07)	44(17.46)	17(32.69)	
Palpable mass	No	223(73.36)	182(72.22)	41(78.85)	0.3253
	Yes	81(26.64)	70(27.78)	11(21.15)	
Incidental finding	No	256(84.21)	208(82.54)	48(92.31)	0.0786
	Yes	48(15.79)	44(17.46)	4(7.69)	
Irregular menstruation	No	275(90.46)	226(89.68)	49(94.23)	0.3094
	Yes	29(9.54)	26(10.32)	3(5.77)	
Postmenopausal bleeding	No	285(93.75)	235(93.25)	50(96.15)	0.4316
	Yes	19(6.25)	17(6.75)	2(3.85)	
Emaciation	No	294(96.71)	248(98.41)	46(88.46)	0.0002*
	Yes	10(3.29)	4(1.59)	6(11.54)	
Abnormal vaginal discharge	No	302(99.34)	250(99.21)	52(100)	0.5192
	Yes	2(0.66)	2(0.79)	0(0)	
Ca125 in normal range(< 35 U/L)	No	249(81.91)	199(78.97)	50(96.15)	0.0034*
	Yes	55(18.09)	53(21.03)	2(3.85)	
CA125group	< 90	112(36.84)	104(41.27)	8(15.38)	0.0004*
	≥90	192(63.16)	148(58.73)	44(84.62)	
Early or late Stage	FIGO I + II	185(60.86)	175(69.44)	10(19.23)	<.0001*
	FIGO III + IV	119(39.14)	77(30.56)	42(80.77)	
FIGO stage[a]	I	141(46.38)	136(53.97)	5(9.62)	<.0001*
	II	44(14.47)	39(15.48)	5(9.62)	
	III	104(34.21)	69(27.38)	35(67.31)	
	IV	15(4.93)	8(3.17)	7(13.46)	
Tumor size group	< 7	80(26.32)	66(26.19)	14(26.92)	0.9130
	≥7	224(73.68)	186(73.81)	38(73.08)	
Pathology Grade	G1	45(24.19)	44(28.03)	1(3.45)	0.0128*
	G2	59(31.72)	49(31.21)	10(34.48)	
	G3	82(44.09)	64(40.76)	18(62.07)	
Pathology type	Endometrioid	186(61.18)	157(62.30)	29(55.77)	0.435
	Clear cell	118(38.82)	95(37.70)	23(44.23)	
Endometriosis	No	235(77.30)	188(74.6)	47(90.38)	0.0134*
	Yes	69(22.70)	64(25.4)	5(9.62)	

Table 1 Clinical and morphological characteristics of patients with or without chemo-resistance *(Continued)*

Variable	Category	Number(%)	Chemo-sensitive(%)	Chemoresistance(%)	P
Side of tumor	Unilateral	212(69.74)	183(72.62)	29(55.77)	0.0160*
	Bilateral	92(30.26)	69(27.38)	23(44.23)	
LN metastasis	No	213(70.07)	195(77.38)	18(34.62)	<.0001*
	Yes	40(13.16)	24(9.52)	16(30.77)	
	unclear	51(16.78)	33(13.1)	18(34.62)	
LN dissection	No	51(16.78)	33(13.1)	18(34.62)	0.0002*
	Yes	253(83.22)	219(86.9)	34(65.38)	
Residual disease	No	231(75.99)	207(82.14)	24(46.15)	<.0001*
	Yes	73(24.01)	45(17.86)	28(53.85)	
TH	No	297(97.7)	246(97.62)	51(98.08)	0.8411
	Yes	7(2.3)	6(2.38)	1(1.92)	
Tubal ligation	No	290(95.39)	243(96.43)	47(90.38)	0.0583
	Yes	14(4.61)	9(3.57)	5(9.62)	
Sterilization surgery	No	283(93.09)	237(94.05)	46(88.46)	0.1481
	Yes	21(6.91)	15(5.95)	6(11.54)	
Endometrial disorder	No	252(82.89)	208(82.54)	44(84.62)	0.7174
	Yes	52(17.11)	44(17.46)	8(15.38)	
Variable endometrial disorder	No	252(82.89)	207(82.14)	45(86.54)	0.7998
	EP	27(8.88)	23(9.13)	4(7.69)	
	EIN	22(7.24)	19(7.54)	3(5.77)	
	EC	3(0.99)	3(1.19)	0(0)	
Breast cancer	No	296(97.37)	248(98.41)	48(92.31)	0.0123*
	Yes	8(2.63)	4(1.59)	4(7.69)	
HT	No	250(82.24)	208(82.54)	42(80.77)	0.7610
	Yes	54(17.76)	44(17.46)	10(19.23)	
DM	No	286(94.08)	236(93.65)	50(96.15)	0.4862
	Yes	18(5.92)	16(6.35)	2(3.85)	

[a]According to the classification system of FIGO staging (2013 version)
Abbreviation: *Ca125* cancer antigen 125, *EM* endometriosis, *LN* lymph node, *TH* total hysterectomy, *EP* endometrial polyps, *EIN* endometrial intraepithelial neoplasm, *EC* endometrial cancer, *HT* hypertension, *DM* diabetic mellitus
*$P < 0.05$

Results

A total of 304 patients diagnosed with EAOC and treated in PUMCH were identified, 52(17.1%) of which were seen with platinum-based drug resistance and the rest 252(82.9%) were in the non-resistant group. Table 1 showed the demographic and clinical characteristics of all the patients. In this study, based on the ROC curve of chemo-resistance, the above continuous variables were grouped by age, tumor size and Ca125 level[age: < 48 or ≥ 48 years; tumor size: < 7 cm or ≥ 7 cm; Ca125: < 90 U/L or ≥ 90 U/L], as seen in Fig. 1. Univariate analysis showed that compared with the non-resistant group, there were more patients with age ≥ 48 years in the chemo-resistant group (71.15% vs 54.76%, $P = 0.0294$), more with symptoms of abdominal distension (32.69% vs 17.46%, $P = 0.0125$) and emaciation (11.54% vs 1.59%, $P = 0.0002$), fewer with normal level of Ca125 (3.85% vs 21.03%, $P = 0.0034$) but more Ca125 < 90 U/L (84.62% vs 58.73%, $P = 0.0004$), more advanced FIGO stage(III + IV) (80.77% vs 30.56%, $P < 0.001$), more high-grade tumor(62.07% vs 40.76%; $P = 0.0128$), fewer coexisting endometriosis (9.62% vs 25.4%, $P = 0.0134$), more bilateral tumors (44.23% vs 27.38%, $P = 0.0160$), more positive LNs (30.77% vs 9.52%, $P < 0.001$), fewer lymphadenectomy (34.62% vs 13.1%, $P = 0.0002$), more residual tumor > 1 cm and more history of breast cancer (7.69% vs 1.59%, $P = 0.0123$). Meanwhile, there was no statistically significant difference seen in menopause status, number of pregnancies and labors, tumor size, histologic type, coexisting endometrial lesions, history of hysterectomy or tubal sterilization and history of diabetes mellitus or hypertension, as showed in Table 1 ($P > 0.05$).

In multivariate analysis however, only FIGO stage ($P = 0.004$), positive LNs ($P = 0.040$), lymph nodes resection ($P = 0.016$) and history of breast cancer ($P = 0.044$) were

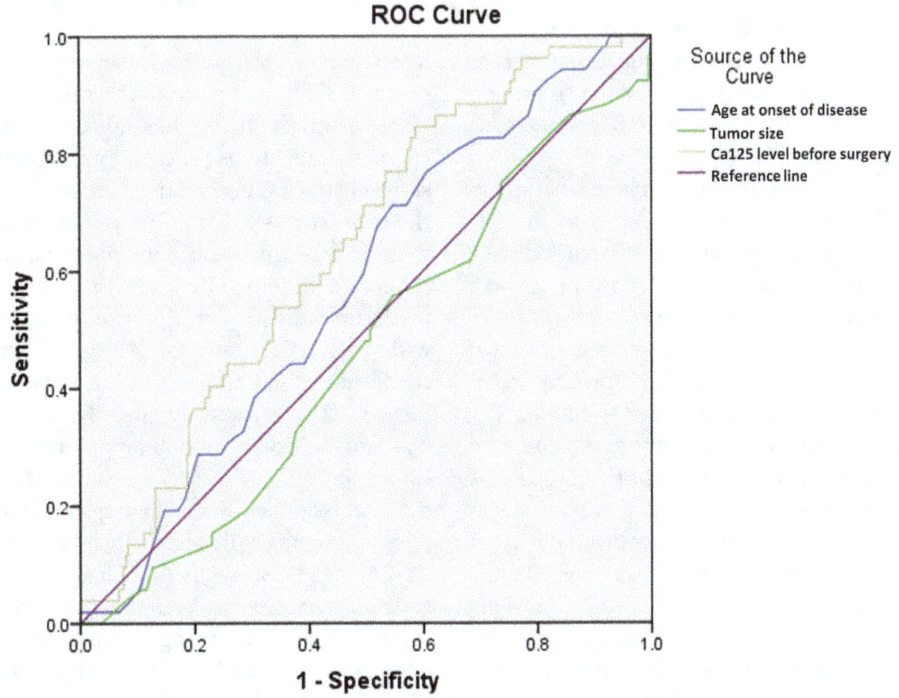

Fig. 1 ROC curve for age of disease onset, tumor size, pre-surgery Ca125 in the occurrence of chemo-resistance

independent risk factors of platinum-based drug resistance, while onset age, initial symptoms, Ca125 level, coexisting endometriosis and residual tumors were not, as seen in Table 2.

Discussion

This study regarded OCCC and ovarian endometrioid carcinoma as a whole of EAOC for the first time and investigated the clinicopathological risk factors of platinum-based chemoresistance. Univariate analysis showed that age, higher level of Ca125, advanced FIGO stage, high-grade tumor, absence of endometriosis, bilateral tumors, lack of lymphadenectomy, positive LNs, residual lesion > 1 cm and history of breast cancer were related to chemoresistance. However, multivariate analysis showed that FIGO stage, lack of lymphadenectomy, positive LNs and history of breast cancer were independent risk factors associated with drug resistance to platinum in patients with such type of EOC.

Table 2 Multivariate analysis of risk factors of chemo-resistance among endometriosis related ovarian cancer patients

	B	S.E.	P	OR(95%CI)
Age	.337	.395	.393	1.4(0.65~ 3.04)
Bloating	−.057	.401	.886	0.94(0.43~ 2.07)
Emaciation	1.447	.791	.067	4.25(0.9~ 20.02)
Ca125 in normal range	.728	.797	.361	2.07(0.43~ 9.87)
EM	−.016	.573	.978	0.98(0.32~ 3.03)
FIGO stage[a]	1.422	.497	.004*	4.15(1.57~ 10.97)
LN metastasis	.980	.477	.040*	2.66(1.05~ 6.78)
LN dissection	1.059	.440	.016*	2.88(1.22~ 6.82)
Residual disease	.396	.405	.328*	1.49(0.67~ 3.29)
Breast cancer	1.851	.918	.044*	6.37(1.05~ 38.49)
Constant	−5.388	1.018	.000	

*The difference reached statistical significance. *P* values were cultivated by Cox regression analysis. The overall test of the above model showed the model was significance, $p < 0.0001$

[a]According to the classification system of FIGO staging (2013 version)

Abbreviation: *Ca125* cancer antigen 125, *EM* endometriosis, *LN* lymph node

A large number of previous studies focused on the drug resistance in OCCC. Some retrospective studies have shown that OCCC was resistant to traditional platinum-based chemotherapy regimens with an objective effective rate of 11–27%, while the response rate of serous adenocarcinoma (SAC) was 73–81%, significantly higher than that of OCCC [5–7]. Utsunomiya et al. found that the effective rate of paclitaxel plus carboplatin (TC) regimen in patients with OCCC was not high either [8]. Rauh-Hain et al. reported that the response rate of 121 OCCC patients treated with first-line platinum-based chemotherapy regimens was 79 and 24% of the patients relapsed within 6 months after the last cycle of chemotherapy of initial treatments [9]. Moreover, their results showed that unsatisfactory cytoreductive surgery and wide dissemination of tumors were significantly associated with platinum resistance by multivariate logistic regression analysis. On the other hand, Liang et al. have reported that advanced stage, poor differentiation, LN positivity, CA125 level > 1000 U/mL and suboptimal cytoreductive surgery would lead to drug resistance or partial sensitivity to chemotherapy during the treatment of OCCC. These results were not in full accord with the findings of this study [10].

The mechanism of drug resistance to chemotherapy in OCCC was complex, which might be related to the low proliferation rate of the tumors, the increase of damage to DNA repair activity, the up-regulation of growth factor signaling pathway and the abnormal expression of microtubule-disaggregated protein, etc. Studies have shown that the high resistance of OCCC to chemotherapy might be related to its low cell proliferation rate [4]. Itamochi et al. reported that the doubling time for tumor cells of OCCC was significantly longer than that of SAC (61.4 vs 29.8 h) [11]. Ki-67 protein was expressed at various stages of the cell cycle, representing the proliferative activity of the cells, and its expression in OCCC was significantly lower than that in SAC. In addition, the Ki-67 labelling index (LI) in patients that are resistant to platinum-based chemotherapy was significantly lower than it in those sensitive (15.3% vs 30.2%) [4]. As known, platinum-based drugs inhibited the proliferation of tumor cells mainly by hindering the replication of DNA. Therefore, the low proliferation rate of OCCC cells enabled them to some extent to be tolerant to platinum-based drugs targeting on DNA, which suggested that the chemoresistance of OCCC might be associated with its low proliferation rate [12].

Previous studies have showed tumors lack of DNA mismatch repair (MMR) system were highly resistant to certain methylated drugs of chemotherapy in vitro [13]. The function of MMR is to correct mistakes in DNA replication and play an important role in the sensitivity of DNA damage factors. MMR deficiency might result from germline mutations of two major MMR genes, such as hMLH1 and hMSH2, as well as epigenetic silencing due to the methylation of the hMLH1 promoter, leading to inactivation of the gene system. Cai et al. reported that the high expression of mutations in hMLH1 and hMSH2 existed in OCCC and was associated with its development [14]. In addition, Niimi K et al. also reported that the expression of DNA damage repair related protein REV7 in OCCC was significantly higher than that in other types of EOCs (73.5% vs 53.4%), and the knockdown of REV gene could induce apoptosis and DNA damage in tumor cells, leading to a significant improvement of chemoresistance to cisplatin in OCCC [15]. On the other hand, Itamochi H et al. reported that the use of CHK inhibitors could improve the drug resistance of OCCC to cisplatin [16], while the main function of cell cycle checkpoint kinase (CHK) was to regulate the synthesis of DNA in tumor cells.

In addition, the up-regulation of growth factor signaling pathway is related to drug resistance in tumor. As cell surface receptor tyrosine kinase, epidermal growth-factor receptor (EGFR) can activate the mitogen-activated protein kinase pathway, thus inhibiting the apoptosis induced by chemotherapy drugs [17]. An immunohistochemical study showed that EGFR could be found in 61% of CCC, and the overexpression of EGFR might be related to chemotherapy resistance and poor prognosis of ovarian cancer [18]. Siddiqui GK et al. reported that in platinum-resistant group, the proportion of patients with high expression of VEGF in tumor tissues was significantly higher than it in the platinum-sensitive group (86% vs 2%), suggesting that the resistance of EOC to platinum-based chemotherapy was related to VEGR expression [19]. Mabuchi S et al. confirmed in vitro that the expression of VEGF in cisplatin-resistant OCCC cell lines was significantly higher than that in cisplatin-sensitive OCCC cell lines, suggesting that the generation of drug resistance might be related to the angiogenesis in the tumors [20]. According to previous literatures, the expression of HER2 in OCCC was much higher than it in other major histological types of EOCs, and tumors with overexpression of HER2 showed low sensitivity to traditional anti-tumor drugs, leading to the poor prognosis of these patients [21, 22].

Studies about the drug resistance in ovarian endometrioid carcinoma was limited. Pylväs-Eerola et al. have reported that the preoperative level of 8-hydroxy-2-deoxyguanosine in patients were significantly associated with chemoresistance of ovarian endometrioid carcinoma, which could be used as a factor for resistance prediction [23].

Our results showed that histologic type indicating OCCC or endometrioid carcinoma was not an independent risk factor of platinum-based drug resistance (55.77% vs 44.23%, $P = 0.435$), which was not consistent with previous studies, suggesting that the platinum-based drug resistance in these two types of tumors might have similarities. More molecular biological researches were expected to explore the molecular mechanism of chemoresistance in EAOC.

Conclusion

This study regarded endometriosis-related OCCC and endometrioid carcinoma as a whole of EAOC for the first time and analyzed the clinicopathological risk factors of platinum-based chemoresistance. Multivariate analysis showed that FIGO stage, positive LNs, lack of lymphadenectomy and history of breast cancer were independent risk factors of drug resistance in patients with EAOC. This finding is of certain value for predicting platinum-based drug resistance in the treatment of EAOC, which may give some instructions for designing individualized chemotherapy regimens. In the future, it is expected to carry out more accurate molecular typing for such patients through molecular biological study, which can be used to guide precise medication of chemotherapy drugs for patients with ovarian cancers.

Methods

This is a retrospective study conducted at Department of Obsterics and Gynecology, Peking Union Medical College Hospital(PUMCH). We identified all the 304 patients who received surgical treatments and postoperative chemotherapy from January 2000 to December 2012, including 118 cases of OCCCs and 186 cases of endometrioid carcinomas confirmed by postoperative histopathology. All patients with EAOC of early stage (stage I and II) have received completed staging surgery; and those of advanced stage (stage III and IV) have undergone optimal CRS, except for those with unresectable tumors who received suboptimal CRS. They all received adjuvant chemotherapy of platinum-based regimens after primary surgery.

The clinicopathologic data of patients with EAOC were collected, including age, initial symptoms, menopause status, number of pregnancies and labors, previous medical complications, preoperative CA125 level, FIGO stage, tumor size, laterality, histologic type, grade, coexisting endometriosis, lymph nodes(LNs) metastasis, lymphadenectomy (the resection of pelvic LNs with or without para-aortic LNs), residual tumor, history of hysterectomy and tubal ligation, coexisting endometrial lesions (including endometrial polyps, atypical hyperplasia and endometrial cancer), history of breast cancer, history of hypertension and diabetes. Platinum-based drug resistance in ovarian cancer was defined as a definite progression or recurrence of disease within 6 months after completing the last cycle of chemotherapy for initial treatments. In this study, we defined ovarian cancer concurrent with endometriosis as the presence of ovarian cancer and endometriosis identified histologically in the same ovary, the presence of endometriosis in one ovary and ovarian cancer in the contralateral ovary, or the presence of ovarian cancer and extraovarian pelvic endometriosis (eg, peritoneal endometriosis).

SPSS 22.0 was used for statistical analysis. Continuous variables were analyzed using an independent-sample t test. Categorical variables were analyzed using χ^2 test or Fisher's exact test. Odds ratio (OR) and 95% confidence interval (CI) were calculated. The effects of clinicopathological characteristics on chemoresistance in EAOC were assessed using logistic regression models through univariate and multivariate analysis. Receiver Operating Characteristic (ROC) curve was constructed to define the optimal cutoff value for stratifying and grouping. All statistical tests were two-sided and differences were considered statistically significant at $P < 0.05$.

Abbreviations

Ca125: Cancer antigen 125; DFS: Disease-free survival; EAOC: Endometriosis-associated ovarian cancer; EAOCCC: Endometriosis-associated ovarian clear cell carcinoma; EAOEC: Endometriosis-associated ovarian endometrioid carcinoma; OS: Overall survival

Acknowledgements

We appreciate the gynecologists at Peking Union Medical College Hospital for their diligent clinical work and precise data recording about the cases we reported in this article.

Funding

This study was funded by National Key R&D Program of China (No.SQ2017YFSF080001) and National Natural Science Foundation of China (No. 81501236).

Authors' contributions

TR and TS make substantial contributions to conception and design, analysis and interpretation of data, and drafting the article. JS has reviewed the pathological slides. WS, YX and JL have designed the study and participate in revising it critically for important intellectual content. KS have contributed to some valuable advice during preparing this paper. All authors read and approved the final manuscript.

Competing interests

The authors declare that they have no competing interests.

Author details

[1]Department of Obstetrics and Gynecology, Peking Union Medical College Hospital, Chinese Academy of Medical Science and Peking Union Medical College, 1 ShuaiFuYuan, DongCheng District, Beijing 100730, China.
[2]Department of Pathology, Peking Union Medical College Hospital, Chinese Academy of Medical Science and Peking Union Medical College, Beijing, People's Republic of China.

References

1. Chan JK, Teoh D, Hu JM, Shin JY, Osann K, Kapp DS. Do clear cell ovarian carcinomas have poorer prognosis compared to other epithelial cell types? A study of 1411 clear cell ovarian cancers. Gynecol Oncol. 2008;109:370–6.
2. Behbakht K, Randall TC, Benjamin I, Morgan AM, King S, Rubin CS. Clinical characteristics of clear cell carcinoma of the ovary. Gynecol Oncol. 1998;70: 255–8.
3. Sugiyama T, Kamura T, Kigawa J, Terakawa N, Kikuchi Y, Kita T, et al. Clinical characteristics of clear cell carcinoma of the ovary. A distinct histologic type with poor prognosis and resistance to platinum-based chemotherapy. Cancer. 2000;88:2584–9.
4. Itamochi H, Kigawa J, Sugiyama T, et al. Low proliferation activity may be associated with chemoresistance in clear cell carcinoma of the ovary[J]. Obstet Gynecol. 2002;100(2):281–7.
5. Mackay HJ, Brady MF, Oza AM, Reuss A, Pujade-Lauraine E, Swart AM, et al. Gynecologic Cancer InterGroup. Prognostic relevance of uncommon ovarian histology in women with stage III/IV epithelial ovarian cancer. Int J Gynecol Cancer. 2010;20:945–52.
6. FC1 K, RC2 W, LY3 Y, et al. Clear cell carcinomas of the ovary have poorer outcomes compared with serous carcinomas: Results from a single-center Taiwanese study. J Formos Med Assoc. 2018;117:117–25.

7. Miyamoto M, Takano M, Goto T, et al. Clear cell histology as a poor prognostic factor for advanced epithelial ovarian cancer: a single institutional case series through central pathologic review [J]. J Gynecol Oncol. 2013;24(1):37–43.
8. Enomoto TKC, Yamasaki M, Kuragaki M, Sagita Y, Otsuki H, Ikegami N, et al. Is clear cell carcinoma and mucinous carcinoma of the ovary sensitive to combination chemotherapy with paclitaxel and carboplatin? Proc Am Soc Clin Oncol. 2003;22:1797.
9. Rauh-Hain AJ, Winograd D, Growdon WB, Schorge JO, Goodman AK, Boruta DM, et al. Prognostic determinants in patients with uterine and ovarian clear cell carcinoma. Gynecol Oncol. 2012;125:376–80.
10. Liang XD, Zeng HX, Zhu HL, Feng YY, Yin LY, Cui H, Wei LH. Prediction of chemoresistance in epithelial ovarian cancer by clinical factors. Zhonghua Yi Xue Za Zhi. 2011;91(29):2030–3.
11. Itamochi H, Kigawa J, Akeshima R, et al. Mechanisms of cisplatin resistance in clear cell carcinoma of the ovary. Oncology. 2002;62:349Y353.
12. Itamochi H, Kigawa J, Terakawa N. Mechanisms of chemoresistance and poor prognosis in ovarian clear cell carcinoma. Cancer Sci. 2008;99:653Y658.
13. Claij N, te Riele H. Microsatellite instability in human cancer: a prognostic marker for chemotherapy? Exp Cell Res. 1999;246:1–10.
14. Cai KQ, Albarracin C, Rosen D, et al. Microsatellite instability and alteration of the expression of hMLH1 and hMSH2 in ovarian clear cell carcinoma. Hum Pathol. 2004;35:552–9.
15. Niimi K, Murakumo Y, Watanabe N, et al. Suppression of REV7 enhances cisplatin sensitivity in ovarian clear cell carcinoma cells. Cancer Sci. 2014; 105(5):545–52.
16. Itamochi H, Nishimura M, Oumi N, et al. Checkpoint kinase inhibitor AZD7762 overcomes cisplatin resistance in clear cell carcinoma of the ovary. Int J Gynecol Cancer. 2014;24(1):61–9.
17. Johnstone RW, Ruefli AA, Lowe SW. Apoptosis. a link between cancer genetics and chemotherapy. Cell. 2002;108:153–64.
18. Fujimura M, Hidaka T, Saito S. Selective inhibition of the epidermal growth factor receptor by ZD1839 decreases the growth and invasion of ovarian clear cell adenocarcinoma cells. Clin Cancer Res. 2002;8:2448–54.
19. Siddiqui GK, Maclean AB, Elmasry K, et al. Immunohistochemical expression of VEGF predicts response to platinum based chemotherapy in patients with epithelial ovarian cancer. Angiogenesis. 2011;14(2):155–61.
20. Mabuchi S, Kawase C, Altomare DA, et al. Vascular endothelial growth factor is a promising therapeutic target for the treatment of clear cell carcinoma of the ovary. Mol Cancer Ther. 2010;9(8):2411–22.
21. Rowinsky EK, Donehower RC, Jones RJ, Tucker RW. Microtubule changes and cytotoxicity in leukemic cell lines treated with taxol. Cancer Res. 1988; 48:4093–100.
22. Rolitsky CD, Theil KS, McGaughy VR, Copeland LJ, Niemann TH. HER-2/neu amplification and overexpression in endometrial carcinoma. Int J Gynecol Pathol. 1999;18:138–43.
23. M P-E, P K, U P. Preoperative serum 8-hydroxydeoxyguanosine is associated with chemoresistance and is a powerful prognostic factor in endometrioid-type epithelial ovarian cancer. BMC Cancer. 2015;15:493.

14

Cross-linked hyaluronan gel inhibits the growth and metastasis of ovarian carcinoma

Ji Pang[1], Pengcheng Jiang[2], Ying Wang[1], Lu Jiang[1], Hai Qian[1], Yan Tao[1], Ruxia Shi[2], Jizong Gao[3], Yongchang Chen[1] and Yan Wu[1*]

Abstract

Background: The recurrence, metastasis and poor prognosis are important characteristics of ovarian carcinoma (OC), which are associated with exfoliation of cells from the primary tumor and colonization of the cells in pelvic cavity. On the other hand, the life quality of the patients undergoing surgical resection of OC was influenced by postoperative adhesions. Therefore, preventing postoperative implant tumor and adhesion may be effective methods to improve OC treatment. HyaRegen Gel, a cross-linked hyaluronan gel (CHAG), has been widely used as an anti-adhesive agent following pelvic operation in clinic. However, whether it can affect the implantation and growth of OC cells or not is still not clear.

Methods: Migration and invasion assays were applied to detect the effect of CHAG on migration and invasion of OC cells. Western blotting was performed to detect the phosphorylation/activation of EGFR and ERK, and the expression of PCNA and MMP7. Pull down assay was used to analyze the effect of CHAG on the activation of small G protein Rac1. Nude mice implantation tumor model was applied to observe the effect of CHAG on implantation tumor of OC cells.

Results: The results of in vitro experiments showed that CHAG suppressed both basic and EGF-induced migration and invasion of OC cells, blocked the activation of EGF-initiated EGFR activation, inhibited downstream signal transduction of EGFR, and decreased expression of proliferation and migration/invasion related proteins. Meanwhile, results of in vivo experiments showed that CHAG not only inhibited the formation of implantation tumor of OC cells but also delayed the of the growth of the tumors.

Conclusions: CHAG inhibited migration, invasion and proliferation of OC cells in vitro, and suppressed development of implantation tumor of OC in vivo. This made it as both anti-tumor and anti-adhesion agents.

Keywords: HyaRegen gel, Ovarian carcinoma, Migration, Invasion, Growth

Background

Ovarian cancer (OC) represents the most lethal malignancy of female reproductive system and the poor prognosis of OC is often attributable to late diagnosis, postoperative metastasis and recurrence [1, 2]. Many factors affect the prognosis, for example, post-operative adhesion [3, 4], malignant cells dropping off from the primary during surgical resection, and then implanting in abdominopelvic cavity. Therefore, taking measures to prevent **abscission of tumour cells** and choosing suitable anti-adhesion produces to reduce postoperative adhesions are equally important for favorable prognosis [5–7].

Hyaluronic Acid (HA) is made up of glucuronic acid and N-acetylglucosamine disaccharide units. It is abundant in the skin and connective tissues, with a turnover time from several hours to a few days according to tissues [8]. HA plays crucial roles in cell motility, cell adhesion, organization of tissue architecture, and cell proliferation processes [9, 10]. Owing to its biological properties, HA has several clinical applications in

* Correspondence: jsdxwuyan@163.com
[1]Department of Physiology, School of Medicine, Jiangsu University, Zhenjiang City, Jiangsu Province 212013, People's Republic of China
Full list of author information is available at the end of the article

aesthetic surgery, dentistry, dermatology, ophthalmology and orthopedics [8]. **Clinical** research showed that injection of hydrogel containing HA and chitosan could serve as an ideal barrier to prevent postoperative tissue adhesion [11]. **A** randomly-controlled trial reported that a new crosslinked gel (CHAG) was efficient and safe in reducing adhesions after gynecologic laparoscopic surgeries in clinical practice [12]. Additionally, absorbable auto-crosslinked hyaluronan gel could prevent intrauterine adhesion (IUA), decrease adhesion severity, and improve menopause postoperatively, indicating that this absorbable gel could be proposed as a barrier for preventing IUA after intrauterine procedures [13]. In a word, hyaluronan might be applied in resection of pelvic tumor for anti-adhesion, but it was still not clear whether the gel might be a potential stimulus for tumor metastasis and growth or not? In other words, is it safe for HA gel to be applied in tylectomy of pelvic tumor? Our previous study showed that CHAG suppressed colonization, growth and metastasis of gastric cancer cells [14]. However, it is still worthy to investigate whether CHAG has the similar effect on female pelvic tumor, such as OC, and whether CHAG is safe enough to be applied in OC operation for preventing post-operatic adhesion. Therefore, the present work was designed to address the above question. Our results showed that CHAG suppressed the migration and invasion of ovarian cancer cells, and delayed the development OC implantation tumor through blocking EGF-stimulated activation of EGFR and its downstream signal transduction.

Methods

Cell lines and mice

Human ovarian cancer cell line A2780 was purchased from CHI Scientific Inc. (Maynard, MA, USA) and human ovarian cancer cell line SKOV3 was purchased from Institute of Cell Biology (Shanghai, China). The cells were cultured in Dulbecco's modified Eagle's medium (DMEM), supplemented with 10% heat-inactivated fetal bovine serum (FBS; Gibco; Thermo Fisher Scientific, Inc., Waltham, MA, USA), 100 U/ml penicillin and 100 μg/ml streptomycin (HyClone; GE Healthcare Life Sciences, Logan, UT, USA), in a humidified incubator at 37 °C and 5% CO_2. Female nude BALB/c mice (with the age of 6 weeks) were purchased from the Animal Center of Yangzhou University (Yangzhou, Jiangsu Province, China) and maintained in the Animal Center of Jiangsu University in compliance with the Guide for the Care and Use of Laboratory Animals (NIH,76 FR 91; May 11, 2011).

Reagents

CHAG was provided by BioRegen Biomedical (Changzhou) Co., Ltd. (Changzhou, Jiangsu Province, China). Antibodies against β-actin (cat. no. sc-4778; dilution, 1:1000), Rac 1 (cat. no. sc-24,567; dilution, 1:500), and matrix metalloproteinases (MMP) 7 (cat. no. sc-80,205; dilution, 1:500) were purchased from Santa Cruz Biotechnology, Inc. (Dallas, TX, USA). The antibodies against proliferating cell nuclear antigen (PCNA; cat. no. #13110; dilution, 1:1000), phosphorylation (p)-EGFR (Tyr1068) (cat. no. #3777; dilution, 1:1000), p-EGFR (Tyr1173) (cat. no. #4407; dilution, 1:1000), p-Akt (Ser473) (cat. no. #4060; dilution, 1:1000) and p-Erk1/2 (Thr202/Tyr204) (cat. no. #4370; dilution, 1:1000) were purchased from Cell Signaling Technology, Inc. (Danvers, MA, USA). Horseradish peroxidase (HRP)-conjugated goat anti-rabbit and goat anti-mouse secondary antibodies (cat. nos. 111–035-003 and 115–035-003; dilution, 1:10,000) were purchased from Jackson Immuno Research Laboratories, Inc. (West Grove, PA, USA). Transwell plates were purchased from Corning Incorporated (Corning, NY, USA). ECM Gel was purchased from Sigma-Aldrich, Inc. (St. Louis, MO, USA). Recombinant Human EGF (rEGF) was purchased from PeproTech, Inc. (Rocky Hill, NJ, USA). Enhanced chemiluminescence (ECL) reagents were from EMD Millipore (Billerica, MA, USA).

Cell migration assay

Cells in logarithmic growth phase were cultured in FBS-free DMEM for 12 h. After trypsin digestion and centrifugation, 5×10^5/mL cells were re-suspended in different concentrations of CHAG in FBS-free DMEM medium. EGF (100 ng/mL) was added to stimulate the migration of the cells. **Three hundred μL** of the above cell suspension was added to the upper chamber of Transwell plate and 500 μL of DMEM containing 10% FBS was added to the lower chamber. The migration time for the cells was 12 h. At the end of the migration, the cells retained on the upper surface the membrane were swapped off and the cells migrated onto the lower surface of the membrane were stained with Giemsa and then counted under inverted microscopy.

Cell invasion assay

Cell invasion assays were same as described in cell migration assay except that the membrane of the upper chamber was coated with 60 μL of 1.125 μg/μL ECM Gel before adding cell suspension and the invasion time for the cells was 24 h.

The model of transplantation tumor of ovarian cancer cells in nude mice and treatment

Specific Pathogen Free (SPF) grade female BALB/c nude mice with weights of 8.76 ± 1.34 g were maintained in a SPF barrier system. In order to increase the rate of tumor formation, 1×10^7 cells suspended in 400 μL of PBS were implanted into one mouse by subcutaneous injection. After 2 weeks, the tumors were collected and ground into cell suspension with glass homogenizer. The dispersed cells were continually cultured to an adequate number. After trypsin digestion, 1×10^7 cells suspended in 400 μL of PBS were implanted into each mouse by intra-peritoneal cavity injection. After 2 h, 400 μL PBS or 400 μL PBS containing **20 μg CHAG** were injected into the peritoneal cavity and the injection was repeated once every week until the 4th weeks. At the end of the experiment, the animals were euthanized, and the tumors were collected and weighed.

Western blotting

The A2780 and SKOV3 cells were accordingly treated and the whole cell lysates were harvested. All procedures of Western blotting were performed following the manufacturer's protocol (Bio-Rad, Hercules, CA). The primary antibodies were incubated over night at 4 °C, and the corresponding secondary antibodies were incubated for 1 h at room temperature. Protein bands were showed by ECL reagents.

"Pull-down" analysis of active small G protein Rac1

The activity of Rac1 was detected by Pull-down method. Cells (3×10^6/mL) were cultured in 10 cm dishes with serum-free DMEM overnight. Then, the cells were treated with 500 μg/mL or 1000 μg/mL CHAG for 1 h and then stimulated with 100 ng/ml EGF for 5 min. Finally, the cells were harvested with lysis buffer. After centrifugation at 12000 g, 4 °C for 10 min, 20 μL of supernatant was used as the control of the loading. The remaining supernatants were incubated with 100 μL of glutathione glucan beads with GST-Pak1 protein binding domain (GST-PBD) at 4 °C for 1 h. Finally, the activated Rac1 bound to the beads and total Rac1 in cell extracts was detected by Western blotting.

Statistical analysis

All experiments were performed in triplicate. Data are expressed as means ± standard deviation (SD). Statistical analysis was performed using a two-tailed ANOVA with SPSS statistical software. Student's t test was performed if equal variance was ascertained in two groups by F test. $P < 0.05$ was considered significant.

Results

CHAG inhibits basic and EGF-induced migration and invasion of ovarian cancer cells

The results of Transwell migration assay showed that compared to the control group, both 500 and 1000 μg/mL CHAG significantly inhibited the migration of A2780 and SKOV3 cells without stimulation of growth factors (Fig. 1a-d, $P < 0.05$). Furthermore, CHAG also inhibited the EGF-induced migration, and especially, 1000 μg/mL CHAG had a significant inhibitory effect (Fig. 1a-d, $P < 0.05$). Similar results were observed in invasion assay (Fig. 1e-h, $P < 0.05$). The above results indicated that CHAG had an inhibitory function on migration and invasion activities of ovarian cancer cells.

CHAG inhibits the growth of implantation tumor originated from ovarian cancer cells

To investigate the effect of CHAG on the in vivo growth of cancer cells, ovarian cancer cells were implanted into the pelvic cavity of nude mouse. CHAG was administrated into pelvic cavity 2 h later, and then the administration was repeated once per week for 4 weeks. At the end of the experiment, the mice were executed and the weights of the transplantation tumors were measured. The results showed that CHAG treatment significantly decreased the weight of transplantation tumor of A2780 and SKOV3 cells (Fig. 2), demonstrating that CHAG had an inhibitory effect on the growth of transplanted ovarian cancer cells.

CHAG inhibits the activation of EGFR and the EGF/EGFR-initiated signalings in ovarian cancer cells

Epidermal growth factor receptor (EGFR) is a key signaling molecule that drives cellular proliferation, migration, and invasion [15]. Some reports showed that high EGFR expression found in ovarian tumors [16] and EGFR signaling was involved in promoting ovarian cancer cell proliferation [17]. However, there is still some conflicting reports. For example, some data favored EGFR as a reliable marker of survival or responsiveness to therapy [18, 19] but others did not [20, 21], and some reports indicated that using EGFR inhibitors in ovarian cancer patient had not shown favorable clinical outcomes [15, 22, 23]. Thus, in this paper, **it was investigated** whether CHAG inhibited the development of ovarian cancer cells via abrogation of activation of EGFR and EGF/EGFR mediated signaling cascades. The result demonstrated both A2780 and SKOV3 expressed EGFR (Additional file 1: Figure S1), and EGF treatment (100 ng/mL, 5 min) led to an increase of Tyr1068 and Tyr1173 phosphorylation of EGFR, and pre-treatment with CHAG (500 and 1000 μg/mL) efficiently inhibited the EGF-induced phosphorylation of EGFR (Fig. 3a, b), indicating that CHAG inhibited EGF-induced activation of EGFR. Additionally, Western blotting results showed that EGF treatment (100 ng/mL, 5 min) caused significant increase of phosphorylation/activation of Akt and ERK, which were main signaling components downstream of EGFR. Treatment with CHAG blocked EGF-induced phosphorylation/activation of Akt and ERK (Fig. 3a, b). These results confirmed that CHAG could inhibit OC cells through blocking activation of EGFR and its downstream signalings.

CHAG inhibits the activation of small G protein Rac1

Small G protein Rac1 is the **chief** member of Rho family which play important role in regulating migration of

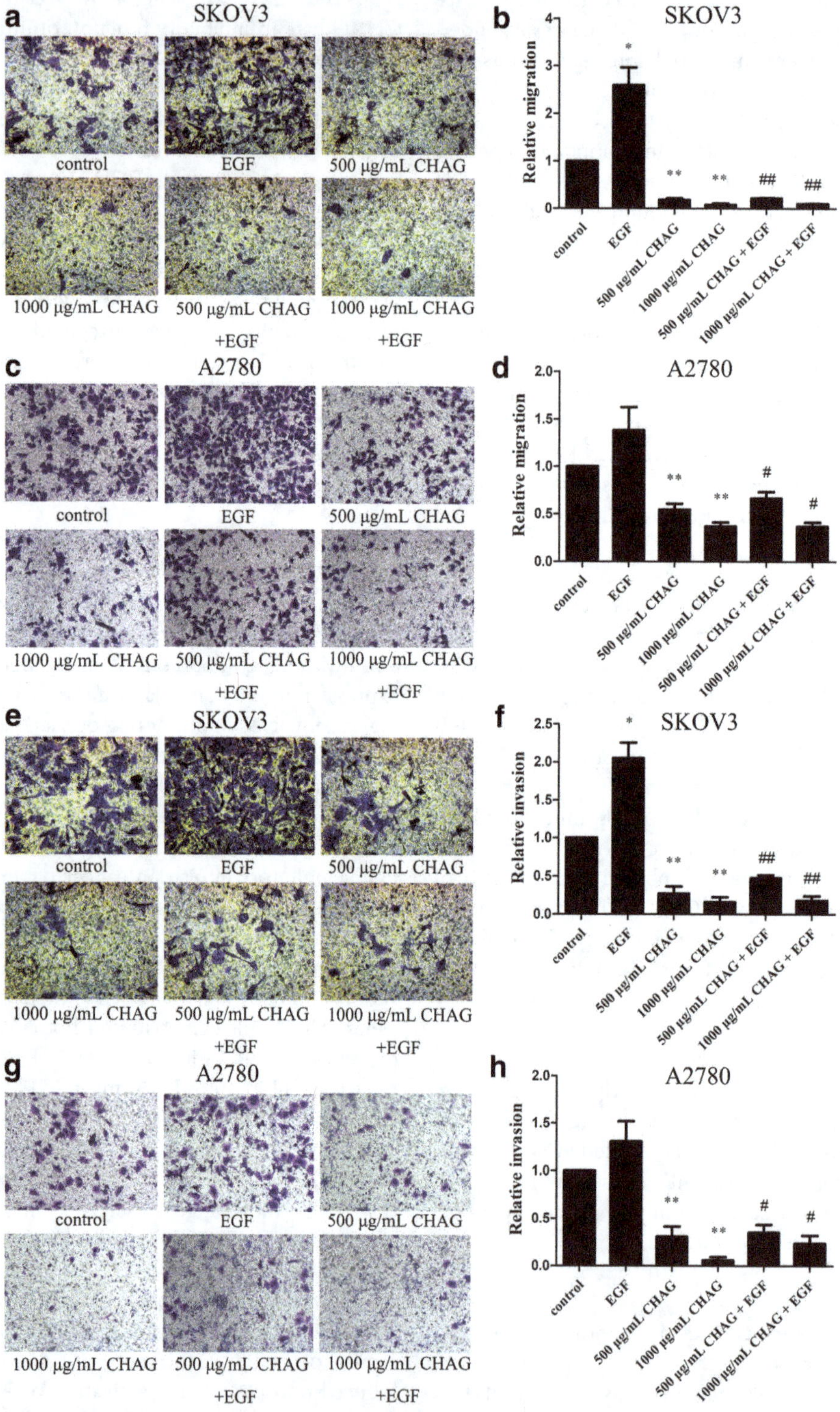

Fig. 1 CHAG inhibits EGF-induced migration and invasion activities of ovarian cancer cells. **a-d** Migration activity of A2780 and SKOV3 cells. **e-h** Invasion activity of A2780 and SKOV3 cells. **a**, **c**, **e** and **g** were representative photomicrographs of cells stained by Giemsa (200×). **b**, **d**, **f** and **h** represent the folds of cells' migration or invasion in the corresponding groups. Data are showed as means ± SD from 3 independent experiments. (*$P < 0.05$, **$P < 0.01$, compared with control group; $^{\#\#}P < 0.01$, compared with EGF group)

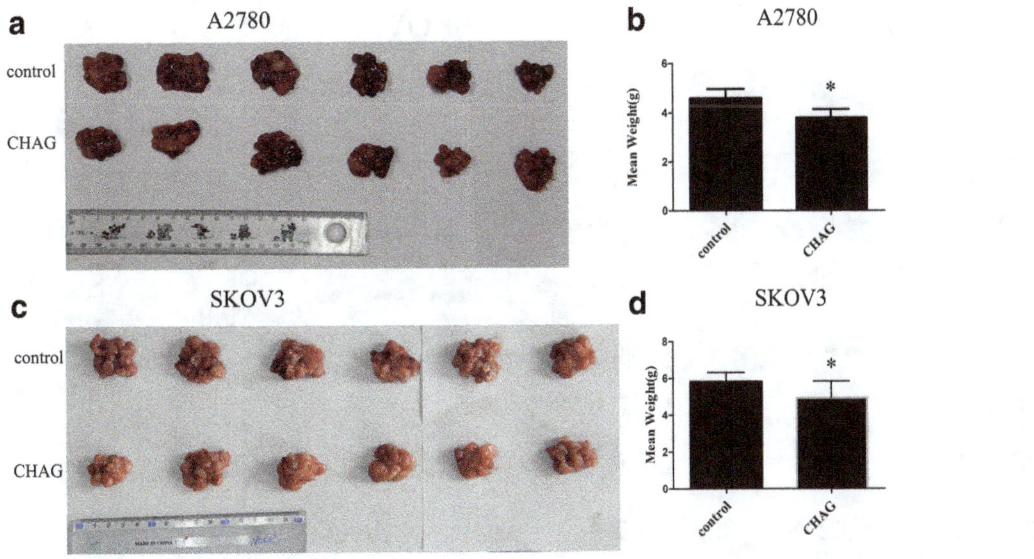

Fig. 2 CHAG inhibits growth of ovarian cancer cell in pelvic cavity. **a** and **c** The tumors from the control and CHAG groups were shown. **b** and **d** The weight of the tumors in corresponding group. The data were shown as means ± SD. (*$P < 0.05$, compared with control group)

cancer cells [24]. Some of EGFR-mediated signal transduction can activate them and thereafter stimulate cell migration [25–27]. Therefore, it is worthy to investigate the inhibitory effect of CHAG on activation of Rac1. In this study, the "Pull-down" assay was performed to detect the level of active (GTP-bound) Rac1. The results showed that treatment with EGF (100 ng/mL, 5 min) increased the amount of GTP-bound/active Rac1. Pretreatment with CHAG efficiently restrained the stimulating effects of EGF on the activation of the small G protein in both A2780 and SKVO3 (Fig. 3g, h).

CHAG inhibits the expression of metastasis and proliferation related proteins.

To get more evidence for the inhibition of CHAG on the migration, invasion and proliferation of OC cells, the proliferation marker, proliferating cell nuclear antigen (PCNA) [28] and tumor-metastasis associated proteins, Matrix metalloproteinase-7 (MMP-7) [29] were detected by Western blotting. The results showed that the expressions of PCNA and MMP7 were increased by EGF treatment (100 ng/mL, 24 h). Applying CHAG (500 or 1000 μg/mL) with EGF at the same time efficiently inhibited EGF-induced expressions of MMP-7 and PCNA (Fig. 3c–f). These results indicated that CHAG could inhibit the expression of migration and proliferation related proteins.

Discussion

OC is one of the major causes of gynecologic cancer-related death, with an overall five-year survival rate of ~45% and an overall 10-year survival rate of 35% in the USA [30]. Currently, the mainstay of OC treatment includes cytoreductive surgery and platinum-based chemotherapy [30]. It is important to perform complete surgery for OC patients, and platinum resistance is the crucial problem in the treatment of these patients. In addition, postoperative tumor metastasis and recurrence cannot be ignored. There are four ways for OC cells to metastasize: direct spreading to the adjacent parts, lymph node metastasizing, blood metastasizing, and planting to other location. During the operation of tumor resection, it is easy to cause tumor cells to fall off and plant into the abdominal cavity or pelvic cavity. In addition to the above problems, adhesion is the most important complication of abdominopelvic surgery, causing some short- and long-term problems, such as infertility, small bowel obstruction and chronic pelvic pain [31]. The main strategies for adhesion prevention in gynecological surgery are focused on improvement of surgical technique and use of anti-adhesive agents, which fall into two major categories: pharmacological agents and barriers [32], and HA is one of them. HA is a naturally component of many body tissues and fluids, where it provides physically supportive and mechanically protective roles [33]. Various combinations of HA have been used for adhesion prevention. However, there were still some unsatisfactory results owing to rapid degradation of native HA. So, modification might be one of the effective ways to prolong the half-life of HA, such as crosslinking modification. In fact, CHAG applied in this paper had been reported to significantly reduce adhesion in abdominopelvic cavity after gynecological laparoscopic surgeries [12, 34]. However, since there was no data elucidating the effect of CHAG on the cells of gynecologic tumor, it is still unclear whether CHAG is safe enough for preventing postoperative adhesion in pelvic surgery of this kind of tumor.

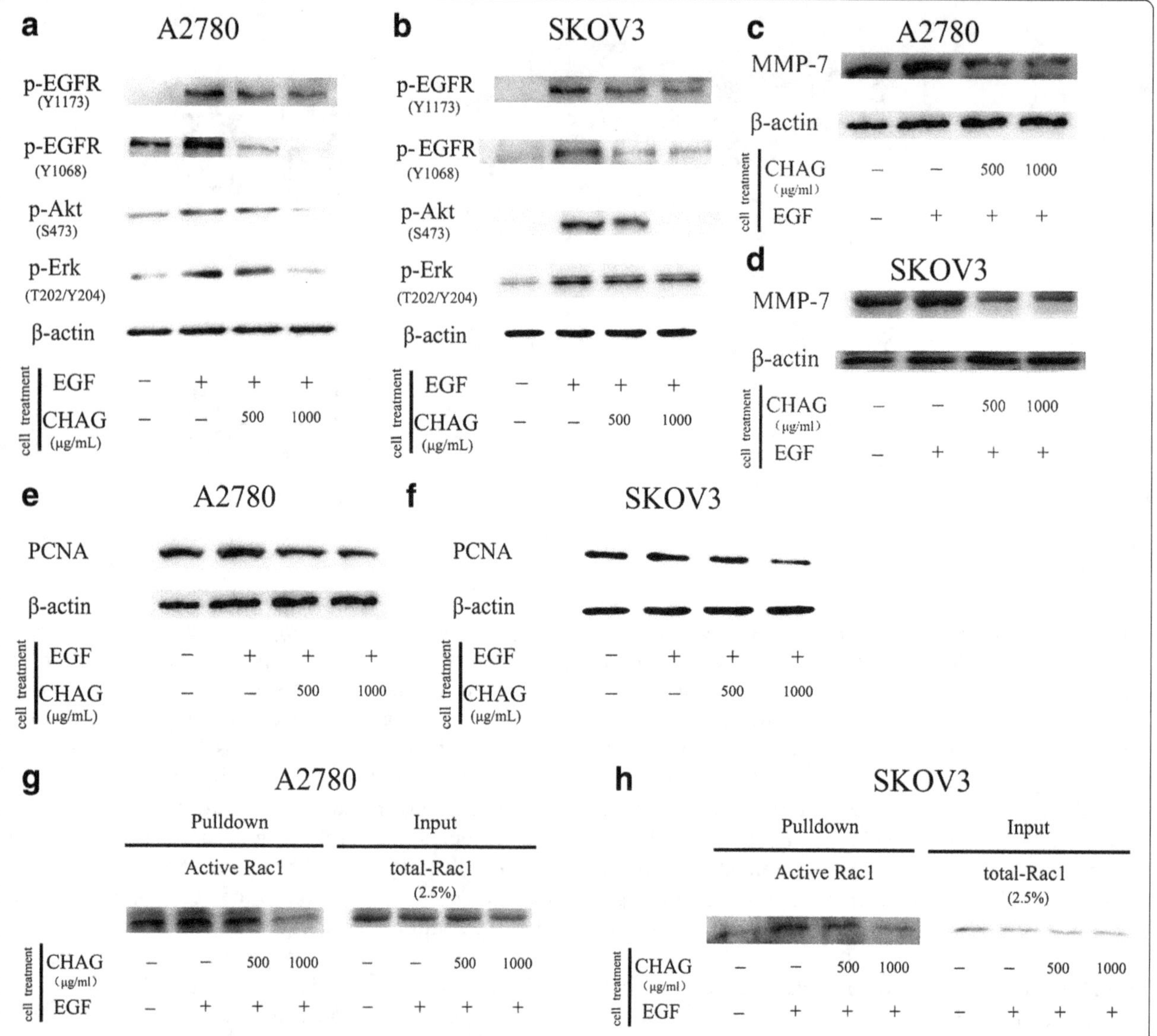

Fig. 3 CHAG blocks activation of EGFR and its downstream signaling molecules, and inhibits EGF-induced expression of MMPs and PCNA in OC cells. **a** and **b** CHAG inhibited phosphorylation/activation of EGFR, Akt and ERK in A2780 and SKOV3 cells. The cells were cultured in serum free DMEM overnight and treated with 500 or 1000 μg/mL CHAG solutions for 1 h and then treated with 100 ng/ml EGF for 5 min. The cellular lysates were subjected to Western blotting. **c** and **d** Detection of the expression of MMP7 in A2780 and SKOV3 cells by Western blotting. In EGF group, the cells were treated with 100 ng/ml EGF for 24 h. In the CHAG + EGF groups, the cells were treated with 500 or 1000 μg/mL CHAG and 100 ng/mL EGF for 24 h. The cells were harvested and the lysates were subjected to Western blotting with anti-MMP7 antibodies. **e** and **f** Western blotting detection of the expression of PCNA in A2780 and SKOV3 cells. The cells were treated same as described in panel **c** and **d**. **g** and **h** CHAG blocked the activation of Rac1. The pull-down results were representatives of three independent experiments

In the in vitro study of this paper, we found that CHAG could inhibit the migration and invasion activities of ovarian cancer cells. And in the in vivo study of this paper, CHAG was administrated 2 h after inoculating ovarian cancer cells into pelvic cavity, which simulated the period that the inoculated cancer cells had been implanted and begun to proliferate in peritoneal cavity. After the first administration, CHAG was administrated weekly until the 4th week, which could simulate the period of mid-term growth of the implantation tumors. The exciting results was that the growth of the transplantation tumors was also efficiently inhibited, indicating that CHAG might be safe to be applied for preventing postoperative adhesion in surgical resection of OC.

In clinical, the effects of HA on tumor are different according to diverse molecular weights. HA synthase (HAS) generates predominantly high molecular weight HA (HMW-HA) with molecular weight between 200 and 2000 kDa, while the degradation generates different-sized

HA polymers (or fragments), such as low molecular weight HA (LMW-HA; < 200 kDa) and HA oligomers [9]. In general, LMW-HA has pro-cancerous effect [35], whereas HMW-HA controls normal homeostasis and displays anti-cancerous activity [34, 35]. Furthermore, there are many controversial findings, which are related to the lack of consensus on size definition, the polydispersity of HA commercial products, and the use of HA from different animal or different tissues. And all the notices should be taken into account whenever a new study on HA is undertaken. The research results of this paper showed that crosslinked hyaluronan, as a HA polymer with boundless molecular weight, had an anti-tumor effects, which was in line with most previous data.

Next, it is worthy to investigate how does CHAG affect proliferation and metastasis activity of cancer cells. Owing to its physical adhesive characteristic, CHAG is speculated to cover the cells and block the interaction between ligands and their receptors. So, the effect of CHAG on the activation of the key growth factor receptor EGFR and its associated signaling molecules were detected. The result indicated that CHAG effectively blocked the EGF-induced phosphorylation/activation of EGFR, inhibited the EGF/EGFR-initiated activation of ERK, Akt and Rac1, and decreased the EGF-induced expression of PCNA and MMP7, suggesting that CHAG inhibited the growth and metastasis of OC cells via blocking the activation of EGFR and subsequent signaling. Our results are similar to the previous research that EGFR is reported to overexpressed in most ovarian cancer [36], and the activation of the EGFR pathway has impact on invasion and metastasis as well as cell survival through the MAPK/ERK, PI3K/AKT and **Rac1** pathways [37–41].

Conclusion

In conclusion, our results demonstrated that CHAG could suppress the development of OC though blocking the activation of EGF-induced activation of EGFR and its downstream signal transduction. This provides evidence for safe application of CHAG in preventing post-operative adhesion of surgical resection of OC.

Abbreviations

CHAG: Cross-linked hyaluronan gel; DMEM: Dulbecco's modified Eagle's medium; EGFR: Epidermal Growth Factor Receptor; GST-PBD: GST-Pak1 protein binding domain; HA: Hyaluronic Acid; HAS: HA synthase; HMW-HA: High molecular weight HA; IUA: Intrauterine adhesion; LMW-HA: Low molecular weight HA; MMP-7: Matrix metalloproteinase-7; OC: Ovarian carcinoma; PCNA: Proliferating cell nuclear antigen; SD: Standard deviation; SPF: Specific Pathogen Free

Funding

This study was supported by grants from the National Natural Science Foundation of China (No. 31771564); the Natural science fund for colleges and universities in Jiangsu Province (No.17KJB310001); the Specialized Research Fund for Senior Personnel Program of Jiangsu University (No.11JDG114); and College student technology innovation project (15A340, 15A341 and 201710299459 W).

Authors' contributions

YCC, JZG and YW: designed the project; JP performed experiments; JP, HQ, YT analyzed the data; YW and YCC wrote the manuscript; LJ, YT, RXS and PCJ contributed to performing data analysis and assisted with manuscript preparation. All authors read and approved the final manuscript.

Competing interests

The authors declare that they have no competing interests.

Author details

[1]Department of Physiology, School of Medicine, Jiangsu University, Zhenjiang City, Jiangsu Province 212013, People's Republic of China. [2]Department of Obstetrics and Gynecology, Changzhou Second People's Hospital Affiliated to Nanjing Medical University, Changzhou City, Jiangsu Province, China. [3]R & D Department, Changzhou BioRegen Biomedical (Changzhou) Co., Ltd., Changzhou City, Jiangsu Province, China.

References

1. Natanzon Y, Goode EL, Cunningham JM. Epigenetics in ovarian cancer. Semin cancer biol 2017.
2. Montagnana M, Benati M, Danese E. Circulating biomarkers in epithelial ovarian cancer diagnosis: from present to future perspective. Ann Transl Med. 2017;5:276.
3. Liu MM, Li PL. Clinical value of anti-adhesion agents used in laparotomy in obstetrics and gynecology. Zhonghua Fu Chan Ke Za Zhi. 2012;47:255–8.
4. Papanikolaou G, Fotopoulou C, Braicu I, Chekerov R, Schmidt SC, Pietzner K, Sehouli J. First surgical experience of intraperitoneal treatment with the trifunctional antibody catumaxomab (anti-EpCam x anti-CD3) for epithelial ovarian cancer. Anticancer Res. 2011;31:2603–8.
5. Fortin CN, Saed GM, Diamond MP. Predisposing factors to post-operative adhesion development. Hum Reprod Update. 2015;21:536–51.
6. Imudia AN, Kumar S, Saed GM, Diamond MP. Pathogenesis of intra-abdominal and pelvic adhesion development. Semin Reprod Med. 2008;26:289–97.
7. Diamond MP. Reduction of postoperative adhesion development. Fertil Steril. 2016;106:994–7. e991
8. Romano CL, De Vecchi E, Bortolin M, Morelli I, Drago L. Hyaluronic acid and its composites as a local antimicrobial/antiadhesive barrier. J Bone Jt Infect. 2017;2:63–72.
9. Jiang D, Liang J, Noble PW. Hyaluronan as an immune regulator in human diseases. Physiol Rev. 2011;91:221–64.
10. Naor D, Sionov RV, Ish-Shalom D. CD44: structure, function, and association with the malignant process. Adv Cancer Res. 1997;71:241–319.
11. Chen CH, Chen SH, Mao SH, Tsai MJ, Chou PY, Liao CH, Chen JP. Injectable thermosensitive hydrogel containing hyaluronic acid and chitosan as a barrier for prevention of postoperative peritoneal adhesion. Carbohydr Polym. 2017;173:721–31.

12. Liu C, Lu Q, Zhang Z, Xue M, Zhang Y, Wang H, Li H, Zhou Y, Li W. A randomized controlled trial on the efficacy and safety of a new crosslinked Hyaluronan gel in reducing adhesions after gynecologic laparoscopic surgeries. J Minim Invasive Gynecol. 2015;22:853–63.
13. Xiao S, Wan Y, Zou F, Ye M, Deng H, Ma J, Wei Y, Tan C, Xue M. Prevention of intrauterine adhesion with auto-crosslinked hyaluronic acid gel: a prospective, randomized, controlled clinical study. Zhonghua Fu Chan Ke Za Zhi. 2015;50:32–6.
14. Lan T, Pang J, Wu Y, Zhu M, Yao X, Wu M, Qian H, Zhang Z, Gao J, Chen Y. Cross-linked hyaluronic acid gel inhibits metastasis and growth of gastric and hepatic cancer cells: in vitro and in vivo studies. Oncotarget. 2016;7:65418–28.
15. Gui T, Shen K. The epidermal growth factor receptor as a therapeutic target in epithelial ovarian cancer. Cancer Epidemiol. 2012;36:490–6.
16. Niikura H, Sasano H, Sato S, Yajima A. Expression of epidermal growth factor-related proteins and epidermal growth factor receptor in common epithelial ovarian tumors. Int J Gynecol Pathol. 1997;16:60–8.
17. Mehner C, Oberg AL, Kalli KR, Nassar A, Hockla A, Pendlebury D, Cichon MA, Goergen KM, Maurer MJ, Goode EL, et al. Serine protease inhibitor Kazal type 1 (SPINK1) drives proliferation and anoikis resistance in a subset of ovarian cancers. Oncotarget. 2015;6:35737–54.
18. Psyrri A, Kassar M, Yu Z, Bamias A, Weinberger PM, Markakis S, Kowalski D, Camp RL, Rimm DL, Dimopoulos MA. Effect of epidermal growth factor receptor expression level on survival in patients with epithelial ovarian cancer. Clin Cancer Res. 2005;11:8637–43.
19. Lassus H, Sihto H, Leminen A, Joensuu H, Isola J, Nupponen NN, Butzow R. Gene amplification, mutation, and protein expression of EGFR and mutations of ERBB2 in serous ovarian carcinoma. J Mol Med (Berl). 2006;84:671–81.
20. Mehner C, Oberg AL, Goergen KM, Kalli KR, Maurer MJ, Nassar A, Goode EL, Keeney GL, Jatoi A, Radisky DC, Radisky ES. EGFR as a prognostic biomarker and therapeutic target in ovarian cancer: evaluation of patient cohort and literature review. Genes Cancer. 2017;8:589–99.
21. Wilken JA, Badri T, Cross S, Raji R, Santin AD, Schwartz P, Branscum AJ, Baron AT, Sakhitab AI, Maihle NJ. EGFR/HER-targeted therapeutics in ovarian cancer. Future Med Chem. 2012;4:447–69.
22. Siwak DR, Carey M, Hennessy BT, Nguyen CT, McGahren Murray MJ, Nolden L, Mills GB. Targeting the epidermal growth factor receptor in epithelial ovarian cancer: current knowledge and future challenges. J Oncol. 2010;2010:568938.
23. Murphy M, Stordal B. Erlotinib or gefitinib for the treatment of relapsed platinum pretreated non-small cell lung cancer and ovarian cancer: a systematic review. Drug Resist Updat. 2011;14:177–90.
24. Donnelly SK, Bravo-Cordero JJ, Hodgson L. Rho GTPase isoforms in cell motility: Don't FRET, we have FRET. Cell Adhes Migr. 2014;8:526–34.
25. Miyamoto Y, Suyama K, Baba H. Recent advances in targeting the EGFR signaling pathway for the treatment of metastatic colorectal cancer. Int J Mol Sci. 2017;18:752.
26. Wertheimer E, Gutierrez-Uzquiza A, Rosemblit C, Lopez-Haber C, Sosa MS, Kazanietz MG. Rac signaling in breast cancer: a tale of GEFs and GAPs. Cell Signal. 2012;24:353–62.
27. Umelo IA, Wever OD, Kronenberger P, Noor A, Teugels E, Chen G, Bracke M, Greve JD. Combined inhibition of rho-associated protein kinase and EGFR suppresses the invasive phenotype in EGFR-dependent lung cancer cells. Lung Cancer. 2015;90:167–74.
28. Jurikova M, Danihel L, Polak S, Varga I. Ki67, PCNA, and MCM proteins: markers of proliferation in the diagnosis of breast cancer. Acta Histochem. 2016;118:544–52.
29. Shiomi T, Okada Y. MT1-MMP and MMP-7 in invasion and metastasis of human cancers. Cancer Metastasis Rev. 2003;22:145–52.
30. Martin Lluesma S, Wolfer A, Harari A, Kandalaft LE. Cancer vaccines in ovarian cancer: how can we improve? Biomedicine. 2016;4:10.
31. Mais V, Angioli R, Coccia E, Fagotti A, Landi S, Melis GB, Pellicano M, Scambia G, Zupi E, Angioni S, et al. Prevention of postoperative abdominal adhesions in gynecological surgery. Consensus paper of an Italian gynecologists' task force on adhesions. Minerva Ginecol. 2011;63:47–70.
32. Pados G, Venetis CA, Almaloglou K, Tarlatzis BC. Prevention of intra-peritoneal adhesions in gynaecological surgery: theory and evidence. Reprod BioMed Online. 2010;21:290–303.
33. Johns DB, Keyport GM, Hoehler F, di Zerega GS. Reduction of postsurgical adhesions with Intergel adhesion prevention solution: a multicenter study of safety and efficacy after conservative gynecologic surgery. Fertil Steril. 2001;76:595–604.
34. Arslan E, Talih T, Oz B, Halaclar B, Caglayan K, Sipahi M. Comparison of lovastatin and hyaluronic acid/carboxymethyl cellulose on experimental created peritoneal adhesion model in rats. Int J Surg. 2014;12:120–4.
35. Wolny PM, Banerji S, Gounou C, Brisson AR, Day AJ, Jackson DG, Richter RP. Analysis of CD44-hyaluronan interactions in an artificial membrane system: insights into the distinct binding properties of high and low molecular weight hyaluronan. J Biol Chem. 2010;285:30170–80.
36. Lafky JM, Wilken JA, Baron AT, Maihle NJ. Clinical implications of the ErbB/epidermal growth factor (EGF) receptor family and its ligands in ovarian cancer. Biochim Biophys Acta. 2008;1785:232–65.
37. Mendelsohn J, Baselga J. The EGF receptor family as targets for cancer therapy. Oncogene. 2000;19:6550–65.
38. Normanno N, De Luca A, Bianco C, Strizzi L, Mancino M, Maiello MR, Carotenuto A, De Feo G, Caponigro F, Salomon DS. Epidermal growth factor receptor (EGFR) signaling in cancer. Gene. 2006;366:2–16.
39. Wang C, Wang W, Liu Y, Yong M, Yang Y, Zhou H. Rac GTPase activating protein 1 promotes oncogenic progression of epithelial ovarian cancer. Cancer Sci. 2018;109:84–93.
40. Gao J, Zhu H, Wan H, Zou X, Ma X, Gao G. Harmine suppresses the proliferation and migration of human ovarian cancer cells through inhibiting ERK/CREB pathway. Oncol Rep. 2017;38:2927–34.
41. Wang Y, Kuang H, Xue J, Liao L, Yin F, Zhou X. LncRNA AB073614 regulates proliferation and metastasis of colorectal cancer cells via the PI3K/AKT signaling pathway. Biomed Pharmacother. 2017;93:1230–7.

15

Determination of sialic acid in saliva by means of surface-enhanced Raman spectroscopy as a marker in adnexal mass patients: ovarian cancer vs benign cases

José de Jesús Zermeño-Nava[1], Marco Ulises Martínez-Martínez[1,4], Ana Laura Rámirez-de-Ávila[1], Aida Catalina Hernández-Arteaga[2], Ma. Guadalupe García-Valdivieso[2*], Alondra Hernández-Cedillo[2], Miguel José-Yacamán[2,3] and Hugo Ricardo Navarro-Contreras[2*]

Abstract

Background: To demonstrate the use of surface-enhanced Raman spectroscopy (SERS) to determine sialic acid (SA) levels in saliva using silver nanoparticles as substrates, in adnexal mass patients scheduled for surgical intervention to remove invasive masses, with the aim to compare SA levels in benign tumor vs ovarian cancer patients.

Methods: Quantification of SA levels was accomplished by measuring their SERS and calibrating with analytical reagent SA. The mean SA concentration in saliva from 37 benign adnexal mass resulted smaller (5.1 mg/dL) than the mean concentration in 15 Ovarium cancer patients (23 mg/dL). The cancer condition was determined by biopsy of the removed adnexal mass. The CA-125 biomarker was also measured. The predictive potential of both biomarkers is discussed, together with the malignity risk index (MRI).

Results: Our results showed a sensitivity/specificity of 80%/100% with a cutoff to distinguish between benign/cancer cases of SA 15.5 mg/dL, as established from a ROC analysis. Our results suggest that SA may be a more useful biomarker than CA-125 to detect ovarian cancer.

Conclusions: Our results suggest that the SA levels measured from saliva may be as good predictors as the MRI index for the presence of ovarian cancer in sensitivity/negative predictive value and outperforms it in specificity/positive predictive value.

Keywords: Sialic Acid, Surface-enhanced Raman, Ag Nanoparticles, Ovarian Cancer

Background

Ovarian cancer is the seventh most common cancer in women worldwide [1, 2]. In 2012 239,000 ovarian cancer cases were reported; which amounts to 4% of all new cases of cancer in women. Ovarian cancer produced approximately 152,000 deaths in 2012. It is the eighth most common cause of cancer death in women across the world [1, 2].

Ovarian cancer (OC), in general do not produce symptoms at early stages. Additionally, there is no early detection method applicable to the general women population, so the disease is generally advanced when it is diagnosed. Ovarian epithelial cancer is the histological type of major incidence, representing almost 90% of reported cases. In more than 70% of all cases, it is usually detected in the advanced clinical stages III and IV. The 5 year survival rate ranges from approximately 30 to 50% depending on the type of ovarian cancer, being the invasive epithelial ovarian cancer the most common, as well as that of the worst prognosis, in phase III-IV patients, which have a 5–20% five year survival rate [3, 4].

* Correspondence: guadalupe.valdivieso@uaslp.mx; hnavarro@uaslp.mx
[2]Coordinación para la Innovación y Aplicación de la Ciencia y la Tecnología (CIACYT), Universidad Autónoma de San Luís Potosí, Álvaro Obregón 64, 78000 San Luis Potosí, SLP, Mexico
Full list of author information is available at the end of the article

This high mortality rate prompts the need to have effective, highly sensitive diagnostics methods to examine women who may have evidence of ovarian cancer, or symptoms who may lead the medical specialist to consider further clinical examination of the involved patient, to discard the existence of ovarian cancer.

For the medical diagnosis, there is a limited set of analysis that may help to detect and diagnose ovarian cancer. Transvaginal ultrasound is the most useful imaging method for routine screening of ovarian cancer, given that this cancer is usually only palpable in advanced stages. The most important biomarker that has proven to be a useful adjunct for ovarian cancer is the protein CA-125, which has been found is produced by more than 90% of advanced epithelial ovarian cancers [3, 4]. Normal values range from 0 to 35 (U/mL). As a result, the CA-125 protein has become the most screened serum marker in laboratory tests for ovarian cancer. However, although CA-125 significantly rises 4 months previous to any clinical manifestation, in almost 50% of the early screenings of positive cases, it results in normal concentration levels [5]. This fact reduces the usefulness of CA-125 as a predictive test for this malignancy. Additionally, for young patients (premenopausal women) there is not any clearly defined cutoff point for this biomarker which can be associated with any malignity risk with certainty.

Considering these limitations, as well as the fact that ovarian cancer is of relative low prevalence, screening of the general sensitive female population for ovarian is not recommended [5], although less than 30% of patients with ovarian cancer are diagnosed at an early curable stage [6]. Instead, an annual gynecological exam with pelvic examination is recommended for preventive health care.

One major problem is that screening methods tend to find a large number of false positive cases. The combined use of transvaginal ultrasound and CA-125 tend to result in a higher sensitivity for ovarian cancer detection, but at an increased rate of false positive results [5, 6]. Unfortunately, malignancy can only be assessed with surgery. These could lead to unnecessary surgery in false cases, with the additional full inconveniency of the probability of complications due to surgery, as well as anxiety caused by false alarming results.

Another biomarker for ovarian cancer screening that has been studied and proposed is the Human Epididymis Protein 4 (HE4) [7]. HE4 is a tumor marker of ovarian cancer, with 80% sensitivity at a cutoff of 150 pmol/L [7]. However, it is not routinely used by the medical professionals in standard medical tests to screen for the presence of this disease.

Saliva has been proposed as an alternative medium to plasma in monitoring biomarkers that may be useful in diagnosis of several human diseases, as well as an element to monitor the etiology of some pathologies or the effects of drugs doses. The simplicity and non-invasiveness of its recollection, the existing positive correlation among multiple substances that are present in serum and saliva, are some of the advantages that this fluid offers as a diagnostic instrument for some human diseases [8, 9].

An important biomarker in saliva is sialic acid (SA), which is a systematic biomarker of systemic inflammation [10], it is a component bound to salivary glycolipids, and to glycoproteins, of which IgA (immunoglobuline A) may be one of the most important, as well as from some other immunologic proteins. SA occupies the interface between a host and pathogenic microorganisms.

Sialic acids are a family of nine-carbon acidic monosaccharides that occur at the end of oligosaccharide chains of mucins, glycoproteins, and glycolipids attached to the cell membranes of all vertebrate organisms [10]; SA emerging from these membranes is continuously shed into the surrounding human fluids. N-acetylneuraminic acid (Neu5AC) is the predominant form of SA and almost the only form found in human body fluids and tissues, among them saliva [10]. It has the chemical formula $C_{11}H_{19}NO_9$. The molecule is composed of a pyranose ring consisting of five carbon atoms and one oxygen atom, to which one N-acetyl, one carboxyl group, and one glycerol ion are attached.

SA is normally detected and calibrated in its concentration in human fluids, by decanting it by an elaborated chemical process to isolate it from other proteins or non-related lipids which are constitutive of these fluids. Followed by comparison of its absorbance at some given wavelengths with standard calibration curves obtained from chemically pure reagents [11, 12]. Recently, we have shown that small amounts of SA in aqueous solution may be easily detected by the alternative method of surface enhanced Raman spectroscopy (SERS) [13], produced by citrate-reduced silver nanoparticles (cit-Ag-NP), with a simplified processing of the saliva sample. We have demonstrated the sensitivity of this method to distinguish between breast cancer patients and healthy control subjects [14]. This is possible as SA is well known to be over expressed in human fluids when there is an ongoing cancer development process. Determination of SA by SERS from cit-Ag-NP is a technological approach that requires fewer reagents, and simplified saliva sample processing. The latter constitutes an advantage that could be useful in clinical diagnosis since it is highly sensitive, fast, and low cost, moreover, the equipment may be portable and results can be obtained in real time.

SERS is a Raman spectroscopic technique that has shown enhancements of the inelastic scattering of the outgoing radiation ranging from 10^6 to 10^{12} in amplification factors from molecules that have been adsorbed in metals [15]. Therefore, SERS has great potential as a molecularly specific analytic probe for highly sensitive detection of weak Raman signals of proteins or other biological analytes with low Raman scattering cross-section or at very low concentrations. The threshold of concentrations detectable may be as low as a single-molecule attached to a Ag-NP [15]. Furthermore, colloidal suspensions of metallic nanoparticles (NP), silver, gold or copper are the most common SERS substrates because they are of easy preparation and have long shelf-lifetime, and high Raman signal enhancement factors [16].

A primary aim of this study is to apply SERS to measure levels of SA in human saliva using colloidal suspension of cit-Ag-NP, and in particular to determine SA levels in saliva of patients to whom adnexal masses in ovary have been observed by ultrasound sonography, and who have been scheduled for surgical removal of the detected tumor.

Hypothesis

The hypothesis is that there may exist a significant difference in SA levels which have been expressed in saliva, as in many other human fluids, between benign tumor cases and ovarian cancer affected patients.

Our main objective was to establish the usefulness of monitoring the SA levels by SERS from cit-Ag-NP, in suspected cases of ovarian cancer, thus adding the SA level tests as another adjunct probe to the diagnosis of ovarian cancer, together with CA-125 and ultrasound imaging. SERS has the advantages of its simplicity and may be extremely useful when it is necessary to monitor the progression of the disease as well as monitor the effectiveness of applied treatments. Our results corroborate that salivary SA concentrations are found to be significantly higher in ovarian cancer patients compared to that of benign adnexal mass patients.

Methods

The study population

Inclusion criteria: Patients attending the service of the Gynecology and Obstetrics at Central Hospital Dr. "Ignacio Morones Prieto" at San Luis Potosí, S.L.P. México, (HCDSLP) during the periods July–December 2017, which were diagnosed by ultrasound to have adnexal tumor masses and that were scheduled for surgical intervention to remove them, with no previous clinical treatment.

Exclusion criteria: any previous cancer diagnosis, second primary cancer, pregnancy, any systemic or circulatory diseases, or periodontal disease.

The study was approved by the HCDSLP Ethics Committee. Written informed consent was obtained from all participants.

Cancer determination

Histological type determined by the Pathology laboratory at the Central Hospital "Dr. Ignacio Morones Prieto" from tumor biopsy.

Data collection

Adnexal tumor patients completed a health questionnaire that included information about systemic health and oral diseases. Blind (regarding the existence of ovarian cancer) determination of the SA concentration (SAC) in saliva and CA-125 in serum were made.

Saliva collection and processing

Before the saliva collection, each participant was required to perform a two-step oral cleansing. The first step consists of a vigorous teeth brushing and the second one involves two subsequent oral rinses with commercial alcohol-free mouthwash. The saliva samples were centrifuged at 6000 rpm (equivalent to 3580 G) for 15 min, and the resulting supernatants were used to determine the concentration of SA.

SERS calibration of SA

The Raman measurements were performed on a Horiba Jobin Yvon XploRA ONE Raman spectrometer coupled to an Olympus BX41 optical microscope, using an excitation green laser 532 nm, with an average power of 20 mW at the sample. The laser beam was focused on the surface of the liquid sample with a 10X objective. The diameter of the laser spot was approximately 8–10 μm. The SERS spectra were collected from the 400 to 1800 cm^{-1} spectral range. The intensity of three Raman shift lines, 1002, 1237 and 1391 cm^{-1}, after fluorescence subtraction, are used to compare with a calibration curve for the SERS obtained from SA Analytical Reagent grade. Next, to record the SERS spectra, 50 μl of a 2.5×10^{-3} M citrate-reduced Ag-NP were placed in an aluminum container, 100 μl in capacity, mixed with 25 μl of the centrifuged saliva sample. An equal volume of a reference SA solution was using in the calibration process previous to any measurement session. Further details on the calibration process are provided in [14].

Data statistical analysis

Continual variables are reported using the median ± interquartile range (IQR) because of the non-normal distribution of some of them, as discussed below. Categorical variables are reported as n and percentage. Non-parametric tests were performed to analyze the continual variables (Mann Whitney U test). The categorical variables were analyzed with the Fisher exact tests. The statistical analysis was carried out with the statistical program R 3.4.3 (R Core Team 2017), and RStudio Version 1.1.423. Receiver operating characteristics (ROC) curves were plotted to calculate the area under the curve and to establish the best point for sensitivity and specificity.

Results and discussion

Fifty-two patients that were diagnosed with adnexal masses scheduled for surgical intervention, age ranging from 25 to 78 years old (average: 41.6 years ±17.3) participated in this study. The characteristics of the patients participating in the project are shown in Table 1. One may see that the histological analysis resulted in 37 patients with benign adnexal masses (mean age and S.D. 36.8 years ±15.3). In 15 patients (mean age and S.D. 51.2 years ±18.7), these masses were ovarian cancer.

A Shapiro test for normality in the distribution of the measured variables was performed. In the test, a significance level below $p < 0.05$ indicates that the variables are not normally distributed. Only body mass index and Menarche were normally distributed, the SA and CA-125 data require a non-parametric statistical analysis. Given the fact that most variables are non-parametric, we proceeded to evaluate the median plus/minus the first and third quartiles (*Q1, Q3*), which are summarized in Table 1 for the relevant parameters SAC and CA-125.

Figure 1 shows the sialic acid concentration (SAC) of each group of patients. Indicated in black, are the SAC of benign adnexal mass (BAMP) affected patients, and in red those in which histology has diagnosed ovarian cancer (OCP). The inset in Fig. 1 shows the boxplot of sialic acid concentration in both groups.

The difference between concentration means of benign adnexal mass patients and positive diagnosis ovarian cancer cases was assessed by a Mann Whitney U test, which has been also summarized in Table 1. A $P \leq 0.05$ value was considered to be statistically significant. The application of the Mann Whitney U test supports the hypothesis that the expression of SA that is present in the saliva of benign and ovarian cancer patients is statistically different.

Table 1 shows that there are no expected statistical differences in the BMI, menarche and gestations variables between the two groups, BAMP and OCP. However, the same analysis indicates that there are significant statistical differences in both CA125 and SAC, between the two groups of patients.

Figure 2 shows the result of a Receiver Operating Characteristic or ROC curve analysis for the sialic acid concentrations between the two group of patients. As always the axes are chosen vertical for Sensitivity (true positive rate), and horizontal 1-Specificity (false positive rate). This analysis performed with the R-Studio program results in that the best threshold to differentiate between BAMP and OCP corresponds to SAC > 15.5 mg/dL, rounded to one decimal digit. The area under the ROC curve is 94.05% for the SAC cutoff proposed. This SAC threshold value corresponds to a sensitivity of 80%, and specificity of 100%. The figure has also included the ROC analysis for the CA-125. This analysis results in a smaller area under the curve of 82.52%, as compared to the SAC. The resultant suggested cutoff from the ROC analysis for the CA-125 is 216.5 U/mL. This is a very high concentration value, corresponding to a high specificity value of 94.5%, but to a poor sensitivity because it fails to identify at least 8 out of the 15 positive cases (more than 50% of the cases).

Figure 3 shows a CA-125 vs SA plot of the benign adnexal mass and ovarian patients, (black and red points, respectively). The Spearman correlation coefficient among CA-125 and SAC is 0.56, indicative of a modest correlation among the expression of these two biomarkers. The blue colored lines depict the standard cutoff concentrations for the CA-125 (horizontal dashed line, 35 U/mL) and the proposed SAC cutoff (vertical dashed line). The

Table 1 Patients that have been diagnosed with adnexal masses characteristics that were included in the study

Mann Whitney U test results	BAMP; *N* = 37		*Q1*	*Q3*	OCP; *N* = 15		*Q1*	*Q3*	*p* value
	Mean	Median			Mean	Median			
CA125 (U/mL)	80.6	34	21	54	1036.3	320	76.6	1662	0.0003
SAC (mg/dL)	5.1	3.2	2.3	7.3	23.0	27.4	18.6	28.5	0.0000
	Median				Median				*p* value
BMI (Kg/m^2)	28		25	32	25		23	27	0.0745
Age Menarche	13.4		12	15	13		12	14	0.7491
	Mean		S.D.		Mean		S.D.		
Gestations	1		2		2		3		0.6524
Age	36.8		15.3		51.2		18.7		0.0148
Pos-menopausal	6 (16.2%)				8 (53.3%)				
Irregular menstruations	6 (16.2%)				2 (13.3%)				
MRI > 200 n (%)	4 (10.8%)				12 (80%)				< 0.0001

The *p* stands for the significance obtained for BAMP benign adnexal mass and OCP ovarian cancer affected patients, under the Mann Whitney U tests

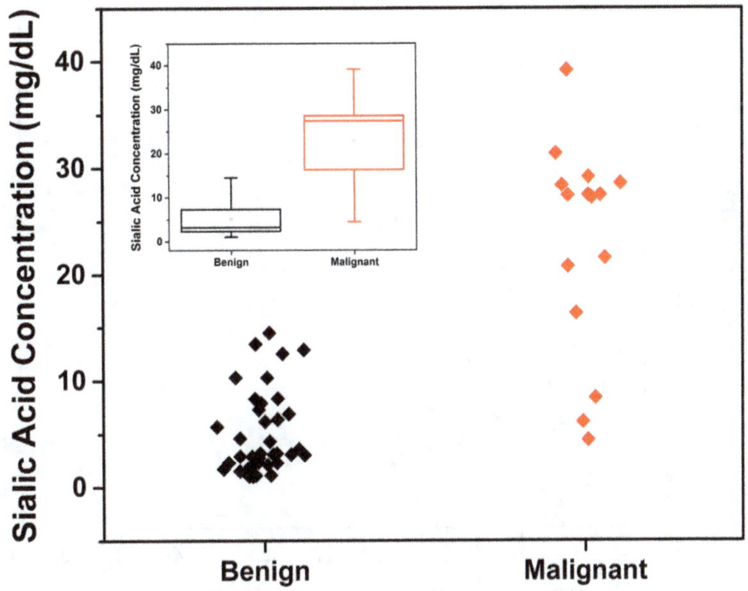

Fig. 1 Cloud plot of sialic acid concentration of each group of patients. Red: ovarian cancer; black: benign adnexal mass. Insert: Box plot of sialic acid concentration, again red: ovarian cancer; black: benign adnexal mass

CA-125 concentrations are plotted on a logarithmic scale, in order to have a better visualization of the spreading in resultant patient concentrations that were determined for this biomarker. From the plot, it is evident that SA under the cutoff provided by the ROC analysis has a better performance than CA-125 to distinguish between benign and ovarian cases. But with respect to detecting true positives, CA-125 in this exercise missed only two positive cases, at the 35 U/ml cutoff, vs 3 for SA, but at the expense of resulting in too many false positives, 15 of them in this study (almost 40% of benign cases), against none for the SA, under the cutoff of 15.5 mg/dL.

Figure 4, presents a comparison between the sensitivities, specificities positive predictive values (PPV) and negative predictive values (NPV) for each test. The Figure includes the cutoff values and confidence intervals for

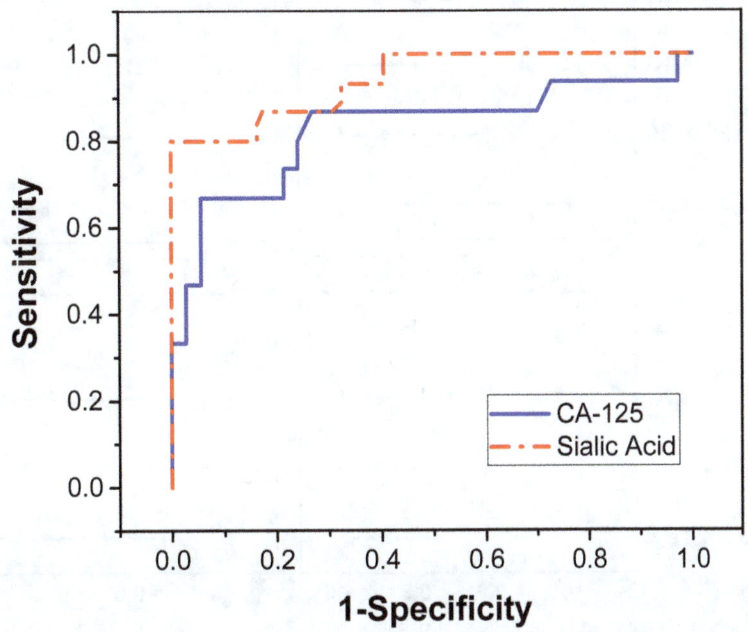

Fig. 2 ROC curve analysis for SA (and CA-125), to optimize the threshold of acid sialic concentrations to distinguish between benign adnexal mass patients, and ovarian cancer patients

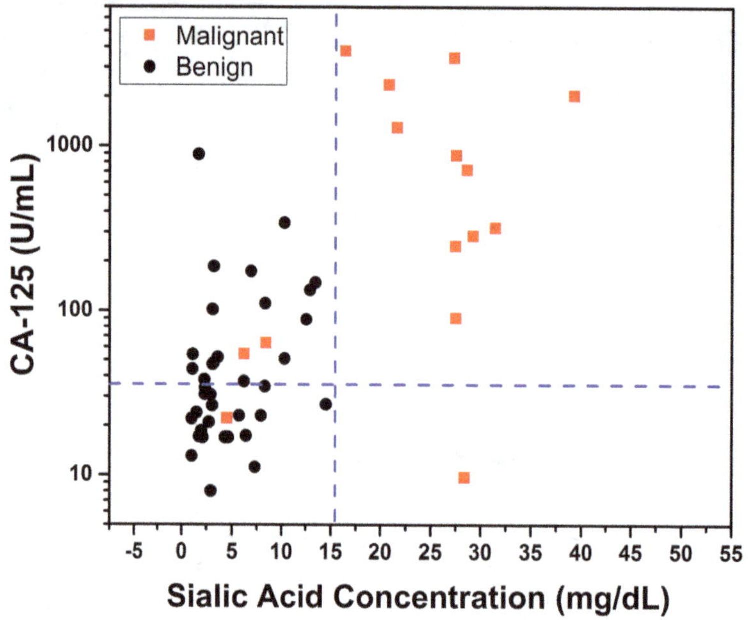

Fig. 3 SA and CA-125 plot, to illustrate how the cutoff values of SA and CA-125 concentrations distinguish between benign adnexal mass patients (black), and ovarian cancer patients (red)

each biomarker, as well as for the calculated MRI. The MRI was calculated following Jacobs et al. [17] $MRI = U \times M \times CA\text{-}125$. In this formula M is the menopausal status score, and U the evaluation of the ultrasound score [17]. The Figure shows how the SAC under the cutoff ROC value of 15.5 mg/dL performs as well as the calculated MRI in sensitivity and negative predictive values and may be even superior in specificity and positive predictive values. The Figure includes the performance of CA-125 under the cutoff values

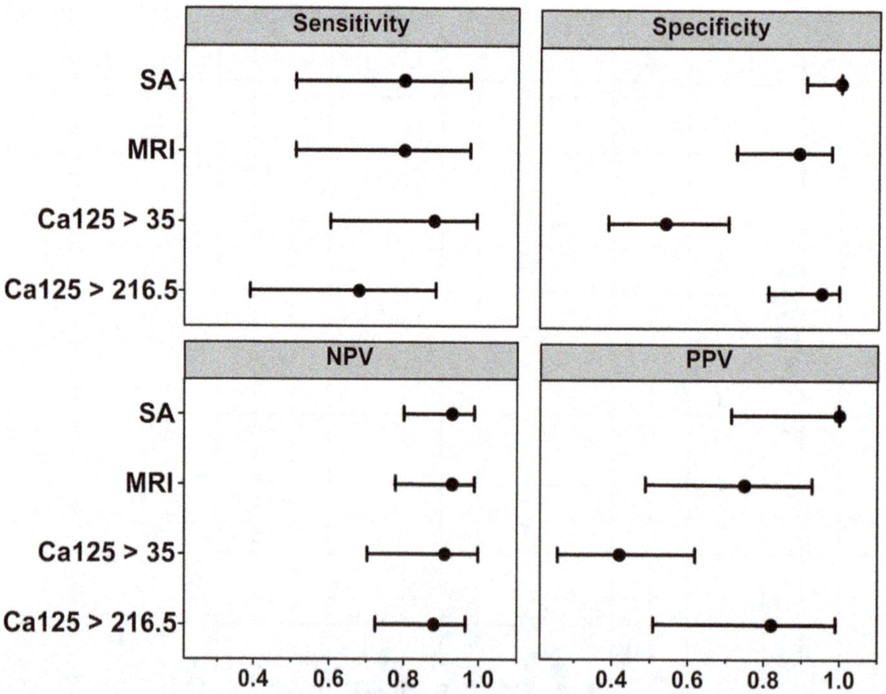

Fig. 4 Sensitivity, specificity, positive predictive value (PPV) and negative predictive value (NPV) for each test. The Figure includes cutoff values and confidence intervals for each biomarker, as well as for the calculated MRI. Abbreviations: SA, sialic acid; MRI, Malignancy risk, index, CA125 > 35, CA-125 larger than 35 U/mL; CA125 > 216.5, CA-125 larger than 216.5 U/mL

of 35 and the best result of the ROC analysis of our data of 216 U/mL.

Discussion

The results indicate that with a cutoff or threshold value of 15.5 mg/dL of the SA concentration measured in saliva we have a 100% specificity (80% sensitivity). These results suggest that we could distinguish before surgery if an adnexal masses patient, as revealed through sonography, is going to have ovarian cancer with high probability, if the patient presents higher SA concentration levels than this cutoff value. Of course this analysis requires that patients are discarded of suffering any systemic or circulatory diseases, advanced periodontitis or from any other primary diagnosed cancer, to circumvent the intrinsic limitation that SA is a nonspecific marker of inflammation.

It is clear that although SA is not a specific marker for ovarian cancer, it should be considered in the clinical scenario of the adnexal mass diagnosed patient, and not in the population in general. In spite of the non-specificity for cancer, the values obtained in the tests suggest that they are sensitive and specific enough to differentiate an inflammatory process against a cancer process, when combined with the clinical evaluation by the medical professional.

It is important to note that in our study, the mean age of the benign adnexal mass group is 36.8 years old which is smaller than the mean age of the ovarian cancer group of age 51.2. It has been reported that the SA levels increases only by 4–5 and 7% in the age groups 50–59 and 60–69, compared to the 20–49 age group, in which the SA levels remain practically the same [18]. Hence, as the mean ages of the two groups fall below < 50 years, any age effect is not expected to affect in any significant way the SAC data of the patients in this study.

The search for malignant tumor markers has been a permanent concern for the professionals of gynecological oncology [18]. In particular for Ovarium cancer Schwartz et al. in 1987, calibrating from absorbance curves, they found that lipid-associated sialic acid (LSA) levels in the serum of patients without any clinical evidence of disease were statistically different, from those patients with evidence of the disease [19]. The medians of LSA that they reported are of 18.4 and 27.2 mg/dL, for those two groups of patients, respectively. Additionally, the Schwartz group [19] found that the simultaneous use of the LSA and CA-125 concentrations enhances significantly the sensitivity for Ovarium cancer detection, from 76% for CA-125 alone to 84% when using information of the two markers combined, with cut off values of LSA > 24 mg/dL and CA-125 > 60 U/mL. A similar improvement is also reported for the specificity of both tests combined. Petru et al. [20], studied also the use of CA-125 and LSA extracted from serum, to test for the increase in sensitivity for diagnosing Ovarium cancer. However, in this study with the determination of both markers no significantly improved sensitivity was reported, in contrast to the use of CA-125 alone. But Petru et al. [20] reports very high sensitivities values for CA-125 (90.2%) for diagnosing Ovarium cancer. These high values have not been replicated by other studies [21–23]. For instance, Li et al. [21], found that the combined determination of SA with hydroxyproline provides a better diagnosis value than either CA-125 or HE4. S. Ghosh [22] discusses in a recent work, how SA in serum may also be used as a clinical predictor for Ovarium cancer. Finally, we add that Thakkar et al. [23] found that protein-bound sialic acid (PBSA) provides the highest overall ability to discriminate between ovarian cancer patients and healthy subjects, in comparison with other glycoproteins in serum [23].

Our present work adds to those previous reports the value of SA as a predictor of possible Ovarium cancer presence in adnexial mass diagnosed patients when it is detected by SERS in saliva in larger concentrations than the cutoff value obtained in our ROC analysis of 15.5 mg/dL. An important problem that our results for SAC in saliva may help to alleviate is the large number of unnecessary surgeries performed during the approach to treat the adnexal lesion. Our study is not a screening test since it was performed in a population with adnexal pathology, however our test of the over expression of SAC in saliva shows a very high specificity. We state the expectation that his may help to significantly decrease the number of unnecesary invasive surgical procedures in the population of these patients.

The present study was by necessity limited to the small group of adnexal mass patients expecting for treatment at HCDSLP during a six month period, and that were scheduled for surgical intervention to remove them. The very promising results for the SERS test determination of SAC from saliva, in specificity and sensitivity for ovarian cancer, determined in this work, suggest that it is necessary to continue the study to include a larger group of patients to corroborate our present results.

A necessary commentary in regards to SERS as a characterization technique of chemical biomarkers is that still has not been readily adopted by the clinical institutions. The only limitation that we perceive is that it is sensitive to the selection of prepared nanoparticles (NP), i.e. metal and full surface coverage of functionalization molecule types required to keep them in suspension, which require a careful study to find the most appropriated to the biomarker in consideration. But once these are established, the NP's are easily reproducible, with repetitive SERS properties.

Conclusions

Our measurements of SA by SERS produced by citrate-reduced silver nanoparticles of ovarian cancer affected patients indicate that these levels are increased with respect to the median SA level in adnexal mass subjects, corroborating previous results in the literature, where SA has been measured by conventional absorbance methods, which require extensive chemical processing of the samples. The threshold to differentiate between benign adnexal mass and Ovarium cancer patients is found to be SAC > 15.5 mg/dL, from a ROC curve analysis. This SA level threshold or cutoff value corresponds to a sensitivity of 80%, and specificity of 100%. Our results suggest that the SA levels that are measured from saliva samples may be as good predictors as the MRI index for the presence of ovarian cancer in sensitivity and negative predictive value and may outperform it in specificity and positive predictive value.

The SERS method requires no chemical elaboration of the saliva samples, and could be useful in clinical diagnosis since it is highly sensitive, fast, inexpensive, the equipment may be portable and results can be obtained in real time. Thus, the SERS method to determine the SA level in saliva may be used as an adjunct test to diagnose the presence of ovarian cancer, distinguishing between benign adnexal mass cases and ovarian cancer, and to assess the efficacy of post-surgical treatment.

Abbreviations

(Q1, Q3): First and third quartiles; BAMP: Benign adnexal mass affected patients; BMI: Body mass index; CA-125: Cancer antigen 125; cit-Ag-NP: Citrate-reduced silver nanoparticles; HCDSLP: Central Hospital Dr. "Ignacio Morones Prieto" at San Luis Potosí; HE4: Human Epididymis Protein 4 (HE4); IgA: Immunoglobuline A; IQR: Interquartile range; LSA: Lipid-associated sialic acid; MRI: Malignity risk index; Neu5AC: N-acetylneuraminic acid (sialic acid); NP: Nanoparticles; NPV: Negative predictive values; OC: Ovarian cancer; OCP: Ovarian cancer patients OCP; PBSA: Protein-bound sialic acid; PPV: Positive predictive values; ROC: Receiver operating characteristics curves; S.D.: Standard deviation; SA: Sialic acid; SAC: Sialic acid concentration; SERS: Surface-enhanced Raman spectroscopy; *U*: Evaluation of the ultrasound score

Acknowledgements

The authors acknowledge the financial support from Consejo Nacional de Ciencia y Tecnología (CONACyT) México, through the Project Problemas Nacionales 2015-01-986, from FAI-UASLP, access to Laboratorio Nacional de Análisis Físicos, Químicos y Biológicos-UASLP, the facilities provided at the Hospital Central de San Luis Potosi. We are also indebted to the Welch Foundation for grant (#AX-1615). ACHA acknowledges the financial support of CONACYT through a Ph.D. scholarship 446208. We wish to thank to Joazet Ojeda Galván for some technical assistance.

Funding

HRNC: Funding from a grant from "Consejo Nacional de Ciencia y Tecnología (CONACyT) México", through the Project Problemas Nacionales 2015-01-986, And from "Fondo de Apoyo a la Investigación" FAI-UASLP.
MJY: Funding from Welch Foundation grant (#AX-1615).
AHA: CONACYT Ph.D. scholarship 446208.

Authors' contributions

JDJZN, drzermenonava@gmail.com. Proposed the subject. Responsible for patient selection and adnexal mass removal surgery. Responsible for all clinical aspects required by the participant patients. MUMM, marcomtzmtz@hotmail.com. Responsable for data statistical analysis. AlrdeÁ, anis.ramirez2887@hotmail.com
Assisted in adnexal mass removal surgery; patients interview and obtaining of consent to participate, recompilation of patients clinical data. Obtention of saliva samples and elaboration of patients data Table. ACHA, aida.arteaga@uaslp.mx. Fabrication of the cit-Ag-NP. Performed the Raman spectroscopy and analyzed spectroscopy results. MGGV*, valdi_95@hotmail.-com. Performed the Raman spectroscopy and analyzed spectroscopy results. Participated in writing parts of the manuscript. AHC, alodella09@gmail.com. Assisted with the Raman spectroscopy and analysis of spectroscopy results. MJY, miguel.yacaman@utsa.edu. Proposed the Project of application of Raman spectroscopy to detect Sialic acid, read and wrote parts of the manuscript, participated in the discussion of results, and of the final conclusions. Hugo Ricardo Navarro-Contreras*, hnavarro@uaslp.mx. Directed the whole Project, coordinated the integration of data; performed their final analysis, defined with Dr. Yacamán the final conclusions, and did the writing of the complete manuscript including all scientific discussion. All co-authors read and discussed the advances of the project, the results and of its recompilation in the manuscript. All authors read and approved the final manuscript.

Authors' information

José de Jesús Zermeño-Nava (JJZN)
B.Sc. Medicine, University of San Luis Potosi (UASLP) 2007. Gynecology and Oncology Specialization National University of Mexico (UNAM) 2011. He is head of the Graduate Medical Specialization in Gynecology Program at Hospital Central of San Luis Potosí and UASLP, and practices medicine at the Gynecology Dpt. Of this the Public Hospital at SLP: His interests are in breast and gynecological cancers.
Marco Ulises Martínez-Martínez (MUMM)
B.Sc. Medicine, University of San Luis Potosí (UASLP) 2004. Rheumatology Specialization 2011, M. Sc. In Clinical Research 2016. Hospital Central of San Luis Potosí and UASLP. His interests are in methodology applied to clinical research.
Ana Laura Rámirez-de-Ávila (ALRA)
B.Sc. Medicine, University of San Luis Potosi (UASLP) 2014. Gynecology and Oncology Specialization Hospital Central of San Luis Potosí and UASLP. 2018. Currently she is doing her master in Clinical research at UASLP, in the subject of sialic acid determination in adnexal mass patients.
Aida Catalina Hernández-Arteaga (ACHA)
B.Sc. in Mathematics 2011, M. Sc. Applied Sciences 2014, Doctoral Student Applied Sciences, University of San Luis Potosi (UASLP), in the subject of sialic acid determination in breast cancer screening public process.
Ma. Guadalupe García Valdivieso (MGGV)
B Sc in Physics 2011, Master in Science in the field of renewable energies, from 2013. Ph.D. In Materials Science and Engineering Autonomous 2017, University of San Luis Potosi (UASLP). Currently she occupies a posdoctoral position in the subject of biomedical application of nanoparticles at CIACYT-UASLP.
Alondra Hernández-Cedillo (AHC)
B.Sc. in Nanotechnology Engineering, 2016, M. Sc. Student (Applied Sciences) University of San Luis Potosi (UASLP), in the subject of sialic acid determination in ovarium and cervical cancer patients.
Miguel José-Yacamán (MJY)
B.Sc. Physics, 1967, M.Sc. Physics, 1968, Ph.D. Materials Science, National University of Mexico (UNAM), Mexico City, 1973. - Post-Doctoral Experience: Department of Metallurgy and Materials Science, University of Oxford, England. 1976–1977. His interests are electron microscopy and its application to materials science and biomedical subjects. He has been the mentor of a whole generation of Materials Engineers and Scientists. He was one of the pioneers of research in nanoparticles in the 70's and 80's before the era of nanotechnology. He demonstrated for the first time that crystal structure existed at nanolevel and that catalysts nanoparticles were indeed nanocrystals. Then in the nanotechnology era he demonstrated the antiviral, anti bacterial and antifungal properties of nanoparticles. His work has had a tremendous

impact in commercial products. Currently he is Professor at the Physics and Astronomy Dpt. at Univ. of Texas at San Antonio, USA.
Hugo Ricardo Navarro-Contreras (HRNC)
Physicist (B. Sc 1971) UASLP, M Sc. CINVESTAV-IPN México 1973. PhD McMaster University, Canada, 1979. Pst-Doctoral Experience: Max Planck Insyitute für Festkörper Forschung, Stuttgart FRG 1984–86. His interests are in optical properties of solid materials, nanomaterials, nanotechnology, and far infrared radiation, as well as in application of nanomaterials in particular to biomedical subjects. Currently, he is Professor and Director of Coordination for Research and Application of Science and Technology, CIACYT at UASLP, SLP, México.

Competing interests

Miguel José-Yacaman has a patent WO2017/015568A1 pending, & a patent MX/a/2017/008084 pending. Both patents are on the application of SERS-NPAg to detect and calibrate SA concentrations.
Hugo Ricardo Navarro-Contreras as a coinventor has a patent WO2017/015568A1 pending, & a patent MX/a/2017/008084 pending. Both patents are on the application of SERS-NPAg to detect and calibrate SA concentrations.
The rest of authors declare that there are no conflicts of interest.

Author details

[1]División de Gineco-Obstetricia, Hospital Central Dr. Ignacio Morones Prieto, Ave. Venustiano Carranza 2395, Zona Universitaria, 78290 San Luis Potosí, SLP, Mexico. [2]Coordinación para la Innovación y Aplicación de la Ciencia y la Tecnología (CIACYT), Universidad Autónoma de San Luís Potosí, Álvaro Obregón 64, 78000 San Luis Potosí, SLP, Mexico. [3]Department of Physics and Astronomy, University of Texas at San Antonio, San Antonio, TX 78249, USA. [4]Hospital General de Zona No.1, Instituto Mexicano del Seguro Social (IMSS), San Luis Potosí, SLP, Mexico.

References

1. World Cancer Research Fund & American Institute for Cancer Research, Ovarian Cancer 2014 Report. http://www.aicr.org/continuous-update-project/reports/ovarian-cancer-2014-report.pdf. (Accessed 10 April 2018).
2. GLOBOCAN 2012. Estimated Cancer incidence, mortality and prevalence worldwide in 2012. International Agency for Cancer Research, World Health Organization. Facts sheets population. (Accessed 10 April 2018). http://globocan.iarc.fr/Pages/fact_sheets_population.aspx. See also NIH, National Institute of Cancer. Cancer Stat Facts: Ovarian Cancer. https://seer.cancer.gov/statfacts/html/ovary.html. (Accessed 10 April 2018).
3. Ferlay J, et al. GLOBOCAN 2012 v1.0, Cancer Incidence and Mortality Worldwide: IARC Cancer Base No. 11. 2013; (Accessed 10 April 2018). http://globocan.iarc.fr/Default.aspx.
4. Jemal A, Clegg LX, Ward E, Ries LA, Wu X, Jamison PM, Wingo PA, Howe HL, Anderson RN, Edwards BK. Annual report to the nation on the status of Cancer, 1975 2001, with a special feature regarding survival. Cancer. 2004; 101:3–27. https://doi.org/10.1002/cncr.20288
5. Jacobs IJ, Menon U, Ryan A, et al. Ovarian cancer screening and mortality in the UK collaborative trial of ovarian Cancer screening (UKCTOCS): a randomized controlled trial. Lancet. 2016;387(10022):945–56. https://doi.org/10.1016/S0140-6736(15)01224-6
6. Verheijen RHM, Zweemer RP. Screening to improve ovarian cancer prognosis? Lancet. 2016;387(10022):921–3. https://doi.org/10.1016/S0140-6736(15)01236-2
7. Molina R, Escudero JM, Augé JM, Filella X, Foj L, Torné A, Lejarcegui J, Pahisa J. HE4 a novel tumor marker for ovarian cancer: comparison with CA 125 and ROMA algorithm in patients with gynecological diseases. Tumor Biol. 2011;32:1087–95. https://doi.org/10.1007/s13277-011-0204-3
8. Pfaffe T, Cooper-White J, Beyerlein P, Kostner K, Punyadeera C. Diagnostic potential of saliva: current state and future applications. Clin Chem. 2011; 57(5):675–87. https://doi.org/10.1373/clinchem.2010.153767
9. Liu J, Duan Y. Saliva: A potential media for disease diagnostics and monitoring. Oral Oncol. 2012;48(7):569–77. https://doi.org/10.1016/j.oraloncology.2012.01.021
10. Schauer R, Kelm S, Reuter G, Roggentin P. In: Rosenberg A, editor. Biology of the Sialic Acids. New York: Plenum Press; 1995. p. 7–49.
11. Spyridaki MHE, Siskos PA. An Improved Spectrophotometric Method for the Determination of Free, Bound and Total N-acetylneuraminic Acid in Biological Fluids. Analytica Chimica Acta. 327 (2016) 277–285. https://doi.org/10.1016/0003-2670(96)00073-6.
12. Aminoff D. Methods for the quantitative estimation of N-Acetylneuraminic acid and their application to hydrolysates of Sialomucoids. J Biochem. 1961; 81:384–92. https://www.ncbi.nlm.nih.gov/pmc/articles/PMC1243351/
13. Feng S, Huang S, Lin D, Chen G, Xu Y, Li Y, Huang Z, Pan J, Chen R, Zeng H. Surface-Enhanced Raman Spectroscopy of Saliva Proteins for the Noninvasive Differentiation of Benign and Malignant Breast Tumors. Int J of Nanomed. 2015;10:537–47. https://doi.org/10.2147/IJN.S71811
14. Hernández-Arteaga A, Zermeño Nava JJ, Kolosovas-Machuca ES, Velázquez-Salazar JJ, Vinogradova E, José-Yacamán M, Navarro-Contreras HR. Diagnosis of Breast Cancer Using Surface-Enhanced Raman Spectroscopy to detect Sialic Acid Concentrations in Human Saliva. Nano Res. 2017;10:3662–70. https://doi.org/10.1007/s12274-017-1576-5
15. Meyer MW, Smith EA. Optimization of Silver Nanoparticles for Surface-Enhanced Raman Spectroscopy of Structurally Diverse Analytes using Visible and Near-Infrared Excitation. Analyst (Royal Soc Chem). 2011;136(17):3542–9. https://doi.org/10.1039/C0AN00851F
16. Munro CH, Smith WE, Garner M, Clarkson J, White PC. Characterization of the surface of a citrate-reduced, Colloid Optimized for Use as a Substrate for Surface-Enhanced Resonance Raman Scattering. Langmuir. 1995;11(10): 3712–20. https://doi.org/10.1021/la00010a021.
17. Jacobs I, Oram D, Fairbanks J, Turner J, Frost C, Grudzinskas JG. A risk of malignancy index incorporating CA-125, ultrasound and menopausal status for the accurate preoperative diagnosis of ovarian cancer. Br J Obstet Gynaecol. 1990;97:922–9. https://doi.org/10.1111/j.1471-0528.1990.tb02448.x
18. Stefenelli N, Klotz H, Engel A, Bauer P. Serum sialic acid in malignant tumors, Bacterial Infections and Chronic Liver Diseases. J Cancer Res Oncol. 1985;109:55–9. https://doi.org/10.1007/BF01884255
19. Schwartz PE, Chambers SE, Chambers JT, Gutmann J, Katopodis N, Foemme R. Circulating tumor markers in the monitoring of gynecologic malignancies. Cancer. 1987;60:353–61. https://doi.org/10.1002/1097-0142(19870801)60:3<353::AID-CNCR2820600312>3.0.CO;2-V
20. Petru E, Sewn BU, Averette HE, Koechli OR, Perras JP, Hilsenbeck S. Comparison of three tumor markers-CA-I 25, lipid-associated acid (LSA), and NB/70K-in monitoring ovarian Cancer. Gynecol Oncol. 1990;38:181–6. https://doi.org/10.1016/0090-8258(90)90037-L
21. Li P, Zhang X, Li T, Wang L, Du L, Yang Y, Li J, Wang HJ, Zhang Y, Wang CX. Combined detection of sialic acid and Hydroxyproline in diagnosis of ovarian Cancer and its comparison with human epididymis protein 4 and carbohydrate antigen. Clin Chim Acta. 2015;439:148–53. https://doi.org/10.1016/j.cca.2014.10.026
22. Ghosh G. Sialic acids: biomarkers in endocrinal cancers. Glycoconj J. 2015;32: 79–85. https://link.springer.com/article/10.1007/s10719-015-9577-7
23. Thakkar T, Patel P, Prajapati N, Kaur R, Nandave M. Serum levels of glycoproteins are elevated in patients with ovarian Cancer. Ind J Clin Biochem. 2014;29(3):345–50. https://link.springer.com/article/10.1007/s12291-013-0380-6

16

Transparency in ovarian cancer clinical trial results

Anna Roberto[*], Silvia Radrezza and Paola Mosconi

Abstract

Background: In recent years the question of the lack of transparency in clinical research has been debated by clinicians, researchers, citizens and their representatives, authors and publishers. This is particularly important for infrequent cancers such as ovarian cancer, where treatment still gives disappointing results in the majority of cases. Our aim was to assess the availability to the public of results in ClinicalTrials.gov, and the frequency of non-publication of results in ClinicalTrials.gov and in PubMed, Embase and Google Scholar. We collected all trials on ovarian cancer identified as "completed status" in the ClinicalTrials.gov registry on 17 January 2017. We checked the availability of the results in ClinicalTrials.gov and systematically identified published manuscripts on results.

Results: Out of 2725 trials on ovarian cancer identified, 752 were classified as "completed status". In those closed between 2008 and 2015, excluding phase I, the frequency of results in ClinicalTrials.gov was 35%. Of the 752 completed studies the frequency of published results in PubMed, Embase or Google Scholar ranged from 57.9% to 69.7% in the last years.

Conclusions: These findings show a lack of transparency and credibility of research. Citizens or patients' representatives, with the medical community, should continuously support initiatives to improve the publication and dissemination of clinical study results.

Keywords: Transparency, Clinical trials, ClinicalTrials.gov, Ovarian cancer, Publication of results

Background

The lack of transparency of clinical research results has long been on the agenda of clinicians [1], researchers, citizens and their representatives [2, 3], authors and publishers [4, 5]. The AllTrials petition on the transparency of clinical data is attracting widespread interest [4], and the "Restoring Invisible and Abandoned Trials" initiative is making public the confidential results about missing and abandoned trials [6]. "Better reporting of better research" is the motto shared by citizens and patients [7], and also underlined recently by members of the European Parliament [8].

To facilitate access to clinical trial information, in 1997 the database ClinicalTrials.gov was developed through the US Food and Drug Administration Modernization Act. This is the world's largest clinical trial registry, public and accessible to citizens [9, 10]. In 2005, the "International Committee of Medical Journal Editors" implemented a policy requiring prospective registration of clinical trials for publication in its member journals [11]. In 2007, the US Food and Drug Administration Amendments Act [FDAAA] required trial results to be reported in ClinicalTrials.gov, within one year from completion and regardless of whether the results had been published [12]. Finally, in 2008, the ClinicalTrials.gov registry expanded its database to include a section reporting basic summary results [13, 14]. Nevertheless, compliance with the reporting of results continued to be lacking, probably because some statutory requirements were ambiguous.

In September 2016, the US Department of Health and Human Services published a final rule to increase the accountability of all clinical research stakeholders by expansion of minimum data sets about legal requirements under FDAAA for trial registration and submission of results. The final rule became effective on 18 January 2017 through those responsible had until 18 April 2017

* Correspondence: anna.roberto@marionegri.it
Laboratory for medical research and consumer involvement, IRCCS Istituto di Ricerche Farmacologiche Mario Negri, Via G. La Masa 19, 20156 Milan, Italy

to become familiar and compliant with it. At the same time, the Nation Institute of Health issued a complementary final policy [15].

Ovarian cancer can be considered a rare disease in comparison with other major oncological killers, even if it is the fifth most common cancer among women. About 65,000 women are diagnosed every year in Europe, and 42,000 die each year [16]. No early diagnosis is available and the results of treatment are still poor for the majority of cases. It is therefore essential that any results of clinical research, positive or negative, be published to permit broad discussion of the different strategies for care.

The aims of this study were to evaluate the availability of basic summary results of registered clinical trials in ovarian cancer in ClinicalTrials.gov, and the frequency of non-publication of results in ClinicalTrials.gov and in PubMed, Embase or Google Scholar.

Methods

From January to September 2017, we examined all completed clinical trials on ovarian cancer registered in ClinicalTrials.gov in terms of the frequency of results published in PubMed, Embase and Google Scholar.

ClinicalTrials.gov database

Using the "advanced search" function of ClinicalTrials.gov we searched for trials on ovarian cancer. Only those listed as "completed status", indicating that the trial was ended normally, were included. All these reports were downloaded as an XML data set (12 January 2017). For each one we considered the following: starting date, study design (observational or interventional), type of study (diagnostic, therapeutic, supportive care, prevention and screening, health services research), country, multicentric (yes or no), funding source (profit or not-for-profit), number of primary outcomes, nature of the primary outcomes, enrolment of participants, and sample size. These variables collected in the ClinicalTrials.gov registration database are described in the Data Element Definitions document issued by the National Library of Medicine [17]. Trials not on ovarian cancer or closed after 2015 were excluded.

PubMed database

For each trial in this analysis, we used the link within ClinicalTrials.gov in order to identify the published article. If this was not possible, we systematically searched for the publication in PubMed, Embase and Google Scholar through the following keywords: trial unique registration number, trial title, principal investigator's name, and treatment. We considered a trial as "published" when a peer-reviewed publication was found, either online or in print, including any data. We then confirmed the publication identity by comparing inclusion and exclusion criteria, trial arms, type of outcomes, treatment and comparator, sample size and primary investigator names in the registration record. For each article the year of publication and the journal, the primary and secondary outcomes, sample size and impact factor (IF) were collected. We examined the correspondence between the journal publication and trial registered, as reported in ClinicalTrials.gov. The outcome correspondence analysis was conducted by IF less or more than 10 and by profit or not-for-profit. Finally, we calculated the mean time to publication of the results.

Basic summary results section in ClinicalTrials.gov

As the section reporting summary results has been available in ClinicalTrials.gov since 2008, we verified whether it had been completed on a subsample of the trials that ended between 2008 and 2015. Phase I trials were not considered as their results are not required to be published in ClinicalTrials.gov [12]. The variables collected in the ClinicalTrials.gov registration database are described in the Basic Results Data Element Definitions document issued by the National Library of Medicine [18]. Generally this section reports descriptive statistics on the characteristics of patients enrolled, and the results for the primary and secondary outcomes.

Statistical analyses

For continuous variables, means, medians and standard deviations were obtained. For categorical variables, proportions were obtained. All descriptive analyses were done using SAS, version 9.4.

Results

As described in the flow-chart (Fig. 1), out of 2725 studies retrieved by the search through ClinicalTrials.gov we identified 1195 with "completed status". The final set, related to ovarian cancer and closed in 2015, comprised 752 completed studies. To examine this database we considered the following groups: 254 completed before 2008; 122 completed Phase I trials closed between 2008 and 2015; 376 other completed studies closed between 2008 and 2015.

Table 1 illustrates the main features of completed studies. Most were Phase II, multicentre trials, conducted in America, for treatment purposes. Safety and efficacy were the most common endpoints, and major were not-for-profit. There was a large amount of missing data for the endpoint classification and center. The mean duration was 4.5 years.

The mean time to journal publication was 2.5 years (SD 1.8, range 1–11) only for reports published after the end of the trials (data not shown).

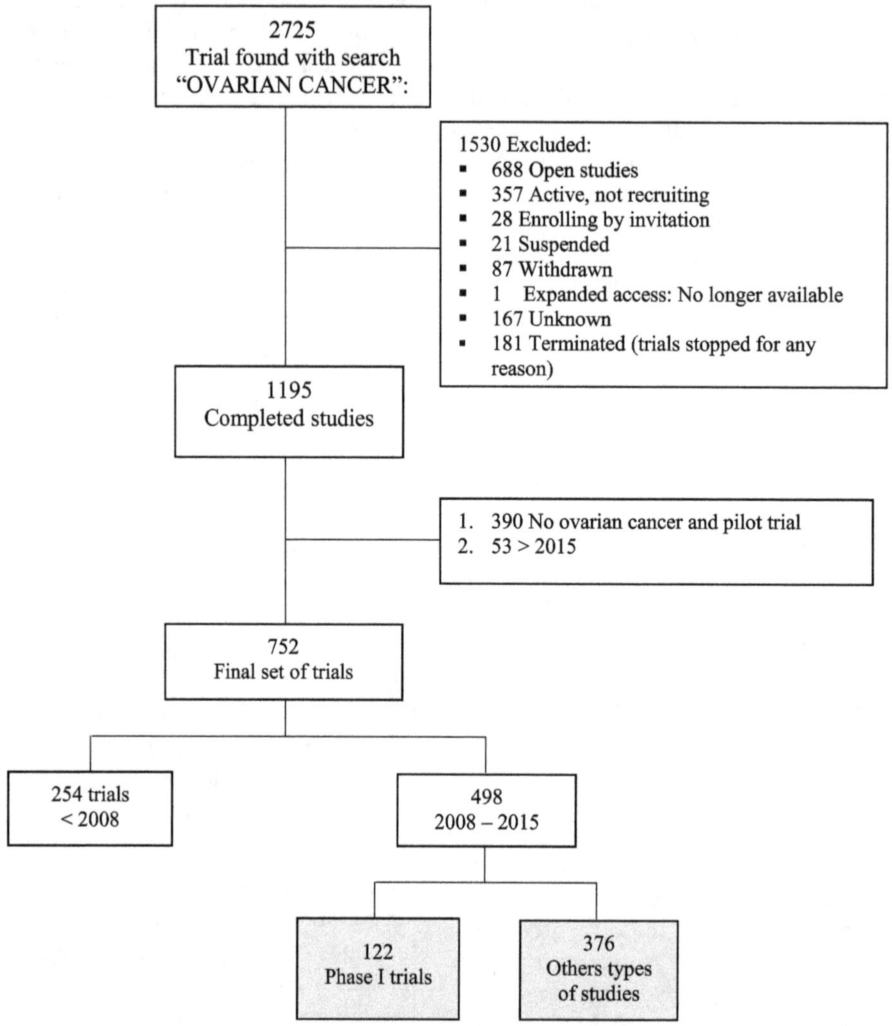

Fig. 1 Flow-chart describing the selection of ovarian cancer trials and the availability of results

Table 2 compares the primary and secondary outcomes reported in published articles and in the trials registered in ClinicalTrials.gov. The frequency of publication of results in the ClinicalTrials.gov section among "other studies" completed between 2008 and 2015 is nearly 35%. For the primary outcome, 51.8% of all trials corresponded, but 37.8% were not declared in ClinicalTrials.gov. The figures for secondary outcome were 39.3% of all trials. In this case, the percentage of secondary outcomes not declared in ClinicalTrials.gov reached 44.5%.

A total of 94 reports of trials completed between 2008 and 2015 did not report results either in ClinicalTrials.gov or in a publication available in PubMed, Embase or Google Scholar (Table 3).

Comparison of the information reported in the published articles and in the results' section of ClinicalTrials.gov (Table 4) shows several discrepancies between what was declared and what was actually published. One hundred and five different journals were found, with an average IF of 10.3 (range 1.5–72.4). For 10 of them no IF was declared. On primary outcomes the correspondence between journal publication and ClinicalTrials.gov trials is similar in both groups (Table 4). Outcome correspondence was less common in the journals with IF≥10. In the high IF journals it was more frequent not to declare primary outcome in ClinicalTrials.gov.

The correspondence for secondary outcomes was similar in both groups. These results suggest that the quality of outcome reported was not significantly influenced by the IF.

We retrieved a total of 463 not-for-profit trials and 289 for profit. Only studies published between 2008 and 2015 were analyzed. The main features such as trial phase, center, purpose, etc., were described and compared (Table 5).

As for the IF, we verified the outcome correspondence between journals and ClinicalTrials.gov not-for-profit and profit trials separately. The correspondence of

Table 1 Main features of the trials reported in ClinicalTrials.gov

ClinicalTrials.gov studies	All (752)		< 2008 (254)		2008–2015 (498)	
	N	%	N	%	N	%
Study phase						
0	3	0.4	–	–	3	0.6
I	186	24.7	67	26.4	119	23.9
I-II	54	7.2	21	8.3	33	6.6
II	313	41.6	114	44.9	199	40.0
II-III	6	0.8	2	0.8	4	0.8
III	67	8.9	21	8.3	46	9.2
IV	7	0.9	2	0.8	5	1.0
Observational	71	9.4	18	7.1	53	10.6
Missing	45	6.0	9	3.5	36	7.2
Center						
Multicenter	393	52.3	106	41.7	287	57.6
Single-center	208	27.7	76	29.9	132	26.5
Missing	151	20.1	72	28.4	79	15.9
Country[a]						
America	489	65.0	195	76.8	294	59.0
Europe	114	15.2	25	9.8	89	17.9
International	99	13.1	17	6.7	82	16.5
Asia	21	2.8	4	1.6	17	3.4
Oceania	3	0.4	–	–	3	0.6
Study purpose[a]						
Treatment	612	81.4	213	83.9	399	80.1
Prevention and screening	20	2.7	6	2.4	14	2.8
Diagnostic	15	2.0	2	0.8	13	2.6
Supportive care	29	3.9	12	4.7	17	3.4
Health services research	5	0.7	1	0.4	4	0.8
Other	34	4.5	4	1.6	30	6.0
Missing	37	5.0	16	6.3	21	4.2
Endpoint classification						
Efficacy	168	22.3	67	26.4	101	20.3
Safety	80	10.6	27	10.6	53	10.6
Safety and efficacy	256	34.0	68	26.8	188	37.8
Other	106	14.1	18	7.1	88	17.7
Missing	142	19.0	74	29.1	68	13.7
Sponsor						
Not-for-profit	463	61.6	189	74.4	274	55.0
Profit	289	38.4	65	25.6	224	45.0
Study duration (years)						
Mean (SD)	4.48 (2.8)		4.12 (2.9)		4.64 (2.7)	
Range	1–24		1–24		1–21	
Number of subjects						
< 50	382	51.6	142	37.2	240	62.8
≥ 50	359	48.5	105	29.3	254	70.8

[a]Some discrepancies in the total are due to missing data; less than 5% of data are missing

Table 2 Trials published and correspondence between outcomes in the publication and ClinicalTrials.gov

	N	%	N	%	N	%	N	%
Results Reported in	All (752)		< 2008 (254)		2008-2015[a] (498)			
					Phase I (122)		Other studies types (376)	
ClinicalTrials.gov	NA		NA		NA		130	34.6
Journal publication	483	64.2	147	57.9	74	60.7	262	69.7
Outcome correspondence	All (483)		< 2008 (147)		Phase I (74)		Other studies types (262)	
Primary Outcome								
Corresponded	249	51.8	40	27.0	37	50.7	172	66.2
Not corresponded	50	10.4	13	8.8	7	9.6	30	11.5
Not declared in ClinicalTrials.gov	182	37.8	95	64.2	29	39.7	58	22.3
Secondary Outcome								
Corresponded	157	39.3	24	19.1	27	41.5	106	50.7
Not corresponded	65	16.2	14	11.1	7	10.8	44	21.1
Not declared in ClinicalTrials.gov	178	44.5	88	69.8	31	47.7	59	28.2

NA, Not applicable
[a]See the number reported in the highlighted boxes in Fig. 1

primary outcomes was similar in both samples with a total correspondence between two sources of 76.2%. For the secondary outcome, however, for profit trials corresponded more closely, with 64.2% vs. 43.2% respectively (Table 6).

Discussion

Several papers indicate a worrisome percentage of clinical trials whose results are not available for clinicians, researchers and citizens or patients [2, 19–23]. To our knowledge this topic is still less deepened in ovarian cancer field. Some publications are consistent with our results showing there is still a general need for transparency in publication of findings. Guo and colleagues reported that 69% of a sample of 35 clinical trials on endometriosis were unpublished [19]. As regards the links between ClinicalTrials.gov and PubMed, Huser and Cimino [20] reported that the majority of 8907 trials (72%] had no structured trial-article link available, and 55% of so-called "silent" trials had no linked results article or even basic summary results. Such underreporting can contribute to biased evidence, with serious consequences for clinical practice, research and, in the end, for patients [21, 24]. Pranic and Marusic [25] report a similar result about 81 eligible trials found in ClinicalTrials.gov between 2009 and 2012. In this sample, the secondary outcomes were left out for 17% at the initial registration and for 19.7% at the last.

Table 3 Results in ClinicalTrials.gov and journal publication for trials ended between 2008 and 2015 (N 376)

	ClinicalTrials.gov	
Journal publication	Yes - *N (%)*	No - *N (%)*
Yes - *N (%)*	110 (29.3)	152 (40.4)
No - *N (%)*	20 (5.3)	94 (25.0)
Total	130 (34.6)	246 (65.4)

Basing on our analysis aimed on ovarian cancer, very high percentages of completed ovarian cancer clinical trials - about a quarter - do not see the light either in the specific results section of ClinicalTrials.gov or in medical journals.

Also important are the inconsistencies between the trials registered and the published primary and secondary outcomes. These inconsistencies are also present in the ClinicalTrials.gov results section. From the viewpoint of citizens or patients a complete results section in a public registry such as ClinicalTrials.gov should offer an easy way to find complete information about all registered clinical trials. On the single level, this could facilitate decision-making on new treatments or even new clinical trials [1, 26]. At the community level, for example for patients' associations, the results could help in identifying uncertainties or answering questions about the effects of treatments and discussing research priorities. From the researchers' point of view the lack of access to all trial results contributes to publication bias [2], to misuse of systematic reviews, meta-analyses and clinical guidelines and, finally, reduces the possibility of designing innovative research. Even more important, from the clinicians' point of view this lack of information on results can lead to an unfair doctor-patient relationship, where advice on care and treatment is not in line with the latest knowledge.

Researchers and sponsors have a great responsibility to report results and data related to their clinical research

Table 4 Correspondence between outcomes in publications and ClinicalTrials.gov, based on Impact Factor

Outcome correspondence based on Impact Factor	Impact factor ≥ 10 (18[a])		Impact factor < 10 (75[a])		Total (93)	
	N	%	N	%	N	%
Primary Outcome						
Corresponded	19	73.1	62	79.5	81	77.9
Not corresponded	2	7.7	11	14.1	13	12.5
Not declared in ClinicalTrials.gov	5	19.2	5	6.4	10	9.6
Secondary Outcome						
Corresponded	11	57.9	36	54.6	47	55.3
Not corresponded	5	26.3	16	24.2	21	24.7
Not declared in ClinicalTrials.gov	3	15.8	14	21.2	17	20.0

[a]Number of journals with IF less than 10 or more according to each subgroup. The same journal could have published several articles

fully, as recently underlined by the new European Medicines Agency regulation on trial publication [27].

Nevertheless, it is not easy to investigate the cause of this marked lack of transparency as many factors can contribute, such as career, market and sponsors, or conflict of interest. Probably until a few years ago some researchers did not even consider the lack of transparency an important issue that could help improve the quality of research and reduce waste. Moreover there was no public opinion movement, such as the AllTrials campaign [4], which could lead to greater transparency. And yet ensuring greater transparency would only need a little effort on the part of researchers, who should be anxious to register publicly their trials and make the results public as required by FDAAA [13]. It also defined criteria and a checklist of mandatory registration data or documents, to register and then to publish results [28]. To guarantee a standard method for reporting results, there are also international guidelines such as CONSORT 2010 (Consolidated Standards of Reporting Results) [29] and ICH E3 (International Conference on Harmonisation of Technical Requirements for Registration of Pharmaceuticals for Human Use) [30].

In addition, to improve the clarity and boost the spread of information, data sharing is encouraged and is considered a new "gold standard" by all scientific stakeholders; several initiatives or projects are planned to increase it. Researchers can, through specific platforms, have access to anonymized patients' data from several clinical trials, and other documentation to conduct further research [31]. As regards the homogenization of procedures to plan and conduct a clinical trial, the European Community has drawn up the New Regulation 536/2014. Its first aim is to improve the transparency of the data collected by all European trials and to make them public. The Regulation also defines the standards to assure the safety and quality of research, fostering collaboration among Member States [32].

Recently, the editors of peer-reviewed journals have become more willing to publish negative trials results and to check the consistency of information to be published with that reported in registers such as ClinicalTrials.gov [25].

Finally, citizens, patients and their associations can all do something to obtain greater transparency in research: for example, associations and public funders can decide to finance only trials which expressly state they will adhere to the rules of transparency.

As ovarian cancer is so infrequent, disclosure of study results is an ethical duty from the moment patients are enrolled, and this should be fully stated in the informed consent form. The latest version of the Declaration of Helsinki exhorts researchers, authors, sponsors, editors and publishers to report and disseminate positive or negative results of clinical research [33]. What patient would be willing to participate in a clinical trial if the data collected will not be useful to anyone - neither the scientific community nor other patients? Associations of citizens or patients could be also more forceful in demanding more transparency in reporting results, and offer their support only to researchers or multicenter groups that guarantee full disclosure.

The sample of trials that did not report the results either in a journal or in the results section in ClinicalTrials.gov amounted to about 30% of those on recurrent platinum-resistant ovarian cancer, and about 30% with advanced ovarian cancer. Only a few trials involved newly-diagnosed women or those in the first line of treatment. Nearly half the trials were Phase II, and one-tenth were observational.

In our sample not only was the results section often missing, but single items required during the registration in ClinicalTrials.gov were often lacking too: for example, the nature of the study, or the endpoint classification. On the other hand, it is worth noting the limited amount of data missing among all the items required

Table 5 Main features of not-for-profit and profit trials ended between 2008 and 2015

ClinicalTrials.gov studies	Not-for-profit 2008–2015 (274)		Profit 2008–2015 (224)	
	N	%	N	%
Study phase				
0	3	16.5	–	–
I	46	19.0	73	33.2
I-II	18	7.4	15	6.8
II	103	42.6	96	43.6
II-III	–	–	4	1.8
III	29	12.0	17	7.7
IV	3	1.2	2	0.9
Observational	40	16.5	13	5.9
Missing	32		4	
Center				
Multicenter	125	58.7	162	78.6
Single-center	88	41.3	44	21.4
Missing	61		18	
Country				
America	178	66.4	116	53.5
Europe	64	23.9	25	11.5
International	16	6.0	66	30.4
Asia	8	3.0	9	4.2
Oceania	2	0.8	1	0.5
Study purpose				
Treatment	196	76.0	203	92.7
Prevention and screening	10	3.9	4	1.8
Diagnostic	8	3.1	5	2.3
Supportive care	15	5.8	2	0.9
Health services research	3	1.2	1	0.5
Other	26	10.1	4	1.8
Missing	16			
Endpoint classification				
Efficacy	71	32.0	30	14.4
Safety	18	8.1	35	16.8
Safety and efficacy	78	35.1	110	52.9
Other	55	24.8	33	15.9
Missing	52		16	
Study duration (years) - Mean (SD)	5.27 (3.00)		3.74 (2.17)	
Number of subjects				
< 50	128	46.7	112	50.0
> =50	143	52.2	111	49.5

Table 6 Correspondence between outcomes in publications and ClinicalTrials.gov among "not-for-profit" vs "profit" studies

Outcome correspondence	Not-for-profit (52)		Profit (58)	
	N	%	N	%
Primary Outcome[a]				
Corresponded	39	76.5	44	75.9
Not corresponded	7	13.7	7	12.1
Not declared in ClinicalTrials.gov	5	9.8	7	12.1
Secondary Outcome[a]				
Corresponded	16	43.2	34	64.2
Not corresponded	12	32.4	11	20.8
Not declared in ClinicalTrials.gov	9	24.3	8	15.1

[a]Some discrepancies in the total are due to missing data

now for registration in the clinical trials whose results were reported both in ClinicalTrials.gov and in a journal. This shows that a high level of data reporting is possible with little extra effort.

The inconsistencies between the trial registered and the published results on primary and secondary outcomes are not to be overlooked; these inconsistencies are also present in the ClinicalTrials.gov results section but also in journals with IF of 10 or more. In fact, a quality analysis based on the IF it does not show any appreciable differences between the two groups. These results are in line with a previous cross-sectional analysis [34] of 96 clinical trials. These trials were published in 2010–2011 in PubMed, in high-impact journals (IF≥10) and the results were registered and reported in ClinicalTrials.gov; nearly all had at least one discrepancy in the cohort, intervention, primary endpoints or results reported in the two sites. In addition, Smith et al. [35] reported disparity for 79% of the registry-publication pairs especially about primary outcomes.

Results that we retrieved were similar for the analysis among not-for-profit and for-profit trials. This implies, that efforts to improve the quality and transparency of data published are still needed especially for secondary outcomes.

At the end of a trial, the analysis should include publication of the results on the basis of the primary outcome on which the trial was designed, and also the sample size. Not disclosing the primary outcome, but only the secondary one, can have a detrimental impact in the scientific community, who do not receive the right information, and on patients who participated in the not properly designed trial. Moreover, future studies can be damaged too as other researchers can may design new trials on the basis of previous uncorrected results. Finally, it is unethical to ask a patient informed consent for to take part in a trial with a defined endpoint, and then not to make the result public.

This analysis has some limitations. Misclassification of clinical trials might have influenced the data collection, as well as the lack of updating by investigators. In addition, the analysis was restricted to the period between 2008 and 2015 and some journal articles might have been missed, considering the time needed for peer review before publication. As concern strengths, this paper adds evidence to the discussion about the lack of transparency of clinical research, showing that the problem is far from solved.

Conclusions

Researchers, clinicians and citizens or patients' representatives need to focus on transparency as an important ethical issue and continuously support initiatives to improve the publication and dissemination of clinical findings. The publication of protocols and statistical analysis plans could be useful to ensure transparency through the investigators themselves should be more compliant or explain discrepancies [36]. In addition, publishers and editors should pay close attention to ensure that information reported in ClinicalTrials.gov is consistent with the information reported in papers submitted.

Abbreviations

FDAAA: Food and Drug Administration Amendments Act; IF: Impact Factor; IRCCS: Istituto di Ricovero e Cura a Carattere Scientifico; SAS: Statistical Analysis Software; XML: Extensible Markup Language

Acknowledgements

We thank the Nerina and Mario Mattioli Foundation. This manuscript is dedicated to the memory of Flavia Bideri, who founded the first Italian ovarian cancer patients' association. We thank Drs. Elena Biagioli and Drs. Chiara Gerardi for their contributions to the discussion. We are grateful to J.D. Baggott for editing.

Funding

This study was supported by internal funds of the IRCCS Istituto di Ricerche Farmacologiche Mario Negri and Nerina and Mario Mattioli Foundation. The funders had no role in the design, data collection and analysis, decision to publish, or preparation of the manuscript.

Authors' contributions

AR, SR and PM contributed equally to this work. All authors read and approved the final manuscript.

Competing interests

The authors declare that they have no competing interest.

References

1. Liberati A. An unfinished trip through uncertainties. BMJ. 2004;328(7438):531.
2. Jones CW, Handler L, Crowell KE, Keil LG, Weaver MA, Platts-Mills TF. Non-publication of large randomized clinical trials: cross sectional analysis. BMJ. 2013;347:f6104.
3. Lomas A. I'm a patient: show me the trial data. BMJ. 2013;346:f2336.
4. Chalmers IGP. All trials must be registered and the results published. BMJ. 2013;346:f105. https://doi.org/10.1136/bmj.f105.
5. Groves T, Godlee F. The European medicines Agency's plans for sharing data from clinical trials. BMJ. 2013;346:f2961.
6. Doshi P, Dickersin K, Healy D, Vedula SS, Jefferson T. Restoring invisible and abandoned trials: a call for people to publish the findings. BMJ. 2013;346: f2865.
7. http://www.equator-network.org/wp-content/uploads/2013/08/4614_3rd-EQUATOR-Annual-Lecture-Hazel-Thornton.pdf. Accessed 4 Apr 2018.
8. Kmietowicz Z. Transparency campaigners welcome new rules for clinical trials in Europe. BMJ. 2014;348:g2579.
9. Food and Drug Administration Modernization Act of 1997. US public law 105-15. (1997, Nov 21); 21 USC 301.
10. Zarin DA, Tse T. Medicine. Moving toward transparency of clinical trials. Science. 2008;319:1340–2.
11. De Angelis C, Drazen JM, Frizelle FA, Haug C, Hoey J, Horton R, et al. Clinical trial registration: a statement from the International Committee of Medical Journal. N Engl J Med. 2004;351:1250–1.
12. Food and Drug Administration Amendments Act of 2007. US public law 110-85. (2007, sept 27); 21 USC 301.
13. ClinicalTrials.gov. FDAAA 801 requirements. National Institutes of Health. https://clinicaltrials.gov/ct2/manage-recs/fdaaa. Accessed 4 Apr 2018.
14. Tse T, Williams RJ, Zarin DA. Reporting "basic results" in ClinicalTrials.gov. Chest. 2009;136:295–303.
15. Zarin DA, Tse T, Williams RJ, Carr S. Trial reporting in — the final rule. N Engl J Med. 2016;375(20):1998–2004.
16. Ferlay J, Steliarova-Foucher E, Lortet-Tieulent J, Rosso S, Coebergh JW, Comber H, et al. Cancer incidence and mortality patterns in Europe: estimates for 40 countries in 2012. Eur J Cancer. 2013;49(6):1374-403. https://doi.org/10.1016/j.ejca.2012.12.027. Epub 2013 Feb 26.
17. Data element definitions http://prsinfo.clinicaltrials.gov/definitions.html. Accessed 4 Apr 2018.
18. Basic results https://prsinfo.clinicaltrials.gov/ResultsDetailedReviewItems.pdf. Accessed 4 Apr 2018.
19. Guo SW, Evers JL. Lack of transparency of clinical trials on endometriosis. Obstet Gynecol. 2013;121:1281–90.
20. Huser V, Cimino JJ. Linking ClinicalTrials.gov and PubMed to track results of interventional human clinical trials. PLoS One. 2013;8:e68409.
21. Hartung DM, Zarin DA, Guise JM, McDonagh M, Paynter R, Helfand M. Reporting discrepancies between the ClinicalTrials.gov results database and peer-reviewed publications. Ann Intern Med. 2014;160:477–83.
22. Mayor S. Half of drug trials with results on ClinicalTrials.gov are not published in journals. BMJ. 2013;347:f7219.
23. Mosconi P, Roberto A. Working together to improve the credibility and transparency of clinical research. BMJ. 2013;347:f7590.
24. Chalmers I, Glasziou P. Avoidable waste in the production and reporting of research evidence. Lancet. 2009;374:86–9.
25. Pranić S, Marušić A. Changes to registration elements and results in a cohort of Clinicaltrials.gov trials were not reflected in published articles. J Clin Epidemiol. 2016;70(Supplement C):26–37.
26. Liberati A. Need to realign patient-oriented and commercial and academic research. Lancet. 2011;378:1777–8.
27. Groves T. Big strides in Europe towards clinical trial transparency. BMJ. 2014; 349:g6276.
28. Zarin DA, Tse T, Williams RJ, Rajakannan T. Update on trial registration 11 years after the ICMJE policy was established. N Engl J Med. 2017;376(4):383–91.
29. Schulz KF, Altman DG, Moher D. CONSORT 2010 Statement: updated guidelines for reporting parallel group randomised trials. BMJ. 2010;340:c332.
30. E3_Guideline.pdf [Internet]. [cited 2018 Mar 14]. Available from: https://www.ich.org/fileadmin/Public_Web_Site/ICH_Products/Guidelines/Efficacy/E3/E3_Guideline.pdf. Accessed 4 Apr 2018.

31. Pansieri C, Pandolfini C, Bonati M. The evolution in registration of clinical trials: a chronicle of the historical calls and current initiatives promoting transparency. Eur J Clin Pharmacol. 2015;71(10):1159–64.
32. Gazzetta Ufficiale dell'Unione Europea L158 [Internet]. [cited 2017 Dec 14]. Available from: http://eur-lex.europa.eu/legal-content/IT/TXT/PDF/?uri=OJ:L:2014:158:FULL&from=IT. Accessed 4 Apr 2018.
33. World Medical Association Declaration of Helsinki: ethical principles for medical research involving human subjects. JAMA. 2013;310:2191–4.
34. Becker JE, Krumholz HM, Ben-Josef G, Ross JS. Reporting of results in clinicaltrials.gov and high-impact journals. JAMA. 2014;311(10):1063–5.
35. Smith SM, Wang AT, Pereira A, Chang RD, McKeown A, Greene K, et al. Discrepancies between registered and published primary outcome specifications in analgesic trials: ACTTION systematic review and recommendations. Pain. 2013;154(12):2769–74.
36. Dwan K, Altman DG, Clarke M, Gamble C, Higgins JPT, Sterne JAC, et al. Evidence for the selective reporting of analyses and discrepancies in clinical trials: a systematic review of cohort studies of clinical trials. PLoS Med. 2014; 11(6):e1001666.

17

Ovarian teratoma in children: a plea for collaborative clinical study

Justyna Łuczak* and Maciej Bagłaj

Abstract

Background: Although teratomas are the most common histologic subtype of childhood ovarian germ cell tumors, their appropriate treatment in this age group still remains unclear. Paucity of research dedicated exclusively to both mature and immature teratomas of the ovary, contribute to decision making difficulties.
Therefore, we decided to review retrospectively our experience in treatment of pediatric ovarian teratomas in order to assess the epidemiology, presenting features, and diagnostic as well as surgical management of these lesions.

Results: The study comprised 58 patients. Fifty percent of patients were between 9 and 15 years old. Mature teratoma was diagnosed in 55(94.83%) patients, while 3(5.17%) patients presented with immature teratoma. Twenty eight (50.91%) girls with mature teratoma had laparotomy and 23 (41.82%) had laparoscopy performed as an initial operative approach. Ovarian tissue sparing technique (preservation of the ovarian tissue of the affected gonad) was applied in only 11.11% of patients operated in the first study period (years 1999–2003) and increased to 40.54% in the second half of our study (years 2004–2016). The extent of gonadal resection was not related with the size of the lesion. Bilateral lesions were noted in 8 patients with mature teratoma. All girls with immature teratoma were subjected to formal laparotomy. Two patients had stage III of the disease and one had stage IV. They underwent at least resection of the affected gonad. Adjuvant chemotherapy was given to all girls with immature teratoma after the surgery.

Conclusions: Under particular conditions ovarian-sparing surgery might be successfully applied in children with mature teratoma. Laparotomy is the treatment of choice in large masses, suspicious for malignancy and if surgical staging is required. High quality prospective multi-institutional studies are required in order to get an objective insight into biology and prognostic factors of teratomas in children.

Keywords: Ovarian teratoma, Ovarian neoplasms, Child

Background

Ovarian teratomas are the most common type of ovarian tumors in children. Nevertheless, some aspects of its pathology, classification and management still remain unclear. Their embryology and genetic basis are not yet understood. Specific concerns regard their malignant potential and therefore the possible use of ovarian-sparing operative techniques and the suitability of chemotherapy in its treatment. According to the recent studies, ovarian-sparing procedures are recommended in case of mature teratoma, on specific conditions [1, 2]. However, variety of tissue architecture in teratomas creates a lot of uncertainty. Such as the significance of grade of immaturity or detection of Yolk sac tumor microfoci. In turn, difficulties in histologic sampling might result in overlooking of some malignant cells, especially in the large tumors. Although surgery remains the mainstay of treatment, the indications for chemotherapy vary between the studies [2–7]. Paucity of research dedicated exclusively to both mature and immature teratomas of the ovary, contribute to decision making difficulties. Therefore, we decided to review our experience of pediatric ovarian teratomas at our institution in order to assess the epidemiology, presenting features, and diagnostic as well as surgical management of these lesions.

Material and methods

We analyzed retrospectively medical files of all consecutive patients aged 0–18 years, who underwent surgical procedures for ovarian teratoma between 1991 and 2016 at the University Department of Pediatric Surgery and Urology in Wroclaw, Poland. The demographic data, presenting

* Correspondence: sitnikjustyna@gmail.com
Pediatric Surgery and Urology Department, Wroclaw Medical University, 52 M. Sklodowskiej – Curie ST, 50-369 Wroclaw, Poland

symptoms and signs, results of laboratory and diagnostic studies (including ultrasound examination, additional imaging studies and tumor markers), details of surgical procedures, and clinical outcomes (including preservation rate), were extracted in each case. Ovarian mass characteristics were evaluated by preoperative imaging (structure and size) or by description of the procedure (size). An ovarian lesion was described arbitrarily as large when its diameter was 10 cm or more in girls aged between 1 and 18 years and 5 cm or more in newborns and infants. Such classification was based on the previous experience of other authors, in order to obtain comparable results [8, 9]. A choice of an operative technique (either laparoscopic or open) depended solely on a surgeon's preference. The extent of gonadal resection was based on intraoperative findings and it ranged from total, when the whole gonad affected by lesion was removed, to partial resection, when at least the remnant of ovarian tissue was preserved. Preservation rates were compared taking into consideration the operative method, the histological type, the size of the mass, the presence of ovarian torsion and the study period (1991–2003 vs 2004–2016). The analyzed data were subjected to the statistical evaluation with Chi square, Kruskal-Wallis and Barttlet test, Pearson's correlation coefficient and logistic regression. The statistical software package EPIINFO Ver. 7.1.1.14 was used for all data analyses.

Results

Epidemiology and presentation

The study comprised 58 patients. The median of age was 12,0 years (SD = 4.2). Fifty percent of patients were between 9 and 15 years old. Mature teratoma was diagnosed in 55(94.83%) patients, while 3(5.17%) patients presented with immature teratoma (age: 8,12 and 15 years old). There were 44 girls (75.86%) with chronic presentation (no symptoms requiring immediate surgical intervention). Fourteen patients (24.14%) presented with acute symptoms (admitted to the hospital as emergency due to relevant pain or/and vomits, fever). Abdominal pain, palpable mass and distension were the most frequent clinical features noted in the whole study group. Palpable mass was the most frequent symptom in girls with chronic presentation (52.27%), while abdominal pain predominated in girls with acute presentation and was noted in 13 of them (92.86%); Fig. 1. The most common intraoperative finding additional to the tumor, in girls with acute presentation, was ovarian torsion (85.71% of patients with acute symptoms; $p = 0.00634$, $\chi^2 = 7.45$, $Rr = 3.83$, $CI = 1.67 \div 8.82$); Table 1. All three patients with immature teratoma presented with chronic symptoms.

Diagnostic studies

Mature teratomas

All of the patients underwent abdominal ultrasound scan (US). It showed a cystic structure in 14 girls (25.45%). A complex ovarian mass was noted in 38 (69.09%) and a solid mass in 2 girls (36.36%). Twenty-eight girls (50.91%) had a large tumor (with a diameter of more than 10 cm). Twenty-one patients (38.18%) had computed tomography (CT) or magnetic resonance(MRI) studies performed preoperatively. In 11

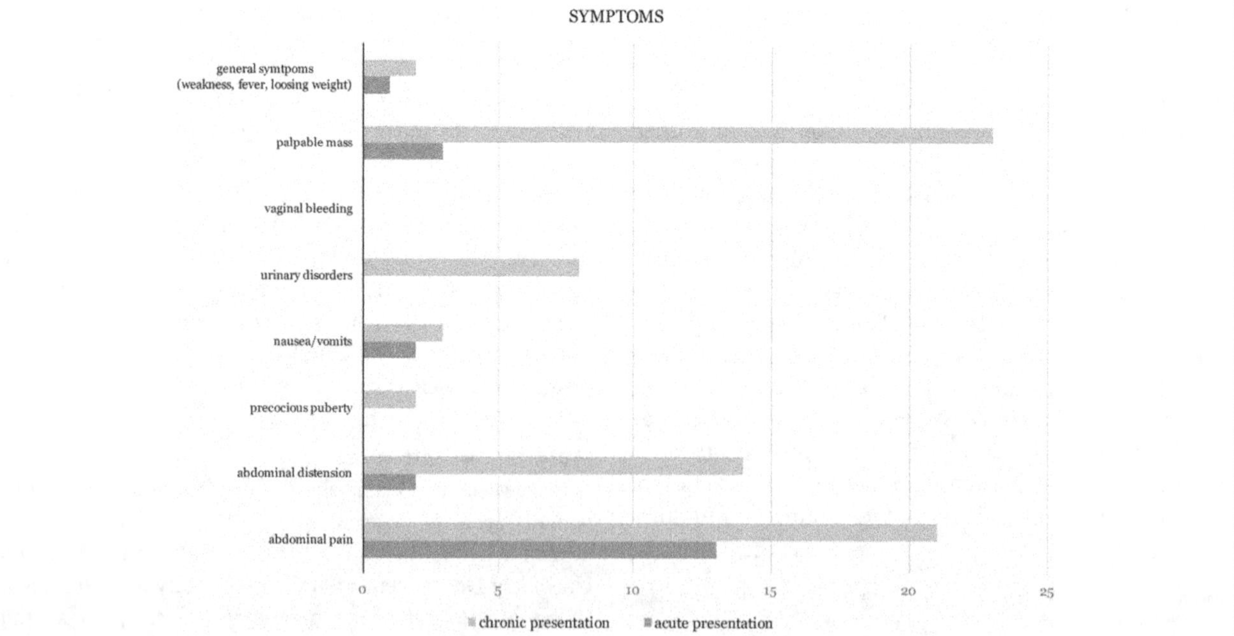

Fig. 1 The most common presented symptoms

Table 1 Comparison of the clinical data between mature and immature teratomas

Overall			
Number of patients	58		
Age(years)	12.0 (9.0÷15.0); sd 4.2		
	Mature teratoma	Immature teratoma	
Number of patients	55	3	
Symptoms			
Acute presentation (number of patients)	14(24.14%)		
Abdominal pain	13		
Palpable mass	3		
Distension	2		
Other	1		
Chronic presentation (number of patients)	44(75.86%)		
Abdominal pain	21		
Palpable mass	23		
Distension	14		
Other	15		
US result			
Solid	2	1	
Complex	38	1	
Cystic	14	0	
Size of the lesion			
Large lesion	28	3	
Lesion that was not described as large	16	0	
Tumor markers			
Positive	5	3	
AFP	1	3	
CA-125	4	0	
Negative	33	0	
Bilateral lesion			
Synchronous	4	0	
Metachronous	2	0	
Ovarian torsion	Mature teratoma	Immature teratoma	*p* value
Acute presentation	7(85.71%)	0	0.00634
Chronic presentation	5(11.36%)	0	

patients this additional examination led to the evaluation of tumor origin or its real structure changing the initial radiological description of the lesion (based on US scan). Statistical analysis revealed linear dependence between the size of the lesion and patient's age (Pearson product-moment correlation coefficient: $r = 0.29$, $N = 53$, $p = 0.039$, Fig. 2). The results of tumor markers evaluation (AFP – alpha-fetaprotein, β-hCG - beta subunit of human chorionic gonadotropin, CA125 - cancer antigen 125, LDH - lactate dehydrogenase) were available for 38 girls (69.09%). They were elevated in 5 girls (9.09%). Only one marker was positive in four patients out of five: CA-125. We noted elevated level of AFP (37.45 ng/ml) in one patient aged 14 (Table 1).

Immature teratomas

Abdominal US showed a complex ovarian lesion and a solid mass in one girl each. A heterogenous structure of one of the lesions was confirmed in CT. One patient had only computed tomography result available, it revealed a complex lesion. Calcifications were observed on imaging in two patients. Large tumor was diagnosed in all three girls. Tumor markers evaluation revealed elevated level of AFP in all girls (186,1680 and 6434 ng/ml).

Treatment

Mature teratomas

Twenty-eight (50.91%) girls had laparotomy and 23 (41.82%) had laparoscopy performed as an initial operative approach. Conversion to open procedure was noted in 4 girls (7.27%). The number of patients operated on with laparoscopy increased from 44.44 to 51.35% in the second part of our study (years 1991–2003 vs 2004–2016). Ovarian tissue sparing technique (preservation of the ovarian tissue of the affected gonad) was applied in only 11.11% of patients operated in the first study period and increased to 40.54% in the second half of our study. The preservation rate was higher in the group of girls in whom laparoscopic technique was chosen. The extent of gonadal resection was not related with the size of the lesion. Moreover, tissue sparing was possible in 32.26% of those with large lesions and 29.17% of girls with lesions not classified as large. The difference was not statistically significant; $p = 0.806$, $\chi 2 = 0.605$ (Table 2). Biopsy procedure was performed in 21 cases and it was negative in all of them.

Immature teratomas

All girls with immature teratoma were subjected to formal laparotomy. Two patients had stage III of the disease and one had stage IV (according to Children's Oncology Group ovarian staging system) [10]. They underwent at least resection of the affected gonad. Biopsy procedure was performed all girls and it was negative in all of them.

Histopathologic findings

Mature teratomas

In 18 cases there was ovarian dermoid cyst diagnosed.

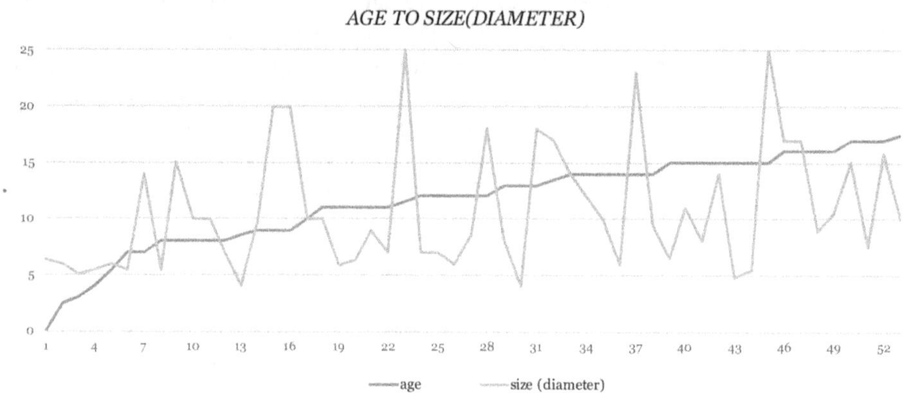

Fig. 2 Patient's age and size of the lesion

Immature teratomas

Grading (according to O'Connor and Norris) was available only in one patient (G1) [11]. No Heifetz lesions were observed.

Final outcome

Mature teratomas

Bilateral, synchronous lesions were noted in 6 patients with mature teratoma. Metachronous disease in the contralateral ovary was observed in two patients with mature teratoma after the first operation within 10 months and 5 years. Respectively (Table 1). Follow-up was possible in 13 patients and lasted between 1 and 12 years. All girls which have at least one ovary have normal menstruation. Some of them (30.77%) reported painful menstruations or are diagnosed with simple cysts (without operative treatment).

Immature teratomas

Adjuvant chemotherapy (protocol TGM 95) was given to all girls with immature teratoma after the surgery. All three patients responded well to the treatment and were disease free after follow-up of 3,4 and 12 years respectively.

Discussion

Teratomas present diverse biological behavior and continue to be the cause of many diagnostically and therapeutically challenging issues. While it is commonly accepted that mature teratomas of the ovary are benign neoplasms, the classification of the immature ones is still discussed. About 25% of all the pediatric GCTs present as tumors with more than one histologic type. In this situation, therapy and prognosis depend on the component with the highest malignancy [12–17]. In accordance with this approach pure immature teratomas were excluded in the recent studies concerning pediatric malignant germ cell tumors. Conversely, patients with malignant germ cell tumors, even when these lesions contained mature teratoma or immature teratoma elements, were not eligible for studies concerning teratomas exclusively [2, 12, 17, 18]. Nevertheless, there are also studies were a lesion was considered as immature teratoma although the pathology report revealed a component of another malignant tumor [19]. Marks of the controversy regarding this topic are also reflected in the nomenclature of these lesions across the studies. The multiplicity of names describing immature teratomas (immature teratoma, malignant teratoma, teratoma with malignant elements, immature teratoma with malignant behavior) renders universally applicable classification of these lesions very difficult [5, 12, 17–21].

All the girls in our study had at least stage III of the disease. In a study from 2012, Schneider et al. ascertain that immature teratomas behave in a malignant fashion only if foci of malignant germ cell elements are present and if they are resected incompletely. According to their paper, tumors containing clusters of yolk sac tumor are

Table 2 Ovarian tissue preservation rates in selected groups of patients

Study period	Overall	Operation method		Large lesion		Torsion	
		Laparoscopy	Laparotomy	–	+	–	+
1991–2016	29.31%	43.48% (27.27% large lesions)	20.00% (75.76% large lesions)	29.17%	32.26%	30.43%	25.00%
				$p = 0.806$			
1991–2003	11.11%	14.28%	7.69%	12.50%	9.09%	7.14%	0.00%
2004–2016	40.54%	56.25%	27.27%	37.50%	45.00%	37.50%	50.00%

likely responsible for the reports that immature teratoma may metastasize [2]. Nevertheless, in some recently published studies immature teratomas are still included in the evaluation of patients with malignant germ cell tumors and even at US National Cancer Institute website reads that "Immature teratomas can exhibit malignant behavior and metastasize" [7, 14, 22, 23]. Therefore, can we definitively classify them as benign?

Another important aspect in attempts to estimate the real nature of these lesions is the importance of the grade of immaturity. In a study published by Malignant Germ Cell Tumor International Collaborative it was revealed that grade was the most important risk factor for relapse in ovarian immature teratoma [6]. However, there is scarceness of papers reporting the use of a detailed grading system and its significance in children has been challenged by some former studies. Additionally, high immaturity itself is not associated with a poor prognosis if the tumor is completely resected [2]. Defining real nature of the lesion is indispensable in choosing optimum management. Obtaining the correct pathology report is crucial here. Clusters of malignant tumor can be easily overlooked and yolk sac tumor components might be very small. Microfoci of yolk sac tumor (Heifetz lesions) are not precisely defined among the studies, thereby classifying a lesion as malignant yolk sac tumor is particularly difficult [2, 5, 12]. Performing a central pathomorphological examination can be helpful in the case of these neoplasms. Perhaps new tumor markers, like the ones discovered by Feng et al. will help eliminate mistakes in pathomorphological diagnoses [24]. Grading was available only in one patient in our study and no Heifetz lesions were observed. This is a retrospective study and we cannot verify the results of the pathology report. Taking into consideration that all immature teratoma cases were of stage III at least, it is questionable if no other malignant components were present.

Despite these unclear pathological aspects, commonly applied diagnostic work-up of ovarian teratomas include physical examination, ultrasound imaging and tumor markers evaluation. In most of the studies the peak incidence of these lesions is reported in early adolescence [2, 12]. It was also confirmed by our study. Symptoms of ovarian teratoma do not differ from those observed in other ovarian masses. Some patients reveal acute symptoms rising suspicion of ovarian torsion. The risk of torsion complicating a case of ovarian teratoma is approximately 3 to 16% in children [2, 25]. Those cases are rarely associated with malignancy. Tsai et al. revealed that young girls tend to have either torsion of a mature cystic teratoma or torsion without underlying condition, while older patients are more likely to present with torsion and a tumor [2, 26]. In our study ovarian torsion was the most common intraoperative finding additional to the tumor in girls with acute presentation. The incidence of ovarian torsion was not higher in older girls (Kruskal-Wallis test, $p = 0{,}765$).

As most of the mature teratomas are slow-growing cystic lesions and there are some common characteristic findings, they are easily recognized on US. Nevertheless, their typical features might be less clear in case of prepubertal girls and when the lesion is large [13, 26, 27]. Our study poses limitations in that respect. The ultrasound description was often very short and we were unable to identify characteristic features for teratoma in each case. Diagnosis of immature type also poses problems. The appearance of the tumor on ultrasound is non-specific, although predominance of solid component is a differentiating factor. Identification of fat, mural nodules and calcified components within the lesion is typical for teratomas. However, there are reports suggesting that typical CT features of teratomas occur more often in mature than in immature lesions. Those findings suggest that CT or MRI imaging might be helpful, rather for staging and assessing of tumor respectability [13, 28, 29].

Alphafetoprotein evaluation is an important prognostic factor in many malignant germ cell tumors treatment protocols and it is also used in follow-up of those patients. Additionally, it is a characteristic marker of yolk sac tumor. Regarding its levels in ovarian teratomas, it was revealed that they are rarely elevated [2, 12]. In the recent Malignant Germ Cell Tumor International Collaborative study regarding ovarian immature teratomas, patients with AFP levels higher than 1000 ng/mL were excluded because this level was considered more likely to indicate malignant elements [6]. However, this approach was questioned by Terenziani et al. who used an AFP level cutoff "high for age" in their study [14]. Another limitation is caused by the vide variation in AFP levels at birth and the variability in its half-time within the first year of life [2]. Multiple publications where cases of immature teratoma are analyzed without taking AFP levels into consideration makes it more difficult to form a credible assessment of this indicator [14, 30, 31]. Only one girl in the immature teratoma group had AFP levels < 1000 ng/mL in our study. Given the results of the recent research this is another factor calling into question the result of pathology report in our cases.

According to the experience of many pediatric surgical centers, surgery remains the mainstay of treatment in ovarian teratomas. Under particular conditions ovarian-sparing surgery might be successfully applied. Preservation of ovarian tissue should be reserved for cases of localized mature teratoma, when there is a plane of dissection between the tumor and the normal ovary [1, 2, 13, 14, 32]. The study by O'Neill et al. revealed that normal ovarian tissue was visualized on follow-up ultrasound after cystectomy even if there was no normal ovarian tissue visible preoperatively [13]. Although incomplete resection is an important risk factor of recurrence, relapse is not inevitable in those cases. The use of laparoscopic techniques in the treatment of ovarian teratomas has its supporters and opponents. If the suspicion of malignancy is low and a surgeon is experienced in minimal invasive surgery, laparoscopic approach might be adequate [2, 6, 7, 12, 15, 21, 33]. Children's Cancer Study Group demonstrated in their study that cyst fluid aspiration or spillage during surgery are not associated with relapse, thereby this factor, claimed by laparoscopy opponents as more often associated with minimal invasive methods, might not have such importance for the final outcome [12, 30]. Our results are promising in that respect. We revealed that the use of laparoscopy increased in time and the preservation rate was higher in the laparoscopy group. Laparotomy is the treatment of choice in large masses, suspicious for malignancy, if surgical staging is required [13]. The preservation rate seemed no to be affected by the size of the lesion in our study.

An important aspect of the management of ovarian teratomas is their recurrence rate and the incidence of bilateral lesions. The recurrence rate after cystectomy vary between 3 to 13%. However, in the study were the recurrence rate was estimated to be of 10% the authors revealed that only 3% of the recurrent cases will require reoperation [13, 34]. There were studies suggesting that women with bilateral or multiple dermoid cysts may include a subgroup of patients with a greater tendency to develop future ovarian germ cell neoplasms. Due to low risk of malignant transformation in case of mature cystic teratomas in children the treatment should be directed on the basis of age, fertility desire or presence of another pelvic pathology rather than the size or bilaterality [35–37]. In the study by O'Neill et al. the biopsy of the contralateral macroscopically normal ovary revealed pathological lesions only in 1.1% of patients. Therefore, preoperative ultrasound in combination with careful inspection of the contralateral ovary at the time of surgery offer a safe alternative to biopsy [13, 38]. Our results support this approach, none of the biopsies was positive in our study. Given the sensitivity of ultrasound in the detection of mature cystic teratomas, annual imaging seems appropriate as a postoperative surveillance. AFP monitoring is not recommended in case of completely resected ovarian teratomas without preoperatively elevated tumor markers [12, 38].

The treatment of immature teratomas poses much more difficulties. Their possible malignant behavior requires appropriate risk classification. Among factors considered as those influencing the prognosis, except the previously mentioned, staging is the next unclear one. Since malignant tumors and benign ones cannot be distinguished based only on intraoperative appearance, there are studies recommending staging in all tumors [2, 39]. However, Billimire et al. revealed that survival appears to have been unaffected by deviations from surgical guidelines when chemotherapy is administrated [39]. Different staging systems across the surgical centers renders evaluation of their significance difficult [2, 6]. Another controversial aspect is the use of chemotherapy. Number of therapeutic options might be found in the literature. To name some of them: chemotherapy for recurrence, only for malignant recurrence, in all cases of stage I grade 2 and higher or only in girls older than 15 [2, 6, 7, 22, 40]. In the German MAKEI study more than half of the children with tumor recurrence after watch and wait strategy had yolk sac tumor in addition to teratoma. It might be one of the main counter-arguments to the results of the studies which did not find evidence that chemotherapy had any significant therapeutic effects in pure teratomas and that it does not decrease relapses in pediatric population [40]. Recently created Malignant Germ Cell Tumor International Collaborative in its publications gathering data from four clinical trials recommends surgery alone for patients with stage I/II, grade 1/2 tumors and suggests conducting of a prospective trial of observation after surgery for patients with grade 2/3, stage II-IV tumors [6]. This approach might be encouraged by the results of Park et al. as they revealed that most stage I malignant ovarian germ cell tumor recurrences can be successfully salvaged by surgery and BEP chemotherapy without compromising the overall survival [22]. Adjuvant chemotherapy according to protocol TGM 95 was given to all girls with immature teratoma in our study group. They all responded well to the therapy but it remains questionable if these were real pure immature teratoma lesions.

Schneider et al. revealed that patients with cytogenetically abnormal immature teratomas often develop recurrence [2]. An optimal consensus treatment strategy should be based on a detailed analysis of all possible factors. In this regard, the above mentioned study shows that we might be still not aware of a number of them. The future molecular research may allow distinguishing low-risk from high-risk patients accurately [15].

Different staging systems, histopathologic classification systems and risk stratification are important factors impeding development of an appropriate treatment protocol [2, 12]. Additional factors include the lack of consistent terminology in the literature and analyzing pediatric and adult patients together [5, 20, 31]. International cooperation seems the only way to progress in the prospective knowledge of prognostic factors for these tumors. It will not be possible without high quality and meticulous diagnostic approach in all participating institutions.

Conclusions

Under particular conditions ovarian-sparing surgery might be successfully applied in children with mature teratoma. Laparotomy is the treatment of choice in large masses, suspicious for malignancy and if surgical staging is required. High quality prospective multi-institutional studies are required in order to get an objective insight into biology and prognostic factors of teratomas in children.

Authors' contributions

JL made substantial contributions to conception and design of this research study as well to acquisition, analysis and interpretation of data. She was responsible for writing and drafting the manuscript. MB he was involved in interpretation of the data, writing and drafting the manuscript as well as revising it critically for important intellectual content. Both authors read and approved the final manuscript.

Competing interests

The authors declare that they have no competing interests.

References

1. Özcan R, Kuruoğlu S, Dervişoğlu S, Eliçevik M, Emir H, Büyükünal C. Ovary-sparing surgery for teratomas in children. Pediatr Surg Int. 2013;29(3):233–7.
2. Schneider DT, Terenziani M, Cecchetto G, Olson TA. Gonadal and extragonadal germ cell tumors, sex cord stromal and rare gonadal tumors. In: Schneider D, Brecht I, Olson T, Ferrari A, editors. Rare tumors in children and adolescents. Pediatric Oncology. Berlin: Springer; 2011. p. 327–402.
3. Ulbright TM. Germ cell tumors of the gonads: a selective review emphasizing problems in differential diagnosis, newly appreciated, and controversial issues. Mod Pathol. 2005;18(Suppl 2):S61–79.
4. Heifetz SA, Cushing B, Giller R, Shuster JJ, Stolar CJ, Vinocur CD, et al. Immature teratomas in children: pathologic considerations: a report from the combined pediatric oncology group/Children's cancer group. Am J Surg Pathol. 1998;22(9):1115–24.
5. Mann JR, Raafat F, Robinson K, Imeson J, Gornall P, Sokal M, et al. The United Kingdom Children's Cancer study Group's second germ cell tumor study: carboplatin, etoposide, and bleomycin are effective treatment for children with malignant extracranial germ cell tumors, with acceptable toxicity. J Clin Oncol. 2000;18(22):3809–18.
6. Pashankar F, Hale JP, Dang H, Krailo M, Brady WE, Rodriguez-Galindo C, et al. Is adjuvant chemotherapy indicated in ovarian immature teratomas? A combined data analysis from the malignant germ cell tumor international collaborative. Cancer. 2016;122(2):230–7.
7. Mangili G, Sigismondi C, Lorusso D, Cormio G, Candiani M, Scarfone G, et al. The role of staging and adjuvant chemotherapy in stage I malignant ovarian germ cell tumors (MOGTs): the MITO-9 study. Ann Oncol. 2017;28(2):333–8.
8. Rogers EM, Casadiego Cubides G, Lacy J, Gerstle JT, Kives S, Allen L. Preoperative risk stratification of adnexal masses: can we predict the optimal surgical management? J Pediatr Adolesc Gynecol. 2014;27(3):125–8.
9. Oltmann SC, Garcia N, Barber R, Huang R, Hicks B, Fischer A. Can we preoperatively risk stratify ovarian masses for malignancy? J Pediatr Surg. 2010;45(1):130–4.
10. PDQ Pediatric Treatment Editorial Board. Childhood Extracranial Germ Cell Tumors Treatment (PDQ®): Health Professional Version. In:PDQ Cancer Information Summaries [Internet]. Bethesda: National Cancer Institute (US); 2002-. https://www.ncbi.nlm.nih.gov/books/NBK65877/. Accessed 18 Aug 2018.
11. O'Connor DM, Norris HJ. The influence of grade on the outcome of stage I ovarian immature(malignant) teratomas and the reproducibility of grading. Int J Gynecol Pathol. 1994;13(4):283–9.
12. Mann JR, Gray ES, Thornton C, Raafat F, Robinson K, Collins GS, et al. Mature and immature extracranial teratomas in children: the UK Children's Cancer study group experience. J Clin Oncol. 2008;26(21):3590–7.
13. O'Neill KE, Cooper AR. The approach to ovarian dermoids in adolescents and young women. J Pediatr Adolesc Gynecol. 2011;24(3):176–80.
14. Terenziani M, Bisogno G, Boldrini R, Cecchetto G, Conte M, Boschetti L, et al. Malignant ovarian germ cell tumors in pediatric patients: The AIEOP (Associazione Italiana Ematologia Oncologia Pediatrica) study. Pediatr Blood Cancer. 2017;64(11)
15. Goebel U, Calaminus G, Schneider DT, Schmidt P, Haas RJ. Management of Germ Cell Tumors in children: approaches to cure. Onkologie. 2002;25:14–2212.
16. Bouffet E, De Lumley LL, Habrand Paris-Igr JL, Lejars Tours O, Martelli Paris H, Perel Bordeaux Y, et al. Strategie thérapeutique des tumeurs germinales malignes extra-cérébrales de l'enfant, TGM 95. Lille Cedex: In: Protocol text: Société Française d'Oncologie Pédiatrique (SFOP); 1994. http://www.oncauvergne.fr/index.php?option=com_content&view=section&layout=blog&id=36&Itemid=118. Accessed 18 Aug 2018.
17. Frazier AL, Hale JP, Rodriguez-Galindo C, Dang H, Olson T, Murray MJ. Revised risk classification for pediatric extracranial germ cell tumors based on 25 years of clinical trial data from the United Kingdom and United States. J Clin Oncol. 2015;33(2):195–201.
18. Billmire DF, Cullen JW, Rescorla FJ, Davis M, Schlatter MG, Olson TA. Surveillance after initial surgery for pediatric and adolescent girls with stage I ovarian germ cell tumors: report from the Children's oncology group. J Clin Oncol. 2014;32(5):465–70.
19. Yanai H, Matsuura H, Kawasaki M, Takada Y, Tabuchi Y, Yoshino T. Immature teratoma of the ovary with a minor rhabdomyosarcomatous component and fatal rhabdomyosarcomatous metastases: the first case in a child. Int J Gynecol Pathol. 2002;21(1):82–5.
20. Fakhr IM, el- Khalil SA, El Baradie TS, Shaalan MA, Shalaby LM, Nassif SL, et al. The role of surgical management in pediatric germ cell tumors (GCTs), NCI case series. J Egypt Natl Canc Inst. 2008;20(1):70–9.
21. L-Y YE, J-J WANG, D-R LIU, G-P DING, L-P CAO. Management of giant ovarian teratoma: a case series and review of the literature. Oncol Lett. 2012;4(4):672–6.
22. Park JY, Kim DY, Suh DS, Kim JH, Kim YM, Kim YT, et al. Outcomes of surgery alone and surveillance strategy in young women with stage I malignant ovarian germ cell tumors. Int J Gynecol Cancer. 2016;26(5):859–64.
23. National Cancer Institute. https://www.cancer.gov (2018). Accessed 18 Aug 2018.
24. Feng S, Huang S, Tong Y, Chen Z, Shen D, Wu D, et al. RNA-binding protein LIN28 is a sensitive marker of pediatric yolk sac tumors. Pediatr Surg Int. 2016; 32(8):819–25.
25. Smith CJ, Bey T, Emil S, Wichelhaus C, Lotfipour S. Ovarian Teratoma with torsion masquerading as intussusception in 4-year-old child. West J Emerg Med. 2008;9(4):228–31.
26. Tsai TC, Wong LY, Wu HP. Ovarian torsion caused by teratoma masquerading as perforated appendicitis in a 5-year-old girl. Pediatr Neonatol. 2011;52(1):51–4.
27. Smorgick N, Maymon R. Assessment of adnexal masses using ultrasound: a practical review. Int J Womens Health. 2014;6:857–63.
28. Alotaibi MO, Navarro OM. Imaging of ovarian teratomas in children: a 9-year review. Can Assoc Radiol J. 2010;61(1):23–8.
29. Sisler CL, Siegel MJ. Ovarian teratomas: a comparison of the sonographic appearance in prepubertal and postpubertal girls. AJR Am J Roentgenol. 1990;154(1):139–41.
30. Yousef Y, Pucci V, Emil S. The relationship between intraoperative rupture and recurrence of pediatric ovarian neoplasms: preliminary observations. J Pediatr Adolesc Gynecol. 2016;29(2):111–6.
31. Chan JK, Gardner AB, Chan JE, Guan A, Alshak M, Kapp DS. The influence of age and other prognostic factors associated with survival of ovarian immature teratoma - a study of 1307 patients. Gynecol Oncol. 2016;142(3): 446–51.
32. Papic JC, Finnell SM, Slaven JE, Billmire DF, Rescorla FJ, Leys CM. Predictors of ovarian malignancy in children: overcoming clinical barriers of ovarian preservation. J Pediatr Surg. 2014;49(1):144–7. discussion 147-8
33. Briones-Landa CH, Ayala-Yáñez R, Leroy-López L, Anaya-Coeto H, Santarosa-Pérez MA, Reyes-Muñoz E. Comparison of laparoscopic vs. laparotomy treatment in ovarian teratomas. Ginecol Obstet Mex. 2010;78(10):527–32.

34. Rogers EM, Allen L, Kives S. The recurrence rate of ovarian dermoid cysts in pediatric and adolescent girls. J Pediatr Adolesc Gynecol. 2014;27(4):222–6.
35. Taskinen S, Urtane A, Fagerholm R, Lohi J, Taskinen M. Metachronous benign ovarian tumors are not uncommon in children. J Pediatr Surg. 2014;49(4):543–5.
36. Anteby EY, Ron M, Revel A, Shimonovitz S, Ariel I, Hurwitz A. Germ cell tumors of the ovary arising after dermoid cyst resection: a long-term follow-up study. Obstet Gynecol. 1994;83(4):605–8.
37. Ayhan A, Bukulmez O, Genc C, Karamursel BS, Ayhan A. Mature cystic teratomas of the ovary: case series from one institution over 34 years. Eur J Obstet Gynecol Reprod Biol. 2000;88(2):153–7.
38. Templeman CL, Hertweck SP, Scheetz JP, Perlman SE, Fallat ME. The management of mature cystic teratomas in children and adolescents: a retrospective analysis. Hum Reprod. 2000;15(12):2669–72.
39. Billmire D, Vinocur C, Rescorla F, Cushing B, London W, Schlatter M, et al. Outcome and staging evaluation in malignant germ cell tumors of the ovary in children and adolescents: an intergroup study. J Pediatr Surg. 2004; 39(3):424–9. discussion 424-9
40. Göbel U, Calaminus G, Schneider DT, Koch S, Teske C, Harms D. The malignant potential of teratomas in infancy and childhood: the MAKEI experiences in non-testicular teratoma and implications for a new protocol. Klin Padiatr. 2006;218(6):309–14.

18

Comparison of stage III mucinous and serous ovarian cancer

Zeliha Firat Cuylan[1], Emine Karabuk[2], Murat OZ[1*], Ahmet Taner Turan[3], Mehmet M. Meydanli[1], Salih Taskin[4], Mustafa Erkan Sari[1], Hanifi Sahin[1], Suat C. Ulukent[5], Ozgur Akbayir[6], Kemal Gungorduk[7], Tayfun Gungor[1], Mehmet F. Kose[2] and Ali Ayhan[8]

Abstract

Background: The purpose of this case-control study was to compare the prognoses of women with stage III mucinous ovarian carcinoma (MOC) who received maximal or optimal cytoreduction followed by paclitaxel plus carboplatin chemotherapy to those of women with stage III serous epithelial ovarian cancer (EOC) treated in the similar manner.

Methods: We performed a multicenter, retrospective review to identify patients with stage III MOC at seven gynecologic oncology departments in Turkey. Eighty-one women with MOC were included. Each case was matched to two women with stage III serous EOC in terms of age, tumor grade, substage of disease, and extent of residual disease. Survival estimates were measured using Kaplan-Meier plots. Variables predictive of outcome were analyzed using Cox regression models.

Results: With a median follow-up of 54 months, the median progression-free survival (PFS) for women with stage III MOC was 18.0 months (95% CI; 13.8–22.1, SE: 2.13) compared to 29.0 months (95% CI; 24.04–33.95, SE: 2.52) in the serous group ($p = 0.19$). The 5-year overall survival rate of the MOC group was significantly lower than that of the serous EOC group (44.9% vs. 66.3%, respectively; $p < 0.001$). For the entire cohort, presence of multiple peritoneal implants (Hazard ratio [HR] 2.39; 95% confidence interval [CI], 1.38–4.14, $p = 0.002$) and mucinous histology (HR 2.28; 95% CI, 1.53–3.40, $p < 0.001$) were identified as independent predictors of decreased OS.

Conclusion: Patients with MOC seem to be 2.3 times more likely to die of their tumors when compared to women with serous EOC.

Keywords: Analyses, survival, Epithelial ovarian cancer, Mucinous adenocarcinoma, Serous cystadenocarcinoma

Introduction

Primary mucinous ovarian carcinoma (MOC) represents a biochemically and genetically distinct subgroup of epithelial ovarian cancer (EOC) [1]. MOC accounts for 3% [2] to 10% [3] of all ovarian carcinomas. Most patients with MOC are diagnosed at an early stage and therefore it confers a favorable prognosis [3]. However, once the disease is advanced, mucinous histology has a poorer outcome compared to the other histologic subgroups [4–7].

* Correspondence: ozmurat@gmail.com
[1]Department of Gynecologic Oncology, Zekai Tahir Burak Women's Health Training and Research Hospital, Faculty of Medicine, University of Health Sciences, Ankara, Turkey
Full list of author information is available at the end of the article

Mucinous histology has consistently been reported as an independent adverse prognostic factor in advanced EOC [6, 8, 9] and the outcomes of MOCs are significantly different from EOCs with serous histology [10]. The reason for poor prognosis of advanced MOC has been suggested to be either the aggressive biology of mucinous tumor or chemoresistance or both [9, 11, 12].

Approximately 14% of all MOCs are diagnosed as stage III disease [7]. Response rates to standard platinum-based chemotherapy are low (12.5–38.5%) among women with MOC, and debulking to minimal or no residual disease (RD) remains the standard of care [13]. It has been reported that overall survival (OS) is 3.8 fold increased in patients who have received optimal cytoreductive surgery

(CRS) compared to the patients who have had suboptimal cytoreduction [14].

We wondered whether the worse prognosis associated with mucinous histology is also valid when age, tumor grade, substage of disease, and extent of RD are matched with serous histology in women with stage III EOC who have undergone primary CRS followed by standard intravenous paclitaxel plus carboplatin chemotherapy. Given the low frequency of stage III MOC, a multicenter effort was essential in order to achieve an adequate number in this case-control study. The objective of this retrospective, multicenter study was to compare prognostic factors of women with stage III MOC to those of women with stage III serous EOC treated in the same fashion.

Methods

After Institutional Review Board approval (IRB Approval Number: 05, Date: November 7th 2017), institutional databases for EOC were utilized to identify eligible cases. The databases consisted of individual patients with EOC who underwent upfront surgery between January 1998 and December 2016 at seven gynecologic oncology departments in Turkey. All patients provided an informed consent at admission for storage of their clinical information and for research use of their clinical data.

The case group consisted of EOC patients with histopathologically confirmed Stage III [15] MOC. We included only the patients with optimal or maximal CRS in the upfront surgery. We excluded the patients who had RD greater than 1 cm. Since the case group included only women having pure mucinous histology; women with mixed histologies including mucinous tumors combined with endometrioid, serous, clear-cell, and/or other histologic types were excluded. The patients who received neoadjuvant chemotherapy, women with synchronous malignancies, and those with incomplete medical records were also excluded from the study.

Using a dependent random sampling method, each case was matched to two patients with serous EOC from a series of 783 women who had undergone maximal or optimal CRS (RD $\leq$ 1 cm) followed by paclitaxel and carboplatin combination chemotherapy for the same period. In the case and control groups, pairs were matched in terms of age at diagnosis (+/− 10 years), year of diagnosis, grade of the tumor (grade 1, 2, or 3), substage (stage $IIIA_1$, $IIIA_2$, IIIB, and IIIC), and extent of RD (maximal vs. optimal debulking). While selecting the patients in the control group, we were blinded to the outcomes of the patients in order to prevent possible patient selection bias.

The following clinical data were extracted from patients' medical, surgical, pathology, and chemotherapy reports: demographic characteristics, preoperative serum cancer antigen 125 (CA 125) levels, type and date of surgical procedure, presence of multiple ($\geq$2) peritoneal implants, ascites status, results of peritoneal washings (negative or positive), appendiceal involvement, omental involvement, size of RD after surgery, stage of disease, time to recurrence, length of follow-up and survival. Pathologic characteristics of the disease were abstracted from original pathology reports. Data were collected from departments with an online standardized form.

Gynecologic oncologists performed all of the operations with the aim of achieving complete cytoreduction. After primary CRS, RD was recorded according to the assessment by the surgical team. Retroperitoneal lymph node dissection was performed after completion of intraabdominal cytoreduction. Number of total lymph nodes (LNs) removed, number of para-aortic LNs removed, and number of pelvic LNs removed and number of metastatic LNs were noted.

All pathologic specimens of the upfront surgery were evaluated and interpreted by expert gynecologic pathologists of the participating institutions with experience in gynecological malignancies but were not reviewed centrally in the current study.MOC was diagnosed after examination of permanent sections. Immunuhistochemical study was performed in women where metastatic tumors could not be excluded. With careful exclusion of noninvasive and metastatic mucinous tumors, women who had final pathologic diagnoses as "primary MOCs" were included in the case group.

The World Health Organization (WHO) criteria were used for histologic classification of the tumors [16, 17]. Architectural grading was defined by standard International Federation of Gynecology and Obstetrics (FIGO) criteria. All tumors were staged according to the FIGO staging system, which was revised in 2014 [15]. In patients treated before 2014, stage was adapted to the FIGO 2014 staging system retrospectively using surgical and pathologic assessment.

All patients (cases and controls) received adjuvant chemotherapy. The standard first line chemotherapy protocol included paclitaxel 175 mg/m^2 plus carboplatin at the dose of area under curve (AUC) 5 or 6 every 21 days for 6 cycles. Targeted agents (i.e. bevacizumab) were not included in the first line chemotherapy. Platinum refractory disease was defined as disease progression on first-line platinum based regimen, whereas platinum resistant disease included patients with tumor progression within 6 months of completion of platinum based chemotherapy.

We followed-up the patients quarterly for the first 2 years, biannually until 5 years, and annually thereafter. The follow-up visits included physical and gynecologic examinations, and serum CA 125 measurements. Each patient was assessed for relapse with imaging studies and serum CA 125 measurements. Treatment of the recurrences (surgery and/or chemotherapy) was applied according to the institutional practices at that time.

Survival data were last calculated on 31st December 2016. The survival status of the patients was determined as alive or dead at the time of the last follow-up visit. Survival status for all the subjects was confirmed by social security death index search.

Maximal cytoreduction was defined as no visible RD left in-situ (microscopic RD) after primary CRS. Optimal cytoreduction was defined as a RD less than or equal to 1 cm maximal diameter of the largest tumor deposit at the end of the primary surgery. Similarly, suboptimal cytoreduction was defined as > 1 cm of RD. Lymphadenectomy was defined as the dissection of pelvic and para-aortic LN's at the same time. Progression-free survival (PFS) was defined as the time, in months, from the primary surgery to the documented recurrence with clinical examination and/or radiologic imaging; or death from any cause, whichever occurred first, or the date of last follow-up for patients remaining alive without recurrence. Patients who had no active disease at the last contact were censored in the PFS analysis. Overall survival (OS) was defined as the time, in months, between the date of primary surgery to the date of death or the last follow-up. Surviving patients were censored at their last known follow-up.

Survival curves were generated using Kaplan-Meier plots and survivals were compared using the log-rank test. The chi-squared test was used for nominal variables. For continuous variables, Student's t-test and the Mann-Whitney U tests were used for continuous variables with and without normal distribution, respectively. Cox logistic regression models were used to determine co-variates affecting survival, and presented as hazard ratios (HRs) with 95% confidence interval (CI), unadjusted or adjusted for all factors. All variables with a p value < 0.05 in the univariate analysis were included in the multivariate analysis. All statistical analyses were performed with the SPSS software version 23.0 (IBM Corp., Armonk, NY, USA). A p value < 0.05 was considered statistically significant.

Results

One hundred and sixty-four women were identified with a postoperative pathology-proven diagnosis of stage III primary MOC at seven participating centers during the study period. We excluded 74 women who had suboptimal CRS, six women who received neoadjuvant chemotherapy, one with synchronous breast cancer and two women with incomplete medical records. Therefore, 81 women with stage III MOC were included in the final analysis. These 81cases were compared to 162 controls with serous EOC who had maximal or optimal CRS followed by paclitaxel plus carboplatin combination chemotherapy.

Table 1 demonstrates the demographic and clinicopathologic characteristics of the study population. Age, menopausal status, presence of multiple peritoneal implants, tumor grade, substage of disease, positive peritoneal cytology, extent of RD, appendiceal involvement, and omental involvement were similar between the cases and controls. Patients with serous EOC were more likely to have elevated median baseline serum CA 125 levels (514 IU/ml vs. 126 IU/ml; $p = 0.022$), ascites (125/162 vs. 42/81; $p < 0.001$), and positive retroperitoneal LNs (116/162 vs. 21/81; $p < 0.001$). The median number of total LNs harvested, the median number of pelvic LNs removed were significantly higher in the serous EOC patients when compared to women with MOC as well as the median number of para-aortic LNs removed (49 vs. 34; $p < 0.001$, 32 vs. 24; $p = 0.003$, and 15 vs. 11; $p <$ 0.001, respectively). In both of the groups, stage $IIIA_1$, $IIIA_2$, IIIB and IIIC disease were noted in 16.1%, 7.4%, 16.0% and 60.5%, respectively.

With a median follow-up of 54 months (range, 5–216 months), the median PFS for women with stage III MOC was 18.0 months (95% CI; 13.8–22.1, SE: 2.13) compared to 29.0 months (95% CI; 24.04–33.95, SE: 2.52) in the serous EOC group ($p = 0.19$) (Fig. 1). The 5-year OS rate of the MOC group was significantly lower than that of the serous EOC group (44.9% vs. 66.3%, respectively; $p < 0.001$) (Fig. 2).

Platinum refractory disease was detected more frequently in the mucinous group ($n = 18$, 22.2%) than in the serous group ($n = 9$, 5.5%) ($p < 0.001$). However, the number of women with platinum resistant disease was comparable between the mucinous and serous groups ($n = 12$ [14.8%] and $n = 21$ [12.9%], respectively, $p = 0.69$).

For the entire cohort, univariate analysis revealed substage of disease (stage $IIIA_1$ vs. other stages) ($p < 0.001$), positive peritoneal cytology ($p = 0.01$), appendiceal involvement ($p < 0.001$), omental involvement ($p < 0.001$), and presence of multiple peritoneal implants ($p < 0.001$) as significant factors for decreased PFS. In multivariate analysis, presence of multiple peritoneal implants (HR 2.1, 95% CI 1.40–3.14; $p < 0.001$) remained as the sole independent risk factor for decreased PFS.

For the entire cohort, univariate analysis revealed substage of disease (stage $IIIA_1$ vs. other stages) ($p = 0.001$), appendiceal involvement ($p < 0.001$), omental involvement ($p < 0.001$), presence of multiple peritoneal implants ($p <$ 0.001), and mucinous histology ($p < 0.001$) as significant factors for decreased OS (Table 2). Multivariate analysis demonstrated presence of multiple peritoneal implants (HR 2.39; 95% CI, 1.38–4.14, $p = 0.002$) and mucinous histology (HR 2.28; 95% CI, 1.53–3.40, $p < 0.001$) as independent predictors of decreased OS (Table 2).

Finally, 81 patients with stage III MOC were separately analyzed. Univariate analysis revealed substage of disease

Table 1 Demographic and clinicopathologic characteristics of the study population ($n = 243$)

Characteristics	MOC Values, n (%)	Serous EOC Values, n (%)	p
Age, y (median, range)	53.9 (18–77)	53.4 (28–81)	0.73
Menopausal status			
Postmenopausal	49 (60.5%)	98 (60.5%)	1.0
Premenopausal	32 (39.5%)	64 (39.5%)	1.0
CA 125 (IU/ml) (median, range)	126 (4–4891)	514 (8–27,580)	0.022
Grade			
1	29 (35.8%)	58 (35.8%)	1.0
2–3	52 (64.2%)	104 (64.2%)	1.0
Stage			
IIIA1	13 (16.1%)	26 (16.1%)	1.0
IIIA2	6 (7.4%)	12 (7.4%)	1.0
IIIB	13 (16%)	26 (16%)	1.0
IIIC	49 (60.5%)	98 (60.5%)	1.0
Debulking			
Optimal	54 (66.7%)	108 (66.7%)	1.0
Maximal	27 (33.3%)	54 (33.3%)	1.0
Ascites			
Present	42 (51.9%)	125 (77.2%)	< 0.001
Absent	39 (48.1%)	37 (22.8%)	
Peritoneal Cytology			
Positive	61 (75.3%)	137 (84.6%)	0.114
Negative	20 (24.7%)	25 (15.4%)	
Number of LNs removed (median, range)	34 (19–96)	49 (21–203)	< 0.001
Pelvic LNs	24 (10–75)	32 (10–101)	0.003
Para-aortic LNs	11 (5–54)	15 (5–102)	< 0.001
Retroperitoneal LN metastases			
Present	21 (25.9%)	91 (56.2%)	< 0.001
Absent	60 (74.1%)	71 (43.8%)	
Appendiceal Involvement			
Present	29 (35.8%)	59 (36.4%)	1.0
Absent	52 (64.2%)	103 (63.6%)	
Omental Involvement			
Present	61 (75.3%)	113 (69.8%)	0.451
Absent	20 (24.7%)	49 (30.2%)	
Peritoneal Involvement			
Present	57 (70.4%)	103 (63.6%)	0.318
Absent	24 (29.6%)	59 (36.4%)	
Status			
Alive	32 (39.5%)	112 (69.1%)	
Dead	49 (60.5%)	50 (30.9%)	
Follow-up, months (median, range)	21 (1–216)	46 (1–121)	

Abbreviations: *n* Number, *LN* Lymph node, *y* year, *MOC* Mucinous Ovarian Carcinoma, *EOC* Epithelial Ovarian Carcinoma, *SD* Standard Deviation

(stage $IIIA_1$ vs. other stages) ($p < 0.001$), omental involvement ($p = 0.004$), and optimal debulking ($p < 0.001$) as significant factors for decreased PFS. In the multivariate Cox regression model, only maximal CRS (HR 0.48; 95% CI, 0.23–0.97, $p = 0.041$) was identified as an independent predictor of increased PFS. For women with stage III MOC, univariate analysis revealed substage of disease (stage $IIIA_1$ vs. other stages) ($p = 0.002$), omental involvement ($p = 0.008$), and optimal debulking ($p < 0.001$) as significant factors for decreased OS (Table 3). In multivariate analysis, only maximal CRS (HR 0.37; 95% CI, 0.16–0.86, $p = 0.021$) remained as an independent predictor of increased OS (Table 3). At the time of reporting, of 81 women with stage III MOC, 49 (60.5%) were dead whereas 32 (39.5%) were alive. The corresponding figures were found to be 50 (30.9%) and 112 (69.1%), respectively in the serous EOC group.

Discussion

Our results indicate that presence of multiple peritoneal implants and mucinous histology seem to be the independent predictors of decreased OS in a cohort of 243 women who have undergone maximal or optimal CRS and found to have either mucinous or serous stage III EOC at the end of final pathology report. Patients with MOC were 2.3 times more likely to die of their tumors when compared to women with serous EOC.

The retrospective nature of the study and lack of central pathology review seem to be the major limitations of the current study. Patients were treated and observed at seven different gynecologic cancer centers. Therefore, we might not have presented the clinical outcomes of the recurrent patients objectively and equally since the treatment of recurrences was not uniform, and changed according to the institutional practices at that time.

It has been reported that the clinical behavior of MOC is distinctly different from serous EOC and the prognosis of MOC is worse when compared to other histologies [6–9, 14, 18–21]. Hess et al. [18] have reported that MOC has a HR of 2.94 for progression and a HR of 3.08 for death in a study of 27 women with stage III/IV MOC. Winter et al. [19] reported that mucinous histology was associated with a worse PFS and OS compared with serous carcinomas in a study including 34 women with stage III MOC. In that study, the median PFS was 10.5 months whereas the median OS was 14.8 months for women with MOC.

In a meta-analysis consisting of 264 women with stage III/IV MOC, Mackay et al. [20] reported that patients with MOC had an increased risk of death (HR 2.66, 95% CI 2.29–3.08) and disease-progression (HR 2.10, 95% CI 1.84–2.41) compared to those with serous carcinoma. Patients with mucinous histology had an estimated median PFS of 7.6 months and a median OS of 14.6 months in that

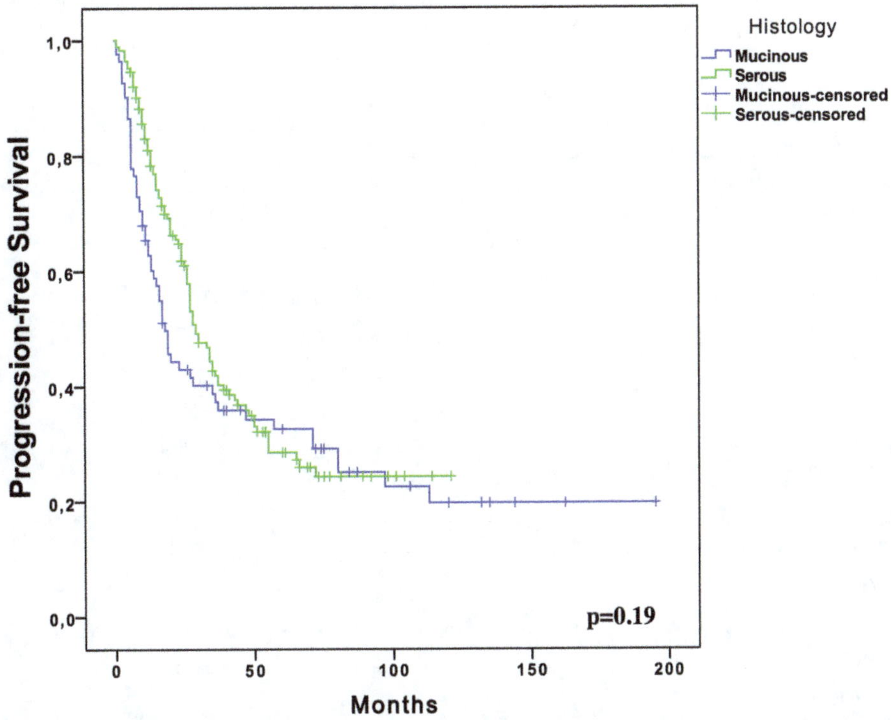

Fig. 1 Kaplan Meier Plots for progression free survival of the women with Stage III mucinous ($n = 81$) and serous ($n = 162$) ovarian cancer

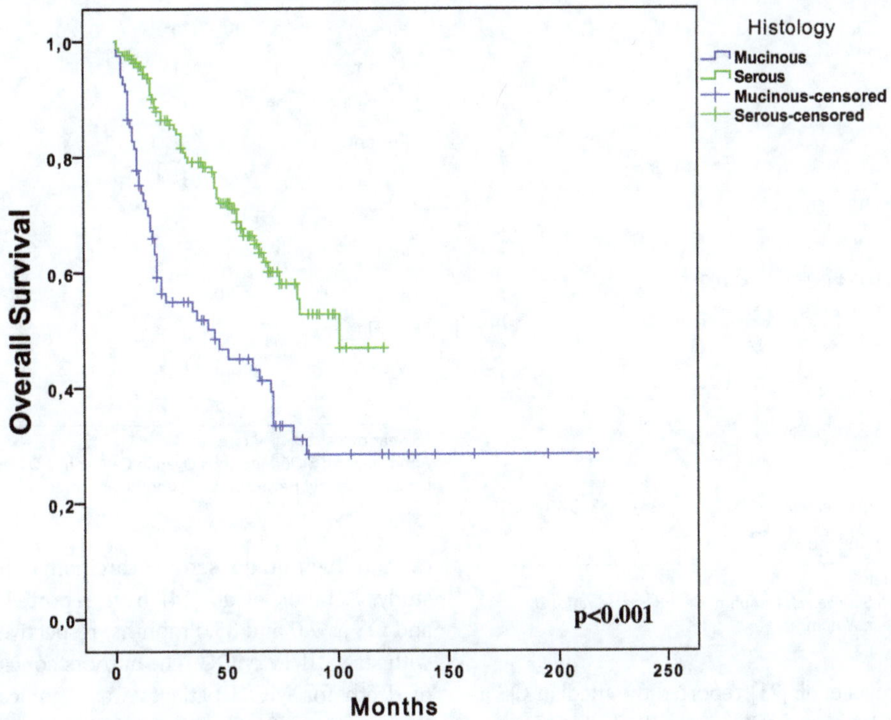

Fig. 2 Kaplan Meier Plots for overall survival of the women with Stage III mucinous ($n = 81$) and serous ($n = 162$) ovarian cancer

Table 2 Univariate and multivariate analyses for overall survival in the entire cohort (stage III mucinous [$n = 81$] and serous [$n = 162$] ovarian carcinoma)

	Univariate analysis OS[a] N of events (%)	p	Multivariateanalysis HR	CI 95%	p
Age, y					
< 52	36/118 (61.7%)	0.163			
≥ 52	47/125 (56.7%)				
Menopausal Status					
Premenopausal	33/96 (56.6%)	0.89			
Postmenopausal	50/147 (60.5%)				
Ca-125(IU/ml)					
< 310	46/121 (56.2%)	0.089			
≥ 310	37/122 (62.2%)				
Grade					
1	33/87 (55.1%)	0.74			
2–3	50/156 (61.5%)				
Ascites					
Present	62/167 (56.2%)	0.371			
Absent	21/76 (66%)				
Retroperitoneal LN metastases					
Present	44/112 (39.2%)	0.646			
Absent	55/131 (41.9%)				
Peritoneal cytology					
Positive	73/198 (56.5%)	0.215			
Negative	10/45 (71.8%)				
Stage					
IIIA1	6/39 (78.4%)	0.001			
IIIA2, IIIB, IIIC	77/204 (55.6%)				
Appendiceal Involvement					
Present	41/88 (45%)	< 0.001			
Absent	42/155 (66.9%)				
Omental Involvement					
Present	71/174 (52%)	< 0.001			
Absent	12/69 (77.6%)				
Peritoneal Involvement					
Present	67/160 (49.2%)	< 0.001	2.39	1.38–4.14	0.002
Absent	16/83 (76.9%)				
Histologic Subtype					
Mucinous	41/81 (44.9%)	< 0.001	2.28	1.53–3.40	< 0.001
Serous	42/162 (66.3%)				

[a]:5-year overall survival rate
Abbreviations: *OS* Overall Survival, *LN* Lymph node, *HR* Hazard ratio, *CI* Confidence interval, *y* Year, *N* number

Table 3 Univariate and multivariate analyses for overall survival in women with stage III mucinous ovarian carcinoma ($n = 81$)

	Univariate analysis OS[a] N of events (%)	p	Multivariate analysis HR	CI 95%	p
Age, y					
< 54	17/39 (52.2%)	0.126			
≥ 54	24/42 (38.1%)				
Menopausal Status					
Premenopausal	15/32 (49%)	0.49			
Postmenopausal	26/49 (42%)				
Ca-125(IU/ml)					
< 126	19/40 (49.2%)	0.42			
≥ 126	22/41 (40.4%)				
Grade					
1	16/29 (36%)	0.98			
2–3	25/52 (48%)				
Ascites					
Present	24/42 (37.4%)	0.174			
Absent	17/39 (52.4%)				
LN metastases					
Present	13/21 (27.9%)	0.433			
Absent	28/60 (50.4%)				
Peritoneal cytology					
Positive	35/61 (36.8%)	0.092			
Negative	6/20 (67.7%)				
Appendiceal Involvement					
Present	18/29 (30.9%)	0.180			
Absent	23/52 (51.9%)				
Omental Involvement					
Present	35/61 (37%)	0.008			
Absent	6/20 (68.4%)				
Stage					
IIIA1	2/13 (83.9%)	0.002			
IIIA2, IIIB, IIIC	39/68 (37%)				
Debulking					
Maximal	6/27 (74.3%)	< 0.001	0.37	0.16–0.86	0.021
Optimal	35/54 (30.1%)				

[a]:5-year overall survival rate
Abbreviations: *MOC* Mucinous Ovarian Carcinoma, *OS* Overall Survival, *LN* Lymph node, *HR* Hazard ratio, *CI* Confidence interval, *y* Years

meta-analysis. Bamias et al. [21] reported the median OS as 15.0 months for 21 women with stage III/IV MOC compared to 45.0 months for 389 women with stage III/IV ovarian high-grade serous carcinoma. In a case-control study, Karabuk et al. [14] have reported the median PFS and OS as 7.0 and 35.0 months, respectively, for 50 women with stage III/IV MOC. The authors concluded that the risk of death for MOC patients was significantly higher than that of serous EOC patients (HR 2.14, 95% CI 1.34–3.42). In the current study, we have found out the median PFS and OS as 18.0 and 45.0 months, respectively, for women with stage III MOC who have undergone maximal or optimal CRS. The corresponding figures were 29.0 and 101.0 months, respectively, for the serous counterpart. There was no significant difference between the cases and the controls in terms of PFS. However, women with MOC were 2.3 times more likely to die of their tumors when compared to patients with serous EOC in the current study. Table 4 compares the findings of the current study with those of previous studies.

Using the Surveillance, Epidemiology and End Results (SEER) database, Schiavone et al. [7] reported that the HR for OS was 1.60 for women with stage III MOC. The 5-year survival rate for women with stage III serous EOC was 33.6% compared with 25.7% for MOC. The corresponding rates were 66.3%, and 44.9%, respectively, in our study. It should be emphasized that the SEER database lacks several important variables such as extent and outcome of initial surgery including the size of RD, type of adjuvant chemotherapy, and recurrence. However, all patients (cases and controls) in the current study underwent maximal or optimal CRS followed by paclitaxel/carboplatin chemotherapy and cases were matched to controls in terms of age, tumor grade, substage of disease, and extent of RD.

Favorable prognostic factors such as younger patient age, lower tumor grade, and less peritoneal carcinomatosis have been reported for women with MOC [9, 22]. However, maximal cytoreduction was identified as the sole independent prognostic factor for increased PFS and OS in the current study. The volume of tumor left after primary CRS depends on the number and the size of the tumor elements [5]. We were not able to define the number of lesions left after initial surgery in this retrospective analysis. The maximal diameter of the largest residual tumor nodule is a very crude estimate of RD [5, 23], but it still gave valuable prognostic information in our study.

Melamed et al. [13] have recently reported that cytoreduction to no gross RD is associated with a hazard reduction of 54% compared to any gross RD in MOCs.. The optimal chemotherapy regimen for MOC has not been clarified yet; so aggressive CRS seems to be the only effective treatment to improve the prognosis in advanced-stage MOC [12]. Our finding associated with maximal cytoreduction as the sole independent prognostic factor for both PFS and OS in women with stage III MOC is in agreement with previous reports [12, 13].

The most important limitation of the current study is the fact that central pathology review was not performed. There is now increasing recognition that many MOCs may in fact be metastatic mucinous neoplasms from other primary sites [7]. Differentiating MOC from gastrointestinal cancer [24, 25], mainly carcinomas of appendix, and colorectal cancer by morphology alone can be difficult. It should be reminded that no patients receiving neoadjuvant chemotherapy were included in the current study and all patients have undergone surgical exploration which commonly would have identified a cancer of gastrointestinal origin. Additionally, immunohistohemical studies were performed in cases where metastatic tumors could not be excluded. Recent data suggests that the application of updated criteria results in reliable histopathological diagnoses based on the cell type [26]. Nevertheless, our study was restricted by the lack of a central pathology review as many previous reports [7, 13, 20, 27].

The major strength of the current study is the inclusion of a relatively large number of patients with stage III MOC. Our study has the advantage that all included patients were treated with the standard paclitaxel/carboplatin regimen. The standard surgery and the standard postoperative adjuvant chemotherapy regimen seem to improve the reliability of our findings and decrease the probable effects of the confounders.

Table 4 Comparison of the findings of the current study with those of previous studies associated with advanced mucinous ovarian carcinoma

Author	Number of women with MOC	Stage of disease	Extent of residual disease	Median PFS (months)	Media OS (months)
Hess, 2004 [18]	27	III, IV	optimal or suboptimal	5.7	12.0
Pectasides, 2005 [27]	47	III, IV	optimal or suboptimal	11.8	33.2
Winter, 2007 [19]	34	III	optimal or suboptimal	10.5	14.8
Bamias, 2010 [8]	24	III, IV	optimal or suboptimal	NR	15.4
Mackay, 2010 [20]	264	III, IV	optimal or suboptimal	7.6	14.6
Bamias, 2012 [21]	21	III, IV	optimal or suboptimal	NR	15.0
Karabuk, 2013 [14]	50	III, IV	optimal or suboptimal	7.0	35.0
Current study	81	III	maximal or optimal	18.0	45.0

Abbreviations: *MOC* mucinous ovarian carcinoma, *PFS* progression-free survival, *OS* overall survival, *NR* not reported

We conclude that women with stage III MOC seem to be 2.3 times more likely to die of their tumors when compared to patients with serous EOC. Maximal cytoreduction seems to be the sole independent prognostic factor for increased OS in women with stage III MOC. As the extent of RD is a modifiable prognostic factor, it seems reasonable to perform maximal CRS whenever possible in order to improve the outcomes of those women.

Acknowledgments
Authors declare that there is neither financial nor academic support or relationships that may pose potential conflict of interest. No funding was required for the study and the preparation of the text. No assistance by individuals other than the authors was required for writing or other purposes.

Funding
There has been no funding for conducting the study and writing the manuscript.

Authors' contributions
ZFC: Conceptualization, Data curation, Investigation, Methodology, Software, Validation, writing – original draft, writing – review & editing. EK: Conceptualization, Data curation, Investigation, Validation: Writing – original draft. MO: Data curation, Formal analysis, Investigation, Methodology, Software, writing – original draft: Writing – review & editing. ATT: Conceptualization, Formal analysis, Methodology, Supervision, Validation. Writing – review & editing. MMM: Conceptualization, Data curation, Formal analysis, Investigation, Methodology, Software, Supervision, Validation, writing – original draft, writing – review & editing. ST: Conceptualization, Formal analysis, Methodology, Software, Supervision, Validation, writing – review & editing. MES: Conceptualization, Methodology, Supervision, Validation, Visualization, writing – review & editing. HS: Data curation, Formal analysis, Investigation, Software. SCU: Data curation, Formal analysis, Methodology, Supervision, Visualization. OA: Data curation, Formal analysis, Methodology, Supervision, Visualization. KG: Data curation, Formal analysis, Investigation, Validation. TG: Conceptualization, Investigation, Methodology, Supervision, Validation, writing – review & editing. MFK: Conceptualization, Investigation, Methodology, Supervision, Validation, writing – review & editing. AA: Conceptualization, Formal analysis, Methodology, Supervision, Visualization, writing – review & editing. All authors read and approved the final manuscript.

Competing interests
The authors declare that they have no competing interests.

Author details
[1]Department of Gynecologic Oncology, Zekai Tahir Burak Women's Health Training and Research Hospital, Faculty of Medicine, University of Health Sciences, Ankara, Turkey. [2]Faculty of Health Sciences, Department of Obstetrics and Gynecology, Acibadem University, Istanbul, Turkey. [3]Department of Gynecologic Oncology, Etlik Zubeyde Hanim Women's Health Training and Research Hospital, Faculty of Medicine, University of Health Sciences, Ankara, Turkey. [4]Division of Gynecologic Oncology, Department of Obstetrics and Gynecology, School of Medicine, AnkaraUniversity, Ankara, Turkey. [5]Department of General Surgery, Kanuni Sultan Suleyman Teaching and Research Hospital, Faculty of Medicine, University of Health Sciences, Istanbul, Turkey. [6]Department of Gynecologic Oncology, Kanuni Sultan Suleyman Teaching and Research Hospital, Faculty of Medicine, University of Health Sciences, Istanbul, Turkey. [7]Department of Gynecologic Oncology, Tepecik Education and Research Hospital, Faculty of Medicine, University of Health Sciences, Izmir, Turkey. [8]Division of Gynecologic Oncology, Department of Obstetrics and Gynecology, Faculty of Medicine, BaskentUniversity, Ankara, Turkey.

References

1. Earp MA, Kelemen LE, Magliocco AM, Swenerton KD, Chenevix-Trench G, Australian Cancer S, Australian Ovarian Cancer Study G, Lu Y, Hein A, Ekici AB, Beckmann MW, Fasching PA, Lambrechts D, Despierre E, Vergote I, Lambrechts S, Doherty JA, Rossing MA, Chang-Claude J, Rudolph A, Friel G, Moysich KB, Odunsi K, Sucheston-Campbell L, Lurie G, Goodman MT, Carney ME, Thompson PJ, Runnebaum IB, Durst M, Hillemanns P, Dork T, Antonenkova N, Bogdanova N, Leminen A, Nevanlinna H, Pelttari LM, Butzow R, Bunker CH, Modugno F, Edwards RP, Ness RB, du Bois A, Heitz F, Schwaab I, Harter P, Karlan BY, Walsh C, Lester J, Jensen A, Kjaer SK, Hogdall CK, Hogdall E, Lundvall L, Sellers TA, Fridley BL, Goode EL, Cunningham JM, Vierkant RA, Giles GG, Baglietto L, Severi G, Southey MC, Liang D, Wu X, Lu K, Hildebrandt MA, Levine DA, Bisogna M, Schildkraut JM, Iversen ES, Weber RP, Berchuck A, Cramer DW, Terry KL, Poole EM, Tworoger SS, Bandera EV, Chandran U, Orlow I, Olson SH, Wik E, Salvesen HB, Bjorge L, Halle MK, van Altena AM, Aben KK, Kiemeney LA, Massuger LF, Pejovic T, Bean YT, Cybulski C, Gronwald J, Lubinski J, Wentzensen N, Brinton LA, Lissowska J, Garcia-Closas M, Dicks E, Dennis J, Easton DF, Song H, Tyrer JP, Pharoah PD, Eccles D, Campbell IG, Whittemore AS, McGuire V, Sieh W, Rothstein JH, Flanagan JM, Paul J, Brown R, Phelan CM, Risch HA, McLaughlin JR, Narod SA, Ziogas A, Anton-Culver H, Gentry-Maharaj A, Menon U, Gayther SA, Ramus SJ, Wu AH, Pearce CL, Pike MC, Dansonka-Mieszkowska A, Rzepecka IK, Szafron LM, Kupryjanczyk J, Cook LS, Le ND, Brooks-Wilson A, Ovarian Cancer Association C (2014) Genome-wide association study of subtype-specific epithelial ovarian cancer risk alleles using pooled DNA. Hum Genet 133 (5): 481–497. doi:https://doi.org/10.1007/s00439-013-1383-3.
2. Prat J. Ovarian carcinomas: five distinct diseases with different origins, genetic alterations, and clinicopathological features. Virchows Arch. 2012;460(3):237–49. https://doi.org/10.1007/s00428-012-1203-5.
3. McGuire V, Jesser CA, Whittemore AS. Survival among U.S. women with invasive epithelial ovarian cancer. Gynecol Oncol. 2002;84(3):399–403. https://doi.org/10.1006/gyno.2001.6536.
4. Omura GA, Brady MF, Homesley HD, Yordan E, Major FJ, Buchsbaum HJ, Park RC. Long-term follow-up and prognostic factor analysis in advanced ovarian carcinoma: the gynecologic oncology group experience. J Clin Oncol. 1991;9(7):1138–50. https://doi.org/10.1200/JCO.1991.9.7.1138.
5. Makar AP, Baekelandt M, Trope CG, Kristensen GB. The prognostic significance of residual disease, FIGO substage, tumor histology, and grade in patients with FIGO stage III ovarian cancer. Gynecol Oncol. 1995;56(2): 175–80.
6. Zaino RJ, Brady MF, Lele SM, Michael H, Greer B, Bookman MA. Advanced stage mucinous adenocarcinoma of the ovary is both rare and highly lethal: a gynecologic oncology group study. Cancer. 2011;117(3):554–62. https://doi.org/10.1002/cncr.25460.
7. Schiavone MB, Herzog TJ, Lewin SN, Deutsch I, Sun X, Burke WM, Wright JD. Natural history and outcome of mucinous carcinoma of the ovary. Am J Obstet Gynecol. 2011;205(5):480 e481–8. https://doi.org/10.1016/j.ajog.2011.06.049.
8. Bamias A, Psaltopoulou T, Sotiropoulou M, Haidopoulos D, Lianos E, Bournakis E, Papadimitriou C, Rodolakis A, Vlahos G, Dimopoulos MA. Mucinous but not clear cell histology is associated with inferior survival in patients with advanced stage ovarian carcinoma treated with platinum-paclitaxel chemotherapy. Cancer. 2010;116(6):1462–8. https://doi.org/10.1002/cncr.24915.
9. Alexandre J, Ray-Coquard I, Selle F, Floquet A, Cottu P, Weber B, Falandry C, Lebrun D, Pujade-Lauraine E, Gineco (2010) Mucinous advanced epithelial

ovarian carcinoma: clinical presentation and sensitivity to platinum-paclitaxel-based chemotherapy, the GINECO experience. Ann Oncol 21 (12): 2377–2381. doi:https://doi.org/10.1093/annonc/mdq257.

10. Massad LS, Gao F, Hagemann I, Powell M. Clinical outcomes among women with mucinous adenocarcinoma of the ovary. Gynecol Obstet Investig. 2016; 81(5):411–5. https://doi.org/10.1159/000441791.
11. Nakayama K, Takebayashi Y, Nakayama S, Hata K, Fujiwaki R, Fukumoto M, Miyazaki K. Prognostic value of overexpression of p53 in human ovarian carcinoma patients receiving cisplatin. Cancer Lett. 2003;192(2):227–35.
12. Shimada M, Kigawa J, Ohishi Y, Yasuda M, Suzuki M, Hiura M, Nishimura R, Tabata T, Sugiyama T, Kaku T. Clinicopathological characteristics of mucinous adenocarcinoma of the ovary. Gynecol Oncol. 2009;113(3):331–4. https://doi.org/10.1016/j.ygyno.2009.02.010.
13. Melamed A, Manning-Geist B, Bregar AJ, Diver EJ, Goodman A, Del Carmen MG, Schorge JO, Rauh-Hain JA. Associations between residual disease and survival in epithelial ovarian cancer by histologic type. Gynecol Oncol. 2017; 147(2):250–6. https://doi.org/10.1016/j.ygyno.2017.08.003.
14. Karabuk E, Kose MF, Hizli D, Taskin S, Karadag B, Turan T, Boran N, Ozfuttu A, Ortac UF. Comparison of advanced stage mucinous epithelial ovarian cancer and serous epithelial ovarian cancer with regard to chemosensitivity and survival outcome: a matched case-control study. J Gynecol Oncol. 2013;24(2):160–6. https://doi.org/10.3802/jgo.2013.24.2.160.
15. Prat J, Oncology FCG. Staging classification for cancer of the ovary, fallopian tube, and peritoneum. Int J Gynaecol Obstet. 2014;124(1):1–5. https://doi.org/10.1016/j.ijgo.2013.10.001.
16. Kurman RJ, Carcangiu, M.L., Herrington, C.S., Young, R.H. (2014) WHO classification of Tumours of female reproductive organs. Fourth edition. Lyon. IARC chapter 1: tumors of the ovary.
17. FAaD T, Devilee P. World health organization Classfication of tumors. Pathology & Genetics of Tumours of the breast and female genital organs. Lyon: IARC (International Agency for Research on Cancer) press; 2003. p. 153–8.
18. Hess V, A'Hern R, Nasiri N, King DM, Blake PR, Barton DP, Shepherd JH, Ind T, Bridges J, Harrington K, Kaye SB, Gore ME. Mucinous epithelial ovarian cancer: a separate entity requiring specific treatment. J Clin Oncol. 2004; 22(6):1040–4. https://doi.org/10.1200/JCO.2004.08.078.
19. Winter WE 3rd, Maxwell GL, Tian C, Carlson JW, Ozols RF, Rose PG, Markman M, Armstrong DK, Muggia F, WP MG, Gynecologic Oncology Group S. Prognostic factors for stage III epithelial ovarian cancer: a gynecologic oncology group study. J Clin Oncol. 2007;25(24):3621–7. https://doi.org/10.1200/JCO.2006.10.2517.
20. Mackay HJ, Brady MF, Oza AM, Reuss A, Pujade-Lauraine E, Swart AM, Siddiqui N, Colombo N, Bookman MA, Pfisterer J, du Bois A, Gynecologic Cancer I. Prognostic relevance of uncommon ovarian histology in women with stage III/IV epithelial ovarian cancer. Int J Gynecol Cancer. 2010;20(6): 945–52. https://doi.org/10.1111/IGC.0b013e3181dd0110.
21. Bamias A, Sotiropoulou M, Zagouri F, Trachana P, Sakellariou K, Kostouros E, Kakoyianni K, Rodolakis A, Vlahos G, Haidopoulos D, Thomakos N, Antsaklis A, Dimopoulos MA. Prognostic evaluation of tumour type and other histopathological characteristics in advanced epithelial ovarian cancer, treated with surgery and paclitaxel/carboplatin chemotherapy: cell type is the most useful prognostic factor. Eur J Cancer. 2012;48(10):1476–83. https://doi.org/10.1016/j.ejca.2011.09.023.
22. Pignata S, Ferrandina G, Scarfone G, Scollo P, Odicino F, Cormio G, Katsaros D, Villa A, Mereu L, Ghezzi F, Manzione L, Lauria R, Breda E, Alletti DG, Ballardini M, Lombardi AV, Sorio R, Mangili G, Priolo D, Magni G, Morabito A. Activity of chemotherapy in mucinous ovarian cancer with a recurrence free interval of more than 6 months: results from the SOCRATES retrospective study. BMC Cancer. 2008;8:252. https://doi.org/10.1186/1471-2407-8-252.
23. Hoskins WJ, McGuire WP, Brady MF, Homesley HD, Creasman WT, Berman M, Ball H, Berek JS. The effect of diameter of largest residual disease on survival after primary cytoreductive surgery in patients with suboptimal residual epithelial ovarian carcinoma. Am J Obstet Gynecol. 1994;170(4):974–9 discussion 979-980.
24. McBroom JW, Parker MF, Krivak TC, Rose GS, Crothers B. Primary appendiceal malignancy mimicking advanced stage ovarian carcinoma: a case series. Gynecol Oncol. 2000;78(3 Pt 1):388–90. https://doi.org/10.1006/gyno.2000.5913.
25. Sehouli J, Kopetsch OJ, Ricke J, Buchmann E, Stengel D, Riess H, Weidemann H, Schaper F, Freiesleben W, Lichtenegger W. Primary mucinous adenocarcinoma of the appendix: a rare entity in the differential diagnosis of ovarian cancer. J Obstet Gynaecol Res. 2000;26(5):333–9.
26. Gilks CB, Ionescu DN, Kalloger SE, Kobel M, Irving J, Clarke B, Santos J, Le N, Moravan V, Swenerton K, Cheryl Brown Ovarian Cancer Outcomes Unit of the British Columbia Cancer A. Tumor cell type can be reproducibly diagnosed and is of independent prognostic significance in patients with maximally debulked ovarian carcinoma. Hum Pathol. 2008;39(8):1239–51. https://doi.org/10.1016/j.humpath.2008.01.003.
27. Pectasides D, Fountzilas G, Aravantinos G, Kalofonos HP, Efstathiou E, Salamalekis E, Farmakis D, Skarlos D, Briasoulis E, Economopoulos T, Dimopoulos MA. Advanced stage mucinous epithelial ovarian cancer: the Hellenic cooperative oncology group experience. Gynecol Oncol. 2005;97(2): 436–41. https://doi.org/10.1016/j.ygyno.2004.12.056.

19

Assessment of Prostaglandin-Endoperoxide Synthase 2 and Versican gene expression profile from the cumulus cells: association with better in vitro fertilization outcomes

Azucena Ocampo[1,3], Jeimy Pedraza[1], Ginna Ortiz[1], Elizabeth Hernández-Pérez[3], Leonardo Porchia[2] and Esther López-Bayghen[1,2*]

Abstract

Background: Current methods for determining superior embryo quality (morphological assessment) are unable to compensate for poor pregnancy outcomes. Due to the importance of the cumulus-oocyte complex and the value of cumulus cells (CCs) as markers of embryo health, we determined the association between the CCs gene expression of the Prostaglandin-Endoperoxide Synthase 2 (PTGS2) and Versican (VCAN) with pregnancy.

Methods: One hundred forty-nine women, suffering from infertility and undergoing IVF, were included in this study (age: 29–46 years; BMI = 25.5 ± 5.0 kg/m^2). Patients underwent a standard IVF protocol. CCs were isolated during oocyte retrieval, and their RNA was isolated using Trizol. The mRNA expression of PTGS2, VCAN, and L19 was measured by qPCR. The PVL index, (PTGS2 + VCAN)*L19$_{normalized}$, was determined for each oocyte. Clinical pregnancy was confirmed by β-hCG and the presence of a fetal heartbeat. Associations were determined by ROC curves or logistic regression.

Results: There was no correlation between the PVL index and morphological scores. Using only single embryo transfers (SETs), we determined that the PVL index was associated with pregnancy (β-hCG: AUC = 0.87, 95%CI: 0.74–1.00) with an optimal cutoff value of 58.2. Using the complete cohort (consisting of SETs, and patients with 2, 3, or 4 embryos transferred), the presence of at least one embryo with a PVL index score ≥ 58.2 was associated with a greater probability of achieving pregnancy (β-hCG: odds ratio = 17.15, 95%CI: 6.82–43.18, $p < 0.001$).

Conclusion: Transferring at least one embryo with a PVL index score ≥ 58.2, generates a higher chance of achieving pregnancy.

Keywords: Prostaglandin-endoperoxide synthase 2, Versican, IVF, Mexico, Cumulus cells

Background

Selection of embryos with a higher implantation potential is a significant challenge in Assisted Reproductive Technology. Currently, embryo selection is based mainly on morphological criteria such as growth rate, early cleavage on Day 2, the degree of fragmentation, and blastocyst formation, to name a few [1]; however, the predictive power of this approach remains limited. With the emergence of "Omics" technologies, new biomarkers can be diagnostic tools and utilized with in vitro fertilization (IVF) to improve oocyte and embryo selection [2].

A key factor in oocyte maturation is the cumulus-oocyte complex (COC), typically found in higher mammals. This complex results from the association between an oocyte and surrounding cumulus cells (CCs) through gap junctions [3]. Moreover, the development of competent oocytes highly depends on the bi-directional communication and interactions between the oocyte and CCs [4]. Several studies have investigated the association between CCs'

* Correspondence: ebayghen@cinvestav.mx
[1]Laboratorio de Investigación y Diagnóstico Molecular, Instituto de Infertilidad y Genética, Ingenes México, Av. IPN 2508, 07360 CDMX, México
[2]Departamento de Toxicología, Centro de Investigación y de Estudios Avanzados del Instituto Politécnico Nacional, Av. IPN 2508, 07360 CDMX, México
Full list of author information is available at the end of the article

gene expression profiles with oocyte competence, embryo quality, and pregnancy outcomes using microarray, reverse transcriptase, and quantitative Real-Time PCR [5–10]. An indirect approach, using CCs RNA transcriptional data, was able to predict embryo quality and pregnancy outcome using gene expression signatures [11]. This raises the question of how can these technologies be used in determining embryo implantation potential. Measuring the expression levels of candidate biomarkers from the CCs can serve as a high-throughput, non-invasive approach to determine oocyte quality and successful pregnancy outcomes [8, 11]. However, there remains a need to determine the optimal usage and practical application of a particular set of genes to monitor and the evaluation of patient factors, such as age, etiology, insulin resistance, etc., that can affect these genes.

Previous studies have shown that Prostaglandin-Endoperoxide Synthase 2 (PTGS2) expression is associated with biological events, such as lesions, inflammation, and proliferation. A recent study demonstrated that up-regulation of PTGS2 in CCs of mice is associated with germinal vesicle to metaphase II (MII) stage transitions and oocyte competency [12]. In treated pigs, increased expression of PTGS2 resulted in improved oocyte competency [13]. In humans, PTGS2 expression in CCs is associated with the development of higher quality embryos [14]. Furthermore, PTGS2 expression levels are associated with good embryo morphology [15]. Many reports have convincingly established PTGS2 in oocyte maturation, nuclear maturation, and cumulus expansion, all predictors of clinical pregnancy [7, 16, 17]. However, even with the numerous studies showing PTGS2 importance, there are no studies to assess the predictability and practical use of PTGS2 levels of the CCs to estimate high-quality embryos that may achieve pregnancy.

Versican (VCAN) is a major component of the COC, located in the extracellular matrix, and its CCs gene expression has been reported as one of the most promising oocyte quality marker [6, 10, 18]. In mice, VCAN augmented a crucial step in embryonic development, cumulus expansion, and promoted the expression of PTGS [19]. In pigs, FSH stimulation increased the expression of VCAN in the CCs, promoting oocyte maturity [20]. In humans, oocyte quality has been positively associated with augmented VCAN expression [19, 21]. Lastly, the increased expression of VCAN at the oocyte stage resulted in a higher probability of pregnancy [10] and live births [18]. However, VCAN expression has yet to assess for its predictability and practical use as a marker of implantation and pregnancy.

Ranking of MII oocytes based on CC-expressed genes can serve as a promising new method for the selection of good quality MII oocytes derived from a pool of oocytes collected from hormone-stimulated IVF treatments in humans [22]. The CC-candidates genes, as potential oocyte quality markers for this study, were selected based on results from previous studies performed on human CCs [5, 14, 15, 18, 23] and were shown to be involved in the process of cumulus expansion, prediction of embryo development, and pregnancy. Therefore, the purpose of this study was to assess the VCAN and PTGS2 gene expression in CCs from individual COC as markers of oocyte quality and predictors of clinical pregnancy, in a manner that could be useful to the IVF laboratory as an extra tool to choose the best combination in number and quality at transfer time.

Results

Participants and study characteristics

One hundred and ninety-eight women that suffer from infertility undergoing IVF in Mexico City, Mexico were selected for this study. Some subjects were lost due to not returning for follow-ups appointments, failure to produce viable oocytes/embryos, failure to collect sufficient RNA from the CCs for analysis, or chose not to be included. CCs RNA was isolated from the individual oocytes for each IVF cycle; however, 2 IVF cycles failed to produce a signal for PTGS2, VCAN, and L19, whereas 9 IVF cycles failed to produce a signal for PTGS2, VCAN, or both, while L19 gene was amplified. Therefore, the study consisted of 31 patients who had a single embryo transferred (SETs), 41 patients with two embryos transferred, 68 patients who had three embryos transferred, and nine patients who had four embryos transferred. Clinical and IVF characteristics are presented in Table 1.

There is no correlation between the PVL index and the embryo morphological assessment scores

A subset of 42 patients agreed to have their complete embryo cohort that consisted of high and low-quality embryos, as determined by morphological assessment, assessed. Of the 384 embryos analyzed, the morphological assessment of these embryos ranged between 0 and 12, whereas the PVL index scores ranged between 35.4 and 80.9. There was no association between the PVL index and the embryo morphological assessment scores ($\rho = -0.013$, $p = 0.831$, Fig. 1).

PTGS2 and VCAN gene expression levels in CCs are associated with clinical pregnancy

Based on their highest morphological score, only high-quality embryos were selected for implantation. Between one and four embryos were transferred per patient (Table 1); however, the effectiveness of the PVL index was assessed using the 31 SETs. ROC analysis determined that the PVL index was highly predictive for implantation (AUC = 0.87, 95% CI: 0.74–1.00, $p = 0.010$, Fig. 2). Using the highest Youden's index, we determined

Table 1 Characteristics of study participants

Category	Value
Sample size (n)	149
Age (years)	37.3 ± 4.9
Body-mass index (kg/m^2)	25.2 ± 4.2
≥7 cells/Day 3 (n)	7.5 ± 1.8
Embryo fragmentation (%)	8.7 ± 4.3
Fertilization rate (%)	65.2 ± 18.0
Embryos transferred (n)	2.4 ± 0.9
1 embryo	31
2 embryos	41
3 embryos	68
4 embryos	9
Pregnancy rate (%)	59.89 ± 13.74
Etiology	
Endometrioma (n)	5
Points of endometriosis (n)	10
Low response (n)	3

that a PVL score ≥ 58.2 was associated with clinical pregnancy (Youden index = 0.769, sensitivity = 100%, and specificity = 76.9%) and was highly accurate (test accuracy = 80.65%, positive predictive value = 45.5%, and negative predictive value =100%).

The effectiveness of the PVL index was also examined in patients with multiple embryos implanted using the 58.2 cutoff value. All IVF cycles ($n = 149$), which consisted of SETs, two embryos transferred, three embryos transferred, and four embryos transferred, were evaluated. To correct for embryo cohorts lacking a completely positive or negative PVL group, we used a modified equation proposed by Ekart et al. and calculated the probability of pregnancy for each IVF cycle. Using logistic regression, a strong association was determined between the probability of pregnancy based on the PVL index and implantation (β-hCG: odds ratio = 11.59, 95%CI: 4.27–31.48, $p < 0.001$), as well as ultra-sound confirmed presence of fetal sac with a heartbeat (odds ratio = 8.40, 95%CI: 3.26–21.63, $p < 0.001$, Table 2).

Interestingly, the implantation of at least one embryo with a PVL index score ≥ 58.2, independent of the total number of embryos implanted, was associated with a greater chance of achieving clinical pregnancy, as determined by β-hCG (Odds Ratio = 17.15, 95%CI: 6.82–43.18, Table 2) and ultra-sound confirmed presence of fetal sac with a heartbeat (Odds Ratio = 16.81, 95%CI: 6.43–43.92, $p < 0.001$, Table 2). Using all 149 IVF cycles, the PVL index was highly accurate (test accuracy = 78.52%, positive predictive value = 76.0%, and negative predictive value =84.4%).

When the group was stratified by age and considering the transfer of at least 1 PVL positive embryo, there was an increased association for women ≥38 years of age for β-hCG (0.6-fold change) and for ultrasound confirmation (2.3-fold change, Table 2). For many of the embryos, PGT

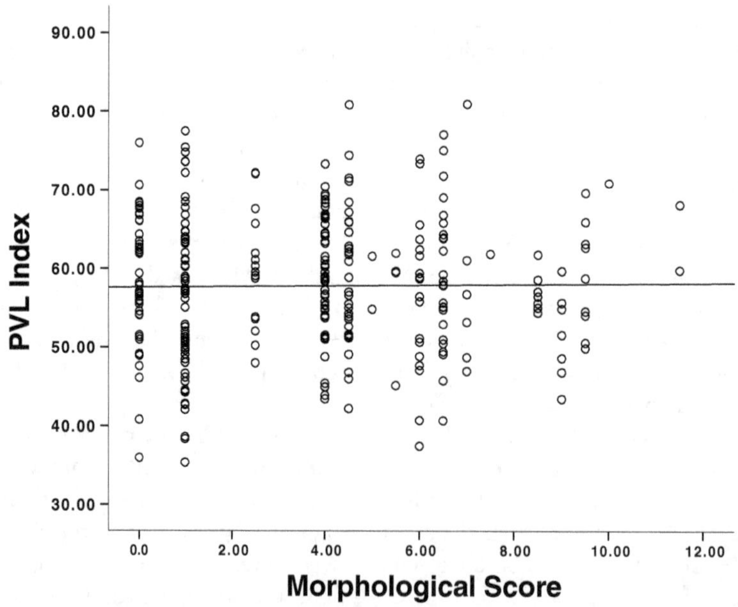

Fig. 1 Correlation between embryo morphological score and the PVL index. For 42 patients, CCs were isolated from an oocyte during a standardized IVF protocol. CCs RNA was isolated using Trizol. Gene expression profile of PTGS2, VCAN, and L19 was determined by qPCR and the PVL index was calculated. Afterwards, oocytes were fertilized and morphological parameters evaluated by a specialized training Embryologist for 384 embryos. The level of association was determined by calculating Spearman's correlation coefficient (ρ)

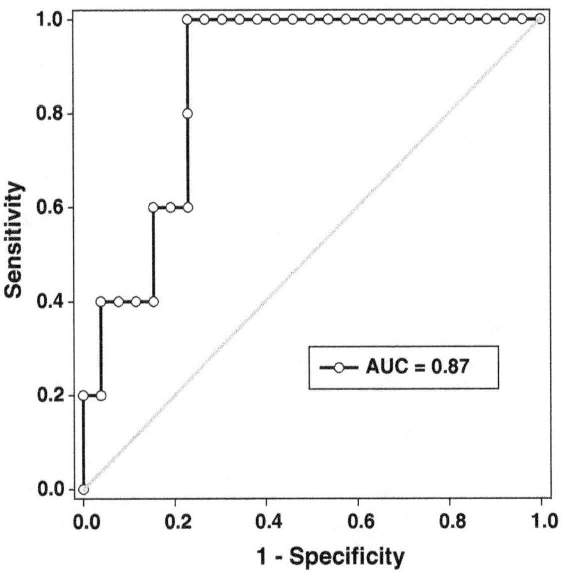

Fig. 2 Receiver operating characteristic curve for the PVL index to clinical pregnancy. 31 single embryos transfers were implanted and pregnancy was confirmed by β-hCG level > 10 mUI/ml on Day 14. The PVL index was determined for each oocyte

was used to confirm the embryos that were transferred were euploid. When stratified by the PGT-confirmed absence of aneuploidy embryos, there was an increased association for β-hCG (6.5-fold change) and for ultrasound confirmation (2.4-fold change) using the probability's raw score. When considering the transfer of at least 1 PVL positive embryo, the fold change could not be determined due to the lack of false negatives for the PGT confirmed euploid embryos. Lastly, 18 subjects were identified with severe etiologies (endometriosis or low response during stimulation) other than infertility. When these patients were stratified, the association between the PVL index and pregnancy was only present in the subjects absent from these etiologies.

Discussion

Gene expression analysis of the CCs can be a valuable tool that allows attaining an estimation of oocyte quality and embryo capabilities, especially in respect to embryo implantation. Different groups have analyzed the CCs transcriptional profile, resulting in the assembly of a group of candidate genes of which only a few have been suggested as genes that could predict oocyte quality and pregnancy success [5–8, 10, 18, 23–25]. For this study, two genes expressed in the CCs were analyzed: PTGS2 and VCAN. Even though both genes have been highly reported in the literature for their association to oocyte quality, to date, neither gene has been included in a single panel profile used to evaluate clinical pregnancy potential for embryos. Here, we show that a high PVL index, which is evaluating the expression of these two genes, resulted in increased clinical pregnancy. Many groups have assessed the gene profile of the CCs, all indicating that both genes, PTGS2 and VCAN, play an important role in oocyte maturation and are relevant indicators of competent oocytes [6, 14, 15, 18]. Gebhardt et al. revealed the presence of a positive correlation with embryonic development and live births. Regardless that Gebhardt et al. proposed PTGS2 and VCAN as candidate genes to measure oocyte quality and embryonic development [18], there is no evidence in the literature to support their practical use in oocyte and embryo selection. In this study, these genes were therefore proposed as the first group of genes that can be used in conjunction with morphological data produced by the IVF laboratory for the selection of embryos to be transferred. A transcriptional profile was generated for the CCs using qPCR data, which allowed us to generate an expression indicator, the PVL index, for the evaluation of oocyte quality and embryo capabilities to implant. Here, only high-quality embryos were selected and transferred. Afterward, their respective PVL index scores were assessed. We determined that the PVL index scores were independent of the morphological assessment. This does demonstrate that the cellular processes vary significantly between similarly scored embryos and posits that alternative tests are required when selecting embryos.

It is imperative to emphasize that until today, no reports establish a cutoff value, based on gene expression, where competent and not competent oocytes/embryos were considered. This study proposes the application of an index that relates the expression of VCAN and PTGS2, as a new tool for the evaluation of pregnancy prediction. Using SETs, which were only high-quality embryos, the PVL index, and measurements of clinical pregnancy presented with a good correlation. This led to establishing a cutoff value for the PVL index of 58.2 (Fig. 2). Afterward, IVF cycles with multiple embryos transferred were assessed, and it was determined that the cutoff value for the PVL index was highly predictive. Unfortunately, there were minimal IVF cycles with completely positive (≥58.2) or completely negative (< 58.2) PVL index score embryos. Therefore, it is difficult to determine if the embryos with the higher PVL index scores are the ones producing the pregnancy when mixed cohorts and several embryos are transferred. Even though, we demonstrated that the implantation of at least one embryo with a PVL score ≥ 58.2 was associated with clinical pregnancy.

Ekart et al. was one of the first groups to propose a new classification and selection system for oocytes, based on the genetic expression shown in the CCs, specifically using molecules involved in the COC interaction that are activated during the second to last phase of foliculogenesis. In addition of developing a mathematical

Table 2 The association between the *probability* and pregnancy determined by β–hCG or USG

Category	Size	OR [a]	95% CI	*p*-value
Pregnancy by β–hCG				
Probability raw score[b]				
Overall	149	11.59	4.27–31.84	< 0.001 *
Patient's age				
< 38 years of age	63	11.46	2.16–60.65	0.004 *
≥ 38 years of age	86	12.41	3.48–44.21	< 0.001 *
Pre-implantation Genetic Testing (PGT)				
No PGT confirmed euploid embryo	104	6.81	2.03–22.86	0.002 *
PGT confirmed euploid embryo	45	51.23	6.46–406.25	< 0.001 *
Patient's health				
No major etiology	131	17.43	5.48–55.44	< 0.001 *
Presence of a major etiology	18	4.48	0.19–104.06	0.350
At least 1 PVL positive embryo [c]				
Overall	149	17.15	6.82–43.18	< 0.001 *
Patient's age				
< 38 years of age	63	13.60	3.71–49.91	< 0.001 *
≥ 38 years of age	86	21.93	5.73–83.94	< 0.001 *
Pre-implantation Genetic Testing (PGT)				
No PGT confirmed euploid embryo	104	9.67	3.54–26.43	< 0.001 *
PGT confirmed euploid embryo	45	N/D		
Patient's health				
No major etiology	131	29.17	10.43–81.56	< 0.001 *
Presence of a major etiology	18	1.20	0.09–15.26	0.888
Pregnancy by Ultrasound confirmation				
Probability raw score [b]				
Overall	149	8.40	3.26–21.63	< 0.001 *
Patient's age				
< 38 years of age	63	3.84	0.92–16.12	0.066
≥ 38 years of age	86	14.79	4.08–53.61	< 0.001 *
Pre-implantation Genetic Testing (PGT)				
No PGT confirmed euploid embryo	104	6.31	1.94–20.50	0.002 *
PGT confirmed euploid embryo	45	21.62	3.53–132.42	0.001 *
Patient's health				
No major etiology	131	10.75	3.77–30.65	< 0.001 *
Presence of a major etiology	18	4.48	0.19–104.06	0.350
At least 1 PVL positive embryo [c]				
Overall	149	16.81	6.43–43.92	< 0.001 *
Patient's age				
< 38 years of age	63	9.48	2.66–33.78	0.001 *
≥ 38 years of age	86	31.63	6.68–149.79	< 0.001 *
Pre-implantation Genetic Testing (PGT)				
No PGT confirmed euploid embryo	104	10.27	3.64–28.96	< 0.001 *
PGT confirmed euploid embryo	45	N/D		

Table 2 The association between the *probability* and pregnancy determined by β-hCG or USG *(Continued)*

Category	Size	OR [a]	95% CI	*p*-value
Patient's health				
No major etiology	131	26.91	9.29–77.94	< 0.001 *
Presence of a major etiology	18	1.20	0.09–15.26	0.888

[a]Crude odds ratio (OR) and 95% confidence intervals (95% CI) were determined using logistic regression. N/D = was not able to be determined. *indicates a significant result, $p < 0.05$ (two-tailed). [b]Probability = $1-(x_{neg}/x_{tot})^n$, where x_{neg} = number of embryos with a PVL index score < 58.2, x_{tot} = total number of transferred embryos, and n = number of embryos with a PVL index score ≥ 58.2. [c]A positive cohort has the probability ≠0.00

tool that can be applied for oocyte selection, their system allows an evaluation of the expression, followed by expression level classification of four genes from the CCs: *hyaluronan synthase 2* (HAS2), *follicle-stimulating hormone receptor* (FSHR), VCAN, and *progesterone receptor*. Combination of the HAS2 and FSHR genes resulted in a predictive value of 80% when applying for the selection of three embryos. However, using this system for a single embryo selection, the predictive value decreased significantly to 48%. Ekart et al. did not include PTGS2 in their gene panel to predict oocyte quality and embryonic development [22]. Even though the PVL index was used to score each embryonic cohort, showing a strong correlation between this index and clinical pregnancy, an additional mathematical analysis was performed to support our findings. The mathematical formula created by Ekart was applied to each embryonic cohort. In theory, this would determine the probability of each embryo to produce a clinical pregnancy, only if this embryo was from an oocyte with a CCs quality index ≥58.2. Undeniably, the probability of pregnancy of a transferred embryo displayed a high correlation with the PVL index and therefore aids us in predicting pregnancy in patients.

Older women have a decreased probability of achieving pregnancy and lower IVF success rates; therefore, exploiting alternative methods to improve IVF outcome remains a key factor. When the cohort was stratified by age, the PVL index was more associated with older women in achieving clinical pregnancy. This posits that using the PVL index could improve the probability of successful implantation for older women.

The implantation of aneuploid embryos is associated with lower IVF success rates and the level of aneuploidy in embryo-cohorts increases with age. In Mexico, older women are suggested to complement IVF with PGT, to assess for aneuploidy; however, the benefits and pitfalls of using of PTGS2 remains under debate. Here, only 30% of the patients opted to have PGT; therefore, it is possible that some of the embryos were genetically compromised, as shown by the decreased diagnostic odds ratio when we examined embryos without confirmed euploidy. Unfortunately, with the embryos that were determined to be euploid, we were unable to determine the diagnostic odds ratio, when at least 1 PVL positive embryo was implanted. This was due to the absence of any false negative results. In other words, the presences of a PVL positive embryo was not associated with failed implantation. This posits that using both the PVL index and PGT would improve IVF outcomes.

Our study has a few limitations. First, we focused on a random set of females with some level of primary and secondary female infertility factor—male factor was not considered. We can only speculate that male factor infertility will not affect the results demonstrated here, as the examined genes are from the CCs and only associated with oocyte health and competence. Second, some of the patients had endometriosis of varying degree, which was probably affecting the implantation results. Endometriosis and its location could affect and explain why some patients did not present with the clinical pregnancy even with good embryos. However, this is outside the scope of the current research and is currently being considered for future studies. Lastly, we cannot be entirely confident if the high PVL scored embryos were the embryos that achieved clinical pregnancy, but SETs results support our confidence in this possibility. This is the preliminary study, and the selection of embryos based on the PVL index is the focus of current and future studies.

Conclusions

The development of new tools, which allow us to obtain an approximation of the state of the oocyte and the embryo, as well as determine the clinical pregnancy potential, is of great importance for IVF treatments. Here, a valuable evaluation system was generated to measure two key genes from the CCs—PTGS2 and VCAN—to relate the ovular state and clinical pregnancy. The PVL index can indicate good quality oocytes that for after fertilization will have the highest probability of achieving clinical pregnancy. This research will allow embryologists and other IVF personnel involved in the selection process to have an alternative test to determine the best embryo to transfer over the current method of embryo morphological assessment.

Methods

Study patients and ethical approval

Women that suffer from infertility, undergoing IVF in Mexico City, Mexico, were asked to participate in this retrospective study (from October 2011 to May 2017). The protocol was approved by the Ethics Committee of the Ingenes Institute (number I/13/2013). Written informed consent was obtained from all patients, conducted in accordance with the Declaration of Helsinki. Patients were clinically evaluated according to a standardized protocol including personal and family clinical history. The patients' height (m) and weight (kg) were measured, and the BMI was calculated as weight divided by the height squared (kg/m^2).

IVF, CC isolation, and pregnancy evaluation

All patients were subjected to controlled ovarian stimulation for ten days with Gonadotropin-releasing hormone agonists and antagonists. Ovarian response was assessed measuring serum estradiol levels, and follicular development was evaluated by ultrasound examination. Oocyte retrieval was conducted 20 h after human chorionic gonadotropin (hCG) administration (10,000 IU Choragon or 6500 IU Ovidrel) with ultrasound guidance. Follicular puncture for oocyte collection was performed under general anesthesia at the end of hormonal stimulation (10–14 days). Transvaginal ultrasound was used to locate mature follicles, and ovulation was induced with hCG. 3–5 ml of follicular fluid containing the oocytes were extracted using a specialized suction system. Follicles aspirated from the patients ranged between 8 and 30. Samples were analyzed using a stereoscopic microscope in order to locate the oocytes, which were kept at 37.5 °C in an atmosphere of 8.3% CO_2 until fertilization. Number and quality of retrieved oocytes were assessed using morphological parameters [granulosa expansion, oocyte maturity (MI, MII, and VG), quality of the cytoplasm, zona pellucida, and polar body]. Oocytes were located, numbered, and separated into drops of HTF-HEPES (Human tubal fluid/(4-(2-hydroxyethyl)-1-piperazineethanesulfonic acid) supplemented with 10% HSA. CCs were removed using a 1-mm needle and isolated using mechanical dispersion. The isolated CCs were preserved in 20 µl of Global Total for Fertilization media (LifeGlobal) and placed into Eppendorf tubes containing 150 µl of Trizol (Ambion, Life Technologies, Carlsbad CA, USA) and stored at − 70 °C until processed. To note, the patient's cumula cells were not pooled; the oocyte and its CCs were analyzed as a corresponding pair.

An Embryologist monitored and recorded information about fertilization, embryo development, embryo morphology, transfer, and pregnancy for each oocyte. Morphological parameters evaluated were weighed into a matrix to rate each oocyte-embryo, with the sum of values obtained on a scale of 0 (low quality) to 12 (high quality). Selection and embryo transfer were done on Day 3 or Day 5 of development according to the embryo morphological assessment, using the criteria established by Istanbul consensus Workshop on Embryo Assessment [26]. The highest quality embryos (morphology) were transferred, and pregnancy was confirmed by β-hCG values > 10 mUI/ml (Day 14) and the presence of a fetal heartbeat, confirmed by ultrasound at 6–8 weeks. The number of embryos transferred (1, 2, 3, or 4) was determined by the number of high-quality embryos achieving full development, patient results from previous attempts, and the opinion of the clinician.

RNA extraction

CCs RNA extraction was carried out using the Trizol® reagent, according to the manufacturer's recommendations. Briefly, CCs samples were processed with 70 µl of chloroform for 5 min at room temperature, followed by centrifugation at 12,500 g for 15 min at 4 °C. The supernatant was transferred to a new tube containing 150 µl isopropanol. Samples were incubated for 10 min at room temperature and centrifuged at 15,000 g for 15 min at 4 °C. The pellet was washed with 100 µl of 75% ethanol and then centrifuged at 12,500 g for 5 min. Pellet was air-dry for 10 min. RNA was re-suspended in 0.1% of DEPC water and quantified by spectrophotometry (Epoch/Biotek, Winooski, VT, USA).

Quantitative reverse transcription- polymerase chain reaction (RT-qPCR)

Primers for PTGS2, VCAN, and Ribosomal Protein L-19 (L19) were designed using the Primer 3 plus v2.0 software. All primer sequences are shown in Table 3. All qPCR reactions were performed using the StepOne Plus apparatus (Applied Biosystems) with the One Step Kappa Syberfast system (KAPA Biosystems, Woburn, MA, USA). PTGS2, VCAN, and L19 genes were quantified in duplicate. Reaction mix was prepared as follows: 5 µl 2X KAPA SYBR® FAST qRT-PCR Master Mix, 0.2 µl ROX, 0.2 µl dUTP (10 mM), 0.2 µl forward and reverse primers (20 pmol), 0.2 µl KAPA RT, 100 ng of RNA sample, and DEPC water for a total volume of 10 µl. qPCR conditions were one cycle of reverse-transcription at 42 °C for 5 min, one cycle of reverse-transcriptase inactivation at 95 °C for 5 min, 40 cycles of amplification at 95 °C for 15 s, 56 °C for 30 s, then 72 °C for 30 s. SYBR Green was used during amplification to construct melting curves that were analyzed to verify if the peaks corresponded with theoretical melting temperatures for each amplicon. All the PCR products were resolved through capillary electrophoresis using the BioAnalyzer Labchip GX (Caliper). The products showed a single band corresponding to the predicted base pair length and a band purity of 95% or higher. Moreover, the bands were cloned and analyzed via sequencing to verify their identity. Sequence identification of the PCR products was confirmed by direct cloning with

Table 3 Primer sequences

Gene	Forward Primer	Reverse Primer
PTGS2	5'-CTGAAGCCCTATGAATCATTT-3'	5'-CATTACCCATAAGTCCTTTCAA-3'
VCAN	5'-TCAGCAAAGGACAATTCAATA-3'	5'-TTTAAAATGTTTTGGGAGCA-3'
L19	5'-TCAGGCTACAGAAGAGGCTTGC-3'	5'-ATCAGCCCATCCTTGATCAGC-3'

the CloneJet system (Fermentas, ThermoFisher, Waltham, MA, USA) and sequencing using the BigDye system. Briefly, the amplicon fragments were purified using the GeneJet Gel Extraction kit and ligated into a pJET1.2/ blunt vector following the manufacturer's protocol. Ligations were transformed into TOP10 competent bacteria and grown in LB medium (Ampicillin, Pisa SA Laboratorios, Mexico; 100 mg/ml) for 16 h at 37 °C. Plasmid DNA was extracted from the bacteria using the mini-prep technique. Amplicon's identity was verified by sequencing using BigDye Terminator v3.1 reagent and the RV primer 3 (3'-CTAGCAAAATAGGCTGTCCC-5') (Applied Biosystems, Foster City, CA, USA). Samples were sequenced with the ABI PRISM 3700 analyzer (Applied Biosystems) and sequences corroborated using Blast software.

PTGS/VCAN/L19 (PVL) index and probability

The PVL index was calculated from the data obtained after processing the isolated CCs of each individual oocyte. L19 was determined to be the optimal housekeeping gene for our system as the variations associated with L19 in a cohort were no larger than 1 C_T in more than 90% of cases. For each patient, the L19 expression was used for normalizing purposes (to the lowest C_T for the patient's oocyte cohort). The index is the sum of the expression levels of PTGS2 and VCAN, normalized by L19.

$$\text{PVL Index} = ([\text{PTGS2}] + [\text{VCAN}])/[\text{L19}]_{\text{normalized}} \quad (1)$$

The probability of pregnancy for each transfer cycle using the PVL index was obtained by the modified formula for random selection described by Ekart et al. [22]:

$$P = 1\text{-}(x^{neg}/x^{tot})^n \quad (2)$$

where P = probability, x^{neg} = number of embryos with a PVL index score < 58.2, x^{tot} = total number of transferred embryos, and n = number of embryos with a PVL index score ≥ 58.2.

Embryo biopsy (day 3 and day 5)

Embryos were assessed for the number of cells, symmetry, and fragmentation. For high-morphological quality embryos, the chromosomal composition was determined using Array Comparative Genomic Hybridization (aCGH). The S-biopsy method was utilized to isolate a blastomere from Day 3 embryos [27]. Briefly, a Hamilton Thorne ZILOS-tk laser (1460 nm, 300 mW) was used to create a funnel in the zona pellucida adjacent to a blastomere. Next, the blastomere was extracted by aspirating the whole embryo with a 140-μm stripper capillary micropipette, leading to the ejection of the blastomere. The blastomere was then placed into a 0.2-μL PCR tube. For Day 5 embryos (expanded blastocyst stage containing 50 to 150 cells), a Hamilton Thorne ZILOS-tk laser was used to create a funnel in the zona pellucida on the opposite side to the inner cell mass. Blastocysts were incubated for a further 2–3 h to allow blastocele expansion and herniation of the trophectoderm cells from the zona pellucida. Afterward, the embryo was placed into 20-μL of Ca^{2+}/Mg^{2+}-free bicarbonate buffered G-PGD medium (cat #10074, Vitrolife). Applying gentle suction with the biopsy pipette (MBB-FP-SM-35, Origio, Malov, Denmark), the trophectoderm cells were encouraged to herniate from the zona pellucida. Trophectoderm cells were dissected from each of the blastocysts using four laser pulses of 3-min duration. 10–15 cells were retrieved, washed, and placed into a 0.2-μL PCR tube.

Whole genome amplification and pre-implantation genetic testing (PGT)

The material obtained from each biopsy was amplified using the SurePlex amplification system (Illumina, San Diego, CA, USA) according to the manufacturer's instructions. PGT was carried out by aCGH using the 24 Sure V3 microarray (Illumina, San Diego, CA, USA) using the protocol described by Fragouli [28, 29]. The amplified DNA was fluorescently labeled (Fluorescence Labelling System, Illumina). The samples were co-precipitated, denatured, and analyzed by array hybridization (for 16 h). A laser scanner (InnoScan 710, Innopsys, Carbonne, France) was used to excite the fluorophores and read the hybridization images. Hybridization images were stored in TIFF format and analyzed by the BlueFuse Multi-Analysis software (Illumina), using the criteria and algorithms recommended by the manufacturer. With this approach, it was possible to determine the chromosome constitution of each embryo.

Statistical analysis

The association between the PVL index and embryo morphological assessment scores was determined by calculating Spearman's rho (ρ). Receiver operating characteristic (ROC) analysis was performed to determine the specificity and sensitivity of the PVL index, by calculating the area under the ROC curve (AUC). The cutoff value was determined calculating the highest Youden Index score: sensitivity + specificity−1. Logistic regression was used to determine the association (Odds Ratio and 95% confidence intervals) between the PVL index and clinical pregnancy. *P*-values < 0.05 (two-tailed) were considered significant. All analyses were carried out using either the Statistical Package for the Social Sciences program, version 22 (SPSS, Chicago, IL) or Sigma Plot software (v. 12.0, San Jose, CA, USA).

Abbreviations

aCGH: array Comparative Genomic Hybridization; AUC: Area under the ROC curve; CCs: Cumulus cells; COC: Cumulus-oocyte complex; FSHR: *Follicle-stimulating hormone receptor*; HAS2: *Hyaluronan synthase 2*; IVF: In vitro fertilization; PGT: Pre-implantation genetic testing; PTGS2: *Prostaglandin-Endoperoxide Synthase 2*; PVL index: (PTGS2 + VCAN)*$L19_{normalized}$; qPCR: Quantitative Reverse Transcription- Polymerase Chain Reaction; ROC: Receiver operating characteristic; SETs: Single embryo transfers; VCAN: *Versican*; β-hCG: Beta human Chorionic Gonadotropin

Acknowledgments

We would like to express our gratitude to the participants of this study, as well to all the personal in IVF lab at Ingenes Institute for their valuable help in CCs collection, particularly Leticia Chiquillo and Paola Olvera Uribe.

Funding

This study was supported in part by grants from the Consejo Nacional de Ciencia y Tecnología (PEI-Conacyt 184497 and 250768).

Authors' contributions

AO, LP, and ELB contributed to the study's design, collection and analysis of the data, and forming conclusions. JP, GM, and EHP contributed to the collection and analysis of the data. ELB and LP prepared the manuscript and contributed to the editing and critical analysis. All authors have knowledge of the manuscript content. All authors read and approved the final manuscript.

Competing interests

The authors declare that they have no competing interests.

Author details

[1]Laboratorio de Investigación y Diagnóstico Molecular, Instituto de Infertilidad y Genética, Ingenes México, Av. IPN 2508, 07360 CDMX, México. [2]Departamento de Toxicología, Centro de Investigación y de Estudios Avanzados del Instituto Politécnico Nacional, Av. IPN 2508, 07360 CDMX, México. [3]Programa de Doctorado en Ciencias Biológicas y de la Salud, División de Ciencias Biológicas y de la Salud, Universidad Autónoma Metropolitana-Iztapalapa, Av. IPN 2508, 07360 CDMX, México.

References

1. Ebner T, Moser M, Sommergruber M, Tews G. Selection based on morphological assessment of oocytes and embryos at different stages of preimplantation development: a review. Hum Reprod Update. 2003;9(3):251–62.
2. Hillier SG. Research challenge: what is the best non-invasive test of oocyte/embryo competence? Mol Hum Reprod. 2008;14(12):665. https://doi.org/10.1093/molehr/gan068gan068.
3. Zhuo L, Kimata K. Cumulus oophorus extracellular matrix: its construction and regulation. Cell Struct Funct. 2001;26(4):189–96.
4. Lourenco B, Sousa AP, Almeida-Santos T, Ramalho-Santos J. Relation of cumulus cell status with single oocyte maturity, fertilization capability and patient age. J Reprod Infertil. 2014;15(1):15–21.
5. Cillo F, Brevini TA, Antonini S, Paffoni A, Ragni G, Gandolfi F. Association between human oocyte developmental competence and expression levels of some cumulus genes. Reproduction. 2007;134:645–50.
6. Adriaenssens T, Wathlet S, Segers I, Verheyen G, De Vos A, Van der Elst J, et al. Cumulus cell gene expression is associated with oocyte developmental quality and influenced by patient and treatment characteristics. Hum Reprod. 2010; 25(5):1259–70. https://doi.org/10.1093/humrep/deq049.
7. Feuerstein P, Cadoret V, Dalbies-Tran R, Guerif F, Bidault R, Royere D. Gene expression in human cumulus cells: one approach to oocyte competence. Hum Reprod. 2007;22(12):3069–77. https://doi.org/10.1093/humrep/dem336.
8. Assou S, Haouzi D, De Vos J, Hamamah S. Human cumulus cells as biomarkers for embryo and pregnancy outcomes. Mol Hum Reprod. 2010; 16(8):531–8. https://doi.org/10.1093/molehr/gaq032.
9. van Montfoort AP, Geraedts JP, Dumoulin JC, Stassen AP, Evers JL, Ayoubi TA. Differential gene expression in cumulus cells as a prognostic indicator of embryo viability: a microarray analysis. Mol Hum Reprod 2008;14(3):157–168. https://doi.org/10.1093/molehr/gam088.
10. Wathlet S, Adriaenssens T, Segers I, Verheyen G, Janssens R, Coucke W, et al. New candidate genes to predict pregnancy outcome in single embryo transfer cycles when using cumulus cell gene expression. Fertil Steril. 2012; 98(2):432–9 e1–4. https://doi.org/10.1016/j.fertnstert.2012.05.007.
11. Assou S, Anahory T, Pantesco V, Le Carrour T, Pellestor F, Klein B, et al. The human cumulus--oocyte complex gene-expression profile. Hum Reprod. 2006 Jul;21(7):1705–19. https://doi.org/10.1093/humrep/del065.
12. Shao L, Chian RC, Xu Y, Yan Z, Zhang Y, Gao C, et al. Genomic expression profiles in cumulus cells derived from germinal vesicle and MII mouse oocytes. Reprod Fertil Dev. 2015. https://doi.org/10.1071/RD15077.
13. Sugimura S, Ritter LJ, Rose RD, Thompson JG, Smitz J, Mottershead DG, et al. Promotion of EGF receptor signaling improves the quality of low developmental competence oocytes. Dev Biol. 2015;403(2):139–49. https://doi.org/10.1016/j.ydbio.2015.05.008.
14. McKenzie LJ, Pangas SA, Carson SA, Kovanci E, Cisneros P, Buster JE, et al. Human cumulus granulosa cell gene expression: a predictor of fertilization and embryo selection in women undergoing IVF. Hum Reprod. 2004;19(12): 2869–74. https://doi.org/10.1093/humrep/deh535.
15. Wathlet S, Adriaenssens T, Segers I, Verheyen G, Van de Velde H, Coucke W, et al. Cumulus cell gene expression predicts better cleavage-stage embryo or blastocyst development and pregnancy for ICSI patients. Hum Reprod. 2011;26(5):1035–51. https://doi.org/10.1093/humrep/der036.
16. Anderson RA, Sciorio R, Kinnell H, Bayne RA, Thong KJ, de Sousa PA, Pickering S. Cumulus gene expression as a predictor of human oocyte fertilisation, embryo development and competence to establish a pregnancy. Reproduction. 2009;138:629–37.
17. Marei WF, Abayasekara DR, Wathes DC, Fouladi-Nashta AA. Role of PTGS2-generated PGE2 during gonadotrophin-induced bovine oocyte maturation and cumulus cell expansion. Reprod BioMed Online. 2014;28(3):388–400. https://doi.org/10.1016/j.rbmo.2013.11.005.
18. Gebhardt KM, Feil DK, Dunning KR, Lane M, Russell DL. Human cumulus cell gene expression as a biomarker of pregnancy outcome after single embryo transfer. Fertil Steril. 2011;96(1):47–52 e2. https://doi.org/10.1016/j.fertnstert.2011.04.033.
19. Dunning KR, Watson LN, Zhang VJ, Brown HM, Kaczmarek AK, Robker RL, et al. Activation of Mouse Cumulus-Oocyte Complex Maturation In Vitro Through EGF-Like Activity of Versican. Biol Reprod. 2015;92(5):116. https://doi.org/10.1095/biolreprod.114.127274.

20. Mito T, Yoshioka K, Noguchi M, Yamashita S, Hoshi H. Recombinant human follicle-stimulating hormone and transforming growth factor-alpha enhance in vitro maturation of porcine oocytes. Mol Reprod Dev. 2013;80(7):549–60. https://doi.org/10.1002/mrd.22190.
21. Tsui KH, Lin LT, Horng HC, Chang R, Huang BS, Cheng JT, et al. Gene expression of cumulus cells in women with poor ovarian response after dehydroepiandrosterone supplementation. Taiwan J Obstet Gynecol. 2014; 53(4):559–65. https://doi.org/10.1016/j.tjog.2014.09.003.
22. Ekart J, McNatty K, Hutton J, Pitman J. Ranking and selection of MII oocytes in human ICSI cycles using gene expression levels from associated cumulus cells. Hum Reprod. 2013;28(11):2930–42. https://doi.org/10.1093/humrep/det357.
23. Assidi M, Dieleman SJ, Sirard MA. Cumulus cell gene expression following the LH surge in bovine preovulatory follicles: potential early markers of oocyte competence. Reproduction. 2010;140(6):835–52. https://doi.org/10.1530/REP-10-0248.
24. Huang Z, Wells D. The human oocyte and cumulus cells relationship: new insights from the cumulus cell transcriptome. Mol Hum Reprod. 2010;16(10): 715–25. https://doi.org/10.1093/molehr/gaq031.
25. Fragouli E, Wells D, Iager AE, Kayisli UA, Patrizio P. Alteration of gene expression in human cumulus cells as a potential indicator of oocyte aneuploidy. Hum Reprod. 2012;27(8):2559–68. https://doi.org/10.1093/humrep/des170.
26. Alpha Scientists in Reproductive M, Embryology ESIGo. The Istanbul consensus workshop on embryo assessment: proceedings of an expert meeting. Hum Reprod. 2011;26(6):1270–83. https://doi.org/10.1093/humrep/der037.
27. Cedillo L, Ocampo-Barcenas A, Maldonado I, Valdez-Morales FJ, Camargo F, Lopez-Bayghen E. A simple, less invasive stripper micropipetter-based technique for day 3 embryo biopsy. Fertility research and practice. 2016;2:13. https://doi.org/10.1186/s40738-016-0027-4.
28. Fragouli E, Katz-Jaffe M, Alfarawati S, Stevens J, Colls P, Goodall NN, et al. Comprehensive chromosome screening of polar bodies and blastocysts from couples experiencing repeated implantation failure. Fertil Steril. 2010; 94(3):875–87. https://doi.org/10.1016/j.fertnstert.2009.04.053.
29. Fragouli E, Alfarawati S, Daphnis DD, Goodall NN, Mania A, Griffiths T, et al. Cytogenetic analysis of human blastocysts with the use of FISH, CGH and aCGH: scientific data and technical evaluation. Hum Reprod. 2011;26(2):480–90. https://doi.org/10.1093/humrep/deq344.

20

Prognostic value of various subtypes of extracellular DNA in ovarian cancer patients

Katarina Kalavska[1,2†], Tomas Minarik[3†], Barbora Vlkova[4], Denisa Manasova[2], Michaela Kubickova[3], Andrej Jurik[3], Jozef Mardiak[1,3], Jozef Sufliarsky[1,3], Peter Celec[4] and Michal Mego[1,2,3*]

Abstract

Background: Patients with ovarian cancer represent a heterogeneous population with a variable prognosis and response to chemotherapy. Plasma DNA has been shown to have a prognostic value in different types of cancer including ovarian carcinoma. Whether total circulating DNA, which can be assessed much easier without knowing the tumor-specific mutations, has similar informative value is currently unknown. The aim of this study was to evaluate the prognostic value of extracellular DNA in advanced ovarian cancer.

Methods: This prospective study included 67 patients (pts) with ovarian cancer treated with 1st line paclitaxel and carboplatin (25 pts) and paclitaxel, carboplatin and bevacizumab (42 pts). Thirty-five patients had optimal surgical debulking before chemotherapy. Extracellular DNA was quantified using real time PCR before administration of chemotherapy (67 pts) and after 6 cycles of chemotherapy (44 pts).

Results: Total extracellular DNA (ecDNA), as well as extracellular DNA of nuclear (nDNA) and mitochondrial origin (mtDNA) significantly ($p < 0.05$) decreased after 6 cycles of chemotherapy (by 54%, 63% and 52%, respectively. Patients with stage I disease had significantly lower mtDNA compared to patients with stage II-IV (8604 vs. 16, 984 ge/mL, $p = 0.03$). Patients with lower baseline nDNA had superior progression-free (HR = 0.35 (0.14–0.86)) and overall survival (HR = 0.18 (0.04–0.77). The prognostic value of nDNA was confirmed independent of tumor stage and confirmed in multivariate analysis.

Conclusions: Our data suggest that ecDNA of both, nuclear and mitochondrial origin could be added to prognostic markers in ovarian cancer. Analysis of ecDNA does not require the knowledge of tumor-specific mutations in contrast to the quantification of tumor-derived ecDNA. Study of the dynamics and cell type-specific source of the ecDNA could shed light on its biology in cancer and might help to direct the treatment of ovarian cancer.

Keywords: Extracellular DNA, Plasma DNA, Ovarian cancer, Prognostic marker

Background

Ovarian cancer represents the most lethal gynecologic malignancy and the fifth most common cause of cancer death in woman [1]. The high mortality of this disease may be due to the lack of early diagnostic and screening methods. Most ovarian cancer patients are diagnosed at an advanced stage of the disease (FIGO Stage III and IV) characterized by widely metastatic disease with 10-year survival rate 5–21% [2]. In contrast, survival rates for patients diagnosed at early stage I (tumor confined to the ovary) are nearly 90% [3]. Thus, patients with ovarian cancer may serve as a heterogeneous population with a variable prognosis and response to chemotherapy. Cancer antigen CA-125 represent frequently used biomarker for predicting prognosis and therapeutic response in ovarian cancer patients. Its levels together with imaging techniques are widely used in patient management. However, sensitivity of current imaging techniques is limited. Therefore, there is an urgent need for development of novel biomarkers effectively predicting therapeutic response and prognosis of patients with ovarian cancer [4–6]. Recently, several studies are focused on

* Correspondence: misomego@gmail.com
†Katarina Kalavska and Tomas Minarik contributed equally to this work.
[1]2nd Department of Oncology, Faculty of Medicine, Comenius University and National Cancer Institute, Klenova 1, 833 10 Bratislava, Slovak Republic
[2]Translational Research Unit, Faculty of Medicine, Comenius University, Bratislava, Slovakia
Full list of author information is available at the end of the article

quantitative analysis of extracellular DNA as on novel non-invasive approach to follow patients after treatment, monitor therapeutic response and promote earlier detection of recurrences in different types of cancer including ovarian carcinoma [7, 8].

Extracellular DNA include double-stranded molecules in the form of short fragments (between 70 and 200 bp) or long fragments up to 21 kb accessible for analysis from plasma or serum of cancer patients [9, 10]. The presence of extracellular DNA in the circulation is explained by releasing of nuclear and mitochondrial DNA by both normal and tumor cells into the circulation through the destruction of apoptic and necrotic cells [9, 11].

Extracellular DNA as a liquid biopsy can also serve as valuable tool revealing tumor genetic changes, including the acquisition of resistance associated mutations during therapy. Various types of DNA alterations (point mutations, microsatellite instabilities, DNA hypermethylations and loses of heterozygosity), identical to the ones detected in the primary tumor tissue, were detected in extracellular DNA [12–14]. The study Gray et al. analyzing extracellular DNA in metastatic melanoma patients showed that lower extracellular DNA levels prior to treatment significantly correlated with response to therapy and prolonged progression free survival, regardless to therapy type. Moreover, detection of circulating mutant *NRAS* preceded radiological detection of disease progression [12]. Similarly, quantitative analysis of tumor associated mutant *BRAF* extracellular DNA revealed that higher overall response rate to BRAF inhibitors and longer progression free survival were seen in melanoma patients with lower concentration of basal mutant *BRAF* extracellular DNA [15, 16]. Tsao et al. also showed correlation between changes in extracellular DNA levels in melanoma patients and their disease status [17]. Fiegl et al. measured *RASSF1A* DNA methylation of extracellular DNA in the serum to monitor response of women with breast cancer and presence of *RASSF1A* methylation 1 year after primary surgery was evaluated as an independent predictor of poor outcome in these patients [18].

Due to significant differences in extracellular DNA levels between ovarian cancer patients before and after chemotherapy, we may suppose that the quantification of plasma DNA might serve as a new method to monitor effect of chemotherapy [19, 20]. Moreover, the extracellular DNA levels also correlate with time of recurrence in these patients [19]. The study Steffensen et al. evaluating 144 patients with epithelial ovarian carcinoma treated with bevacizumab showed significant association between high levels of extracellular DNA and shorter progression free survival and overall survival [21]. In addition, the treatment efficacy in ovarian carcinoma may be also monitored by detection of mutations in extracellular DNA. It was showed that 12 of 27 ovarian carcinoma patients had mutations of p53 in the cancer tissue. In 2 of those 12 cases identical mutations in the DNA of their preoperative plasma were detected. Interestingly, mutant DNA was undetected in after surgery follow-up of these two patients with p53 mutations in their extracellular DNA; however, in one case, the p53 mutation resurfaced 16 months after surgery [22]. Moreover, the predictive value of extracellular DNA was also revealed by studies showing that very high pre-operative plasma levels of extracellular *RAB25* were significantly associated with decreased patients' survival. Therefore, plasma levels of cfDNA may represent an independent predictor of death from ovarian cancer [4, 23].

Kamat et al. used an orthotopic ovarian cancer mouse model to determine the relationship between the kinetics of tumor-specific extracellular DNA and tumor growth. They found that extracellular DNA levels closely correlated with tumor burden and varied during treatment with two separate therapeutic regimens (cytotoxic chemotherapy and anti-angiogenic treatment with monoclonal antibodies). Specifically, the extracellular DNA levels rapidly declined after an initial rise. The peak in ecDNA levels was associated with an increase in the rate of apoptosis in treated ovarian tumors [11].

The higher abundance and shorter length of mitochondrial genome (mtDNA) as opposed to nuclear genome allow the suggestion that the amount of circulating extracellular mtDNA should be higher than extracellular nuclear DNA. Thus quantification of the extracellular mtDNA may increase sensitivity of this method [24, 25]. Moreover, presence of mtDNA in circulation may inform on cellular stress and cellular senescence [26]. The study Zachariah et al. showed that levels of extracellular mtDNA and nuclear DNA in plasma of patients with epithelial ovarian cancer were significantly elevated in comparison to healthy controls amd patients with benign ovarian lesions. However, no correlation between extracellular mtDNA a nuclear DNA was found [24].

Whether total circulating DNA, which can be assessed much easier without knowing the tumor-specific mutations, has similar informative value is currently unknown. The aim of this study was to evaluate the prognostic value of the quantity of extracellular DNA in advanced ovarian cancer.

Results

Patients' characteristics

Patients' characteristics are shown in Table 1. This prospective study included 67 patients with ovarian cancer treated with 1st line paclitaxel and carboplatin (25 pts) and paclitaxel, carboplatin and bevacizumab (42 pts). Thirty-five patients had optimal surgical debulking before

Table 1 Patients' characteristics

	N	%	Total extracellular DNA ng/mL median	*p*-value	Extracellular nuclear DNA ge/mL median	*p*-value	Extracellular mitochondrial DNA ge/mL median	*p*-value
All patients	67	100.0	8.3		2266		16,526	NA
Surgical Debulking								
Optimal	35	52.2	8.26	0.35	1944	0.13	11,422	0.09
Suboptimal	32	47.8	8.94		2584		20,297	
Histology								
Serous	53	79.1	9	0.31	2422	0.63	16,526	0.70
Other	14	20.9	6.16		1919		13,117	
Grade								
1 and 2	14	20.9	7.63	0.47	2083	0.49	16,470	0.90
3	41	61.2	8.32		2266		15,646	
Unknown	12	17.9						
Stage								
1	12	17.9	5.3	0.58	1862	0.45	8604	0.16
2	7	10.4	8.26		2422		16,526	
3	43	64.2	9		2455		17,575	
4	5	7.5	9.7		1736		16,413	
Stage								
1	12	17.9	5.3	0.19	1862	0.18	8604	0.03
2 to 4	55	82.1	9		2438		16,984	
		0.0						
Chemotherapy								
paclitaxel+carboplatin	25	37.3	6.26	0.21	1893	0.19	14,314	0.76
paclitaxel+carboplatin +bevacizumab	42	62.7	9.17		2447		16,755	

chemotherapy (less than 1 cm residual disease). Thirty three tumors with serous histology in our study were grade 3. Six patients with serous histology had stage I disease (grade 2 had 1 patient, grade 3 had 3 patients and 2 patients had unknown grading). Six patients had endometrioid tumors (three grade 3, two grade 2, one patient had unknown grading), one of them had stage I, one stage II and 4 had stage III, 4 patients had clear cell carcinoma, all grade III, 3 of them had stage I and the last had stage III. Three patients had mucinous carcinoma, two had stage I and one had stage III disease (1 patient grade 1, 2 patients had unknown grading). One patient had undifferentiated carcinoma, grade III, stage III.

Extracellular plasma DNA was quantified using real time PCR before administration of chemotherapy (67 pts) and after 6 cycles of chemotherapy (44 pts).

Association between cfDNA and patients/tumor characteristics

Total extracellular DNA (ecDNA), as well as extracellular DNA of nuclear (nDNA) and mitochondrial origin (mtDNA) significantly ($p < 0.05$) decreased after 6 cycles of chemotherapy (by 54%, 63% and 52%, respectively) (Table 2). Discrepancy between number of samples before treatment ($n = 67$) and after the 6 cycles of chemotherapy ($N = 44$) was due to logistic reason and was not related to disease/patient's characteristic, only 3 of 67 patients experienced disease progression before 6 cycles of chemotherapy. Patients with stage I disease had significantly lower mtDNA compared to patients with stage II-IV (8604 vs. 16, 984 ge/mL, $p = 0.03$). Pretreatment

Table 2 Comparison between pre-treatment and matched post-treatment extracellular DNA ($N = 44$)

	Pre-treatmnet (median)	After-treatment (median)	*p*-value
Total extracellularDNA (ng/mL)	7.4	3.4	0.002
Extracellular nuclear DNA (ge/mL)	2163.5	791.0	0.004
Extracellular mitochondrial DNA (ge/mL)	12,304.0	5915.5	0.001

Table 3 Prognostic value of pre-treatment extracellular DNA

Variable	PFS			OS		
	HR	95% CI	*p*-value	HR	95% CI	*p*-value
Total extracelular DNA	0.62	0.25–1.53	0.28	0.27	0.06–1.24	0.09
Extracellular nuclear DNA	0.35	0.14–0.86	0.02	0.18	0.04–0.77	0.06
Extracellular mitochondrial DNA	0.83	0.34–2.00	0.67	0.57	0.13–2.55	0.45

level of all cfDNA subtypes were significantly higher at baseline before chemotherapy compared to levels after 6 cycles of chemotherapy (Table 1).

Prognostic value of cfDNA

Median follow-up for all patients was 19.9 months (range: 0.2–34.2 months). Patients with lower baseline nDNA had superior progression-free (HR = 0.35 (0.14–0.86)) and overall survival (HR = 0.18 (0.04–0.77) (Table 3), while baseline total ecDNA and mtDNA were not prognostic for PFS nor for OS. In opposite patients with higher posttreatment mtDNA, but not total and nDNA, had inferior PFS compared to patients with lower posttreatment mtDNA (Table 4).

In multivariate analysis, the prognostic value of baseline nDNA was confirmed independent of tumor stage and debulking status (Table 5) while posttreatment mtDNA were not independent from tumor stage (data not shown).

Discussion

The presence of cfDNA within the plasma was initially reported by Mandel and Metais in 1948 [27, 28]. Currently there is a great interest in the potential use of cfDNA in many different areas of biomedical research, including cancer biomarker research [4, 29, 30]. Interestingly, cfDNA may serve as a surrogate marker in monitoring of NETs (neutrophil extracellular traps) playing role as procoagulant and prothrombotic factor in thrombosis. The study of Demers et al. revealed that malignant neutrophils are more prone to NET formation. This elevated sensitivity to NET generation suggests that malignant process through a systemic effect on the host can lead to increased NET formation and cancer-associated thrombosis [31]. Several studies have demonstrated that cancer patients have generally higher levels of total cfDNA (from both normal and malignant cells) compared to healthy individuals [23, 31, 32]. However, it is not yet clear whether the majority of cfDNA present in plasma of cancer patients is tumor-derived [33, 34]. The proportion of cfDNA originated from tumor tissue is not only associated by the state and size of the tumor [35], but also by clearance, degradation, lymphatic circulation, and other physiological blood processing tumor [6, 36, 37] Circulating tumor DNA (ctDNA) is characterized by specific genetic alterations such as methylation or mutation present in DNA of malignant cells [8]. Many studies have evaluated prognostic value of both cfDNA and ctDNA and investigated their role as a marker of response to therapy [13, 14, 19, 20]. Although reported data are abundant, results differ among studies. To the best our knowledge, only two meta-analyses have shown the diagnostic accuracy of quantitative analysis of cfDNA is at least the same as the conventional biomarkers for diagnosis of lung cancer [29, 38] and hepatocellular carcinoma [29, 36]. Moreover, meta-analysis published by Ocana et al. showed correlation between the high levels of cfDNA and the worse survival in solid tumors [37]. Screening biomarkers potentially used in diagnosis of ovarian cancer have been widely studied, but only few have satisfactory specificity and sensitivity for clinical applications [4]. Therefore, improving of early detection methods and finding of novel diagnostic biomarkers for ovarian cancer is highly warranted.

Table 4 Prognostic value of post-treatment extracellular DNA

Variable	PFS			OS		
	HR	95% CI	*p*-value	HR	95% CI	*p*-value
Total extracellular DNA(ng/mL)	1.23	0.41–3.68	0.72	0.88	0.14–5.4	0.89
Extracellular nuclear DNA (ge/mL)	0.7	0.23–2.16	0.51	0.97	0.16–5.83	0.97
Extracellular mitochondrial DNA (ge/mL)	3.45	1.16–10.24	0.04	0.41	0.07–2.49	0.27

Table 5 Multivariate analysis of factors associated with progression free survival

Variable	Progression-free survival (HR (95% C.I.), *P* – value)
Stage	
Stage IV vs. stage I	5.20 (0.44–61.89), *P* = 0.19
Stage III vs. stage I	2.18 (0.22–21.45), *P* = 0.50
Stage II vs. stage I	1.34 (0.08–22.94), *P* = 0.84
Debulking	
Suboptimal vs. optimal	1.79 (0.57–5.62). *P* = 0.32
Pre-treatment extracellular nuclear DNA (ng/mL)	
High vs. Low	3.11 (1.03–9.45). *P* = 0.045

In present translational study, we sought to define the prognostic value of various subtypes of cfDNA in ovarian cancer patients. The total ecDNA, as well as DNA and mtDNA was significantly decreased after 6 cycles of chemotherapy (by 54%, 63% and 52%, respectively). We also found that ovarian cancer patients with stage I disease had significantly lower mtDNA compared to patients with stage II-IV. Moreover, patients with lower baseline nDNA had superior progression-free survival. Patients with optimal debulking had better PFS and OS compared to patients with suboptimal debulking, interestingly, statistically significant difference in pre-chemotherapy extracellular DNA was not detected between optimally debulked and suboptimally debulked patients. In multivariate analysis was the prognostic value of nDNA confirmed independent of tumor stage and tumor debulking.

Recently, the quantitative analysis of circulating cf. DNA in ovarian cancer patients has attracted increasing attention. The meta-analysis published by Zhou et al. showed that quantitative analysis of cfDNA has poor sensitivity (0.70 (95% CI, 0.65–0.74) but acceptable specificity (0.90 (95% CI, 0.87–0.93) for diagnosis of ovarian cancer [29]. Data obtained in our study indicate that ecDNA of both, nuclear and mitochondrial origin could be added to prognostic markers in ovarian cancer. ecDNA as a prognostic marker has currently been evaluated in several solid tumors [39–42]. In patients with non-small cell lung cancer was found significant correlation between tumor progression and increasing plasma DNA [43]. Wei and colleagues reported the association between surgical resection of the tumor and significant decline in the Epstein-Barr virus (EBV) DNA copy numbers in nasopharyngeal carcinoma patients [40]. Moreover, significantly elevated pre-therapy plasma EBV DNA levels were also detected as a predictor of clinical outcome in nasopharyngeal carcinoma patients with early stage of disease [42]. The study Kamat et al. reported that preoperative levels of cfDNA were significantly increased in ovarian cancer patients compared to patients with benign ovarian disease and healthy controls. Moreover, high levels of ecDNA were associated with high-grade and high-stage of disease [4]. These data are consistent to our results, where ovarian cancer patients with stage I disease had significantly lower mtDNA when compared to patients with stage II-IV. Patients with lower baseline nDNA had superior progression-free and overall survival. On the other hand, although the study Zachariah et al. have reported increased levels of both ecDNA and mtDNA in patients with ovarian cancer compared to healthy controls, the association between ecDNA and prognosis was not confirmed [24]. Disparity between the extracellular mt DNA, nDNA and total DNA may be explained by different release mechanisms in the events of cell turnover in circulation [24]. In addition, our study also showed significant decline of ecDNA, as well as nDNA and mtDNA after 6 cycles of chemotherapy. Similar results were seen in study Kamat et al. using an orthotopic mouse model of ovarian cancer. In this study they have demonstrated that tumor-specific cfDNA correlated with tumor burden and levels decreased in response to chemotherapy [11]. Another study analyzing 144 patients with epithelial ovarian cancer treated with bevacizumab showed significantly shorted PFS and OS in patients with high levels of cfDNA in the blood [21]. Interestingly, it was showed that absolute amounts of cfDNA analyzed in cancer patients vary between different studied and whether the DNA is isolated by plasma-based or serum-based assays. cfDNA derived from plasma samples showed higher level of sensitivity but lower level of specificity. While Zhou et al. concluded that the best source for reliable cfDNA detection cannot be determined by current evidence; Thijssen et al. supposed that cfDNA isolated from plasma samples better reflects the in vivo levels of cfDNA [29, 44]. Furthermore ROC curves of cfDNA presented by Shao et al. revealed that the sensitivity and specificity of serum cfDNA levels were 88.9 and 89.5%, while cfDNA combined with CA125 and HE-4 impoved sensitivity up to 91.67% [45]. Storage of cfDNA (EDTA or citrate) and centrifugation speed by isolation of cfDNA may also affect detection levels of cfDNA [41, 46]. These factors may also represent the limitations of our study. In addition, our study did not compare the diagnostic value of cfDNA with other diagnostic markers (eg. CA125), thus could not compare its diagnostic accurancy with clinically used diagnostic markers for ovarian cancer.

Conclusions

In conclusion, our data suggest that ecDNA of both, nuclear and mitochondrial origin could be added to prognostic markers in ovarian cancer, however further studies with larger sample size are needed to define their role in the context of existing prognostic markers. Analysis of ecDNA does not require the knowledge of tumor-specific mutations in contrast to the quantification of tumor-derived ecDNA. Study of the dynamics and cell type-specific source of the ecDNA could shed light on its biology in cancer and might help to direct the treatment of ovarian cancer.

Methods

Patients

Into this translational study were included 67 patients with ovarian cancer treated with first line chemotherapy from February 2014 to March 2016 in the National Cancer Institute in Slovakia. Patients with concurrent malignancy other than non-melanoma skin cancer in the previous 5 years were excluded. All patients were chemo-naïve. Median time between last surgery and blood draw for analysis was 20 days (range: 7–108 days). All patients were treated with primary cytoreductive surgery, no patients with neoadjuvant chemotherapy were included. In all patients, data regarding age, tumor histology, clinical stage, type/number of metastatic sites and delivery of systemic therapy were recorded and compared with extracellular DNA levels. The study was approved by the Institutional Review Board (IRB) of the National Cancer Institute of Slovakia. All patients enrolled into this study gave informed consent.

Plasma isolation

Total venous peripheral blood volume (12 mL) was collected in EDTA-treated tubes and centrifuged at 1000 g for 10 min at room temperature within 2 h of venipuncture. To avoid cellular contamination, plasma was carefully harvested and centrifuged again at 1000 g for 10 min at room temperature. The cell-free plasma samples were cryopreserved at − 80 °C until further analyses.

Circulating plasma DNA measurement

Plasma samples were re-centrifuged at 16000×g and 4 °C to pellet the cellular debris. The final supernatant (200 μl) was used for plasma ecDNA isolation (QIAamp DNA Blood Mini Kit, Qiagen, Hilden, Germany). The concentration of total ecDNA was measured fluorometrically using Qubit 2.0 Fluorometer and the dsDNA HS Assay kit (Thermo Fisher Scientific, Wilmington, DE, USA). Real time PCR targeting the nuclear beta globin gene and the mitochondrial cytochrome b gene was used for the quantification of ecDNA of nuclear and mitochondrial origin as described previously [31]. The QuantiTect SYBR Green PCR Kit (Qiagen, Hilden, Germany) and the MasterCycler RealPlex cycler (Eppendorf, Hamburg, Germany) were used the real time PCR analysis. The efficiency of both reactions was between 90 and 110% and the resulting Ct values were used for the calculation of genome equivalents (GE) per ml of plasma. All PCR products were checked using the melting curve analysis to ensure a single product was amplified.

Statistical analysis

The characteristics of the cohort were summarized using the median (range) for continuous variables and frequency (percentage) for categorical variables. Normality of distribution was tested using the Kolmogorov-Smirnoff test. For normally distributed data, differences between the groups were tested using the Student *t*-test or analysis of variance (ANOVA) with corrections according to Bonferroni or Tamhane depending on the homogeneity of variance. The nonparametric Mann-Whitney *U* test was used for non-normally distributed data. Pearson or Spearman correlations test was used according to the normality of data. Categorical data were tested using the Fisher's exact test or Chi square test.

Median follow-up period was calculated as a median observation time among all patients and among those still alive at the time of their last follow-up. Progression-free survival (PFS) was calculated from the date of the starting treatment with chemotherapy to the date of progression or death or the date of the last adequate follow-up. Overall survival (OS) was calculated from the date of starting treatment with chemotherapy to the date of death or last follow-up. Survival rates were estimated using the Kaplan-Meier product limit method and were compared with the log-rank test to determine significance. cfDNA level data were dichotomized into high and low groups based on the cfDNA level median value of all samples. A multivariate Cox proportional hazards model for PFS and OS was used to assess differences in outcome on the basis of cfDNA level, debulking status and stage of disease. All *p*-values presented are two-sided and were considered significant if less than 0.05. Statistical analyses were performed using NCSS 2007 software (Hintze J, 2007, Kaysville, UT, USA).

Acknowledgements

We would like to acknowledge our collaborators Mrs. Alzbeta Jancikova and Mrs. Zlatica Pekova from Department of Oncology, National Cancer Institute of Slovakia for administration support and Mrs. Daniela Jantekova from the Population Registry of Slovak Republic for help with updating patients' database.

Funding

This publication is the result of the implementation of project no. APVV-16-0010 funded by the Slovak Research and Development Agency.

Authors' contributions

All the authors participated in the conception and design, acquisition, analysis and interpretation of data. K-K and M-M drafted the article and all authors revised it critically for important intellectual content. All the authors give the final approval of the version to be published. K-K and T-M share first authorship.

Competing interests

The authors declare that they have no competing interests.

Author details

[1]2nd Department of Oncology, Faculty of Medicine, Comenius University and National Cancer Institute, Klenova 1, 833 10 Bratislava, Slovak Republic. [2]Translational Research Unit, Faculty of Medicine, Comenius University, Bratislava, Slovakia. [3]National Cancer Institute, Bratislava, Slovakia. [4]Institute of Molecular Biomedicine, Faculty of Medicine, Comenius University, Bratislava, Slovakia.

References

1. Siegel RL, Miller KD, Jemal A. Cancer statistics, 2015. CA Cancer J Clin. 2015; 65(1):5–29.
2. Jelovac D, Armstrong DK. Recent progress in the diagnosis and treatment of ovarian cancer. CA Cancer J Clin. 2011;61(3):183–203.

3. Ahmed FY, Wiltshaw E, A'Hern RP, Nicol B, Shepherd J, Blake P, Fisher C, et al. Natural history and prognosis of untreated stage I epithelial ovarian carcinoma. J Clin Oncol. 1996;14:2968–75.
4. Kamat AA, Baldwin M, Urbauer D, Dang D, Han LY, Godwin A, et al. Plasma cell-free DNA in ovarian cancer: an independent prognostic biomarker. Cancer. 2010;116(8):1918–25.
5. Berek J, Hacker N. Practical gynecologic oncology. 3rd ed. Philadelphia: Lippincott Williams & Wilkins; 2000.
6. Francis G, Stein S. Circulating cell-free tumour DNA in the Management of Cancer. Int J Mol Sci. 2015;16(6):14122–42.
7. Murtaza M, Dawson SJ, Tsui DW, Gale D, Forshew T, Piskorz AM, et al. Non-invasive analysis of acquired resistance to cancer therapy by sequencing of plasma DNA. Nature. 2013;497(7447):108–12.
8. Marzese DM, Hirose H, Hoon DS. Diagnostic and prognostic value of circulating tumor-related DNA in cancer patients. Expert Rev Mol Diagn. 2013;13(8):827–44.
9. Schwarzenbach H, Hoon DS, Pantel K. Cell-free nucleic acids as biomarkers in cancer patients. Nat Rev Cancer. 2011;11(6):426–37.
10. Traver S, Assou S, Scalici E, Haouzi D, Al-Edani T, Belloc S, et al. Cell-free nucleic acids as non-invasive biomarkers of gynecological cancers, ovarian, endometrial and obstetric disorders and fetal aneuploidy. Hum Reprod Update. 2014;20(6):905–23.
11. Kamat AA, Bischoff FZ, Dang D, Baldwin MF, Han LY, Lin YG, et al. Circulating cell-free DNA: a novel biomarker for response to therapy in ovarian carcinoma. Cancer Biol Ther. 2006;5(10):1369–74.
12. Gray ES, Rizos H, Reid AL, Boyd SC, Pereira MR, Lo J, et al. Circulating tumor DNA to monitor treatment response and detect acquired resistance. Oncotarget. 2015;6(39):42008–18.
13. Bettegowda C, Sausen M, Leary RJ, Kinde I, Wang Y, Agrawal N, et al. Detection of circulating tumor DNA in early- and late-stage human malignancies. Sci Transl Med. 2014;6:224ra24.
14. Heitzer E, Ulz P, Geigl JB. Circulating tumor DNA as aliquid biopsy for cancer. Clin Chem. 2015;1:112–23.
15. Ascierto PA, Minor D, Ribas A, Lebbe C, O'Hagan A, Arya N, et al. Phase II trial (BREAK-2) of the BRAF inhibitor dabrafenib (GSK2118436) in patients with metastatic melanoma. J Clin Oncol. 2013;31:3205–11.
16. Sanmamed MF, Fernandez-Landazuri S, Rodriguez C, Zarate R, Lozano MD, Zubiri L, et al. Quantitative cell-free circulating BRAFV600E mutation analysis by use of droplet digital PCR in the follow-up of patients with melanoma being treated with BRAF inhibitors. Clin Chem. 2015;61:297–304.
17. Tsao SC, Weiss J, Hudson C, Christophi C, Cebon J, Behren A, et al. Monitoring response to therapy in melanoma by quantifying circulating tumour DNA with droplet digital PCR for BRAF and NRAS mutations. Sci Rep. 2015;5:11198.
18. Fiegl H, Millinger S, Mueller-Holzner E, Marth C, Ensinger C, Berger A, et al. Circulating tumor-specific DNA: a marker for monitoring efficacy of adjuvant therapy in cancer patients. Cancer Res. 2005;65:1141–5.
19. Cheng X, Zhang L, Chen Y, Qing C. Circulating cell free and circulating tumor cells, the "liquid biopsies" in ovarian cancer. J Ovarian Res. 2017;10(1): 75. https://doi.org/10.1186/s13048-017-0369-5.
20. Capizzi E, Gabusi E, Grigioni AD, De Iaco P, Rosati M, Zamagni C, et al. Quantification of free plasma DNA before and after chemotherapy in patients with advanced epithelial ovarian cancer. Diagn Mol Pathol. 2008; 17(1):34–8.
21. Steffensen KD, Madsen CV, Andersen RF, Waldstrom M, Adimi P, Jakobsen A. Prognostic importance of cell-free DNA in chemotherapy resistant ovarian cancer treated with bevacizumab. Eur J Cancer. 2014;50(15):2611–8.
22. Otsuka J, Okuda T, Sekizawa A, Amemiya S, Saito H, Okai T, et al. Detection of p53 mutations in the plasma DNA of patients with ovarian cancer. Int J Gynecol Cancer. 2004;14(3):459–64.
23. No JH, Kim K, Park KH, Kim YB. Cell-free DNA level as a prognostic biomarker for epithelial ovarian cancer. Anticancer Res. 2012;32(8):3467–71.
24. Zachariah RR, Schmid S, Buerki N, Radpour R, Holzgreve W, Zhong X. Levels of circulating cell-free nuclear and mitochondrial DNA in benign and malignant ovarian tumors. Obstet Gynecol. 2008;112(4):843–50.
25. Chiu RW, Chan LY, Lam NY, Tsui NB, Ng EK, Rainer TH, et al. Quantitative analysis of circulating mitochondrial DNA in plasma. Clin Chem. 2003;49: 719–26.
26. Yu M. Circulating cell-free mitochondial DNA as a novel cancer biomarker: opportunities and challenges. Mitochondrial DNA. 2012;23(5):329–32.
27. Ebell MH, Culp MB, Radke TJ. A systematic review of symptoms for the diagnosis of ovarian Cancer. Am J Prev Med. 2015. https://doi.org/10.1016/j.amepre.2015.09.023.
28. Mandel P. Metais P. C R Seances Soc Biol Fil. 1948;142(3–4):241–3.
29. Zhou Q, Li W, Leng B, Zheng W, He Z, Zuo M, et al. Circulating cell free DNA as the diagnostic marker for ovarian Cancer: a systematic review and meta-analysis. PLoS One. 2016;11(6):e0155495.
30. Karampini E, McCaughan F. Circulating DNA in solid organ cancers-analysis and clinical application. QJM. 2016;109(4):223–7.
31. Nawroz H, Koch W, Anker P, Stroun M, Sidransky D. Microsatellite alterations in serum DNA of head and neck cancer patients. Nat Med. 1996;2:1035–7.
32. Wu TL, Zhang D, Chia JH, Tsao K, Sun CF, Wu JT. Cell-free DNA: measurement in various carcinomas and establishment of normal reference range. Clin Chim Acta. 2002;321:77–87.
33. Stroun M, Maurice P, Vasioukhin V, Lyautey J, Lederrey C, Lefort F, et al. The origin and mechanism of circulating DNA. Ann N Y Acad Sci. 2000;906:161–8.
34. Anker P, Mulcahy H, Chen XQ, Stroun M. Detection of circulating tumor DNA in the blood (plasma/serum) of cancer patients. Cancer Metastasis Rev. 1999;18:65–73.
35. Cheng X, Zhang L, Chen Y, Qing C. Circulating cell-free DNA and circulating tumor cells, the "liquid biopsies" in ovarian cancer. J Ovarian Res. 2017;10:75.
36. Liao W, Mao Y, Ge P, Yang H, Xu H, Lu X, et al. Value of quantitative and qualitative analyses of circulating cell-free DNA as diagnostic tools for hepatocellular carcinoma: a meta-analysis. Medicine. 2015. https://doi.org/10.1097/MD.0000000000000722.
37. Ocana A, Diez-Gonzalez L, Garcia-Olmo DC, Templeton AJ, Vera-Badillo F, Jose Escribano M, et al. Circulating DNA and survival in solid tumors. Cancer Epidemiol Biomark Prev. 2016;25(2):399–406.
38. Zhang R, Shao F, Wu X, Ying K. Value of quantitative analysis of circulating cell free DNA as a screening tool for lung cancer: a meta-analysis. Lung Cancer. 2010;69(2):225–31.
39. Malkasian GD Jr, Knapp RC, Lavin PT, Zurawski VR Jr, Podratz KC, Stanhope CR, et al. Preoperative evaluation of serum CA125 levels in premenopausal and postmenopausal patients with pelvic masses: discrimination of benign from malignant disease. Am J Obstet Gynecol. 1988;159:341–6.
40. Wei WI, Yuen AP, Ng RW, Kwong DL, Sham JS. Quantitative analysis of plasma cell-free Epstein-Barr virus DNA in nasopharyngeal carcinoma after salvage nasopharyngectomy: a prospective study. Head Neck. 2004;26:878–83.
41. Chiu RWK, Poon LLM. Effects of blood-processing protocols on fetal and total DNA quantification in maternal plasma. Clin Chem. 2001;47:1607–13.
42. Leung SF, Chan AT, Zee B, Ma B, Chan LY, Johnson PJ, et al. Pretherapy quantitative measurement of circulating Epstein-Barr virus DNA is predictive of posttherapy distant failure in patients with early-stage nasopharyngeal carcinoma of undifferentiated type. Cancer. 2003;98:288–91.
43. Gautschi O, Bigosch C, Huegli B, Jermann M, Marx A, Chassé E, et al. Circulating deoxyribonucleic acid as a prognostic marker in non-small cell lung cancer patients undergoing chemotherapy. J Clin Oncol. 2004;22:4157–64.
44. Thijssen MA, Swinkles DW, Ruers TJ, de Kok JB. Difference between free circulating plasma and serum DNA in patients with colorectal cancer metastasis. Anticancer Res. 2002;22:421–5.
45. Shao X, He Y, Ji M, Chen X, Qi J, Shi W, et al. Quantitative analysis of cell-free DNA in ovarian cancer. Oncol Lett. 2015;10:3478–82.
46. Shao XF, Ji M, Chen XF, Qi J, Shi W, Zhu ZL, et al. Evaluation of cell-free DNA detection in supplementary diagnosis of ovarian cancer. Chin J Clin Lab Sci. 2014;32(11):821–4.

Mitochondrial membrane depolarization enhances TRAIL-induced cell death in adult human granulosa tumor cells, KGN, through inhibition of *BIRC5*

Julie A. MacDonald, Niharika Kura, Carleigh Sussman and Dori C. Woods*

Abstract

Background: Cellular metabolic changes that accompany malignant transformation have been heralded as hallmark features of cancer. However, metabolic signatures between neoplasms can be unique, allowing for distinctions in malignancy, invasion and chemoresistance between cancer types and subtypes. Mitochondria are central metabolic mediators, as cellular bioenergetics veers from oxidative phosphorylation to glycolysis. Herein, we evaluate the role of mitochondria in maintenance of cellular metabolism, proliferation, and survival in the adult granulosa tumor cell line, KGN, as well as three epithelial ovarian cancer cell lines to determine distinctions in specific features.

Results: Notably, KGN cells were susceptible to TRAIL- and cisplatin-induced death following pretreatment with the metabolic inhibitor FCCP, but not oligomycin A. Collapse of mitochondrial membrane potential was found concomitant with cell death via apoptosis, independent from extrinsic canonical apoptotic routes. Rather, treatment with FCCP resulted in elevated cytochrome c release from mitochondria and decreased responsiveness to *BIRC5*. Following knockdown of *BIRC5*, mitochondrial membrane depolarization further sensitized KGN cells to induction of apoptosis via TRAIL.

Conclusions: These results indicate an essential role, distinct from metabolism, for mitochondrial membrane potential in KGN cells to sense and respond to external mediators of apoptotic induction.

Keywords: Granulosa cell tumor, KGN, Mitochondria, Metabolism, TRAIL, BIRC5

Background

Among the subtypes of ovarian cancer, granulosa cell tumors (GCTs) of the ovary are relatively rare in occurrence, representing only approximately 2–5% of all ovarian neoplasms, yet represent the most common sex cord tumors [1]. This heterogeneous classification includes tumors derived from the stroma, rete ovarii, and developing ovarian follicles [1]. GCTs can be categorized as either adult (> 95%) or juvenile (< 5%) types, with adult GCTs (aGCTs) harboring a somatic missense mutation in the *FOXL2* gene, ($FOXL2^{C134W}$), which is not present in the rarer juvenile subtype [2]. Arguably pathogenic, the mechanisms by which $FOXL2^{C134W}$ drive tumorigenesis are not well characterized, but set this tumor type apart from not only the juvenile subtype, but ovarian cancers of epithelial origin as well [2–5]. Due to the relative paucity of information regarding the etiology, progression, and molecular properties of aGCTs given their comparatively infrequent manifestation, the prevailing therapeutic strategies used to treat aGCTs are derived from those used in treatment of more common epithelial ovarian cancers (EOCs), despite the distinct phenotype of aGCTs [6, 7]. Among the stark differences that distinguish GCTs from EOCs is the capacity of aGCTs to exhibit steroidogenesis associated with gonadotropin-responsiveness, categorizing aGCTs as endocrine tumors [4]. Consequently, unlike EOCs which

* Correspondence: d.woods@northeastern.edu
Laboratory for Aging and Infertility Research, Northeastern University, Boston, MA 02115, USA

can remain asymptomatic and evade detection until late-stage, the elevated estrogen synthesized by aGCTs initiates symptoms characteristic of estrogen excess, including menorrhagia and endometrial hyperplasia [8], resulting in earlier clinical detection than other ovarian cancers. However, recurrence is common and often delayed, with relapses occurring between 6– and 30–years from the initial diagnosis [9]. Accordingly, additional characterization of the aGCT response, as compared to EOCs, is an important consideration for the treatment of aGCTs.

Recent evidence from a number of cancer types highlights the cellular metabolic properties of tumor cells as a potential mediator of cancer growth and progression, metastasis, and evasion of chemotherapeutic-induced cell death. In cancer cells, a distinctive and near-universal trait is a metabolic switch in carbohydrate metabolism from oxidative phosphorylation (OXPHOS) to glycolysis [10]. While most normal cells generate ATP primarily from OXPHOS in aerobic conditions, tumor cells are more likely to synthesize ATP via conversion of glucose to lactate, and consequently exhibit a reduction in OXPHOS activity [11]. Although this metabolic shift to aerobic glycolysis at first glance appears to decrease energetic efficiency, it is believed the upregulation of glycolysis is a key step in carcinogenesis, providing a growth advantage to malignant cells capable of surviving a hypoxic microenvironment [12]. Malignant transformation is known to be associated with other alterations in mitochondrial function as well. For example, in normal cells a high mitochondrial membrane potential ($\Delta\psi_m$) reflects mitochondrial respiration and generation of ATP, whereas mitochondria in cancer cells demonstrate an aberrant $\Delta\psi_m$ [13]. These types of alterations in mitochondrial function specifically in cancer cells have raised prospects for therapeutic targeting of mitochondria in cancer cells. Notably, metabolic profiles defining OXPHOS vs glycolytic status for aGCT cells, as well as EOCs, have yet to be well- reported [14–17].

We have previously reported on the efficacy of the naturally occurring cytokine, tumor necrosis factor-related apoptosis-inducing ligand (TRAIL), to promote cell death in aGCTs under specific conditions [18, 19]. This is of particular interest, as evidence from primary cultured ovarian granulosa cells have demonstrated that under normal conditions, healthy granulosa cells are inherently resistant to TRAIL-induced apoptosis [20]. However, while treatment of aGCTs with TRAIL in combination with therapeutic agents such as cisplatin or proteasome inhibitors enhances TRAIL-induced cell death, this action is mediated largely through upregulation of death receptors (e.g., DR4 or DR5), and downstream effectors, such as p53, are not impacted [18, 19]. DR4 and DR5 are members of the tumor necrosis factor receptor (TNFR) superfamily [21], and are characterized by multiple cysteine-rich domains present within the extracellular domain, in addition to an intracellular death domain (DD) [22]. Following activation through TRAIL-binding, the DD links with Fas-associated death domain (FADD) protein, resulting in the formation of the apoptosis-inducing signaling complex (DISC) [23], which subsequently leads to activation of caspase-8, which cleaves bid and triggers the release of cytochrome c from the mitochondria into the cytosol [24], triggering the caspase cascade that ultimately results in cellular apoptosis. However, the ability of TRAIL to readily induce apoptosis is diminished, as the TRAIL-induced caspase cascade is opposed by pro-survival proteins, namely the inhibitor of apoptosis (IAP) family, which includes Survivin, also called baculoviral inhibitor of apoptosis repeat-containing 5 (BIRC5). Notably, BIRC5 is a potent inhibitor of caspase activation, and when present, actively promotes cell survival through inhibition of caspase-induced apoptosis. Moreover, and perhaps not surprisingly, BIRC5 levels are elevated in tumors as compared to normal tissues [25]. Additionally, BIRC5 is thought to play an important role in mediating aerobic glycolysis in cancer cells through suppression of OXPHOS, which occurs, at least in part, through inhibition of respiratory complex-I [26].

The disruption of mitochondria-driven metabolism, as well as mitochondria-mediated pro-apoptotic cascades, has been well-characterized in many models of cancer, although not yet including aGCTs. A better understanding of the molecular characteristics of aGCT metabolism, as well as the response to traditional therapeutics, could serve to inform novel therapies which specifically target aGCTs. Herein, we evaluated the metabolic profile of three human EOC cell lines, SKOV3, OVCAR3, and Kuramochi, as well as KGN, a well-established human aGCT cell line heterozygous for the *FOXL2*^{C134W} mutation. Through the use of metabolic inhibitors, we investigated the role of KGN metabolism in survival following treatment with either TRAIL or cisplatin, and determined an essential role for $\Delta\psi m$ in the opposition of pro-apoptotic signals.

Results

Metabolism of ovarian cancer cell lines and impact of metabolic inhibitors on adult granulosa tumor cell line (KGN) culture viability

Epithelial ovarian cancer cell lines assayed for total cellular ATP content following a 6-h incubation with glycolysis inhibitor, 2-deoxy-d-glucose (2-DG), or oxidative phosphorylation inhibitor, oligomycin A, were heterogeneous in metabolic profiles (Fig. 1). SKOV3 cells demonstrated reduced ATP content as compared to vehicle treated cells following a high dose of 2-DG, indicating

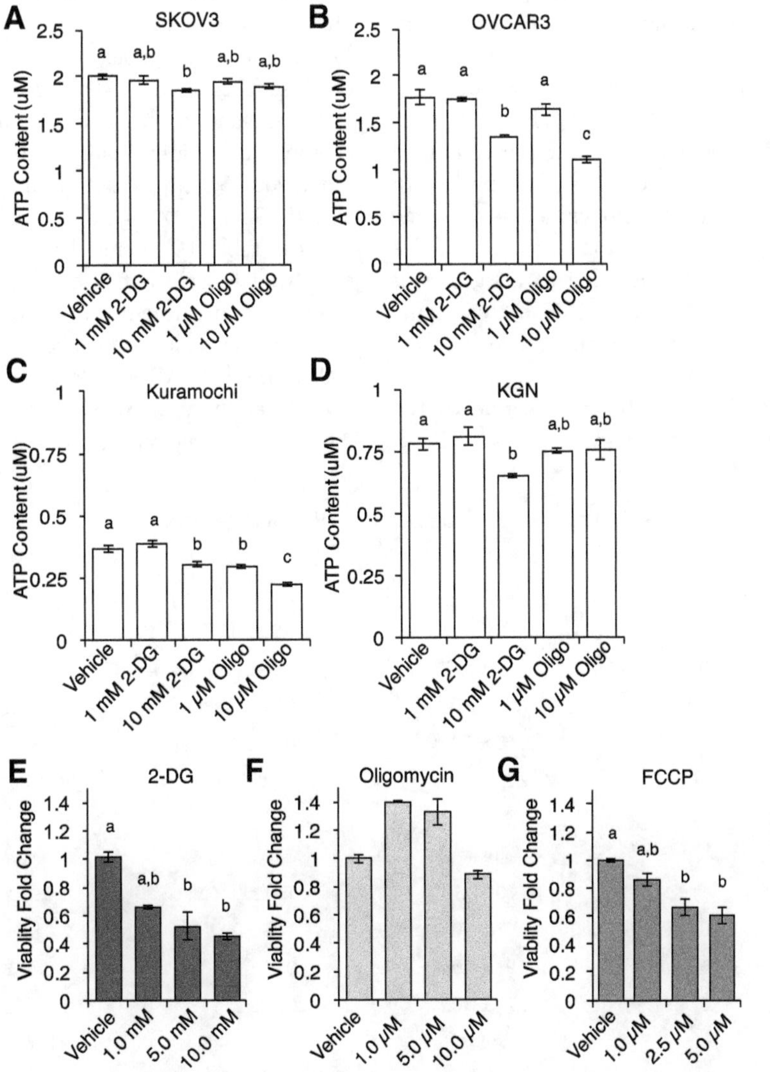

Fig. 1 Metabolism of ovarian cancer cell lines and impact of metabolic inhibitors on adult granulosa tumor cell line (KGN) culture viability. Dynamics of metabolism of ovarian cancer cell lines was analyzed through disruption of both glycolysis and oxidative phosphorylation (OXPHOS). Total cellular ATP content was analyzed following 6-h treatments with glycolysis inhibitor 2-deoxy-d-glucose (2-DG) or OXPHOS inhibitor, oligomycin A (Oligo), where indicated conditions annotated with different letters indicates statistical significance between conditions of at least $P < 0.05$. **a** SKOV3 cells had significantly reduced total cellular ATP following treatment with 10 mM 2-DG. **b** OVCAR3 cells and (**c**) Kuramochi cells decreased in ATP content following treatment with high doses of both 2-DG and Oligo. **d** KGN cells had a significant decrease in total cellular ATP levels after treatment with 10 mM 2-DG. **e** Treatment with 5 mM and 10 mM 2-DG over 24 h significantly decreased KGN culture viability, as measured by MTS assay. **f** Treatment with oligomycin A for 24 showed no changes in KGN culture viability, whereas treatment with the respiratory chain uncoupler carbonyl cyanide-4-(trifluoromethoxy)phenylhydrazone (FCCP; **g**) significantly decreased culture viability at both 2.5 μM and 5.0 μM after 24 h

glycolytic metabolism (Vehicle: 1.99 ± 0.03 μM; 10 mM 2-DG: 1.85 ± 0.02 μM, $P < 0.05$; Fig. 1a). Treatment with either inhibitor resulted in a reduction in ATP content in both OVCAR3 and Kuramochi (OVCAR3: Vehicle: 1.77 ± 0.08 μM; 10 mM 2-DG: 1.36 ± 0.01, $P < 0.01$; 10 μM Oligomycin: 1.11 ± 0.03, $P < 0.01$, $n = 3$; Fig. 1b. Kuramochi: Vehicle: 0.37 ± 0.01 μM; 10 mM 2-DG: 0.30 ± 0.01, $P < 0.01$; 10 μM Oligomycin: 0.22 ± 0.01, $P < 0.01$, $n = 3$; Fig. 1c). In KGN, total cellular ATP content was significantly decreased as compared to vehicle-treated controls following a 6-h incubation with the glycolysis inhibitor 2-DG (Vehicle: 0.78 ± 0.02 μM; 10 mM 2-DG: 0.65 ± 0.01 μM, $P < 0.05$, $n = 3$), with no change in samples treated with the oxidative phosphorylation inhibitor oligomycin A (10 μM Oligomycin A; 0.75 ± 0.04 μM, $n = 3$), consistent with glycolytic metabolism (Fig. 1d).

Culture viability of KGN cells was assayed using a MTS assay following 24-h treatments with metabolic inhibitors. Following treatment with 2-DG (Fig. 1e), viability of KGN cells was significantly reduced as compared to vehicle controls at both 5 mM and 10 mM doses (5 mM: 0.52 ± 0.12-fold change, $P < 0.05$; 10 mM: 0.45 ± 0.06-fold change, $P < 0.01$, $n = 3$). However, after 24-h treatments with oligomycin A, viability remained unchanged ($n = 9$; Fig. 1f). Interestingly, treatment with carbonyl cyanide-4-(trifluoromethoxy)phenylhydrazone (FCCP; Fig. 1g), a metabolic inhibitor which uncouples $\Delta\psi_m$ from ATP synthesis [27], also led to a significant reduction in culture viability following 24-h treatments at 2.5 μm and 5.0 μM as compared to vehicle controls (2.5 μM: 0.66 ± 0.06-fold change, $P < 0.01$; 5.0 μM: 0.60 ± 0.06-fold change, $P < 0.01$, $n = 9$), of note due to the otherwise glycolytic nature of the cells.

Metabolic inhibitors sensitize KGN cells to cytotoxicity via TRAIL or cisplatin

Pretreatment with metabolic inhibitors FCCP or oligomycin A sensitized KGN cells, which are otherwise predominately resistant, to cell death induction by TRAIL or the chemotherapeutic cisplatin (Table 1). Following pretreatment with 5.0 μM FCCP, KGN cells treated with either TRAIL (50 and 100 ng mL^{-1}; Table 1A) or cisplatin (1 and 10 μM; Table 1B), demonstrated reduced cell viability as compared to vehicle-treated controls. Additionally, oligomycin A pretreatment sensitized KGN cells to significant decreases in culture viability following treatment with 100 ng ml^{-1} TRAIL (Table 1C) or 10 μM cisplatin (Table 1D). When these assays were performed in the ovarian epithelial carcinoma cell lines SKOV3 (Table 2), Kuramochi

Table 1 Metabolic inhibition sensitize KGN cultures to cytotoxicity via TRAIL and cisplatin

A		TRAIL			
		Untreated	50 ng/mL	100 ng/mL	ANOVA
FCCP (μM)	Vehicle	1.00 ± 0.01[a]	0.83 ± 0.06[a*]	0.97 ± 0.04[a]	0.0206
	1.0	0.94 ± 0.02[a]	0.84 ± 0.06[a,b]	0.85 ± 0.04[a,b]	0.1921
	2.5	0.74 ± 0.05[b]	0.74 ± 0.04[b]	0.74 ± 0.04[b]	0.9967
	5.0	0.68 ± 0.05[b]	0.44 ± 0.02[c]	0.49 ± 0.06[c*]	0.0327
ANOVA		2.30E-06	2.82E-06	7.48E-08	
B		Cisplatin			
		Untreated	1 μM	10 μM	ANOVA
FCCP (μM)	Vehicle	1.00 ± 0.10[a]	1.21 ± 0.16[a]	0.98 ± 0.06[a]	0.3321
	1.0	0.93 ± 0.07[a]	1.03 ± 0.12[a]	0.81 ± 0.03[b]	0.1766
	2.5	0.91 ± 0.03[a]	0.97 ± 0.16[a]	0.79 ± 0.01[b]	0.4927
	5.0	0.79 ± 0.03[a]	0.89 ± 0.08[a]	0.59 ± 0.03[c*]	0.0155
ANOVA		0.1798	0.427	0.0005	
C		TRAIL			
		Untreated	50 ng/mL	100 ng/mL	ANOVA
Oligomycin (μM)	Vehicle	1.00 ± 0.05[a]	1.15 ± 0.08[a]	0.96 ± 0.02[a]	0.1381
	1.0	0.99 ± 0.08[a]	1.01 ± 0.03[a]	0.81 ± 0.01[b]	0.0511
	2.5	1.00 ± 0.07[a]	0.97 ± 0.01[a]	0.82 ± 0.02[b*]	0.0368
	5.0	1.06 ± 0.02[a]	0.97 ± 0.03[a]	0.83 ± 0.02[b*]	0.0013
ANOVA		0.8191	0.0827	0.0013	
D		Cisplatin			
		Untreated	1 μM	10 μM	ANOVA
Oligomycin (μM)	Vehicle	1.00 ± 0.05[a]	0.85 ± 0.04[a]	0.65 ± 0.07[a]	0.0144
	1.0	1.08 ± 0.06[a]	1.03 ± 0.08[a]	0.84 ± 0.02[b]	0.0548
	2.5	1.03 ± 0.03[a]	1.05 ± 0.07[a]	0.83 ± 0.02[b*]	0.0293
	5.0	0.98 ± 0.02[a]	0.94 ± 0.03[a]	0.77 ± 0.06[b*]	0.0206
ANOVA		0.4821	0.161	0.0802	

Resistance of KGN cultures to cell death inducing agents TRAIL or cisplatin was analyzed through inhibition of OXPHOS using oligomycin A and a mitochondrial membrane potential uncoupler, FCCP, using MTS viability assays. Results are presented as fold change to vehicle treated control cultures with differing letters indicating significant ($p < 0.05$) changes in viability with treatment of inhibitor, and asterisks (* $p < 0.05$) indicating significant changes in viability with treatment of cytotoxic agent. (**A**) Sequential treatment with FCCP and TRAIL resulted in decreases in culture viability over control samples. (**B**) Culture viability also decreased with FCCP treatment prior to addition of cisplatin. (**C**) Oligomycin A pretreatment sensitized KGN cells to both TRAIL and (**D**) cisplatin

Table 2 Metabolic inhibitors sensitize SKOV3 cultures to cytotoxicity via TRAIL or cisplatin

A		TRAIL			
		Untreated	50 ng/mL	100 ng/mL	ANOVA
FCCP (μM)	Vehicle	1.00 ± 0.02[a]	0.90 ± 0.06[a]	0.93 ± 0.02[a]	0.1901
	1.0	0.98 ± 0.04[a]	0.85 ± 0.04[a*]	0.90 ± 0.02[a]	0.0448
	2.5	0.94 ± 0.03[a]	0.75 ± 0.04[a**]	0.79 ± 0.01[b**]	0.0011
	5.0	0.91 ± 0.02[a]	0.69 ± 0.03[b**]	0.72 ± 0.02[b**]	7.16E-05
ANOVA		0.1335	0.0143	1.28E-06	
B		Cisplatin			
		Untreated	1 μM	10 μM	ANOVA
FCCP (μM)	Vehicle	1.00 ± 0.01[a]	0.95 ± 0.07[a]	1.07 ± 0.04[a]	0.2609
	1.0	0.96 ± 0.04[a,b]	0.85 ± 0.03[a]	0.99 ± 0.04[a]	0.1036
	2.5	0.85 ± 0.00[b,c]	0.91 ± 0.05[a]	0.95 ± 0.04[a]	0.2008
	5.0	0.80 ± 0.02[c]	0.78 ± 0.04[a]	0.88 ± 0.02[b]	0.1185
ANOVA		0.0012	0.1549	0.0384	
C		TRAIL			
		Untreated	50 ng/mL	100 ng/mL	ANOVA
Oligomycin (μM)	Vehicle	1.0 ± 0.04[a]	0.97 ± 0.04[a]	0.95 ± 0.02[a]	0.5931
	1.0	0.90 ± 0.01[a]	0.85 ± 0.01[a]	0.80 ± 0.01[b**]	0.006
	2.5	0.96 ± 0.04[a]	0.82 ± 0.05[a]	0.81 ± 0.00[b]	0.0483
	5.0	0.86 ± 0.03[a]	0.82 ± 0.08[a]	0.84 ± 0.04[b]	0.9093
ANOVA		0.0507	0.2121	0.0062	
Cisplatin					
		Untreated	1 μM	10 μM	ANOVA
Oligomycin (μM)	Vehicle	1.00 ± 0.03[a]	0.88 ± 0.09[a]	0.94 ± 0.02[a]	0.3459
	1.0	0.92 ± 0.02[a]	0.85 ± 0.01[a*]	0.84 ± 0.01[b*]	0.0129
	2.5	0.91 ± 0.02[b]	0.84 ± 0.03[a]	0.89 ± 0.01[a]	0.1578
	5.0	0.91 ± 0.00[b]	0.88 ± 0.03[a]	0.84 ± 0.03[b]	0.2232
ANOVA		0.0279	0.9114	0.0135	

Resistance of SKOV3 cultures to cell death inducing agents TRAIL or cisplatin was analyzed through inhibition of OXPHOS using oligomycin A and a mitochondrial membrane potential uncoupler, FCCP, using MTS viability assays. Results are presented as fold change to vehicle treated control cultures with differing letters indicating significant ($p < 0.05$) changes in viability with treatment of inhibitor, and asterisks indicating significant (* $p < 0.05$; ** $p < 0.01$) changes in viability with treatment of cytotoxic agent (**A**) Pretreatment with FCCP sensitized SKOV3 cultures to TRAIL, (**B**) but not cisplatin. (**C**) Culture viability was decreased with oligomycin A treatment prior to TRAIL, (**D**) as well as cisplatin

(Table 3), and OVCAR3 (Table 4), the trend of metabolic inhibition increasing sensitivity to cytotoxic agents was repeated, but was inconsistent between the cell lines. In SKOV3 cultures, cell viability was reduced following oligomycin A pretreatment, and subsequent treatment with either TRAIL or cisplatin (Table 2C-D), whereas pretreatment with FCCP sensitized cells to TRAIL (Table 2A), but not cisplatin (Table 2B). FCCP treatment also resulted in decreased viability in Kuramochi when treated in combination with TRAIL (Table 3A), but not with cisplatin (Table 3B). Interestingly, when treated with oligomycin A (Table 3C-D), Kuramochi cultures increased in viability, with the only significant decrease in cisplatin treated cells observed after pretreatment with 2.5 μM of oligomycin A (Table 3D). The OVCAR3 cell line was previously reported as TRAIL-sensitive [28], which was repeated herein (Table 4A, C), as well as a demonstrated sensitivity to cisplatin without metabolic inhibition (Table 4B, D). However, pretreatment with both FCCP and oligomycin further sensitized OVCAR3 cells to cisplatin treatment (Table 4B,D).

Combinatorial treatment with FCCP and TRAIL induces apoptosis and disrupts both cellular metabolism and $\Delta\psi_m$

Cells treated with the combination of FCCP and TRAIL were analyzed for extracellular expression of phosphatidylserine by antibody labeling with Annexin V to determine apoptotic induction (Fig. 2). Co-labeling with DAPI (Fig. 2a) indicated a high culture viability in vehicle control and single treatment wells (~ 85–90% viable, similar to that observed utilizing the MTS assays), with significant increases in both apoptotic cells

Table 3 FCCP pretreatment sensitize Kuramochi cultures to TRAIL and oligomycin A increases baseline Kuramochi culture viability

A		TRAIL			
		Untreated	50 ng/mL	100 ng/mL	ANOVA
FCCP (μM)	Vehicle	1.00 ± 0.08^{a}	1.00 ± 0.06^{a}	0.94 ± 0.07^{a}	0.7702
	1.0	$0.89 \pm 0.03^{a,b}$	$0.72 \pm 0.03^{b*}$	$0.74 \pm 0.03^{a*}$	0.009
	2.5	$0.74 \pm 0.03^{b,c}$	0.67 ± 0.02^{b}	$0.60 \pm 0.02^{b*}$	0.0233
	5.0	0.66 ± 0.02^{c}	0.58 ± 0.06^{b}	0.57 ± 0.05^{b}	0.3392
ANOVA		0.0035	0.0009	0.002	
B		Cisplatin			
		Untreated	1 μM	10 μM	ANOVA
FCCP (μM)	Vehicle	1.00 ± 0.06^{a}	0.97 ± 0.13^{a}	1.11 ± 0.02^{a}	0.5124
	1.0	0.89 ± 0.01^{a}	0.82 ± 0.10^{a}	0.85 ± 0.01^{b}	0.6946
	2.5	0.99 ± 0.09^{a}	0.78 ± 0.08^{a}	0.75 ± 0.01^{c}	0.0941
	5.0	0.90 ± 0.01^{a}	0.74 ± 0.10^{a}	$0.78 \pm 0.04^{b,c}$	0.23
ANOVA		0.3707	0.4635	7.78E-06	
C		TRAIL			
		Untreated	50 ng/mL	100 ng/mL	ANOVA
Oligomycin (μM)	Vehicle	1.00 ± 0.02^{a}	0.96 ± 0.14^{a}	1.08 ± 0.03^{a}	0.5539
	1.0	1.37 ± 0.00^{b}	1.15 ± 0.07^{a}	1.26 ± 0.07^{a}	0.093
	2.5	1.38 ± 0.12^{b}	1.14 ± 0.15^{a}	1.31 ± 0.04^{a}	0.353
	5.0	1.36 ± 0.05^{b}	1.19 ± 0.16^{a}	1.25 ± 0.05^{a}	0.535
ANOVA		0.0082	0.6272	0.0503	
D		Cisplatin			
		Untreated	1 μM	10 μM	ANOVA
Oligomycin (μM)	Vehicle	1.00 ± 0.01^{a}	0.99 ± 0.01^{a}	1.01 ± 0.02^{a}	0.6714
	1.0	$1.46 \pm 0.18^{a,b}$	1.29 ± 0.16^{a}	1.62 ± 0.03^{b}	0.3404
	2.5	1.83 ± 0.06^{b}	$1.21 \pm 0.04^{a**}$	$1.55 \pm 0.09^{b,c*}$	0.0014
	5.0	1.23 ± 0.08^{a}	1.10 ± 0.04^{a}	1.13 ± 0.02^{a}	0.2911
ANOVA		0.003	0.1401	4.23E-05	

Resistance of Kuramochi cultures to cell death inducing agents TRAIL or cisplatin was analyzed through inhibition of OXPHOS using oligomycin A and a mitochondrial membrane potential uncoupler, FCCP, using MTS viability assays. Results are presented as fold change to vehicle treated control cultures with differing letters indicating significant ($p < 0.05$) changes in viability with treatment of inhibitor, and asterisks indicating significant (* $p < 0.05$; ** $p < 0.01$) changes in viability with treatment of cytotoxic agent. (A) Pretreatment with FCCP resulted in reduced culture viability following treatment with TRAIL, (B) but not cisplatin. (C) Oligomycin treatment increased culture viability, when compared to vehicle, but did not sensitize Kuramochi cultures to TRAIL. (D) Pretreatment with 2.5 μM oligomycin A sensitized Kuramochi cultures to decrease viability following cisplatin treatment

($DAPI^{+}/FITC^{+}$; purple) as well as nonviable cells ($DAPI^{+}/FITC^{-}$; blue) following both FCCP and TRAIL (Fig. 2c). DAPI-positive events also increased when evaluating changes in global cellular metabolism utilizing the dye resazurin, which fluoresces when reduced, indicative of actively respiring cells [29] (Fig. 2b, d). These trends also occurred in the ovarian epithelial carcinoma line Kuramochi (Fig. 2e, f), but there were no statistical differences in apoptotic induction seen in SKOV3 cells following treatment with FCCP and TRAIL (Fig. 2g, h).

To confirm induction of apoptosis in KGN cells following treatment with FCCP and TRAIL, cells were fixed and evaluated for cytochrome c release via immunocytochemistry (Fig. 3). ATPB was used as an identifying marker for mitochondria (Fig. 3a, c), and cells were scored as having released cytochrome c via loss of colocalization with ATPB (Fig. 3b, c). In vehicle treated and TRAIL treated cells there was a low percentage of cells scored as having released cytochrome C (9.49 ± 0.98%, 10.79 ± 1.60%, respectively), but in both FCCP treated and dual treated cells there were significant increases in the population of cells with diffuse cytochrome c localization (59.05 ± 5.39%, $P < 0.05$, 58.17 ± 15.65%, $P < 0.05$, respectively, Fig. 3d).

As an additional characterization of apoptosis, $\Delta\psi_m$ was measured as the relative fluorescence of the $\Delta\psi_m$ dependent dye: JC-1. Following $\Delta\psi_m$-dependent accumulation within mitochondria, JC-1 J-aggregates fluoresce at ~ 590 nm (orange-red), whereas background fluorescence of JC-1 monomers fluoresce at ~ 525 nm

Table 4 FCCP and oligomycin pretreatment sensitize OVCAR3 cultures to cisplatin treatment

A		TRAIL			
		Untreated	50 ng/mL	100 ng/mL	ANOVA
FCCP (μM)	Vehicle	1.00 ± 0.12^{a}	$0.12 \pm 0.01^{a,b,c*}$	$0.07 \pm 0.02^{a*}$	0.0001
	1.0	0.98 ± 0.09^{a}	$0.21 \pm 0.06^{a,b*}$	$0.06 \pm 0.01^{a*}$	0.0001
	2.5	0.77 ± 0.08^{a}	$0.06 \pm 0.05^{a,b,c*}$	$0.00 \pm 0.02^{a,b*}$	0.0001
	5.0	0.70 ± 0.03^{a}	$0.01 \pm 0.02^{a,c*}$	$-0.02 \pm 0.01^{b*}$	5.89E-07
ANOVA		0.0929	0.0436	0.0087	
B		Cisplatin			
		Untreated	1 μM	10 μM	ANOVA
FCCP (μM)	Vehicle	1.00 ± 0.07^{a}	1.16 ± 0.03^{a}	$0.79 \pm 0.03^{a*}$	0.0052
	1.0	$0.84 \pm 0.02^{a,b}$	$0.89 \pm 0.02^{b*}$	$0.60 \pm 0.01^{b*}$	8.79E-05
	2.5	$0.70 \pm 0.01^{b,c}$	$0.79 \pm 0.02^{b,c*}$	$0.52 \pm 0.01^{b,c*}$	7.98E-05
	5.0	0.54 ± 0.03^{c}	0.57 ± 0.02^{d}	$0.40 \pm 0.00^{d*}$	0.0015
ANOVA		0.0002	1.22E-06	2.47E-06	
C		TRAIL			
		Untreated	50 ng/mL	100 ng/mL	ANOVA
Oligomycin (μM)	Vehicle	1.00 ± 0.01^{a}	$0.09 \pm 0.02^{a*}$	$0.14 \pm 0.01^{a*}$	2.90E-08
	1.0	0.94 ± 0.03^{a}	$0.01 \pm 0.00^{a*}$	$0.07 \pm 0.00^{b*}$	6.04E-05
	2.5	0.89 ± 0.05^{a}	$0.01 \pm 0.02^{a*}$	$0.08 \pm 0.01^{b*}$	3.19E-06
	5.0	0.78 ± 0.08^{a}	$0.06 \pm 0.02^{a*}$	$0.09 \pm 0.01^{a*}$	5.10E-05
ANOVA		0.0988	0.0629	0.0091	
D		Cisplatin			
		Untreated	1 μM	10 μM	ANOVA
Oligomycin (μM)	Vehicle	1.00 ± 0.02^{a}	1.10 ± 0.05^{a}	$0.91 \pm 0.03^{a*}$	0.0385
	1.0	0.91 ± 0.04^{a}	$1.09 \pm 0.03^{a*}$	0.80 ± 0.03^{a}	0.0031
	2.5	0.92 ± 0.02^{a}	$1.08 \pm 0..02^{a}$	0.83 ± 0.05^{a}	0.1875
	5.0	0.90 ± 0.05^{a}	0.99 ± 0.03^{a}	0.87 ± 0.02^{a}	0.0864
ANOVA		0.2729	0.1875	0.2136	

Resistance of OVCAR3 cultures to cell death inducing agents TRAIL or cisplatin was analyzed through inhibition of OXPHOS using oligomycin A and a mitochondrial membrane potential uncoupler, FCCP, using MTS viability assays. Results are presented as fold change to vehicle treated control cultures with differing letters indicating significant ($p < 0.05$) changes in viability with treatment of inhibitor, and asterisks indicating significant (* $p < 0.05$) changes in viability with treatment of cytotoxic agent. (**A,C**) OVCAR3 cultures are sensitive to cell-death via TRAIL. (**B,D**) OVCAR3 cultures were significantly sensitive to treatment with cisplatin, however pretreatment with both FCCP and oligomycin further decreased culture viability

(green), and the proportion of such populations (JC-1 red:JC-1 green ratio) analyzed via flow cytometry (Fig. 4). Not surprisingly, KGN cells (Fig. 4a) treated with the $\Delta\psi_m$ uncoupler FCCP had a significant decrease (Fig. 4b; 39 ± 7% relative to vehicle treated cells, $n = 3$, $P < 0.01$) in the JC-1 red:JC-1 green ratio, however, this effect was also in cells treated with TRAIL alone (29 ± 14%, $n = 3$, $P < 0.01$), as well as in combination (FCCP and TRAIL together: 25 ± 9%, $n = 3$, $P < 0.01$), indicative of a collapse in $\Delta\psi_m$ associated with apoptotic induction. In SKOV3 cells FCCP treatment alone did not significantly decrease the JC-1 red:JC-1 green ratio (Fig. 4c, d), however single treatment with TRAIL did decrease $\Delta\psi_m$ (62 ± 7% relative to vehicle, $n = 3$, $P < 0.05$) and was further decreased following dual treatment (50 ± 7%, $n = 3$, $P < 0.01$). No significant changes in $\Delta\psi_m$ were observed in Kuramochi cells under the same conditions (Fig. 4e, f; ANOVA $P = 0.19$). These data collectively indicate distinct cell-specific responses to alterations in $\Delta\psi_m$.

Inhibition of BIRC5 sensitizes KGN cells to TRAIL-induced apoptosis following mitochondrial membrane depolarization

Following treatment, KGN cells were collected for gene expression analysis of *MDR1, DR4, DR5, and BIRC5* (Fig. 5). The mRNA expression of the ATP dependent efflux pump, *MDR1* was significantly downregulated following all treatment conditions (Fig. 5a, FCCP: 0.41 ± 0.08- fold change, $n = 3$, $P < 0.05$; TRAIL: 0.42 ± 0.12-fold change, $n = 3$, $P < 0.05$; FCCP and TRAIL: 0.30 ±

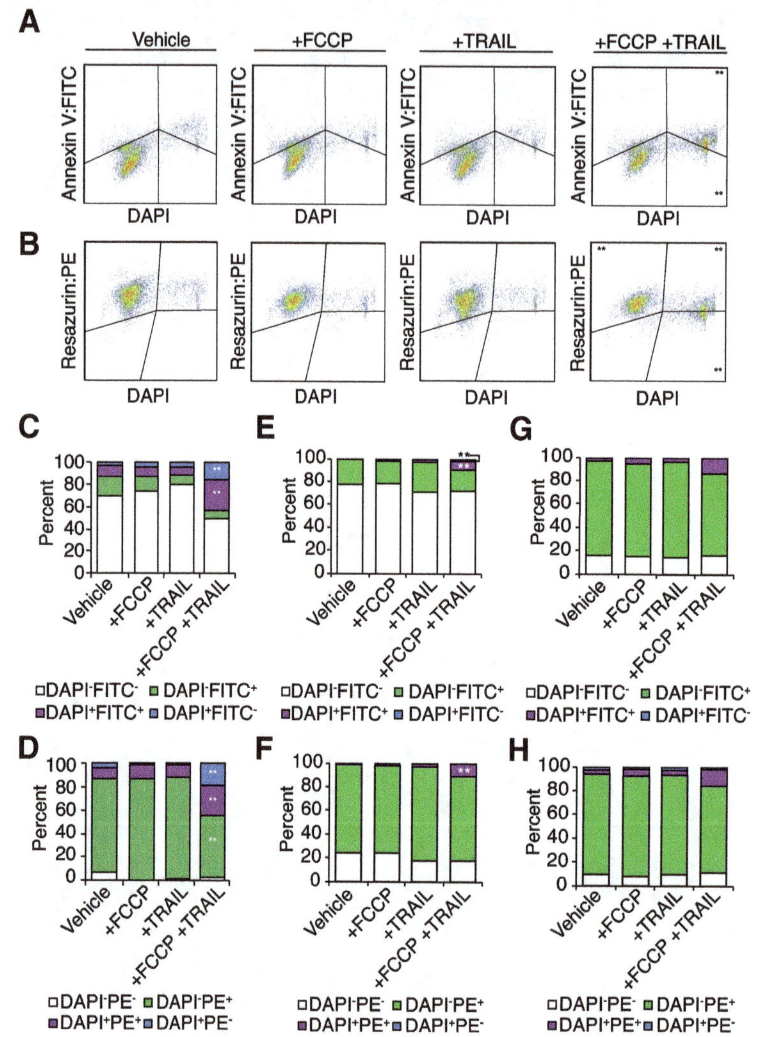

Fig. 2 Dual treatment with FCCP and TRAIL induces apoptosis and disrupts cellular metabolism. Dual treated cells were analyzed for extracellular expression of phosphatidylserine by antibody labeling with Annexin V (AnnexinV:FITC), the fluorescent metabolic dye resazurin (Resazurin:PE), and viability probe DAPI to determine apoptotic induction. **a** Co-labeling with AnnexinV:FITC and DAPI indicated high viability in control wells, with significant increases in both apoptotic cells ($DAPI^+FITC^+$; purple) as well as nonviable cells ($DAPI^+FITC^-$; blue) following both FCCP and TRAIL (**c**: $n = 3$ ANOVA $p < 0.001$**). **b** The increase in $DAPI^+$ events was also present when evaluating changes in global cellular metabolism, indicative of both respiring non-viable cells, as well as non-respiring non-viable cells. Additionally, there was a significant decrease in viable and metabolically active cells ($DAPI^-PE^+$; green) only after dual treatment with FCCP and TRAIL (**d**: $n = 3$ ANOVA $p < 0.001$**.) **e** In Kuramochi cultures, there was significant increases in both apoptotic cells as well as nonviable cells following treatment with both FCCP and TRAIL in the Kuramochi cell line ($n = 3$ ANOVA $p < 0.001$**), as well as (**f**) nonviable respiring cells ($n = 3$, ANOVA $p < 0.001$**). **g**, **h** SKOV3 cultures had no significant changes in apoptotic induction or metabolic modulation following treatment with FCCP and TRAIL

0.13- fold change, $n = 3$, $P < 0.01$). Of the primary receptors for extrinsic activation of apoptosis by TRAIL, *DR4* (Fig. 5b) and *DR5* (Fig. 5c), only *DR4* mRNA was significantly upregulated by treatment with TRAIL alone (1.79 ± 0.09-fold change, $n = 3$, $P < 0.05$). On the other hand, *BIRC5*, a negative regulator of apoptosis, was significantly upregulated following treatment with TRAIL (Fig. 5d; 2.17 ± 0.14-fold change, $n = 3$, $P < 0.01$), and this upregulation was prevented when pretreated with FCCP (0.76 ± 0.25-fold change, $n = 3$). To determine if loss of this negative regulator would additionally sensitize KGN to apoptosis, we completed a knockdown of *BIRC5* (Fig. 5e), which resulted in significant enhancement of the FCCP and TRAIL dual treatment effect (Fig. 5f; scRNA: 0.43 ± 0.06-fold change to scRNA vehicle; siRNA: 0.23 ± 0.01-fold change to scRNA vehicle, $n = 3$, $P < 0.05$).

Discussion and conclusions

Inherent in studies of ovarian cancer is the caveat of the disease's high degree of heterogeneity in presentation. Because aGCTs represent a small proportion of clinical diagnoses under the umbrella term of "ovarian cancer" many clinical

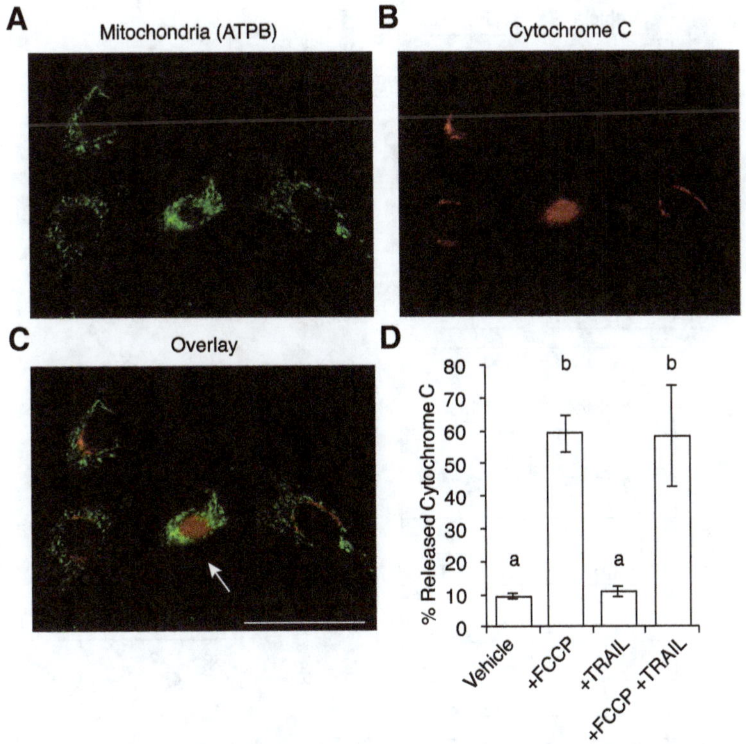

Fig. 3 Cytosolic localization of cytochrome c following dual treatment with FCCP and TRAIL indicates induction of apoptosis in KGN cells. Cytochrome c release was assayed via immunocytochemistry to detect induction of apoptosis. Following treatment with FCCP and/or TRAIL, cells were fixed and immunolabeled with antibodies against (**a**) the mitochondrial marker ATPB (green) and (**b**) cytochrome C (red). In addition, cells were also labeled with DAPI to visualize the cell nuclei and establish random fields of view for imaging. **c** Representative image indicating a cell (white arrow) scored as having released cytochrome C due to the loss of colocalization with ATPB. **d** Vehicle treated and TRAIL treated cells contained a small percentage of cells with released cytochrome C whereas both FCCP treated and FCCP and TRAIL treated cells showed significant increases in the percentage of cells exhibiting released cytochrome C (59.05 ± 5.39%, $P < 0.05$, 58.17 ± 15.65%, $P < 0.05$, respectively. Differing letters indicate significance). Scale bar indicates 50 μm

treatment paradigms are developed in context of epithelial adenocarcinomas [7], with a limited number of small clinical studies specifically targeting aGCTs [30]. While prognosis following stage I detection is excellent [7], high rates of recurrence of aGCTs necessitates a further evaluation of the molecular characterization of these tumors, which are likely distinct from epithelial carcinomas [7]. These data represent a characterization of the metabolic profile of KGN cells as a valuable model for aGCTs, with comparative assays run using epithelial-origin tumor derived cell lines instructive in demonstrating the heterogeneous response to treatments, even at the basic level of cells in vitro.

KGN cells were found to be primarily glycolytic, in both short-term responses to ATP production as well as over longer proliferation assays utilizing inhibitors against glycolysis, oxidative phosphorylation, or $\Delta\psi_m$. Treatment with FCCP was surprisingly effective in inhibiting proliferation in otherwise glycolytic cells, implicating a role for $\Delta\psi_m$ outside of metabolism. In fact, pretreatment with FCCP, a proton ionophore which uncouples oxidation from phosphorylation within mitochondria via export of H^+ ions [27], sensitized cells to TRAIL or cisplatin, more effectively than treatment with oligomycin A, which specifically inhibits oxidative phosphorylation by blocking the F0 subunit of ATP synthase [31]. We confirmed dual treatment was inducing apoptosis, rather than slowing proliferation rates, through Annexin V labeling, with significant increases in apoptosis occurring only in cells treated with both FCCP and TRAIL in combination. When evaluating cytochrome c as an upstream mediator of apoptotic induction, we found significantly higher rates of cytochrome c release in both the FCCP single treatment and dual treated cells, suggesting FCCP treatment is sensitizing cells to further induction via uncoupling $\Delta\psi_m$. Interestingly, the $\Delta\psi_m$ probe JC-1 indicated that both FCCP and TRAIL single treatments were each sufficient to depolarize $\Delta\psi_m$, which indicates a balance between extrinsic signaling, as TRAIL alone is insufficient to induce cell death, and intrinsic regulation, as FCCP alone is sufficient to decrease cell proliferation but not to induce apoptosis. Additionally, we found the IAP, BIRC5, to be essential in this balance, as treatment with TRAIL significantly increased *BIRC5* expression, however this response was lost upon

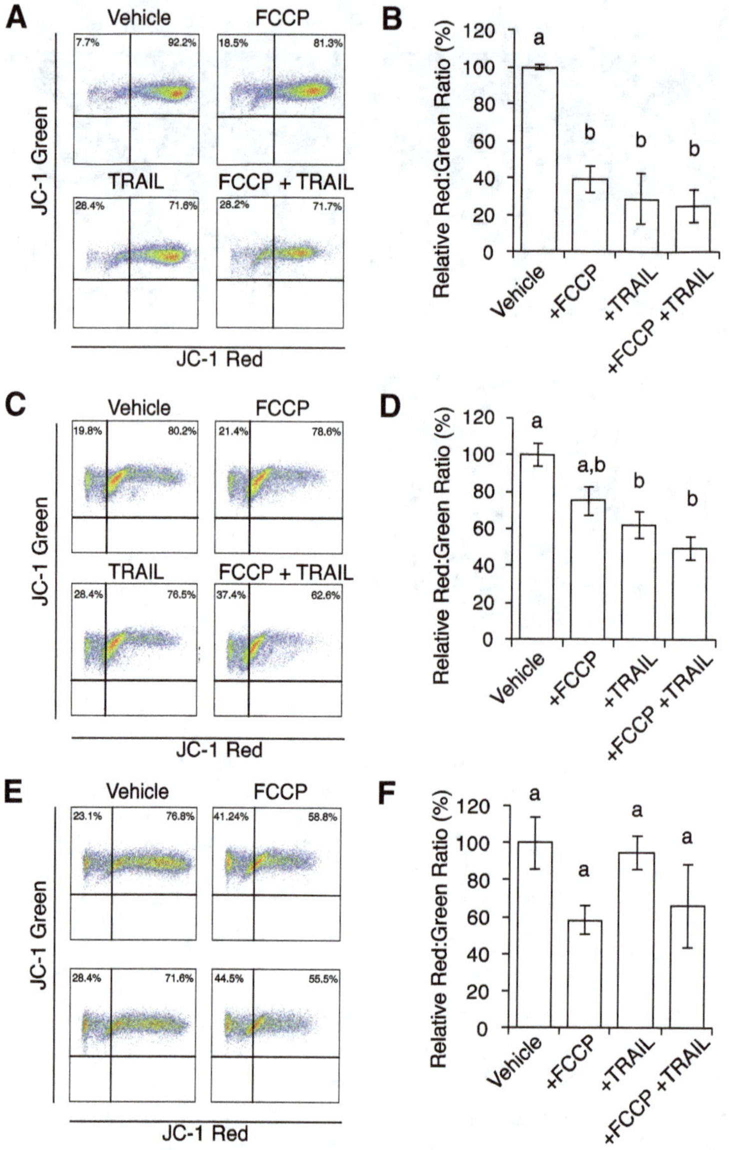

Fig. 4 KGN and SKOV3, but not Kuramochi, cells exhibit decreased mitochondrial membrane potential ($\Delta\psi_m$) following dual treatment with FCCP and TRAIL. Flow cytometry was used to detect changes in $\Delta\psi_m$ using the fluorescent dye, JC-1. **a** $\Delta\psi_m$ independent JC-1 monomers fluoresce at ~ 525 nm (green) throughout the cell, while $\Delta\psi_m$ dependent JC-1 polymers form following accumulation within mitochondria and fluoresce at ~ 595 nm (orange-red), allowing quantitation of $\Delta\psi_m$ as the JC-1 red:JC-1 green ratio, representative plots of KGN culture. **b** Quantitation of the JC-1 red:JC-1 green ratio in KGN culture exhibited a decreased $\Delta\psi_m$ across all conditions tested (FCCP: 39 ± 7% relative to vehicle treated cells, with differing letters indicating statistical significance. **c**, **d** In SKOV3 cells FCCP treatment did not significantly decrease the JC-1 red:JC-1 green ratio, however single treatment with TRAIL decreased $\Delta\psi_m$, and was further decreased following treatment with both FCCP and TRAIL (**e**, **f**) In Kuramochi cells, no significant changes in $\Delta\psi_m$ were observed under the same conditions

pretreatment with FCCP. A knockdown of *BIRC5* prior to treatment further sensitized cells to apoptotic induction. These data indicate an essential role for both $\Delta\psi_m$ and *BIRC5* in KGN cell response to TRAIL as summarized in Fig. 6. These data present the first molecular characterization of $\Delta\psi_m$ in KGN cells and its essential role in the inhibition of pro-apoptotic signaling, independent of a metabolic role. Such findings suggest the development of new therapeutic strategies targeting $\Delta\psi_m$ to more specifically treat aGCTs, in comparison to EOCs. Although there is limited clinical data focused solely on aGCTs, others have also described glycolytic signatures [32], with promising initial studies in mural models of GCTs [33], however the GCT field remains sparse, in comparison to EOCs. The availability of the KGN cell line to model aGCTs in vitro provides an important opportunity to characterize new basic research strategies, such as deciphering the role played by

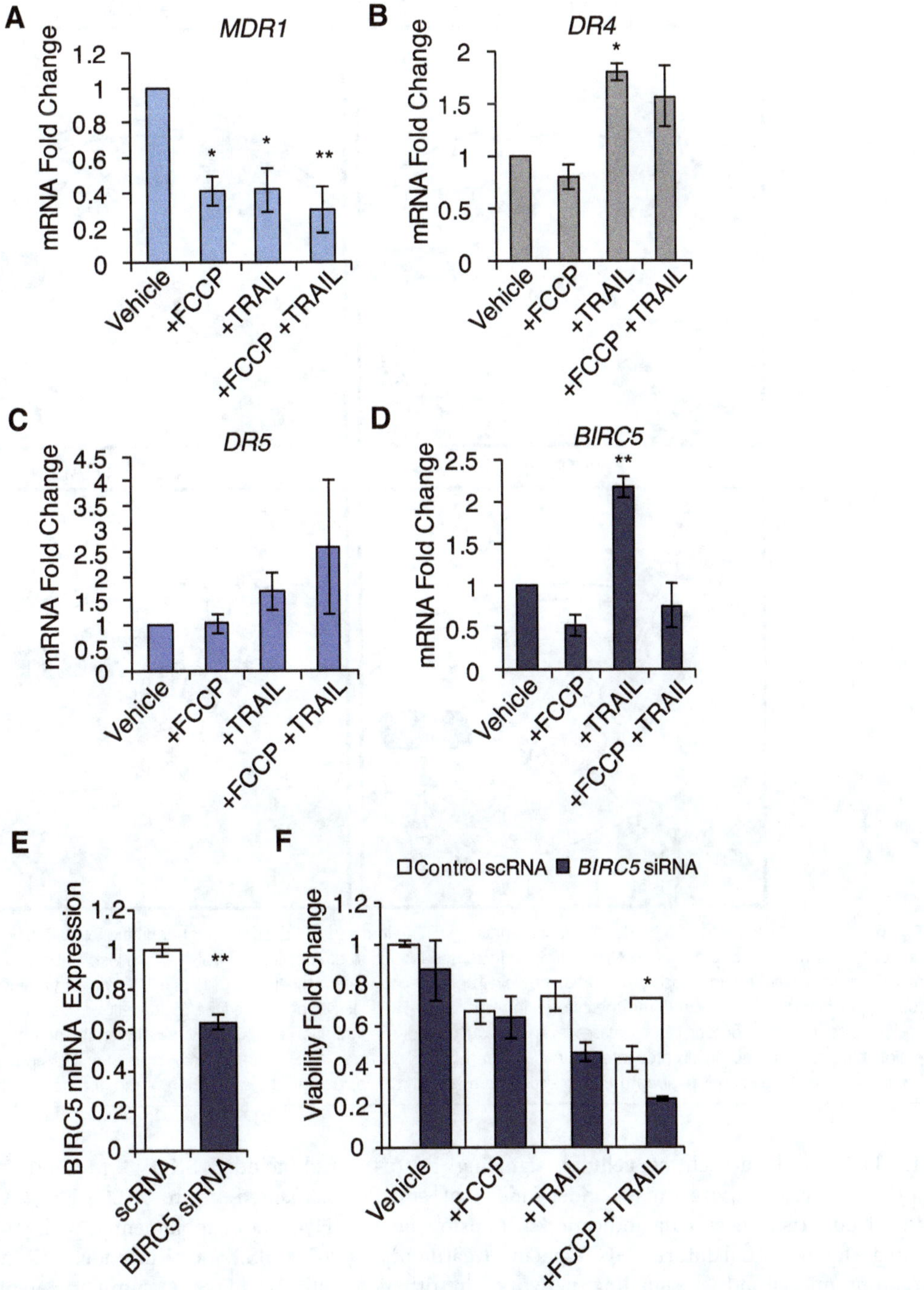

Fig. 5 Inhibition of BIRC5 sensitizes KGN cells to TRAIL-induced apoptosis following mitochondrial membrane depolarization. Gene expression analysis of *MDR1*, *DR4*, *DR5*, and *BIRC5* following treatment with FCCP and/or TRAIL. **a** Expression of the ATP dependent efflux pump, *MDR1*, which conveys multidrug resistance, was downregulated following all treatment conditions, asterisks indicate significance with regard to vehicle treated cells- $P < 0.05$* and $P < 0.01$**. **b** *DR4* was significantly upregulated by treatment with TRAIL alone, but the secondary receptor for TRAIL, *DR5* (**c**), showed no change in expression ($P = 0.42$). **d** The negative regulator of apoptosis, *BIRC5*, was significantly upregulated following treatment with TRAIL, however when pretreated with FCCP this response was lost. **e** A knockdown of *BIRC5* (64.0 ± 3.3% mRNA expression, 48 h post treatment, $n = 3$, $P < 0.01$**) prior to treatment (**f**) led to a significant enhancement of apoptosis induction by dual treatment with FCCP and TRAIL

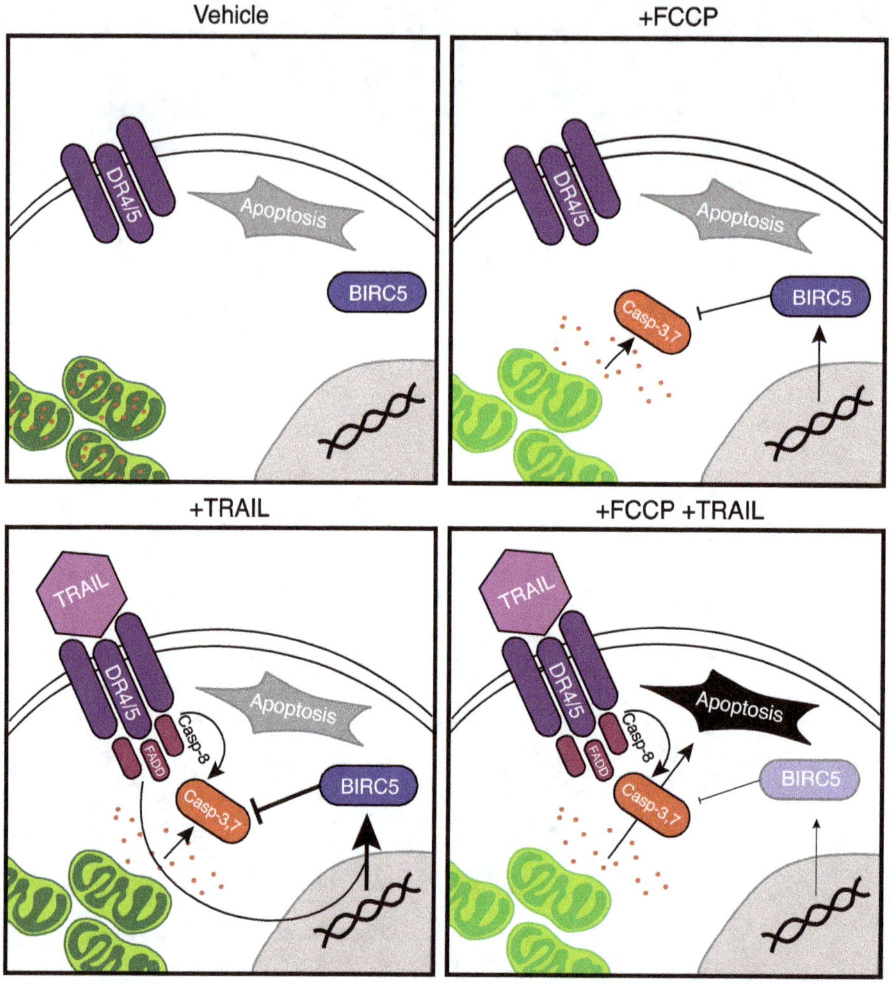

Fig. 6 Summary mechanism of $\Delta\psi_m$ depolarization enhances TRAIL-induced cell death through inhibition of BIRC5. Proposed mechanism depicting the interplay of $\Delta\psi_m$ and TRAIL resulting in increased induction of apoptosis in KGN cells. In viable and metabolically active cells, mitochondria (green) retain cytochrome c (red), however upon depolarization by either FCCP, or TRAIL (violet) binding with its receptors DR4/5 (purple), cytochrome c is released into the cytosol. In response to TRAIL activation of the DR4/5 intracellular death domain (DD) to form FADD and activate the pro-apoptotic caspase cascade, an upregulation of the inhibition of apoptosis protein family member, BIRC5 (blue), is induced, maintaining cell survival. In cells pretreated with FCCP, or those following a knockdown of *BIRC5* expression, pro-apoptotic signals overcome pro-survival signaling to induce apoptosis, suggesting an essential role for $\Delta\psi_m$ in the opposition of pro-apoptotic signals

mitochondria as a hub of cellular signaling in response to cytotoxic treatment, independent of small clinical cohorts. These data indicate a promising new strategy for potential future aGCT-specific treatments, targeting mitochondrial signaling networks in otherwise glycolytic cells.

Methods

Cell culture and media conditions

The adult-type human ovarian GCT line, KGN [34], were generously provided by Drs. Nishi and Yanase (Kyushu University, Japan), and maintained in DMEM/Ham's F12 (Corning) supplemented with 10% FBS (Peak Serum), as described previously [18]. Ovarian epithelial adenocarcinoma cell lines were purchased from ATCC and included: SKOV3, McCoy's 5a (Gibco) medium supplemented with 10% FBS; OVCAR3, RPMI-1640 (HyClone) supplemented with 0.01 mg ml^{-1} insulin and 20% FBS; and Kuramochi, RPMI-1640 supplemented with 10% FBS. A summary of previously published reports [35–37] which robustly characterize the EOCs of interest in regard to histological subtype and mutational profiles inclusive of seven common oncogenes is provided as Additional file 1: Table S1. All cells were routinely subcultured and maintained at 37 °C in a humidified atmosphere of 5% CO_2, 95% air.

ATP content analysis

Cells were plated as 1×10^4 cells per well in a 96-well plate in cell type specific media. 18 h after plating, culture media was supplemented to include the metabolic inhibitors 2-deoxy-d-glucose (2-DG; Acros Organics) or oligomycin A (Cayman Chemical) to final concentrations as indicated in the figures (0.2% DMSO vehicle). 6 h following treatment, cells were lysed as per the manufacturer's protocol for the Promega™ CellTiter-Glo™ 2.0 Assay. Total cellular ATP content was calculated using a standard curve of serially diluted ATP (Roche Applied Science) ranging from 0.5 nM to 5.0 μM. Significance was determined between groups via ANOVA, with post hoc Tukey HSD analysis for three experimental replicates, using the One-way ANOVA (ANalysis Of VAriance) with post-hoc Tukey HSD (Honestly Significant Difference) Test Calculator for comparing multiple treatments available at astatsa.com.

Culture viability via MTS assay

Cells were plated as 1×10^4 cells per well in a 96-well plate in cell-type specific media. For single treatment experiments, 24 h after plating, culture media was supplemented to include metabolic inhibitors 2-DG, oligomycin A, or carbonyl cyanide-*4*-(trifluoromethoxy)-phenylhydrazone (FCCP; Tocris) (0.02% DMSO vehicle for oligomycin A and FCCP). For dual treatment experiments, inhibitors were supplemented and cells were pre-incubated for 1 h at 37 °C, 5% CO_2, 95% air prior to further treatment with the cytotoxic agents TRAIL (EMD Millipore) or cisplatin (EMD Millipore). Treated plates were incubated for a further 20-h incubation, at which time the Promega™ CellTiter 96™ AQ_{ueous} One Solution Cell Proliferation Assay (MTS) reagent was added to each well and incubated for an additional 3 h at 37 ° C, 5% CO_2, 95% air for color development via formazan production prior to assessment of color change. The samples were normalized to blank media control wells and assayed against vehicle control cells, using Biotek Synergy H1 plate reader. All data are presented as fold-change relative to untreated controls, with significance determined between groups via ANOVA, with post hoc Tukey HSD.

Flow cytometry analysis of Annexin V and $\Delta\psi_m$

Cells were plated as 1.25×10^5 cells per well in a 6-well plate, and 24 h following plating FCCP was added to a final concentration of 5.0 μM and preincubated for 1 hour prior to the addition of 50 ng ml^{-1} TRAIL, and returned to the incubator for an additional 20-h incubation. Cells were collected and prepared for analysis of apoptosis via binding Annexin V to extracellular phosphatidylserine, or for analysis of $\Delta\psi_m$ using the fluorescent dye, JC-1, by flow cytometry. For experiments examining apoptotic induction, additional cells were prepared as an induced necrosis control following incubation with 2 mM H_2O_2 for 4 hours prior to labeling. Cells were labeled for 15 min at 37 °C, 5% CO_2, 95% air per the manufacturer's recommendation, with the metabolic dye resazurin (Acros Organics) at a final concentration of 500 nM and a FITC-conjugated monoclonal antibody against Annexin V (Invitrogen; clone: VAA-33), and maintained on ice until analysis. Immediately prior to analysis, DAPI (4′,6-Diamidino-2-Phenylindole, Dihydrochloride; Sigma) was added to a final concentration of 200 ng ml^{-1}. All gates for flow cytometry analysis were set utilizing single color stained control samples. For experiments examining $\Delta\psi_m$, cell suspensions were stained with 2.0 μM JC-1 (Marker Gene) for 15 min at 37 °C, 5% CO_2. Stained cells were washed with 1x PBS (Gibco), maintained on ice, and 200 ng ml^{-1} DAPI (Sigma) was added immediately prior to analysis. All gates for flow cytometry analysis were set utilizing unstained control samples. Analyses were completed using a BD FACSAria III. The JC-1 Red: JC-1 Green ratio was determined.

Immunocytochemistry of cytochrome c release

Cells were grown on glass coverslips and treated with FCCP and TRAIL, as described above, were fixed in 2% formaldehyde (Electron Microscopy Sciences) and permeabilized in 0.25% Triton-X (Sigma). After washing, coverslips were blocked in 5% BSA (Jackson Immuno Research Labs) for 1 hour at room temperature (22 °C), and washed with PBS. A mouse monoclonal antibody to the beta subunit of ATP synthase (ATBP; Abcam; ab14730, 1 μg ml^{-1}), a mitochondrial protein, and a rabbit oligoclonal antibody to cytochrome c (Invitrogen; 710,627, 5 μg ml^{-1}) were diluted in 1% BSA and coverslips were incubated overnight at 4 °C. After washing with PBS, species specific secondary antibodies (Goat anti-mouse Alexa488, Invitrogen; Goat anti-rabbit Alexa568, Invitrogen) were diluted 1:500 in 1% BSA and coverslips were incubated for 1 hour at room temperature (22 °C). After washing, cells were incubated with 200 ng ml^{-1} DAPI for 10 min at room temperature (22 °C), and mounted onto slides using Prolong Gold (Life Technologies). Fields of view were randomly selected and focused at the nuclear plane using DAPI labeling, ($n = 98–250$ cells per condition), imaged, and scored according to localization of cytochrome c as either densely colocalized with ATPB-positive mitochondria or diffuse localization in the cytoplasm, indicative of release from mitochondria. Counts were normalized to total number of nuclei, with representative images presented.

Gene expression analysis

For all gene expression analyses, cultures were treated as described above, and total RNA was isolated using RNazol®RT (Molecular Research Center). One microgram of isolated RNA per sample was treated with DnaseI (Thermo Fisher Scientific) to remove potential genomic DNA contamination, followed by first strand cDNA synthesis using a RevertAid RT kit (Thermo Fisher Scientific). Quantitative analysis of *Multi-Drug Resistance Gene 1* (*MDR1,* also referred to as *P-gp, ABCB1,* or *CD243;* assay ID: Hs00184500_m1), *Death Receptor 4 (DR4,* also referred to as *TRAILR1* or *TNFRSF10A*; assay ID: Hs00269492_m1), *Death Receptor 5* (*DR,* also referred to as *TRAILR2* or *TNFRSF10B*; assay ID: Hs00366278_m1), and *BIRC5* (assay ID: Hs00977611_g1) expression was completed using TaqMan gene expression assays (Applied Biosystems) with the reference gene *beta-2-microglobulin* (*B2M*; assay ID: Hs99999907_m1) using TaqMan™ Fast Advanced Master Mix (Life Technoliges) and a StepOnePlus™ Real-Time PCR System (Applied Biosystems), under parameters recommended by the manufacturer for TaqMan gene expression assays. In brief, each reaction was run with 250 nM of 6-FAM™ dye-labeled TaqMan® MGB probe for each gene of interest, 250 nM of 6-VIC® dye-labeled TaqMan MGB probe for *B2M,* and 50 ng of synthesized cDNA in technical duplicates for 40 cycles at an annealing temperature of 60C using fast ramp rate experimental parameters.

BIRC5 knockdown

KGN cells were reverse transfected using Lipofectamine LTX with a commercially available dicer-substrate siRNA construct against *BIRC5* (IDT; Design ID: hs.Ri.-BIRC5.13.1) or non-targeting control (IDT; Negative Control SdiRNA # 51–01–14-03) at time of plating, and the culture viability was assessed by MTS assay as previously described. *BIRC5* mRNA knockdown was confirmed by qRT-PCR, as described above, 48 h following transfection.

Funding

This material is based upon work supported by the National Science Foundation under grant number 1750996 to D.C.W.

Authors' contributions

DCW and JAM designed the project and wrote the manuscript, with input from all other authors. JAM designed experimental protocols. JAM, NK, and CS performed experiments and analyzed the data. All authors read and approved the final manuscript.

Competing interests

The authors declare that they have no competing interests.

References

1. Truman AM, Johnson AL, Woods DC. Granulosa Cell Tumors. In: Schwab M, editor. Encyclopedia of Cancer. 4th revise. Berlin: Springer-Verlag Berlin and Heidelberg GmbH & co.; 2016.
2. Shah S, Köbel M, Senz J, Morin R, Clarke B, Wiegand K, et al. Mutation of FOXL2 in granulosa-cell tumors of the ovary. N Engl J Med. 2009;360(26): 2719–29.
3. Leung D, Fuller P, Chu S. Impact of FOXL2 mutations on signaling in ovarian granulosa cell tumors. Int J Biochem Cell Biol. 2016;72:51–4.
4. Jamieson S, Fuller PJ. Molecular pathogenesis of granulosa cell tumors of the ovary. Endocr Rev. 2012;33(1):109–44.
5. Köbel M, Gilks C, Huntsman D. Adult-type granulosa cell tumors and FOXL2 mutation. Cancer Res. 2009;69(24):9160–2.
6. Schumer ST, Cannistra SA. Granulosa cell tumor of the ovary. J Clin Oncol. 2003;21(6):1180–9.
7. Colombo N, Parma G, Zanagnolo V, Insinga A. Management of ovarian stromal cell tumors. J Clin Oncol. 2007;25(20):2944–51.
8. Segal R, DePetrillo AD, Thomas G. Clinical review of adult granulosa cell tumors of the ovary. Gynecol Oncol. 1995;56:338–44.
9. Miller K, McCluggage WG. Prognostic factors in ovarian adult granulosa cell tumour. J Clin Pathol. 2008;61(8):881–4.
10. Vander Heiden MG, Cantley LC, Thompson CB, Mammalian P, Exhibit C, Metabolism A. Understanding the Warburg effect: the metabolic requirements of cell proliferation. Science. 2009;324(5930):1029–33.
11. Koppenol WH, Bounds PL, Dang CV. Otto Warburg's contributions to current concepts of cancer metabolism. Nat Rev Cancer. 2011;11(5):325–37.
12. Gatenby RA, Gillies RJ. Why do cancers have high aerobic glycolysis? Nat Rev Cancer. 2004;4(11):891.
13. Bonnet S, Archer SL, Allalunis-Turner J, Haromy A, Beaulieu C, Thompson R, et al. A mitochondria-K+ channel axis is suppressed in cancer and its normalization promotes apoptosis and inhibits cancer growth. Cancer Cell. 2007;11(1):37–51.
14. Schmidt M, Kammerer U, Segerer S, Cramer A, Kohrenhagen N, Dietl J, Voelker H. Glucose metabolism and angiogenesis in granulosa cell tumors of the ovary: activation of Akt, expression of M2PK, TKTL1 and VEGF. Eur J Obstet Gynecol Reprod Biol. 2008;139(1):72–8.
15. Dier U, Shin DH, Hemachandra LMP, Uusitalo LM, Hempel N. Bioenergetic analysis of ovarian cancer cell lines: profiling of histological subtypes and identification of a mitochondria-defective cell line. PLoS One. 2014;9(5): e98479.
16. Xintaropoulou C, Ward C, Wise A, Marston H, Turnbull A, Langdon SP. A comparative analysis of inhibitors of the glycolysis pathway in breast and ovarian cancer cell line models. Oncotarget. 2015;6(28):25677–95.
17. Sun L, Yin Y, Clark LH, Sun W, Sullivan SA, Tran AQ, et al. Dual inhibition of glycolysis and glutaminolysis as a therapeutic strategy in the treatment of ovarian cancer. Oncotarget. 2017;8(38):63551–61.
18. Woods DC, Liu HK, Nishi Y, Yanase T, Johnson AL. Inhibition of proteasome activity sensitizes human granulosa tumor cells to TRAIL-induced cell death. Cancer Lett. 2008;260(1):20–7.
19. Woods DC, Alvarez C, Johnson AL. Cisplatin-mediated sensitivity to TRAIL-induced cell death in human granulosa tumor cells. Gynecol Oncol. 2008; 108(3):632–40.
20. Johnson AL, Ratajczak C, Haugen MJ, Liu HK, Woods DC. Tumor necrosis factor-related apoptosis inducing ligand expression and activity in hen granulosa cells. Reproduction. 2007;133(3):609–16.
21. Ashkenazi A. Targeting death and decoy receptors of the tumour-necrosis factor superfamily. Nat Rev Cancer. 2002;2(6):420–30.
22. Chinnaiyan AM, O'Rourke K, Tewari M, Dixit VM. FADD, a novel death domain-containing protein, interacts with the death domain of Fas and initiates apoptosis. Cell. 1995;81(4):505–12.
23. Peter ME. Programmed cell death: apoptosis meets necrosis. Nature. 2011; 471(7338):310–2.
24. Deveraux Q, Roy N, Stennicke H, Van Arsdale T, Zhou Q, Srinivasula S, et al. IAPs block apoptotic events induced by caspase-8 and cytochrome c by direct inhibition of distinct caspases. EMBO J. 1998;17(8):2215–23.
25. Sah NK, Khan Z, Khan GJ, Bisen PS. Structural, functional and therapeutic biology of survivin. Cancer Lett. 2006;244(2):164–71.
26. Ausserlechner MJ, Hagenbuchner J. Mitochondrial survivin–an Achilles' heel in cancer chemoresistance. Mol Cell Oncol. 2016;3(2):e1076589.
27. Benz R, McLaughlin S. The molecular mechanism of action of the proton ionophore FCCP (carbonylcyanide p-trifluoromethoxyphenylhydrazone). Biophys J. 1983;41(3):381–98.

28. Lane D, Côté M, Grondin R, Couture M, Piché A. Acquired resistance to TRAIL-induced apoptosis in human ovarian cancer cells is conferred by increased turnover of mature caspase-3. Mol Cancer Ther. 2006;5(3):509–21.
29. O'brien J, Wilson I, Orton T, Pognan F. Investigation of the Alamar blue (resazurin) fluorescent dye for the assessment of mammalian cell cytotoxicity. FEBS J. 2000;267(17):5421–6.
30. Raspagliesi F, Martinelli F, Grijuela B, Guadalupi V. Third-line chemotherapy with tyrosine kinase inhibitor (imatinib mesylate) in recurrent ovarian granulosa cell tumor: case report. J Obstet Gynaecol Res. 2011;37(12):1864–7.
31. Penefsky HS. Mechanism of inhibition of mitochondrial adenosine triphosphatase by dicyclohexylcarbodiimide and oligomycin: relationship to ATP synthesis. Proc Natl Acad Sci. 1985;82(6):1589–93.
32. Miyazawa M, Yasuda M, Fujita M, Hirabayashi K, Hirasawa T, Kajiwara H, Muramatsu T, et al. Granulosa cell tumor with activated mTOR-HIF-1α-VEGF pathway. J Obstet Gynaecol Res. 2010;36(2):448–53.
33. Tsoi M, Laguëëlle MN, Boyer A, Paquet M, Nadeau MÈ, Boerboom D. Anti-VEGFA therapy reduces tumor growth and extends survival in a murine model of ovarian granulosa cell tumor. Transl Oncol. 2013;6(3):226–33.
34. Nishi Y, Yanase T, Mu YM, Oba K, Ichino I, Saito M, et al. Establishment and characterization of a steroidogenic human granulosa-like tumor cell line, KGN, that expresses functional follicle-stimulating hormone receptor. Endocrinology. 2001;142(1):437–45.
35. Domcke S, Sinha R, Levine DA, Sander C, Schultz N. Evaluating cell lines as tumour models by comparison of genomic profiles. Nat Commun. 2013;4: 2126.
36. Hernandez L, Kim MK, Lyle LT, Bunch KP, House CD, Ning F, et al. Characterization of ovarian cancer cell lines as in vivo models for preclinical studies. Gynecol Oncol. 2016;142(2):332–40.
37. Beaufort CM, Helmijr JC, Piskorz AM, Hoogstraat M, Ruigrok-Ritstier K, Besselink N, et al. Ovarian cancer cell line panel (OCCP): clinical importance of in vitro morphological subtypes. PLoS One. 2014;9(9):e103988.

Does a poor-quality embryo have an adverse impact on a good-quality embryo when transferred together?

Jiaheng Li[1†], Mingze Du[1†], Zhan Zhang[1*], Yichun Guan[1], Xingling Wang[1], Xiao Zhang[2], Jing Liu[1], Zhouhui Pan[1], Bijun Wang[1] and Wenxia Liu[1]

Abstract

Background: In some in vitro fertilization (IVF) or intracytoplasmic sperm injection (ICSI) cycles, we may consider transferring one poor-quality embryo with one good-quality embryo. Previous studies have indicated that the poor-quality embryo transferred with a good-quality embryo does not negatively affect the clinical pregnancy rate or live birth rate. The purpose of this study was to evaluate pregnancy outcomes and neonatal outcomes in this context.

Methods: This was a retrospective study that included 1646 cycles from our centre. Patients were divided into two groups (group A: one good-quality embryo was transferred with one poor-quality embryo; group B: two good-quality embryos were transferred). The primary outcomes were the clinical pregnancy rate and live birth rate. Additionally, we investigated the implantation rate, ectopic pregnancy rate, abortion rate, multiple pregnancy rate, birthweight and gestational age.

Results: We found that there were no differences in the clinical pregnancy rate and live birth rate between group A and group B. However, the implantation rate and multiple pregnancy rate were higher in group B than in group A.

Conclusions: The poor-quality embryo does not have a significant influence on the good-quality embryo when transferred together.

Keywords: Embryo quality, Live birth rate, Clinical pregnancy rate, Neonatal outcome

Background

The frequency of the use of assisted reproductive technology is increasing. Globally, the number of fresh cycles has increased by 6.4% between 2008 and 2010, and the number of frozen embryo transfer cycles has increased by 27.6% [1]. Double-embryo transfers (DETs) still hold a dominant position despite the increasing number of single-embryo transfer (SET) procedures. In Europe, the rates of SET and DET were 22.4% and 53.2%, respectively, in 2008 and 31.4% and 56.3%, respectively, in 2012 [2, 3]. A meta-analysis found that the live birth rate was lower for SET than for DET, while the live birth rate of a repeated SET (two cycles of SET) was not different from that of a DET [4]. In another meta-analysis, SET reduced the probability of a live birth by 38% and of multiple births by 94%. However, the cumulative live birth rate remained unchanged [5]. Although DET has a higher multiple birth rate than SET, DET also has a higher live birth rate per cycle than SET.

Additionally, the quality of the embryo influences the results of assisted reproductive technology treatment [6–8]. A good-quality embryo is predictive of a better outcome than a poor-quality embryo. However, we cannot guarantee that all embryos are good-quality embryos. What should be done with a poor-quality embryo in assisted reproductive technology treatments? One study indicated that the poor quality of one embryo may influence the quality of another embryo [9]. The blastocyst rate is indeed decreased due to the influence of a poor-quality embryo. Regarding embryo transfer into the uterus, one study pointed out that a poor-quality embryo

* Correspondence: zhangzhan1616@126.com
†Jiaheng Li and Mingze Du contributed equally to this work.
[1]The Reproduction Center, The Third Affiliated Hospital of Zhengzhou University, 7 Kangfuqian Road, Zhengzhou 450052, Henan, People's Republic of China
Full list of author information is available at the end of the article

would affect a good-quality embryo in DET [10]. This study also found that the implantation rates were higher in the control group (transferred two good-quality embryos or one good-quality embryo) than in the study group (transferred one good-quality embryo and one poor-quality embryo). Although previous studies have discussed these problems, the sample sizes have been small. Additionally, previous studies did not discuss the birthweight, gestational age and abortion rate. Therefore, whether we should transfer a poor-quality embryo with a good-quality embryo needed to be evaluated again.

The aim of our research was to determine whether we should transfer a poor-quality embryo with a good-quality embryo.

Methods

Study design

This retrospective study was approved by the Ethics Committee of the Third Affiliated Hospital of Zhengzhou University. All patients who underwent in vitro fertilization (IVF) or intracytoplasmic sperm injection (ICSI) at the reproduction centre of the Third Affiliated Hospital of Zhengzhou University between January 2012 and December 2015 were included in this study. Patients who underwent transfer of one or two cleavage-stage embryos were included in our study. We divided these patients into two groups: group A comprised cycles in which one poor-quality embryo was transferred with one good-quality embryo, and group B comprised cycles in which two good-quality embryos were transferred. The outcomes we analysed were the implantation rate, the clinical pregnancy rate, the ectopic pregnancy rate, the abortion rate, the live birth rate, the number of foetuses, birthweight, gestational age, and the incidence of low birth weight and preterm birth.

Clinical pregnancy was diagnosed by transvaginal ultrasound of at least one gestational sac or definitive clinical signs of pregnancy. Live birth was defined as one or more new-borns after 20 completed weeks of gestation. Ectopic pregnancy was defined as a pregnancy that did not occur inside the uterine cavity. Low birth weight was defined as a newborn weight less than 2500 g. Preterm birth was defined as a gestational age of less than 37 weeks.

Embryo quality

Embryo quality was determined according to a ranking system. Class I embryos were defined as those with six to ten cells on day 3 and < 5% embryo fragmentation. Class II embryos were defined as those with six to ten cells on day 3 and 5–20% embryo fragmentation. Class III embryos were defined as those with uneven cell size, irregular cell morphology, and embryo fragmentation from 21% to 49%. Class IV embryos were defined as those with extremely uneven cell size, a large number of intracellular vacuoles, arrest of embryonic development or embryo fragmentation of over 50%. Class I embryos and Class II embryos were defined as good-quality embryos. Class III embryos were defined as poor-quality embryos, and Class IV embryos were defined as unavailable embryos.

Inclusion criteria

The inclusion criteria were as follows: fresh IVF/ICSI cycles occurring between January 2012 and December 2015, and patients aged ≤35 years.

Exclusion criteria

The exclusion criteria were as follows: patients with uterine malformations, patients using donor oocytes, patients who opted for PGD/PGS, and patients with vanishing twins.

Statistical analysis

The objective of this study was to determine the influence of a poor-quality embryo on a good-quality embryo. The primary outcomes were the clinical pregnancy rate and live birth rate. The secondary outcomes of the study were the implantation rate, the abortion rate, the ectopic pregnancy rate, the multiple pregnancy rate, birthweight and gestational age. Analyses were performed using SPSS (Statistical Package for the Social Sciences) 22.0. We used chi-square tests to evaluate categorical variables. For continuous variables, we used Student's t-test or the Mann-Whitney test. Logistic regression was performed for live birth and clinical pregnancy using the following variables: maternal age, male age, insemination method, type of infertility, duration of infertility, body mass index, reason for infertility, endometrial thickness and type of cycle. All p values less than 0.05 were considered statistically significant.

Results

We included 1646 cycles in the present study. A total of 1200 cycles involved transfers of two good-quality embryos (group B), and 446 cycles involved transfers of one poor-quality embryo with one good-quality embryo (group A). Body mass index, the reason for infertility, the cause of infertility, male age, endometrial thickness and the insemination method were not significantly different between group A and group B (Table 1). However, we found that male age was lower in group B than in group A ($p = 0.01$). Regarding the outcome of assisted reproductive technology treatment, we found that only the implantation rate was different between group A and group B. Group B had a higher implantation rate (54.8% vs 49.2%, $P = 0.01$) than group A (Table 2). Additionally, group A had a lower multiple pregnancy rate than group B (41.3% vs 33.6%, $P = 0.02$). However, we did not find other differences in

Table 1 Basic information of patients in the two groups

	Group A (*n* = 446)	Group B (*n* = 1200)	*P*
Maternal age (y)	29.0 ± 3.8	28.6 ± 3.2	0.05
Body mass index (kg/m^2)	22.9 ± 3.3	22.7 ± 3.1	0.17
Duration of infertility (y)	3.5 ± 2.5	3.4 ± 2.5	0.35
Male age (y)	30.5 ± 4.8	29.9 ± 4.6	0.01
Type of infertility			0.47
Primary infertility	266 (59.6%)	692 (57.7%)	
Secondary infertility	180 (40.4%)	508 (42.3%)	
Cause of infertility			0.12
Tubal disease	248 (55.6%)	688 (57.3%)	
Male factor	110 (24.7%)	297 (24.8%)	
Endometriosis	62 (13.9%)	176 (14.7%)	
Unexplained	26 (5.8%)	39 (3.3%)	
Endometrial thickness (mm)	11.4 ± 2.3	11.3 ± 2.2	0.33
Insemination method			0.81
IVF	326 (73.1%)	870 (72.5%)	
ICSI	120 (26.9%)	330 (27.5%)	

the clinical pregnancy rate, the ectopic pregnancy rate, the abortion rate, the live birth rate, birthweight, gestational age, and the incidence of low birth weight or preterm birth. To adjust for confounding factors, we used logistic regression to investigate whether a poor-quality embryo affected a good-quality embryo in terms of the clinical pregnancy rate and live birth rate. We did not observe any differences in the primary outcomes (Table 3).

Table 2 Clinical and neonatal outcomes in the two groups

	Group A (*n* = 446)	Group B (*n* = 1200)	*P*
Implantation rate	49.2% (439/892)	54.8% (1314/2400)	0.01
Clinical pregnancy rate	71.3% (318/446)	74.7% (896/1200)	0.17
Ectopic pregnancy rate	1.3% (4/318)	2.7% (24/896)	0.15
Abortion rate	8.8% (28/318)	9.7% (87/896)	0.64
Live birth rate	64.1% (286/446)	65.4% (785/1200)	0.63
Number of foetuses			0.02
Singleton	190 (66.4%)	461 (58.7%)	
Twin	96 (33.6%)	324 (41.3%)	
Birthweight			
Singleton	3346 ± 545	3318 ± 563	0.67
Twin	2596 ± 402	2567 ± 436	0.40
Low birth weight			
Singleton	4.2% (8/190)	4.8% (22/461)	0.76
Twin	35.4% (68/192)	39.0% (253/648)	0.36
Gestational age			
Singleton	38.8 ± 1.5	38.7 ± 1.8	0.42
Twin	36.5 ± 1.9	36.4 ± 1.9	0.86
Preterm birth			
Singleton	7.9% (15/190)	5.9% (27/461)	0.34
Twin	39.6% (38/96)	36.4% (118/324)	0.57

Discussion

A poor-quality embryo can provide a chance to achieve pregnancy. However, a previous study suggested that transfer of a poor-quality embryo would lead to a reduction in the clinical pregnancy rate and live birth rate. However, there were no differences between transfer of a poor-quality embryo and transfer of a good-quality embryo in terms of the abortion rate, pregnancy complications, maternal complications or neonatal complications [6]. In another study, authors found that a poor-quality embryo may affect a good-quality embryo in vitro [9]. Therefore, we wondered whether a poor-quality embryo had an adverse influence on a good-quality embryo. Two experts have previously discussed this topic. One expert suggested that the poor-quality embryo would influence the pregnancy rate and implantation rate [11], and the other expert indicated that transfer of one poor-quality embryo with one good-quality embryo resulted in a lower implantation rate than transfer of two good-quality embryos [10]. However, those researchers did not find a difference in the clinical pregnancy rate, live birth rate, abortion rate, ectopic pregnancy rate or multiple pregnancy rate.

Compared with groups that underwent transfer of one good-quality embryo, group A and group B had higher

Table 3 Logistic regression of clinical pregnancy and live births

Predictors	AOR[a] (95%CI)	*P*
Clinical pregnancy		
Maternal age	0.959 (0.922–0.996)	0.032
Body mass index	1.031 (0.995–1.069)	0.094
Duration of infertility	0.886 (0.685–1.147)	0.359
Type of infertility	0.952 (0.750–1.208)	0.686
Male age	0.991 (0.957–1.026)	0.612
Endometrial thickness	1.098 (1.044–1.155)	< 0.001
Group C	0.839 (0.655–1.076)	0.166
Live birth		
Maternal age	0.936 (0.895–0.980)	0.005
Body mass index	1.003 (0.971–1.037)	0.843
Duration of infertility	1.065 (0.838–1.355)	0.605
Type of infertility	1.067 (0.856–1.329)	0.563
Male age	1.008 (0.976–1.042)	0.615
Endometrial thickness	1.096 (1.046–1.148)	< 0.001
Group	0.952 (0.755–1.200)	0.676

AOR adjusted odds ratios

[a]Adjusted for maternal age, male age, insemination method, type of infertility, duration of infertility, body mass index, reason for infertility and endometrial thickness

clinical pregnancy rates and live birth rates. However, we did not observe differences between group A and group B. Hence, the poor-quality embryo may not affect these outcomes. After adjusting for confounding factors, we did not find that the conditions of the two groups had any influence on the outcomes. Consistent with a previous article, we did not find evidence that the poor-quality embryo affected the live birth rate or pregnancy rate. Additionally, we found that the implantation rate was lower in group A than in group B, although two previous articles had indicated that good-quality embryos were easier to implant and develop than poor-quality embryos. However, we found that the multiple pregnancy rate was higher in group B. In other studies, the multiple pregnancy rate was not significantly different between patients who underwent different embryo transfer schemes. We hypothesized that a high implantation rate was related to a high multiple pregnancy rate. After all, a good-quality embryo has a higher chance of implantation and development than a poor-quality embryo [7, 8]. Regarding the abortion rate and ectopic rate, there were no differences between the two groups. We also specifically investigated the birthweight, gestational age, and incidence of low birth weight and preterm birth. However, after dividing pregnancies into singletons and twins, we found no differences in these outcomes. Hence, the poor-quality embryo did not influence birthweight or gestational age.

In summary, we found that only the implantation rate and multiple pregnancy rate were different between group A and group B. We did not find significant differences in the other parameters. A high multiple pregnancy rate is associated with high risks of infant death, low birth weight, deformational plagiocephaly, and other problems [12]. To reduce the risk of a multiple pregnancy, we should consider the conditions of group A as an alternative transfer scheme with no difference in the live birth rate compared to that in group B.

The clinical pregnancy rate (74.7% vs 71.3%, $P = 0.17$) and live birth rate (65.4% vs 64.1%, $P = 0.63$) were higher in group B than in group A; however, the difference was not statistically significant. We tried our best to reduce the influence of confounding factors by optimizing the inclusion and exclusion criteria. However, our study has several limitations. First, this study was a retrospective study, and perhaps a randomized controlled trial would be more persuasive. Second, the criteria for the evaluation of embryo quality were subjective. Finally, additional big-data research studies and a systematic review are required to confirm these findings.

Conclusion

The poor-quality embryo does not significantly influence the good-quality embryo when transferred together.

Abbreviations

DET: Double-embryo transfer; ICSI: Intracytoplasmic sperm injection; IVF: In vitro fertilization; SET: Single-embryo transfer

Funding

This research study did not receive any funding.

Authors' contributions

ZZ proposed the design ideas. LJH and DMZ checked the data and constructed the tables. LJH, DMZ, WXL, GYC, LJ, PZH, WBJ and LWX wrote the manuscript. All authors approved the final version of this article. LJH and DMZ contributed equally to this paper.

Competing interests

All authors have declared that they have no competing interests.

Author details

[1]The Reproduction Center, The Third Affiliated Hospital of Zhengzhou University, 7 Kangfuqian Road, Zhengzhou 450052, Henan, People's Republic of China. [2]Waterstone Clinic, Lotamore House, Tivoli, Cork, Ireland.

References

1. Dyer S, et al. International Committee for Monitoring Assisted Reproductive Technologies world report: Assisted Reproductive Technology 2008, 2009 and 2010. Hum Reprod. 2016;31:1588–609. https://doi.org/10.1093/humrep/dew082.
2. Ferraretti AP, et al. Assisted reproductive technology in Europe, 2008: results generated from European registers by ESHRE. Human Reprod. 2012;27: 2571–84. https://doi.org/10.1093/humrep/des255.
3. Calhaz-Jorge C, et al. Assisted reproductive technology in Europe, 2013: results generated from European registers by ESHRE. Human Reprod. 2017; 32:1957–73. https://doi.org/10.1093/humrep/dex264.
4. Pandian, Z., Marjoribanks, J., Ozturk, O., Serour, G. & Bhattacharya, S. Number of embryos for transfer following in vitro fertilisation or intra-cytoplasmic sperm injection. Cochrane Database Syst Rev. 2013:Cd003416. doi:https://doi.org/10.1002/14651858.CD003416.pub4.
5. Gelbaya TA, Tsoumpou I, Nardo LG. The likelihood of live birth and multiple birth after single versus double embryo transfer at the cleavage stage: a systematic review and meta-analysis. Fertil Steril. 2010;94:936–45. https://doi.org/10.1016/j.fertnstert.2009.04.003.
6. Oron G, Son WY, Buckett W, Tulandi T, Holzer H. The association between embryo quality and perinatal outcome of singletons born after single embryo transfers: a pilot study. Human Reprod. 2014;29:1444–51. https://doi.org/10.1093/humrep/deu079.
7. Giorgetti C, et al. Embryo score to predict implantation after in-vitro fertilization: based on 957 single embryo transfers. Human Reprod. 1995;10: 2427–31.
8. Ziebe S, et al. Embryo morphology or cleavage stage: how to select the best embryos for transfer after in-vitro fertilization. Human Reprod. 1997;12: 1545–9.
9. Tao T, Robichaud A, Mercier J, Ouellette R. Influence of group embryo culture strategies on the blastocyst development and pregnancy outcome. J Assist Reprod Genet. 2013;30:63–8. https://doi.org/10.1007/s10815-012-9892-x.
10. Wintner EM, et al. Does the transfer of a poor quality embryo together with a good quality embryo affect the in vitro fertilization (IVF) outcome? J Ovarian Res. 2017;10:2. https://doi.org/10.1186/s13048-016-0297-9.
11. El-Danasouri I, et al. Effect of transferring a morphologically impaired embryo with a good quality embryo on the pregnancy and implantation rates. Eur Rev Med Pharmacol Sci. 2016;20:394–8.
12. Elster N. Less is more: the risk of multiple births. Fertil Steril. 2000;74:617–23.

23

Identification of core genes in ovarian cancer

Wenyu Li[1†], Zheran Liu[2†], Bowen Liang[3†], Siyang Chen[3], Xinping Zhang[3], Xiaoqin Tong[3], Weiming Lou[3], Lulu Le[1], Xiaoli Tang[4*] and Fen Fu[1*]

Abstract

Background: Epithelial ovarian cancer is one of the most severe public health threats in women. Since it is still challenging to screen in early stages, identification of core genes that play an essential role in epithelial ovarian cancer initiation and progression is of vital importance.

Results: Seven gene expression datasets (GSE6008, GSE18520, GSE26712, GSE27651, GSE29450, GSE36668, and GSE52037) containing 396 ovarian cancer samples and 54 healthy control samples were analyzed to identify the significant differentially expressed genes (DEGs). We identified 563 DEGs, including 245 upregulated and 318 downregulated genes. Enrichment analysis based on the gene ontology (GO) functions and Kyoto Encyclopedia of Genes and Genomes (KEGG) pathways showed that the upregulated genes were significantly enriched in cell division, cell cycle, tight junction, and oocyte meiosis, while the downregulated genes were associated with response to endogenous stimuli, complement and coagulation cascades, the cGMP-PKG signaling pathway, and serotonergic synapse. Two significant modules were identified from a protein-protein interaction network by using the Molecular Complex Detection (MCODE) software. Moreover, 12 hub genes with degree centrality more than 29 were selected from the protein-protein interaction network, and module analysis illustrated that these 12 hub genes belong to module 1. Furthermore, Kaplan-Meier analysis for overall survival indicated that 9 of these hub genes was correlated with poor prognosis of epithelial ovarian cancer patients.

Conclusion: The present study systematically validates the results of previous studies and fills the gap regarding a large-scale meta-analysis in the field of epithelial ovarian cancer. Furthermore, hub genes that could be used as a novel biomarkers to facilitate early diagnosis and therapeutic approaches are evaluated, providing compelling evidence for future genomic-based individualized treatment of epithelial ovarian cancer.

Keywords: Ovarian cancer, Meta-analysis, Differentially expressed genes

Introduction

Ovarian cancer is the most lethal gynecological cancer in the world and a general term which contains some cancers derived from various tissues [1]. Epithelial ovarian cancer is the most common and representative histological types in primary ovarian cancer and is the primary cause of deaths in female cancer patients in North America and over 100,000 deaths every year worldwide [2]. High-grade serous carcinoma (HGSC) is the most lethal subtype in the epithelial ovarian cancer, and most of them are diagnosed in an advanced stage [3]. The standard treatment for ovarian cancer is maximal cytoreductive surgery and platinum-based chemotherapy [4]. Although ovarian cancer actively responds to the initial anticancer therapy, nearly 75% of patients may relapse within two years and cannot be treated with the available chemotherapy drugs [5, 6]. Meanwhile, metastasis within the peritoneal cavity and resistance to chemotherapy are the leading causes of the high mortality rate associated with ovarian cancer, because this cancer is often diagnosed in late clinical stages as what has been mentioned above [5]. Thus, identifying new targets for treatment and seeking effective

* Correspondence: xltangmail@163.com; FF.NCU@hotmail.com
[†]Wenyu Li, Zheran Liu and Bowen Liang contributed equally to this work.
[4]School of Basic Medical Science, Nanchang University, Nanchang, Jiangxi 330031, People's Republic of China
[1]The Second Affiliated Hospital of Nanchang University, Nanchang, Jiangxi 330031, People's Republic of China
Full list of author information is available at the end of the article

chemotherapy drugs are crucial for overcoming drug resistance in advanced ovarian cancer [7].

Thus far, many genetic factors, such as *BRCA1, BRCA2, P53 (TP53), KRAS, PIK3CA, CTNNB1*, and *PTEN*, have been correlated with ovarian cancer [8]. In recent years, many studies have shown promise for gene-targeted therapies in ovarian cancer [9–11]. The poly-ADP-ribose polymerase (PARP) inhibitor olaparib, a targeted therapeutic drug approved by the Food and Drug Administration, is used to treat ovarian cancer patients with BRCA1 and BRCA2 mutations. Olaparib has also been used as maintenance therapy for patients with platinum-sensitive recurrent BRCA-mutated ovarian cancer [12]. Therefore, gene-targeted therapies provide a new possibility for the personalized treatment of ovarian cancer patients.

However, the lack of large-scale studies for the identification of differentially expressed genes (DEGs) in ovarian cancer limits the reliability of previous results and makes it difficult to screen potential targets. DNA microarray analysis is a systematic and global approach to analyze genomic expression profiles and physiological mechanisms in diseases [13, 14]. High-throughput microarray experiments have been used to analyze gene expression patterns and identify potential target genes in ovarian cancer [15].

To fill the gap regarding the identification of DEGs in ovarian cancer, we performed this meta-analysis to identify DEGs between ovarian cancer and healthy control tissues and aimed to provide a powerful tool to investigate microarray datasets by integrating data from multiple studies. An important advantage of this large-scale analysis lies in the reduction of discrepancies among different study conditions; additionally, this analysis combines the results from previous studies to assess an existing problem from a novel perspective [16]. it is worth noting that although ovarian cancer is known as a series of different molecular and histological diseases [17], we aim to uncover those common genes across different molecular subtypes of epithelial ovarian cancer. Genes discovered in meta-analyses generally overlap with genes identified in various studies, indicating increased reliability [18]. The present meta-analysis aimed to identify DEGs between ovarian tissues and control tissues. In addition, we attempted to identify potential core genes associated with epithelial ovarian cancer and to investigate some possible related mechanisms.

Materials and methods

Selection of microarray datasets for the meta-analysis

According to the Preferred Reporting Items for Systematic Reviews and Meta-Analyses (PRISMA) guidelines published in 2009, we performed a comprehensive search of Gene Expression Omnibus (GEO) databases from the National Center for Biotechnology Information (NCBI, http://www.ncbi.nlm.nih.gov/geo/). The keywords "ovarian neoplasms" and "ovarian cancer" were used in our search. The datasets were required to meet the following criteria: (1) the samples had to be from the Affymetrix Human Genome U133A Array platform or Affymetrix Human Genome U133 Plus 2.0 Array platform; (2) the study organisms had to be *Homo sapiens*; (3) the datasets had to contain ovarian cancer and normal ovarian tissue samples; and (4) the number of normal ovarian tissue samples had to be greater than three. Studies were excluded if (1) they were cell line studies; (2) they involved dual-channel arrays; (3) they did not have literature traceability; (4) they were DNA methylation studies; (5) they were miRNA-based studies; and (6) they lacked cases and controls. The data from the original studies were selected by two independent analysts. Any disagreement between the two analysts was solved by consultation with a third analyst.

Meta-analysis of multiple microarray datasets

From the GEO database, we downloaded Ovarian files (.CEL) of microarray datasets that met the inclusion criteria. A total of 13,294 common genes were obtained by integrating the genes from seven datasets using the R statistical software (http://www.r-project.org/). Then, we performed a meta-analysis of gene expression profiles of the 13,294 common genes according to combined *p*-values and Z scores using R statistical software. Combined p-values (pval_test) included the test-statistic and p-value. The meta-analysis of common genes was conducted by the MAMA, mataMA, affyPLM, CLL and RankProd packages. In performing two meta-analysis with R statistical software, combined p-values method (where the threshold was an absolute value more than 5) and Z-scored meta-analysis (where the threshold was an absolute value more than 7) were used as the cutoff criteria, and a list of DEGs (up- or downregulated) was identified.

GO annotations and KEGG pathway enrichment analysis

Identifying the biological characteristics of DEGs is vital. Based on the results of the meta-analysis, the most significant DEGs were evaluated by enrichment analyses. Then, gene ontology (GO) annotations and Kyoto Encyclopedia of Genes and Genomes (KEGG) pathway enrichment analyses were conducted to identify the most significant DEGs using the WEB-based GEne SeT AnaLysis Toolkit (http://www.webgestalt.org/option.php) with a significance threshold of false-discovery rate (FDR) less than 0.1.

PPI network construction

The Search Tool for the Retrieval of Interacting Genes (STRING) database (http://string-db.org) displays information on protein-protein interactions (PPIs) [19]. We charted a PPI network of DEGs using STRING with confidence score more than 0.7 as the significance cutoff criterion to acquire an in-depth understanding and predict the cellular functions and biological behaviors of the identified DEGs. Further, PPI networks were visualized utilizing the Cytoscape software [19].

Selection of hub genes and modules

CentiScaPe 2.1 was used to calculate the degree, closeness, and betweenness of the PPI network. The degree of a node is the average number of edges (interactions) incident on the node [20]. According to the degree of a node, we identified the hub genes. The Molecular Complex Detection (MCODE) software was employed to select the most important clustering modules of PPI networks in Cytoscape with degree cutoff = 2, node score cutoff = 0.2, k-core = 2, and max. Depth = 100. Furthermore, KEGG pathway enrichment analysis was conducted for DEGs in every module using the WEB-based GEne SeT AnaLysis Toolkit with a significance threshold of FDR less than 0.1.

Survival analysis using hub genes

The Kaplan-Meier plotter (KM plotter, http://kmplot.com/analysis/) was used to display the relevance of the identified genes regarding patient survival using 1816 ovarian cancer samples. Gene expression data and relapse-free and overall survival (OS) information were downloaded from the GEO (Affymetrix microarrays only), the European Genome-phenome Archive (EGA) and the Cancer Genome Atlas (TCGA) databases. Hazard ratios (HRs) with 95% confidence intervals and log-rank *p*-value were calculated and displayed on the plot.

Results

Identification of upregulated or downregulated DEGs through the meta-analysis

According to the inclusion criteria, the following seven GEO datasets from the NCBI were obtained: GSE6008, GSE18520, GSE26712, GSE27651, GSE29450, GSE36668, and GSE52037 (see "Materials and Methods", Fig. 1). A total of 396 ovarian cancer samples and 54 normal ovarian tissue samples were analyzed. The GEO Platform Files (GPLs) from the seven datasets were obtained using Affymetrix gene chips (Table 1).

We identified common genes across all datasets and performed a meta-analysis of multiple gene expression profiles using two platforms according to combined *p*-values and Z scores. According to the combined *p*-values (the threshold was 5) and Z scores (the limit was 7), 563 DEGs including 245 upregulated and 318 downregulated genes were identified (Additional file 1: Table S1 and Additional file 2: Table S2). The overlapping DEGs based on the combined *p*-values and Z scores are shown in Fig. 2.

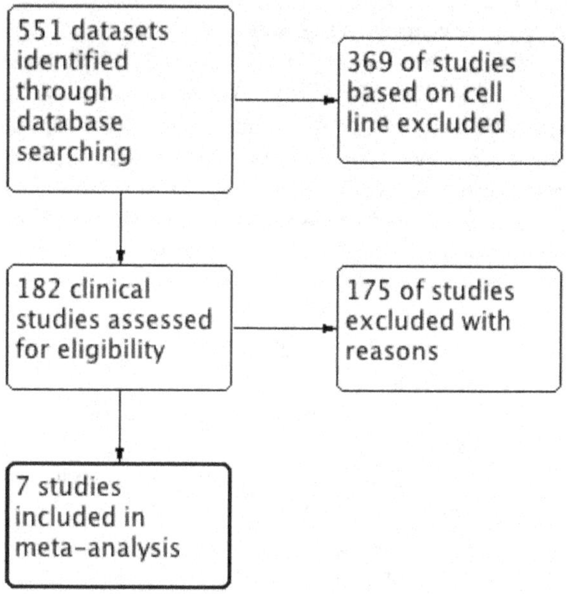

Fig. 1 Selection procession of microarray datasets for meta-analysis

GO term and KEGG pathway enrichment analyses

To further investigate the functions of the DEGs, we separately classified the upregulated and downregulated genes into functional GO and KEGG categories and then performed pathway enrichment analyses with a significance threshold less than 0.05. The top five terms enriched in each category were selected according to the *p*-value.

For biological processes, GO analysis results showed that the upregulated DEGs were separately enriched in 'cell division' (GO:0051301), 'cell-cell junction' (GO:0005911) and 'enzyme binding' (GO:0019899), whereas and the downregulated DEGs were enriched in 'response to endogenous stimulus' (GO:0009719), 'extracellular space' (GO:0005615) and 'RNA polymerase II transcription factor activity, and 'sequence-specific DNA binding' (GO:0000981, Table 2).

The most enriched KEGG pathway term for the upregulated DEGs was 'cell cycle' (KEGG:04110) and for the downregulated DEGs was 'complement and coagulation cascades' (KEGG:04610, Table 3).

Hub gene and module screening from the PPI network

First, we determined the PPI network of the DEGs. The PPI network consisted of 275 nodes and 770 edges with a confidence score of more than 0.7 based on the STRING database. The top 12 hubs with degree centrality more than 29 were screened from the PPI network as hub genes. These hub genes included Cyclin-dependent kinase 1 (*CDK1*), DNA topoisomerase 2-alpha (*TOP2A*), cell-division cycle protein 2 (*CDC20*), G2/mitotic-specific cyclin-B2 (*CCNB2*), baculoviral inhibitor of apoptosis repeat-containing 5 (*BIRC5*), ubiquitin-conjugating enzyme E2 C2 (*UBE2C*), budding uninhibited by benzimidazoles 1

Table 1 Characteristic of individual studies retrieved from Gene Expression Omnibus for meta-analysis

Dataset	Samples	Case/Control	Country	PMID	Platforms	Gene#	Gene chip
GSE6008	103	99/4	USA	16,452,189/ 19,843,521/ 17,418,409/ 27538791	GPL96	13,909	Affymetrix Human Genome U133A Array
GSE18520	63	53/10	USA	19,962,670	GPL570	22,838	Affymetrix Human Genome U133 Plus 2.0 Array
GSE26712	195	185/10	USA	18,593,951/25944803	GPL96	13,909	Affymetrix Human Genome U133A Array
GSE27651	41	35/6	USA	21,451,362	GPL570	22,838	Affymetrix Human Genome U133 Plus 2.0 Array
GSE29450	20	10/10	USA	21,754,983	GPL570	22,838	Affymetrix Human Genome U133 Plus 2.0 Array
GSE36668	8	4/4	Norway	23,029,477	GPL570	22,838	Affymetrix Human Genome U133 Plus 2.0 Array
GSE52037	20	10/10	USA	24,666,724	GPL570	19,257	Affymetrix Human Genome U133 Plus 2.0 Array

(*BUB1*), non-SMC condensin I complex subunit G (*NCAPG*), Ribonucleoside-diphosphate reductase subunit M2 (*RRM2*), Kinesin-like protein (*KIF2C*), centromere protein A (*CENPA*), and maternal embryonic leucine zipper kinase (*MELK*).

Moreover, the top 2 significant modules were obtained from the PPI network of DEGs using the MCODE software (Fig. 3). Then, KEGG pathway enrichment analyses of the genes in these two modules were performed using the WEB-based GEne SeT AnaLysis Toolkit (Additional file 3: Table S3). The results demonstrated that the genes in module 1 were mainly associated with cell cycle, oocyte meiosis and the p53 signaling pathway, while the genes in module 2 were primarily in tight junction proteins, leukocyte transendo thelial migration, hepatitis C, and cell adhesion molecules (CAMs). The top 12 hub genes belonged to module 1 and confirmed the critical pathways associated with ovarian cancer. In conclusion, these essential genes provide new ideas for the treatment of ovarian cancer.

KM plots for hub genes

The prognostic information of the 12 hub genes is freely available in http://kmplot.com/analysis/. The results demonstrated that the expression of *CDK1* (203213_at, HR 1.27 (1.11–1.46), $p = 6 \times 10^{-4}$), *TOP2A* (201291_s_at, HR 1.27 (1.11–1.44), $p = 3.9 \times 10^{-4}$), *CCNB2* (202705_at, HR 1.15 (1.22–1.81), $p = 0.049$), UBE2C (202954_at, HR 1.28 (1.12–1.47), $p = 3.8 \times 10^{-4}$), *BUB1* (209642_at, HR 1.26 (1.08–1.46), $p = 2.9 \times 10^{-3}$), *NCAPG* (218663_at, HR 1.26 (1.09–1.46), $p = 1.9 \times 10^{-3}$), *RRM2* (201890_at, HR 1.17 (1.03–1.34), $p = 1.7 \times 10^{-2}$), *KIF2C* (209408_at, HR 1.15 (1.01–1.32), $p = 3.8 \times 10^{-2}$) and *CENPA* (204962_s_at, HR 1.23 (1.08–1.41), $p = 2.4 \times 10^{-3}$) was negatively associated with the OS of epithelial ovarian cancer patients (Fig. 4 and Additional file 4: Figure S1).

Discussion

The problematic diagnosis in an early stage and recurrence and resistance to current chemotherapeutic agents are the leading causes of high mortality in ovarian cancer based on data from The Surveillance, Epidemiology, and End Results (SEER) Program of the National Cancer Institute [21]. Therefore, the development of novel therapies for ovarian cancer is of great urgency. Previous research has proven that ovarian cancer is caused by the activation of oncogenes and the inactivation of cancer suppressor gene [22]. With continued advancements in high-throughput technologies,

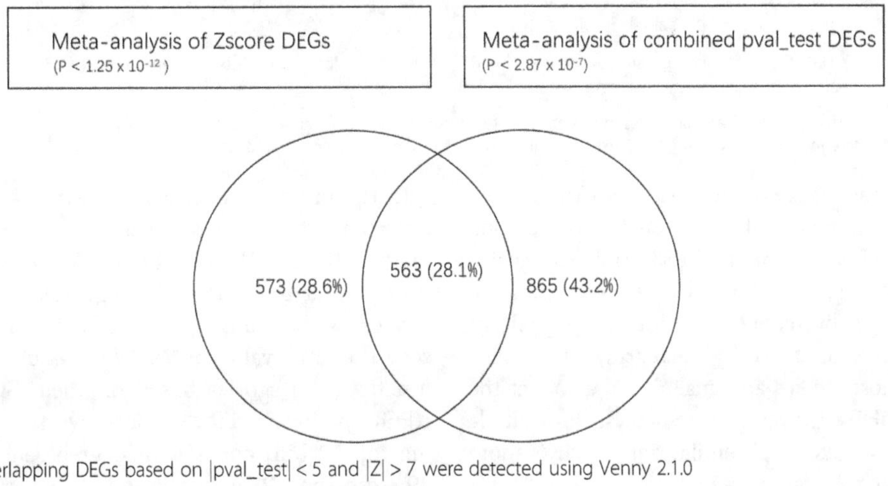

Fig. 2 The 563 overlapping DEGs based on |pval_test| < 5 and |Z| > 7 were detected using Venny 2.1.0

Table 2 GO analysis of differentially expressed genes

Category	Term	O	C	E	R	*P* Value
Up-regulated						
GOTERM_BP_DIRECT	GO:0051301~cell division	32	553	7.28	4.40	1.64E-12
	GO:0051276~chromosome organization	33	597	7.86	4.20	2.48E-12
	GO:0000819~sister chromatid segregation	19	215	2.83	6.71	6.47E-11
	GO:0007059~chromosome segregation	23	329	4.33	5.31	7.00E-11
	GO:0000278~mitotic cell cycle	40	972	12.79	3.13	9.53E-11
GOTERM_CC_DIRECT	GO:0005911~cell-cell junction	28	626	7.05	3.97	4.55E-10
	GO:0030054~cell junction	39	1357	15.28	2.55	4.45E-08
	GO:0000777~condensed chromosome kinetochore	10	101	1.14	8.79	2.05E-07
	GO:0000776~kinetochore	11	130	1.46	7.52	2.52E-07
	GO:0043296~apical junction complex	11	130	1.46	7.52	2.52E-07
GOTERM_MF_DIRECT	GO:0019899~enzyme binding	44	1756	22.14	1.99	6.09E-06
	GO:0098632~protein binding involved in cell-cell adhesion	14	288	3.63	3.86	1.79E-05
	GO:0098631~protein binding involved in cell adhesion	14	293	3.69	3.79	2.17E-05
	GO:0042802~identical protein binding	35	1330	16.77	2.09	2.39E-05
	GO:0098641~cadherin binding involved in cell-cell adhesion	13	277	3.49	3.72	5.15E-05
Down-regulated						
GOTERM_BP_DIRECT	GO:0009719~response to endogenous stimulus	62	1536	25.89	2.40	5.06E-11
	GO:0071495~cellular response to endogenous stimulus	53	1190	20.06	2.64	5.06E-11
	GO:0009725~response to hormone	42	832	14.02	3.00	1.65E-10
	GO:0032870~cellular response to hormone stimulus	34	608	10.25	3.32	8.17E-10
	GO:1901700~response to oxygen-containing compound	55	1445	24.35	2.26	6.68E-09
GOTERM_CC_DIRECT	GO:0005615~extracellular space	49	1385	17.58	2.79	3.25E-11
	GO:0005578~proteinaceous extracellular matrix	21	347	4.40	4.77	3.59E-09
	GO:0031012~extracellular matrix	25	503	6.39	3.92	6.13E-09
	GO:0042995~cell projection	42	1806	22.93	1.83	7.75E-05
	GO:0005925~focal adhesion	15	390	4.95	3.03	1.44E-04
GOTERM_MF_DIRECT	GO:0000981~RNA polymerase II transcription factor activity, sequence-specific DNA binding	31	652	10.49	2.95	6.92E-08
	GO:0003700~transcription factor activity, sequence-specific DNA binding	42	1203	19.36	2.17	1.53E-06
	GO:0001071~nucleic acid binding transcription factor activity	42	1204	19.38	2.17	1.56E-06
	GO:0000982~transcription factor activity, RNA polymerase II core promoter proximal region sequence-specific binding	19	342	5.50	3.45	2.96E-06
	GO:0001228~transcriptional activator activity, RNA polymerase II transcription regulatory region sequence-specific binding	17	323	5.20	3.27	2.00E-05

If there are more than five pathways in this category, the top five are selected according to the *P* value
O number of genes in this category in the user gene list, *E* expected number of genes in this category, *R* concentration ratio

some genetic alterations associated with ovarian cancer, such as specific mutations in KRAS, loss-of-function mutations in PTEN, mutations in TP53, modifications in BRCA1/2, and changes in homologous recombination genes, have been uncovered [23]. Although a significant amount of data were produced by microarray studies, the sample sizes of most studies are small and may affect the identification of DEGs. However, meta-analysis of multiple microarray datasets makes the identification of DEGs more reliable by increasing the sample size.

In the present study, we performed a meta-analysis to determine the DEGs between ovarian cancer and normal ovarian tissues. We identified 563 DEGs, including 245 upregulated and 318 downregulated DEGs, in ovarian tissues by combining *p*-values (cutoff value of 5) and Z scores (cutoff value of 7). We classified the DEGs into functional categories based on their GO functions and KEGG pathways. Furthermore, we screened the following top 12 hub nodes with degree centrality more than 29 from the PPI network as hub genes: *CDK1, TOP2A,*

Table 3 KEGG enrichment analysis of differentially expressed genes

Term	C	O	E	R	*P* Value	Genes
Up-regulated						
hsa04110: Cell cycle	124	11	1.90	5.79	2.64E-06	E2F3, SFN, MCM4, BUB1, BUB1B, TTK, YWHAZ, CCNE1, CCNB2, CDK1, CDC20
hsa04530: Tight junction	139	9	2.13	4.22	0.00026240	CLDN4, CLDN3, CLDN7, TJP3, KRAS, LLGL2, PRKCI, CLDN10, MAGI1
hsa04114: Oocyte meiosis	124	8	1.90	4.21	0.00059620	ITPR3, BUB1, YWHAZ, CCNE1, CCNB2, CALML4, CDK1, CDC20
hsa01230: Biosynthesis of amino acids	75	6	1.15	5.22	0.00096638	PSAT1, IDH2, PFKP, PKM, PYCR1, TPI1
hsa00051: Fructose and mannose metabolism	33	4	0.51	7.91	0.00151933	PFKP, SORD, TPI1, TSTA3
Down-regulated						
hsa04610: Complement and coagulation cascades	79	7	1.42	4.93	0.00051053	PROCR, CFH, TFPI, THBD, C1S, C4BPB, C7
hsa04022: cGMP-PKG signaling pathway	168	10	3.02	3.31	0.00084616	AKT3, ADCY2, EDNRA, AKT2, GATA4, ITPR1, KCNJ8, MEF2C, PLN, RGS2
hsa04726: Serotonergic synapse	113	8	2.03	3.94	0.00092536	DUSP1, GNG4, GNG11, HTR2B, ITPR1, MAOA, MAOB, TRPC1
hsa04550: Signaling pathways regulating pluripotency of stem cells	142	9	2.55	3.53	0.00098921	AKT3, AKT2, APC, ID3, IL6ST, WNT4, TBX3, LEFTY2, KLF4
hsa04270: Vascular smooth muscle contraction	121	8	2.18	3.68	0.00144356	CALCRL, ADCY2, EDNRA, ITPR1, PPP1R12B, PLA2G1B, PLA2G5, CALD1

If there are more than five pathways in this category, the top five are selected according to the *P* value
O number of genes in this category in the user gene list, *E* expected number of genes in this category, *R* concentration ratio

CDC20, CCNB2, BIRC5, UBE2C, BUB1, NCAPG, RRM2, KIF2C, CENPA, and *MELK*. Additionally, we obtained two top significant modules from PPI networks of DEGs using MCODE analysis. Genes in module 1 were mainly associated with cell cycle, oocyte meiosis and the p53 signaling pathway, while genes in module 2 were primarily enriched in tight junction proteins, leukocyte transendothelial migration, hepatitis C, and CAMs.

Among the top 12 hub genes, nine hub genes were associated with poor OS in epithelial ovarian cancer patients. Based on GO functional analysis, KEGG pathway analysis, and survival analysis, we found that *CDK1, TOP2A*, and *UBE2C* might be the core genes contributing to the development of epithelial ovarian cancer at the molecular level.

CDK1 plays a vital role in the regulation of the cell cycle by modulating the centrosome. CDK1 not only promotes G2-M transition but also regulates G1 progression and G1-S transition by binding with multiple interphase cyclins [24, 25] In ovarian cancer, the expression of CDK1 is significantly associated with survival status, histological grade, FIGO stage, lymph node metastasis, and metastasis in epithelial ovarian cancer patients [26].

TOP2A is a nuclear enzyme involved involved in cell division and the cell cycle. TOP2A controls topological states of DNA by transiently breaking and subsequently rejoining of DNA strands [27]. Additionally, TOP2A is a direct molecular target of topoisomerase inhibitor, and its upregulation has been reported in several cancers including lung, nasopharyngeal, esophageal, gallbladder, hepatocellular, colorectal, breast, endometrial, pancreatic and ovarian cancer [28–31].

UBE2C, an essential factor of the anaphase-promoting complex/cyclosome (APC/C), is required for the destruction of mitotic cyclins and cell cycle progression [32]. The N-terminal extension of UBE2C contributes to the regulation of APC/C activity for substrate selection and checkpoint control [33]. UBE2C, the exclusive partner of APC/C, participates in the degradation of the APC/C target protein family by initiating the formation of a Lys11-linked ubiquitin chain. Thus, UBE2C plays a vital role in the destruction of mitotic cyclins and other mitosis-related substrates. During early mitosis, the APC is activated through cyclin B/Cdk1-dependent phosphorylation and binding of its activator CDC20. During metaphase, UBE2C degrades securin and cyclin B by APC/C^{CDC20} to promote progression to anaphase [34]. UBE2C is significantly upregulated in several types of cancer including bladder, breast, brain, cervical, esophageal, colorectal, liver, lung, nasopharyngeal, prostate (late-stage), pancreatic, thyroid, stomach, and ovarian cancer [33]. UBE2C is associated with tumor progression. I. van Ree et al. identified UBE2C as a prominent proto-oncogene that contributes to whole chromosome instability and tumor formation over a wide range of overexpression levels [35].

In our study, in addition to *UBE2C* upregulation, *CDC20, CDK1*, and *CCNB2* are overexpressed. Combined with the above results, it is logic to assume that the interaction among UBE2C, CDC20, CDK1, and CCNB2 may play a vital role in the formation and development of ovarian cancer. Overexpression of *UBE2C* was associated with poor OS for ovarian

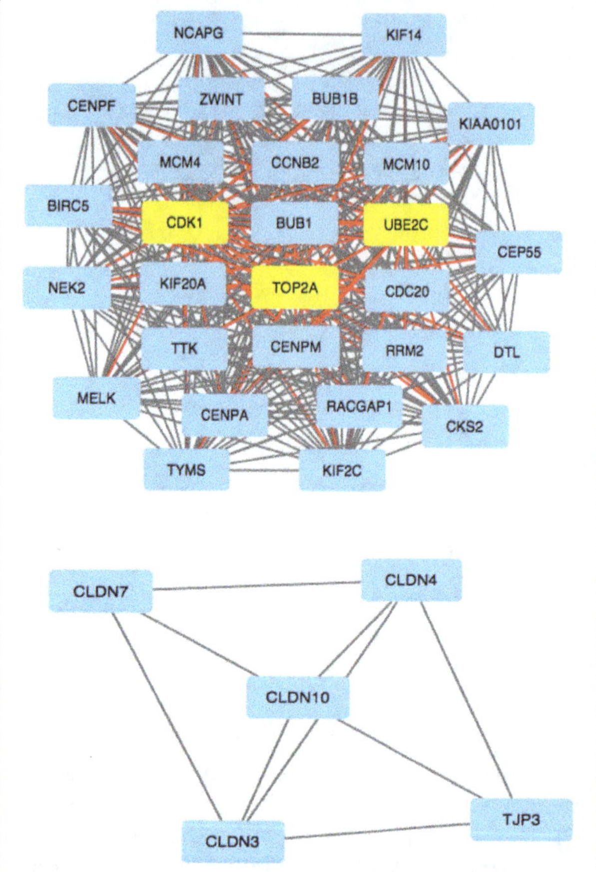

Fig. 3 2 modules obtained from PPI network of DEGs using the MCODE software. The top 12 hub genes were all in the module 1

cancer patients, and thus UBE2C might be a promising prognostic molecular biomarker and therapeutic target for ovarian cancer. It is worth to emphasize that though a series of distinct molecular and histologic subtypes of ovarian cancer exists and each subtype has different tumor microenvironment. The present research mainly focuses on those common pathways of epithelial ovarian cancer. Yet we have analyzed the corresponding gene expression data acquired from GSE9891 and the results shows that 11 out of 12 hub genes (expression data of CDK1 cannot be found in the datasets GSE9891) are significantly up-regulated (Additional file 5: Figure S2, Additional file 6: Figure S3, Additional file 7: Figure S4, Additional file 8: Figure S5, Additional file 9: Figure S6, Additional file 10: Figure S7, Additional file 11: Figure S8, Additional file 12: Figure S9, Additional file 13: Figure S10, Additional file 14: Figure S11 and Additional file 15: S12, Additional file 16: Table S4) in all of the molecular subtypes (differential, immunoreacted, proliferation and mesenchymal) comparing to control group. Subsequent researches will be conducted to investigate the role each hub gene played in each subtype of ovarian cancer,

Besides, we consider the protein expression of these hub genes might be instructive to the further study. The protein expression data of hub genes is acquired from the Human Protein Atlas for evaluation. The protein expressions of 5 hub genes (CDK1, TOP2A, CDC20, NCAPG, and MELK) are significantly up-regulated in ovarian cancer compared to normal tissues (Additional file 17: Table S5.). Also, we have done a chi-square analysis to explore the relationship between the expression of 12 hub genes and the metastasis of ovarian cancer. The results show none of these genes has connections to the cancer metastasis ($P > 0.05$). Overall, the present study was designed to identify DEGs through integrated bioinformatics analysis to find potential biomarkers and predict the development and prognosis of ovarian cancer. However, to obtain more accurate correlation results, we need to performed a series of validation experiments. In conclusion, this study provides robust evidence for future genomic-based individualized treatment of ovarian cancer.

Conclusion

Until now, a large-scale meta-analysis identifying DEGs was absent from the ovarian cancer literature. Our study

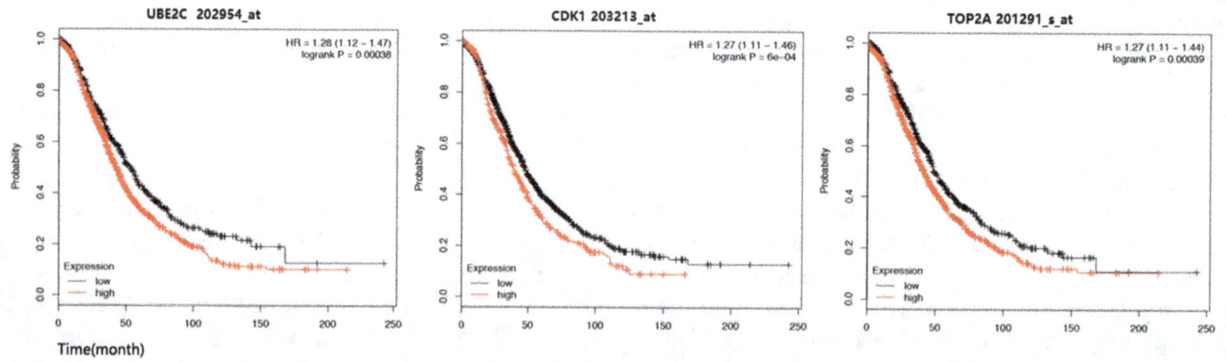

Fig. 4 Top 3 genes (*CDK1*, *TOP2A* and *UBE2C*) significantly correlates with poor OS of ovarian cancer

systematically validated previous studies and filled the gap regarding a large-scale meta-analysis in the field of ovarian cancer. Moreover, our meta-analysis identified three specific genes, namely, *CDK1*, *TOP2A* and *UBE2C*, which may be potential targets of ovarian cancer. Thus, this study provides convincing evidence for future genomic individualized treatment of epithelial ovarian cancer.

Additional files

Additional file 1: Table S1. Information of 245 upregulated DEGs. (XLSX 49 kb)

Additional file 2: Table S2. Information of 318 downregulated DEGs. (XLSX 59 kb)

Additional file 3: Table S3. KEGG pathway enrichment analyses of the genes in the two modules using the WEB-based GEne SeT AnaLysis Toolkit. (XLSX 13 kb)

Additional file 4: Figure S1. The Kaplan-Meier plots of 9 hub gene selected from PPI network are associated with poor prognosis of ovarian cancer patients. (TIF 893 kb)

Additional file 5: Figure S2. The difference of BIRC5 expression level in four molecular subtypes of epithelial ovarian cancer to control group. (PDF 5 kb)

Additional file 6: Figure S3. The difference of BUB1 expression level in four molecular subtypes of epithelial ovarian cancer to control group. (PDF 5 kb)

Additional file 7: Figure S4. The difference of CCNB2 expression level in four molecular subtypes of epithelial ovarian cancer to control group. (PDF 4 kb)

Additional file 8: Figure S5. The difference of CDC20 expression level in four molecular subtypes of epithelial ovarian cancer to control group. (PDF 5 kb)

Additional file 9: Figure S6. The difference of CENPA expression level in four molecular subtypes of epithelial ovarian cancer to control group. (PDF 5 kb)

Additional file 10: Figure S7. The difference of KIF2C expression level in four molecular subtypes of epithelial ovarian cancer to control group. (PDF 5 kb)

Additional file 11: Figure S8. The difference of MELK expression level in four molecular subtypes of epithelial ovarian cancer to control group. (PDF 4 kb)

Additional file 12: Figure S9. The difference of NCAPG expression level in four molecular subtypes of epithelial ovarian cancer to control group. (PDF 5 kb)

Additional file 13: Figure S10. The difference of RRM2 expression level in four molecular subtypes of epithelial ovarian cancer to control group. (PDF 5 kb)

Additional file 14: Figure S11. The difference of TOP2A expression level in four molecular subtypes of epithelial ovarian cancer to control group. (PDF 5 kb)

Additional file 15: Figure S12. The difference of UBE2C expression level in four molecular subtypes of epithelial ovarian cancer to control group. (PDF 5 kb)

Additional file 16: Table S4. The difference of 11 hub genes expression changes in four molecular subtypes of epithelial ovarian cancer to normal tissues. (XLSX 9 kb)

Additional file 17: Table S5. The protein expression changes of hub genes in the ovarian cancer. (XLSX 9 kb)

Abbreviations

APC/C: Anaphase-promoting complex/cyclosome; BIRC5: Baculoviral inhibitor of apoptosis repeat-containing 5; BUB1: Budding uninhibited by benzimidazoles 1; CAMs: Cell adhesion molecules; CCNB2: G2/mitotic-specific cyclin-B2; CDC20: Cell-division cycle protein 2; CDK1: Cyclin-dependent kinase 1; CENPA: Centromere protein A; DEGs: Differentially expressed genes; EGA: The European Genome-phenome Archive; FDR: False-discovery rate; GEO: Gene Expression Omnibus; GO: Gene ontology; GPLs: The GEO Platform Files; HGSC: High-grade serous carcinoma; HRs: Hazard ratios; KEGG: Kyoto Encyclopedia of Genes and Genomes; KIF2C: Kinesin-like protein; KM plotter: Kaplan-Meier plotter; MCODE: Molecular Complex Detection; MELK: Maternal embryonic leucine zipper kinase; NCAPG: Non-SMC condensin I complex subunit G; NCBI: National Center for Biotechnology Information; OS: Overall survival; PARP: Poly-ADP-ribose polymerase; PPIs: Protein-protein interactions; PRISMA: Systematic Reviews and Meta-Analyses; RRM2: Ribonucleoside-diphosphate reductase subunit M2; SEER: The Surveillance, Epidemiology, and End Results; TCGA: The Cancer Genome Atlas; TOP2A: DNA topoisomerase 2-alpha; UBE2C: Ubiquitin-conjugating enzyme E2 C2

Acknowledgements

Thanks to Prof. Deng Libin for providing the technical help and writing assistance.

Funding

This work was supported by the National Natural Science Foundation of China (Grant No. #81760504 to F Fu) and the Natural Science Foundation of Jiangxi Province (Grant No. #20171BAB205109 to X. Tang).

Authors' contributions

FF and XT conceived of the concept. WLi, ZL and BL made substantial contributions to data collection and interpretation of results; WLou, SC, XZ, XT and LL analyzed the data; ZL and BL wrote the manuscript. WLi assisted with manuscript preparation. All authors read and approved the final manuscript.

Competing interests

The authors declare that they have no competing interests.

Author details

[1]The Second Affiliated Hospital of Nanchang University, Nanchang, Jiangxi 330031, People's Republic of China. [2]Queen Mary School, Medical College of Nanchang University, Nanchang, Jiangxi 330031, People's Republic of China. [3]School of Public Health, Nanchang University, Nanchang, Jiangxi 330031, People's Republic of China. [4]School of Basic Medical Science, Nanchang University, Nanchang, Jiangxi 330031, People's Republic of China.

References

1. Desai A, Xu J, Aysola K, et al. Epithelial ovarian cancer: an overview. World J Transl Med. 2014;3(1):1-8.
2. Ferlay J, Soerjomataram I, Dikshit R, et al. Cancer incidence and mortality worldwide: sources, methods and major patterns in GLOBOCAN 2012. Int J Cancer. 2015;136(5):E359–86.
3. Bast RC Jr, Hennessy B, Mills GB. The biology of ovarian cancer: new opportunities for translation. Nat Rev Cancer. 2009;9(6):415.
4. Cortez AJ, Tudrej P, Kujawa KA, Lisowska KM. Advances in ovarian cancer therapy. Cancer Chemother Pharmacol. 2018;81:17–38.

5. Banno K, Yanokura M, Iida M, et al. Application of MicroRNA in diagnosis and treatment of ovarian cancer. Biomed Res Int. 2014;2014(3):232817.
6. Agarwal R, Kaye SB. Ovarian cancer: Strategies for overcoming resistance to chemotherapy. Nat Rev Cancer. 2003;3:502–16.
7. Norouzi-Barough L, Sarookhani MR, Sharifi M, Moghbelinejad S, Jangjoo S, Salehi R. Molecular mechanisms of drug resistance in ovarian cancer. J Cell Physiol. 2018;233:4546–62.
8. Lech A, Daneva T, Pashova S, Gagov H, Crayton R, Kukwa W, et al. Ovarian cancer as a genetic disease. Front Biosci. 2013;18:543–63.
9. An J, Lv W, Zhang Y. LncRNA NEATI contributes to paclitaxel resistance of ovarian cancer cells by regulating ZEBI expression via miR-194. Onco Targets Ther. 2017;10:5377–90.
10. Morgan RD, Clamp AR, Evans DGR, Edmondson RJ, Jayson GC. PARP inhibitors in platinum-sensitive high-grade serous ovarian cancer. Cancer Chemother Pharmacol. 2018;81:647–58.
11. Vetter MH, Hays JL. Use of targeted therapeutics in epithelial ovarian cancer: a review of current literature and future directions. Clin Ther. 2018;40:361–71.
12. Johnson N, Liao JB. Novel therapeutics for ovarian cancer: the 11th Biennial Rivkin Center Ovarian cancer Research Symposium. Int J Gynecol Cancer. 2017;27(9S):S14–9.
13. Spies M, Dasu MRK, Svrakic N, Nesic O, Barrow RE, Perez-Polo JR, et al. Gene expression analysis in burn wounds of rats. Am J Physiol Regul Integr Comp Physiol. 2002;283(4):R918–30.
14. Guo QM. DNA microarray and cancer. Curr Opin Oncol. 2003;15:36–43.
15. Cheung HW, Cowley GS, Weir BA, Boehm JS, Rusin S, Scott JA, et al. Systematic investigation of genetic vulnerabilities across cancer cell lines reveals lineage-specific dependencies in ovarian cancer. Proc Natl Acad Sci. 2011;108(30):12372–7.
16. Chee M, Yang R, Hubbell E, et al. Accessing genetic information with high-density DNA arrays. Science. 1996;274(5287):610–4.
17. Vaughan S, Coward JI, Bast RC Jr, et al. Rethinking ovarian cancer: recommendations for improving outcomes. Nat Rev Cancer. 2011;11(10):719.
18. Hong F, Breitling R, McEntee CW, Wittner BS, Nemhauser JL, Chory J. RankProd: a bioconductor package for detecting differentially expressed genes in meta-analysis. Bioinformatics. 2006;22(22):2825–7.
19. Szklarczyk D, Franceschini A, Wyder S, Forslund K, Heller D, Huerta-Cepas J, et al. STRING v10: protein-protein interaction networks, integrated over the tree of life. Nucleic Acids Res. 2015;43(D1):D447–52.
20. Scardoni G, Tosadori G, Faizan M, et al. Biological network analysis with CentiScaPe: centralities and experimental dataset integration. F1000Res. 2015;139(3):1-9.
21. Cronin KA, Lake AJ, Scott S, Sherman RL, Noone AM, Howlader N, et al. Annual report to the nation on the Status of Cancer, part I: National cancer statistics. Cancer. 2018;124(13):2785-800.
22. Di Men C, Liu QN, Ren Q. A prognostic 11 genes expression model for ovarian cancer. J Cell Biochem. 2018;119(2):1971–8.
23. Previs RA, Sood AK, Mills GB, Westin SN. The rise of genomic profiling in ovarian cancer. Expert Rev Mol Diagn. 2016;16:1337–51.
24. Lindqvist A, Rodríguez-Bravo V, Medema RH. The decision to enter mitosis: feedback and redundancy in the mitotic entry network. J Cell Biol. 2009;185: 193–202.
25. Diril MK, Ratnacaram CK, Padmakumar VC, Du T, Wasser M, Coppola V, et al. Cyclin-dependent kinase 1 (Cdk1) is essential for cell division and suppression of DNA re-replication but not for liver regeneration. Proc Natl Acad Sci. 2012;109(10):3826–31.
26. Xi Q, Huang M, Wang Y, Zhong J, Liu R, Xu G, et al. The expression of CDK1 is associated with proliferation and can be a prognostic factor in epithelial ovarian cancer. Tumor Biol. 2015;36(7):4939–48.
27. Md AS, Md S, Mazharol HM, et al. Inhibition of DNA topoisomerase type IIα(TOP2A) by mitoxantrone and its halogenated derivatives: a combined density functional and molecular docking study. Biomed Res Int. 2016;2016(5):12.
28. Zhou Z, Liu S, Zhang M, Zhou R, Liu J, Chang Y, et al. Overexpression of topoisomerase 2-alpha confers a poor prognosis i pancreatic adenocarcinoma identified by co-expression analysis. Dig Dis Sci. 2017;62(10):2790–800.
29. Ito F, Furukawa N, Nakai T. Evaluation of TOP2A as a predictive marker for endometrial cancer with taxane-containing adjuvant chemotherapy. Int J Gynecol Cancer. 2016;26(2):325–30.
30. Erriquez J, Becco P, Olivero M, Ponzone R, Maggiorotto F, Ferrero A, et al. TOP2A gene copy gain predicts response of epithelial ovarian cancers to pegylated liposomal doxorubicin. Gynecol Oncol. 2015;138(3):627–33.
31. Chen T, Sun Y, Ji P, Kopetz S, Zhang W. Topoisomerase IIalpha in chromosome instability and personalized cancer therapy. Oncogene. 2015; 34(31):4019–31.
32. Yamaguchi M, VanderLinden R, Weissmann F, Qiao R, Dube P, Brown NG, et al. Cryo-EM of mitotic checkpoint complex-bound APC/C reveals reciprocal and conformational regulation of ubiquitin ligation. Mol Cell. 2016;63(4): 593–607.
33. Xie C, Powell C, Yao M, et al. Ubiquitin-conjugating enzyme E2C: a potential cancer biomarker. Int J Biochem Cell Biol. 2014;47:113–7.
34. Rape M, Reddy SK, Kirschner MW. The processivity of multiubiquitination by the APC determines the order of substrate degradation. Cell. 2006;124(1):89–103.
35. Van Ree JH, Jeganathan KB, Malureanu L, Van Deursen JM. Overexpression of the E2 ubiquitin-conjugating enzyme UbcH10 causes chromosome missegregation and tumor formation. J Cell Biol. 2010;188(1):83–100.

24

DAXX promotes ovarian cancer ascites cell proliferation and migration by activating the ERK signaling pathway

Sheng-Bing Liu, Xue-Ping Lin, Ying Xu, Zhong-Fei Shen and Wei-Wei Pan*

Abstract

Background: The death-domain-associated protein (DAXX) was originally identified as a protein that binds to the transmembrane death receptor FAS and enhances both FAS-induced and transforming growth factor-β-dependent apoptosis. In a previous study, we found that nude mice injected with DAXX-overexpressing cells (ES-2-DAXX) accumulated large concentrations of first-generation ascites cells (I ascites cells). The role of DAXX in the development of ascites is unknown. The aim of this study was to analyze the effect of DAXX on proliferation and migration of ascites cells in ovarian cancer in vitro and in vivo.

Methods: Nude mice were housed in cages with a 14:10 h light:dark cycle; water and food were provided ad libitum. ES-2-DAXX cells (1×106) were injected intraperitoneally into athymic nude mice (8-week-old female mice). After 4 weeks, I ascites cells were collected. The I ascites cells were injected intraperitoneally into athymic nude mice (8-week-old female mice). After 4 weeks, II ascites cells were collected and cultured. Ascites cell survival, migration, and colony formation were measured using colony formation and cell growth assays. Immunofluorescent staining revealed the co-localization of DAXX and promyelocytic leukemia protein (PML) in ascites cell nuclei. Western blotting and immunohistochemistry showed that extracellular signal-related kinase (p-ERK) 1/2 and CEBP-β were highly expressed in tumor tissues formed by II ascites cells. Through immunoprecipitation, we also found that DAXX can interact with CEBP-β.

Results: DAXX enhanced ascites cell survival, migration, and colony formation. DAXX and PML nuclear foci dramatically increased in a passage-dependent manner in ascites cells, DAXX promoted the tumor growth of ascites cells in vivo, increased ascites cell proliferation in vivo, and enhanced ascites cell survival and migration by activating the ERK signalling pathway and integrating with CEBP-β.

Conclusions: DAXX can interact with CEBP-β. DAXX can induce ovarian cancer ascites formation by activating the ERK signal pathway and binding to CEBP-β.

Keywords: DAXX, Ascites cell, Cell proliferation, Cell migration

Introduction

Ovarian cancer is the fifth most common cause of death in women, and the second most common gynecological cancer worldwide [1]. Serous ovarian cancer is the most common subtype; most patients present with late-stage tumor and dissemination of tumor implants throughout the peritoneal cavity [2]. Ascites creates a protective environment for ovarian tumor cells that inhibit drug-induced apoptosis [3, 4]. Ascites is described as heterogeneous fluids that display marked differences in their levels of soluble factors; some of these factors can potentially activate an array of signaling pathways [5].

Ascites formation is an important problem in patients with ovarian cancer. The development of ascites is a hallmark symptom of late-stage ovarian cancer, and biologically active factors within the fluid can affect disease progression and interfere with anti-tumor vaccination strategies [6, 7]. The mechanism of ovarian cancer ascites formation is unknown. In a previous study, we found that DAXX-overexpressing cells (ES-2-DAXX) accumulated

* Correspondence: wwpan@mail.zjxu.edu.cn
College of Medicine, Jiaxing University, Jiaxing 314001, China

large concentrations of ascites cells [8]. Based on these data, we found that DAXX-overexpression-induced ascites cells had an increased colony number and migration ability in vitro. We further demonstrated that the ERK pathway was activated in DAXX-overexpression-induced ascites cells. We also found that DAXX interacted with CEBP-β in DAXX-overexpression-induced ascites cells. Our results indicated that DAXX promotes ovarian cancer ascites cell proliferation by activating the ERK pathway and directly binding to CEBP-β.

Methods

Reagents and cell culture

ES-2 cells (human ovarian cancer cell lines) purchased from the ATCC (Manassas, VA, USA) were cultured in DMEM (Dulbecco's Modified Eagle's Medium) which contains 10% fetal bovine serum and 1% penicillin-streptomycin solution (Hyclone, GE Healthcare, Little Chalfont, UK) at 37 °C in a humidified 5% CO_2 incubator.

Plasmids and Daxx-overexpressing ovarian cancer cell lines

The plasmid of pLEGFP-*Daxx* which encode the full-length *Daxx* sequence and HA-CEBP-β were kindly provided by Zhejiang University Professor Fan Heng-yu. Overexpressed ES-2-DAXX cells were established using the methods described previously [8].

Ascites cells and xenograft models

Nude mice were housed in cages with a 14:10 h light:dark cycle; water and food were provided ad libitum. The NIH Guides for the Care and Use of Laboratory Animals were used as all animal protocols. ES-2-DAXX (The abbreviation of ES-2-DAXX cells is ES-DAXX in all figures.) (1×10^6) were injected intraperitoneally into athymic nude mice (8-week-old female mice), ovarian cancer ascites cells in vivo were obtained through the above experiments.- After 4 weeks, ascites cells were collected and centrifuged at 157 g for 10 min. The acellular fractions were cultured in DMEM which contained 10% fetal bovine serum mediums and 1% penicillin-streptomycin in a humidified 5% CO_2 incubator at 37 °C. These cells were designated I ascites cells.The I ascites cells (1×10^6) were injected intraperitoneally into athymic nude mice (8-week-old female mice). After 4 weeks, II ascites cells were collected and cultured. Nude mice were injected with the BrdU solution to a concentration of 100 mg/kg. Two hours later, primary tumor, ovaries, and intestinal masses were collected from athymic nude mice, these primary tumor and organs were fixed with 4% formalin and made into slices (5-μm thick), then the slices were stained with HE (hematoxylin and eosin) staining.

Colony formation assay

Single ascites cell suspensions were prepared and seeded. Colonies were counted after 10 days in 60-mm dishes. The dishes were cultured in triplicate in a 5% CO_2 humidified incubator at 37 °C.

Transwell migration assay

For the transwell migration assay, 24-well plate inserts with 8-μm pore filters, the migration was assessed with BioCoat Matrigl (BD Biosciences, San Jose, CA, USA). 5×10^4cells was added to serum-free medium and suspended in a transwell. Ascites cells stably transfected with DAXX at the upper surface of the transwells were removed after cells were incubated for 24 h at 37 °C. Migrated cells were stained with H&E staining and rinsed with double distilled water, then the transwells were air-dried. The positive cells were counted by ImagePro Plus 6.0 software.

Cell growth assay

Cell proliferation was assessed by MTT assay. Ascites cells were cultured and seeded in plates, the cell densities of the 96-well plates was 3×10^3 cells/well. After the cell adhered to the wall, the 96-well plates was added 20 μl /well MTT solution (5 mg/ml in PBS) and was put into incubator in 37 °C for 4 h. Absorbance value was tested using micro-plate reader at 490 nm.

Soft agar colony formation assay

Cells were cultured using the method of Hamburger and Salmon with modifications. 1.5 ml of 0.5% agar were prepared in 6-well. Cells were suspended in 1.5 ml of 0.35% agar containing $1 \times$ cell culture medium and 10% fetal bovine serum and poured over these underlayers. The final cell concentration in each culture was 0.5×10^3 cells/ml. Triplicate cultures were used for each experiment. The plates were placed in a 5% CO_2 humidified incubator at 37 °C. Colonies were counted at 2 to 3 weeks after plating using an Omnicon FAS II Image Analysis System.

Immunohistochemistry

Paraffin-embedded human ovarian tumor tissues were obtained from the Jiaxing Maternity and Child Health Care Hospital, China. The archived human ovarian tumor tissues used in the experiments had the Jiaxing University Institutional Review Board approval. 5-μm sections were made, referring to ABC kit (Vector Laboratories, Burlingame, CA, USA), sections stained includes the following aspects: deparaffinized, rehydrated, and antigen retrieval, after the sections were incubated in H_2O_2 (0.3%) for 10 min, the sections were incubated in 10% goat serum for 30 min. Then the sections stained with affinity-purified anti-BrdU, anti-DAXX (Sigma Aldrich,

St. Louis, MO, USA), anti-p-AKT, anti-p-ERK (Cell Signaling Technology, Danvers, MA, USA), and anti-CEBP-β (Santa Cruz Biotechnology, Dallas, TX, USA) antibodies (1:200 dilution), The antibodies were incubated for 1 h. After washing with PBS, the sections were incubated with a secondary antibody for 30 min and washed again with PBS before incubation with avidin-biotin complex (ABC) solution. The sections were stained through DAB (diaminobenzidine) (DAB substrate kit, Vector Laboratories) staining.

Immunofluorescence

Nude mouse tumor tissues were gained to make microtome section, the tissues embedded in OCT compound (Sakura Finetek USA, Torrance, CA, USA) after fixed in 4% paraformaldehyde, then Leica CM1850 cryomicrotome (Leica Microsystems) was used to slice. Ascites cells of nude mouse were washed with PBS after the cells were seeded on coverslips for 24 h, then ascites cells were fixed and permeabilized, 5% BSA was used as blocking reagent. The ascites cells were incubated with primary antibodies at room temperature for 1 h. The sections of ascites cells were stained through DAPI.

RNA extraction and real-time RT–PCR analysis

Total RNA was extracted from cultured cells using Trizol reagent (Invitrogene), according to the manufacturer's instructions. Real-time PCR analysis was performed using TB Green Premix qPCR kit (TaKaRa, Japan) and an Applied 7300 Real-Time PCR System. Relative mRNA levels were determined by normalizing to the endogenous *Gapdh* mRNA.

Gapdh:5′-gcctggagaaacctgccaagtatg-3′; 5′-gagtgggagttgctgttgaagtcg-3′;
CEBP-β: 5′-gacaagcacagcgacgagta-3′; 5′-agctgctccaccttcttctg-3'
Fog2: 5′-tggggacacacagtcagaga-3′; 5′-cctcagagatggccttcgta-3′
Tff1: 5′-gaaggtcatgtcaagggaggt-3′; 5′-atgagcttgcaccacgttct-3'

Western blotting

The proteins extracted from ascites cells were separated by SDS-PAGE and transferred to PVDF membranes, then the membranes were incubated with 5% BSA for 1 h at room temperature. The membranes were incubated with primary antibodies for 1 h at room temperature and the horseradish peroxidase-conjugated goat anti - rabbit antibodies were used as second antibodies (Cell Signaling Technology). After incubated for 1 h at room temperature, the membranes were washed with TBST. Bound antibodies were visualized through ECL Western Blotting chemiluminescence reagent kit (Amersham, GE Healthcare).The primary antibodies dilution was1:1000, antibodies which were tested included DAXX (Sigma Aldrich), ERK, CEBP-β, p-ERK and β-actin (Cell Signaling Technology).

Immunoprecipitation

To detect protein-protein interactions, the vector HA-CEBP-βwere transfected into ascites cells. After transfection, Ascites cells were lysed 48 h using NP-40 buffer. The lysates were centrifuged at 13,000×*g* for 25 min. By using anti-HA M2 affinity beads (Sigma Aldrich) for 4 h at 4 °C, immunoprecipitation was performed. The NTEN buffer was boiled in loading buffer (4 × SDS) after the beads were washed in NTEN buffer, then separated by electrophoresis (SDS-PAGE). The membranes were incubated with antibodies included DAXX, CEBP-β, and β-actin after incubated with 5% BSA.

Statistical analysis

The in vitro assays results were repeated for three times. The statistical techniques employed for analysis are one-way ANOVA using GraphPad Prism statistical software (GraphPad Prism, La Jolla, CA, USA) and two-tailed T-tests. To consider $p < 0.05$ as statistically significant.

Results

DAXX enhances ascites cell survive, migration, and colony formation

To investigate the role of DAXX in ascites cells, we developed first- and second-generation ovarian cancer ascites cells (I ascites cells and II ascites cells) with stable green fluorescent protein (GFP)-DAXX expression. First, we investigated the role of DAXX in ascites cell survive, migration, and colony formation. As shown in Fig. 1a–b, II ascites cells grew faster than the parental GFP-DAXX overexpression cells, as assessed by MTT assays. The role of DAXX on ascites cell migration was also determined. We found that overexpressed DAXX markedly promoted ascites cells migration (Fig. 1c–d). Furthermore, DAXX expression in ascites cells strongly promoted colony formation (Fig. 1e–f). Notably, one important criterion distinguishes malignant cancer cells from "normal" cells is their ability to grow in soft agar. 3D cell cultures are well documented to better mimic the in vivo situation than monolayer cell culture on plastic [9–11]. Then, we compared the cell growth of ES-2-DAXX cells, I ascites cells and II ascites cells under soft agar and anchorage-independent conditions (in cell suspension). We found that II ascites cells showed a significantly stronger growth potential than ES-2-DAXX cells in soft agar and suspension (Fig. 1g–h). These results demonstrate that DAXX promoted ascites cell proliferation and migration in a passage-dependent manner.

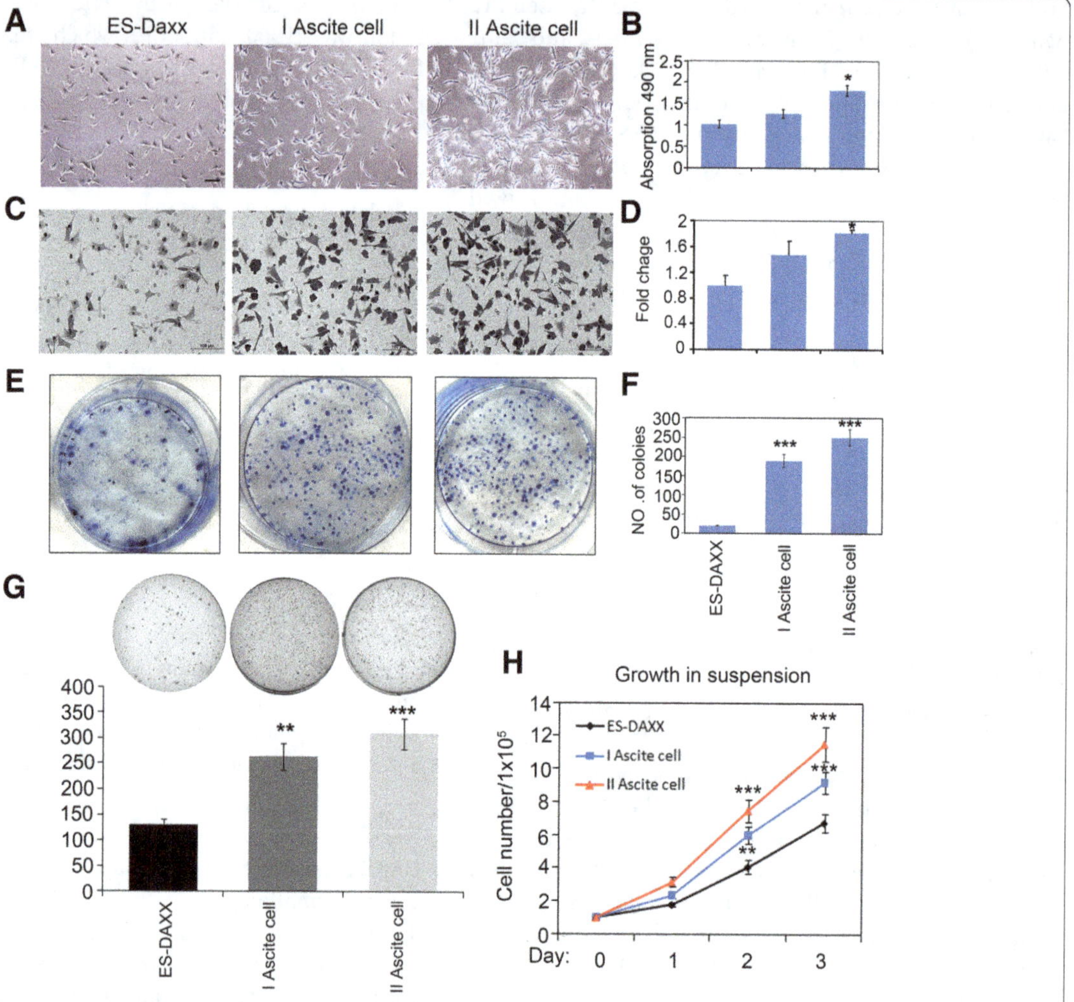

Fig. 1 DAXX enhances ascites cell colony formation and migration. **a–b** DAXX-induced ascites cell proliferation. Ascites cells were seeded into 96-well plates (3,000 cells/well) overnight, and then assessed by an MTT assay. Scale bar, 50 μm. **c–d** Transwell experiment to determine the migration capability of ascites cells and their derivatives (GFP-DAXX-overexpressing ascites cells). Cells were added to transwells and allowed to migrate for 12 h. Cells at the upper surface of the membrane were removed with cotton swabs, and cells on the bottom surface were stained with hematoxylin and eosin. Scale bar, 100 μm. **e–f** Colony formation assay for the growth of ascites cells with DAXX overexpression. Colony numbers were counted after 10–14 days. * $p < 0.05$; ***, $p < 0.0001$. **g** DAXX overexpression promotes anchorage-independent growth of ascite cells in vitro. Soft-agar colony-formation assay was performed and the colonies were stained with crystal violet for quantification. **h** DAXX overexpression promoted cell proliferation in suspension (detachment) conditions. Cells (1×10^5) were plated in 6-well culture dishes and cell number was determined with trypan blue staining. Three replicates were included. The error bars represent s.d. ns ($p > 0.05$); *** $p < 0.001$. Student's t-test was applied

DAXX and promyelocytic leukemia protein (PML) nuclear foci dramatically increase in a passage-dependent manner in ascites cells

To explore the role of DAXX on ascites cells, we harvested and cultured ascites cells in DMEM medium (Fig. 2a). Western blot examination revealed that the ascites cells were positive for GFP-DAXX (Fig. 2b), which illustrated that ascites cells were derived from the parental ES-Daxx cells. Through immunostaining, we found that DAXX nuclear aggregation significantly increased in a passage-dependent manner (Fig. 2c). In our previous study, we found that DAXX co-localized with PML in ovarian cancer cells and mouse ovarian surface epithelium (mOSE) [12]. Here, we sought to quantify PML expression in ascites cells through immunofluorescence staining. We found that PML exhibited nuclear location in ascites cells; this distribution was consistent with DAXX in ascites cells nuclei (Fig. 2d–e).

DAXX promotes the tumor growth of ascites cells in vivo

We also detected the role of DAXX in promoting the tumorigenic and metastatic capabilities of ascites cells. Female nude mice were injected intraperitoneally with either parental ES-2-DAXX cells or ascites cells. As shown in Fig. 3a–b, the average weight of the abdominal solid tumors formed by II ascites cells was approximately

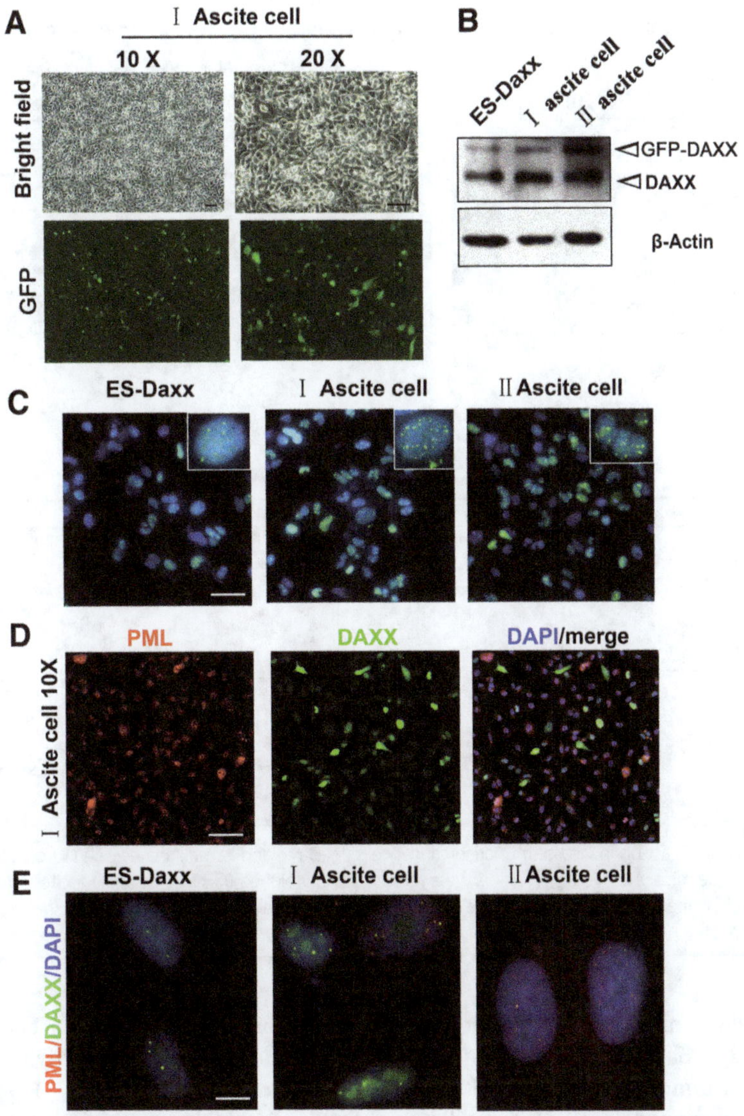

Fig. 2 DAXX and PML nuclear localization in ascites cells. **a** Ascites cell morphology using brightfield and GFP microscopy (10 × and 20× magnification, respectively). **b** Western blot results for DAXX overexpression in ascites cells. **c** Ascites cells were harvested from nude mice and cultured in vitro. Fluorescence microscopy showing the localization of overexpressed DAXX (green) in ascites cells stably transfected with GFP-DAXX. Nuclei were stained with 4′,6-diamidino-2-phenylindole (DAPI; blue). *Scale bar*, 50 μm. **d** Immunofluorescence results for promyelocytic leukemia protein (PML) foci formation in ascites cells. *Scale bar*, 50 μm. **e** Immunofluorescence results for PML, DAXX and DAPI in ES-Daxx, I and II ascites cells. *Scale bar*, 10 μm

threefold greater than the average weight of the control formed by the parental ES-2-DAXX cells. The ascites formation time decreased in a passage-dependent manner (Fig. 3c). Examination of the peritoneal cavities of mouse that injected II ascites cells showed a significant and dispersed distribution of tumor exposites in the ovary and intestine (Fig. 3d).

DAXX increases ascites cell proliferation in vivo

To illuminate the role of DAXX on ascites cells proliferation, we observed GFP expression. Fluorescence microscopy showed that the most of the tumor cells were derived from ES-2-DAXX ascites cells (Fig. 4a). Immunohistochemical examinations showed that DAXX and PML were all significantly expressed in ascites cell-derived tumors (Fig. 4b). Next, we measured bromodeoxyuridine (BrdU) levels through immunohistochemical staining. We found that BrdU was present in high concentrations in ascites cell-derived tumors (Fig. 4c). These results showed that DAXX promotes ascites cell proliferation in vivo.

DAXX enhances ascites cell survival and migration by activating the ERK signaling pathway and integrating with CEBP-β

To understand how DAXX expression promoted ascites cells growth, we measured p-ERK1/2 and p-AKT

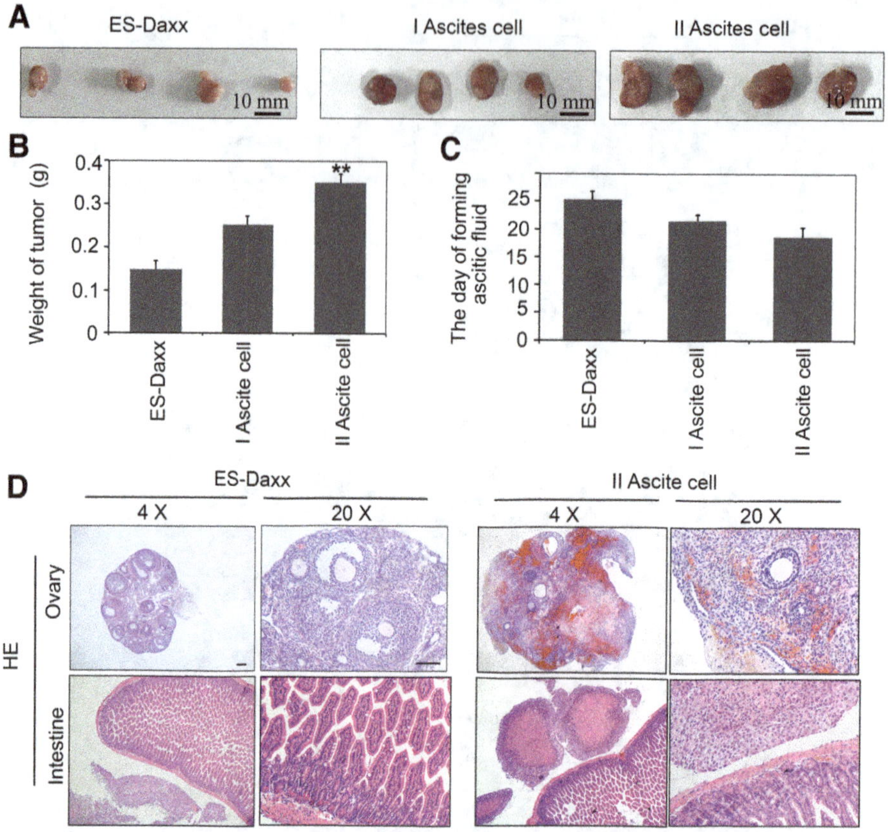

Fig. 3 DAXX promotes ascites cell metastasis in vivo. **a–b** Ovarian cancer cells (ES-Daxx) and I and II ascites cells (10^{6}cells for each) were implanted intraperitoneally into different nude mice. After 20 days, tumors were removed and weighed ($n = 5$). **c** Quantify ascites formation time (d). **d** ES-Daxx and II ascites cells were injected intraperitoneally into nude mice (10^{6} cells/mouse). HE staining showing cells metastasis to the intestine and ovary 3 weeks later. *Scale bar*, 250 μm

expression in ascites cells tumors using immunohistochemistry. As shown in Fig. 5a–b, p-ERK1/2 was highly expressed in II ascites cell tumors. However, p-AKT was found to be minimally expressed in II ascites cell tumors. In order to confirm these results, we measured p-ERK1/2 expression in ascites cells using a western blot. We found that p-ERK1/2 and CEBP-β were highly expressed in a passage-dependent manner (Fig. 5c). A previous study showed that CEBP-β directly interacts with DAXX [13]. Next, we investigated the interaction between DAXX and CEBP-β by co-immunoprecipitation in ascites cells. As shown in Fig. 5d, DAXX was found to be co-immunoprecipitated with CEBP-β. After confirming that DAXX interacts with CEBP-β in ovarian cancer ascites cells, we investigated the expression of CEBP-β in human ovarian cancer tissues by immunohistochemistry (Fig. 5e). We found that CEBP-β and DAXX were significantly expressed in human ovarian cancer tissues (Fig. 5e). To confirm the function of CEBP-β, we detect CEBP-β target gene TFF1 and Fog2 expression in ES-2-DAXX cells, I ascites cells and II ascites cells. We found that II ascites cells decrease TFF1 and Fog2 expression (new Fig. 5f). The results showed that CEBP-β transcriptional activity were increased in a passage-dependent manner. These results suggest that DAXX integrated with CEBP-β and promoted ascites cells survival and migration.

Discussion

Ovarian cancer is the most lethal tumor of all human gynecological malignancies. It is estimated that 220,000 new cases of ovarian cancer and 140,000 deaths are reported every year [14]. Due to the lack of symptoms and adequate screening methods in early stages, more than 60% of patients are diagnosed with advanced stages of ovarian cancer [15]. Ovarian cancer has a specific transmission pattern that is different from other malignancies. Tumors generally diffuse in abdominal cavity; even after recurrence, it is mostly confined to the peritoneal cavity, where it can carry out immune-suppressive activity [16]. Furthermore, for effective immune therapy, identification of the tumor antigen is required; for cellular immune therapy, the epitope recognized by T-cells must be identified.

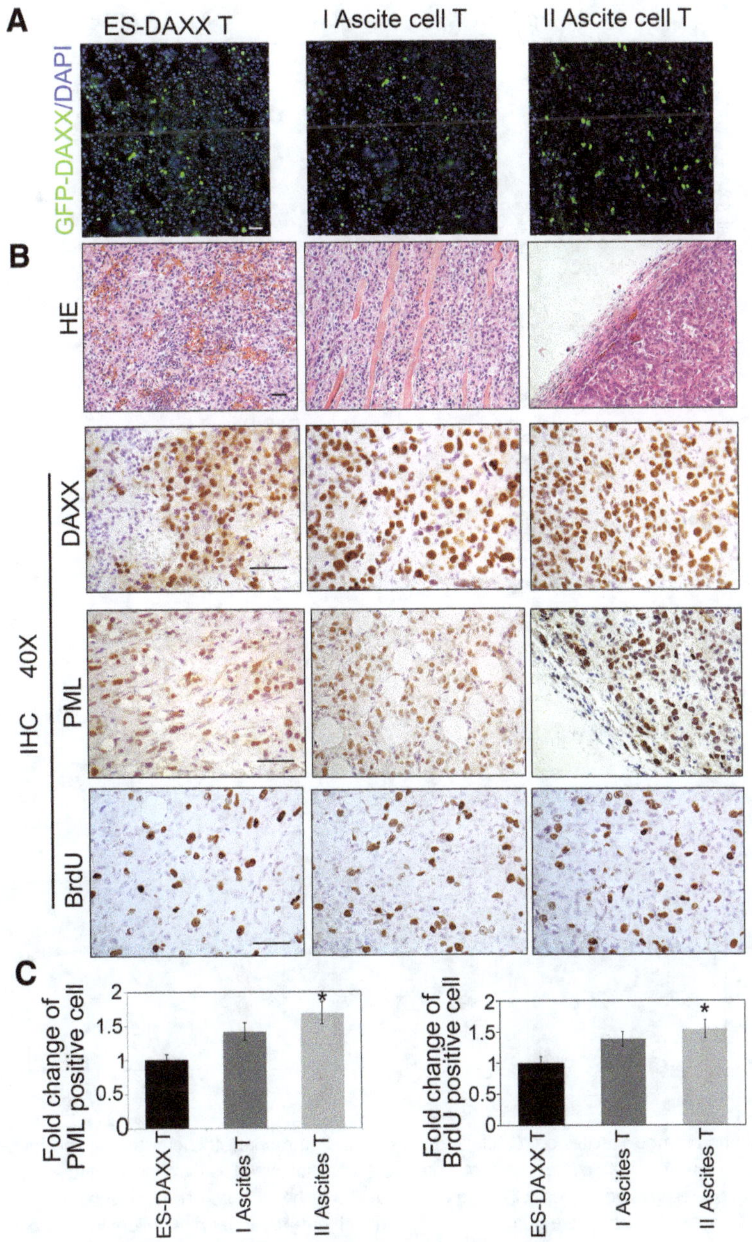

Fig. 4 DAXX promotes ascites cell proliferation in vivo. **a** Cryosections were prepared from tumor tissues derived from GFP-DAXX-overexpressing ascites cells. **b** HE and Immunohistochemistry staining for DAXX, PML, and BrdU in representative DAXX-overexpressingascites cells. *Scale bar*, 50 µm. **c** Quantify PML and BrdU positive cells in B. *, $p < 0.05$

DAXX can be either a pro- or anti-apoptotic factor, depending on the cell type [17]. DAXX was initially identified as a cytoplasmic molecule that links Fas signaling to the c-Jun N-terminal kinase (JNK) pathway via apoptosis signal-regulating kinase 1 (ASK1) [18]. In addition to its role in the cytoplasm, DAXX acts as a transcriptional co-repressor in the nuclear compartment. DAXX has been found to be associated with multiple proteins involved in transcriptional repression, such as HDAC1, DNA methyltransferase 1 (DMNT1), and α-thalassaemia/mental retardation syndrome X-linked (ATRX) [19–21]. DAXX also suppresses the activity of several transcription factors, including ETS1, Pax3, glucocorticoid receptor (GR), and p53 [22–25]. DAXX-dependent recruitment of H3.3 into PML-NBs both in proliferating cells, thus establishing PML-NBs as important assembly points for newly synthesized H3.3 histones and regulated gene expression. H3.3 is found enriched at active genes, centromeric heterochromatin, and telomeres, and has been proposed to

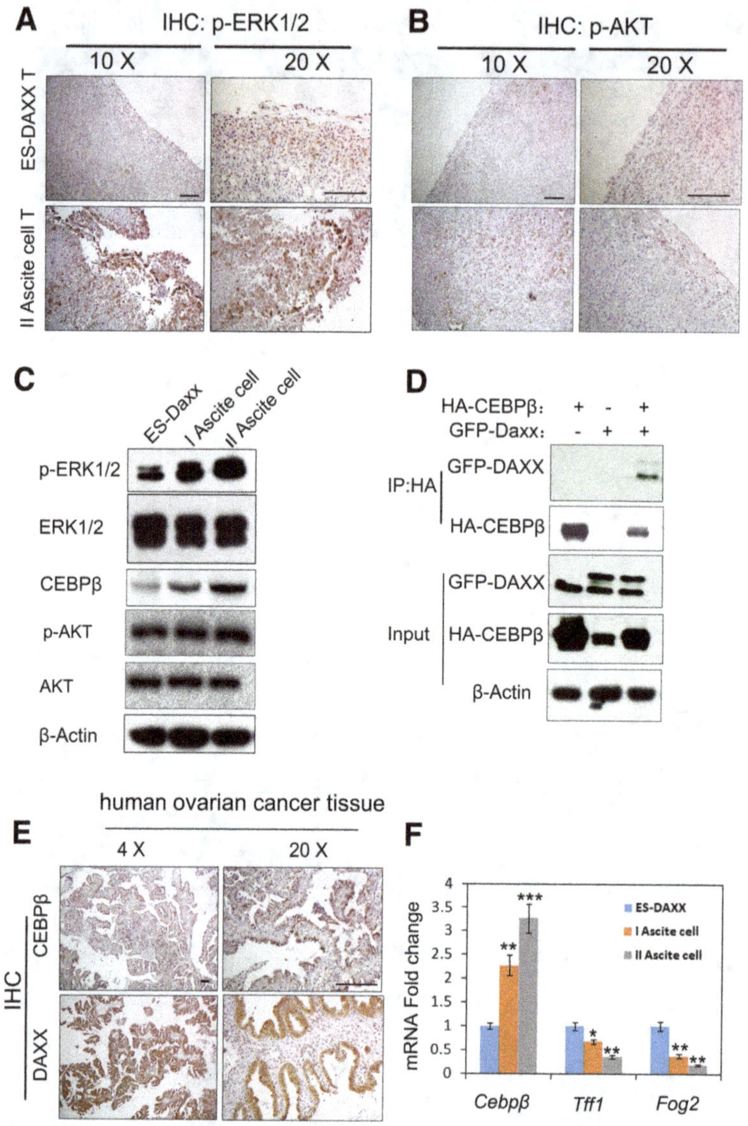

Fig. 5 DAXX binds to CEBP-β and promotes ascites cell proliferation in vivo. **a–b** Immunohistochemistry staining for p-ERK1/2 and p-AKT in mouse tumor tissue. *Scale bar*, 200 μm. **c** DAXX-overexpressing ascites cells were subjected to immunoblotting analysis with antibodies against the indicated proteins. **d** DAXX-overexpressing ascites cells were transfected with the indicated combinations of plasmids encoding HA-CEBP-β. Cells were lysed after 24 h, and protein extracts were immunoprecipitated with anti-HA antibodies, followed by SDS-PAGE and western blotting. **e** Immunohistochemical analysis of DAXX and CEBP-β levels in human ovarian tumor tissue samples ($n = 10$). Sections were counterstained with hematoxylin and eosin. *Scale bar*, 200 μm. **f** *Cebpβ*, *Tff1* and *p16* mRNA expressions in ES-Daxx, I and II ascites cells were determined by Q-PCR

act as important carrier of epigenetic information [26]. In our previous study, we found that DAXX was significantly expressed in human ovarian cancer tissue and weakly expressed in normal ovarian tissue. Female athymic nude mice were injected intraperitoneally with ES-2-DAXX cells or DAXX silencing cell (ES-2 shDAXX). Nude mice that injected ES-DAXX cells accumulated large amounts of ascites. These results showed that DAXX-overexpression played important role in ovarian cancer ascites forming [8]. In this study, we found that ES-2-DAXX cells promoted ascites cells proliferation and migration. DAXX co-localized with PML in ovarian cancer cells nuclei. DAXX and PML nuclear foci dramatically increase in a passage-dependent manner in ascites cells. This result showed that the co-localization of DAXX and PML maybe increased ascites cell-related gene expression by epigenetic regulation and promoted ascites forming.

It is well known that ascites-induced signaling events trigger the activation of both the ERK1/2 and AKT pathways. MAPK pathways is present in all cancer cells and regulates cell differentiation, proliferation, migration, apoptosis, and inflammation [27, 28]. In mammals, the activation of the MAPK/ERK pathway requires Ras, a single G protein recruited by receptor and non-receptor tyrosine kinases [29]. Activation of the ERK1/2 pathway is also involved in tumor cell survival by coupling survival stimuli to transcription factors controlling gene expression. For example, higher levels of phospho-ERK1/2 in ovarian cancer cells were found to be associated with an increased resistance to cisplatin [30]. Our results also showed that DAXX induced ovarian cancer ascites cell proliferation through ERK activation. These results were consistent with a previous study [31].

Phosphatidylinositol-4,5-bisphosphate 3 kinase (PI3K)/AKT may be a key pathway in the regulation of cell survival under anchorage-independent stress [32]. Previous studies demonstrating AKT activation by ascites cells prompted us to investigate whether AKT was also involved in DAXX-overexpression-induced ascites. We measured the phosphorylation of AKT in tumor tissues by immunohistochemistry, and found that AKT was not activated in DAXX-overexpression-induced ascites cells. These results indicated that ERK1/2, but not AKT, plays a major role in DAXX-overexpression-induced ascites cell proliferation.

CEBP-β is involved in tissue-specific gene expression and participates in fundamental cellular processes such as proliferation and differentiation [33]. In addition, CEBP-β is capable of increasing the expression of several target genes including genes coding for cytokines such as IL-6, IL-4, IL-5 and TNFα and genes coding for drug resistance such as ABCC2 and ABCB1 [34, 35]. Our results clearly demonstrated that DAXX interacts with CEBP-β in ascites cells. This indicated that DAXX-CEBP-β promotes ascites cells growth by stimulating ascites formation, altering the components of the ascites or having any other chemokines inside the ascites that leads to such cell growth promotion. A further delineation of the mechanistic link between DAXX and CEBP-β should allow a better understanding of DAXX functions in ovarian cancer ascites cells.

Conclusions

DAXX can induce ovarian cancer ascites formation by activating the ERK signal pathway and binding to CEBP-β.

Abbreviations

ASK1: Apoptosis signal-regulating kinase 1; ATRX: α-thalassaemia/mental retardation syndrome X-linked; CEBP-β: CCAAT/enhancer-binding protein-β; DAXX: Death-domain-associated protein; DMEM: Dulbecco's Modified Eagle's Medium; DNMT1: DNA methyltransferase 1; ERK: Extracellular signal-related kinase; GR: Glucocorticoid receptor; HDAC1: Histone deacetylase 1; MAPK: Mitogen-activated protein kinase; mOSE: Mouse ovarian surface epithelium; PML: Promyelocytic leukemia protein

Acknowledgements

We thank Dr. Heng-Yu Fan of Zhejiang University for the plasmid of pLEGFP-*Daxx* which encodethe full-length *Daxx* sequence and HA-CEBP-β.

This work was supported by The Natural Science Foundation of Zhejiang Province (LY17H160060, LQ13H160020). National Natural Science Foundation of China (81402162).

Funding

The Natural Science Foundation of Zhejiang Province (LY17H160060, LQ13H160020). National Natural Science Foundation of China (81402162).

Authors' contributions

PW-W made substantial contributions to the study conception and conceived of the study, performed experiments, interpreted data and corrected the manuscript. LS-B designed the study and wrote the manuscript, corrected the manuscript and critically revised the manuscript. LX-P analyzed the characteristics of the images and interpreted morphological data. XY and SZ-F performed experiments and wrote specific sections of the manuscript. LS-B and PW-W designed the study and participated in the revision of the manuscript. All the authors read and approved the final manuscript.

Authors' information

Where the work was performed: Laboratory of molecular biology, college of medicine, Jiaxing University.

Competing interests

The authors declare that they have no competing interests.

References

1. Ozols RF, Bookman MA, Connolly DC, Daly MB, Godwin AK, Schilder RJ, Xu X, Hamilton TC. Focus on epithelial ovarian cancer. Cancer Cell. 2004;5:19–24.
2. Bast RC Jr, Hennessy B, Mills GB. The biology of ovarian cancer: new opportunities for translation. Nat Rev Cancer. 2009;9:415–28.
3. Lane D, Robert V, Grondin R, Rancourt C, Piché A. Malignant ascites protect against TRAIL-induced apoptosis by activating the PI3K/Akt pathway in human ovarian carcinoma cells. Int J Cancer. 2007;121:1227–37.
4. Lane D, Goncharenko-Khaider N, Rancourt C, Piché A. Ovarian cancer ascites protects from TRAIL-induced cell death through αvβ5 integrin-mediated focal adhesion kinase and Akt activation. Oncogene. 2010;29:3519–31.
5. Ahmed N, Riley C, Oliva K, Rice G, Quinn M. Ascites induces modulation of 6β1 integrin and urokinase plasminogen activator receptor expression and associated functions in ovarian carcinoma. Br J Cancer. 2005;92:1475–85.
6. Giuntoli RL, Webb TJ, Zoso A, Rogers O, Diaz-Montes TP, Bristow RE, Oelke M. Ovarian cancer-associated ascites demonstrates altered immune environment: implications for antitumor immunity. Anticancer Res. 2009;29:2875–84.
7. Yigit R, Figdor CG, Zusterzeel PL, Pots JM, Torensma R, Massuger LF. Cytokine analysis as a tool to understand tumour–host interaction in ovarian cancer. Eur J Cancer. 2011;47:1883–9.
8. Pan WW, Zhou JJ, Liu XM, Xu Y, Guo LJ, Yu C, Shi QH, Fan HY. Death domain-associated protein DAXX promotes ovarian cancer development and chemoresistance. J Biol Chem. 2013;288:13620–30.
9. Dolznig H, Rupp C, Puri C, et al. Modeling Colon Adenocarcinomas in Vitro: A 3D Co-Culture System Induces Cancer-Relevant Pathways upon Tumor Cell and Stromal Fibroblast Interaction. Am J Pathol. 2011;179:487–501.
10. Fischbach C, Kong HJ, Hsiong SX, et al. Cancer cell angiogenic capability is regulated by 3D culture and integrin engagement. Proc Natl Acad Sci U S A. 2009;106:399–404.
11. Pickl M, Ries CH. Comparison of 3D and 2D tumor models reveals enhanced HER2 activation in 3D associated with an increased response to trastuzumab. Oncogene. 2009;28:461–8.
12. Pan WW, Yi FP, Cao LX, Liu XM, Shen Z, Bu Y, Xu Y, Fan HY, Song FZ. DAXX silencing suppresses mouse ovarian surface epithelial cell growth by inducing senescence and DNA damage. Gene. 2013;526:287–94.

13. Wethkamp N, Klempnauer KH. Daxx is a transcriptional repressor of CCAAT/enhancer-binding protein β. J Biol Chem. 2009;284:28783–94.
14. Innao P, Pothisuwan M, Pengsa P. Does human epididymis protein 4 (HE4) have a role in prediction of recurrent epithelial ovariancancer. Asian Pac J Cancer Prev. 2016;17:4483–6.
15. Jelovac D, Armstrong DK. Recent progress in the diagnosis and treatment of ovarian cancer. CA Cancer J Clin. 2011;61(3):183–203.
16. Auer K, Bachmayr-Heyda A, Sukhbaatar N, Aust S, Schmetterer KG, Meier SM, Gerner C, Grimm C, Horvat R, Pils D. Role of the immune system in the peritoneal tumor spread of high grade serous ovarian cancer. Oncotarget. 2016;7:61336–54.
17. Chen LY, Chen JD. DAXX silencing sensitizes cells to multiple apoptotic pathways. Mol Cell Biol. 2003;23:7108–21.
18. Yang X, Khosravi-Far R, Chang HY, Baltimore D. DAXX, a novel Fas-binding protein that activates JNK and apoptosis. Cell. 1997;89:1067–76.
19. Li H, Leo C, Zhu J, Wu X, O'Neil J, Park EJ, Chen JD. Sequestration and inhibition of DAXX-mediated transcriptional repression by PML. Mol Cell Biol. 2000;20:1784–96.
20. Muromoto R, Sugiyama K, Takachi A, Imoto S, Sato N, Yamamoto T, Oritani K, Shimoda K, Matsuda T. Physical and functional interactions between DAXX and DNA methyltransferase 1-associated protein, DMAP1. J Immunol. 2004;172:2985–93.
21. Ishov AM, Vladimirova OV, Maul GG. Heterochromatin and ND10 are cell-cycle regulated and phosphorylation-dependent alternatenuclear sites of the transcription repressor DAXX and SWI/SNF protein ATRX. J Cell Sci. 2004;117:3807–20.
22. Li R, Pei H, Watson DK, Papas TS. EAP1/DAXX interacts with ETS1 and represses transcriptional activation of ETS1 target genes. Oncogene. 2000;19:745–53.
23. Lehembre F, Müller S, Pandolfi PP, Dejean A. Regulation of Pax3 transcriptional activity by SUMO-1-modifiedPML. Oncogene. 2001;20:1–9.
24. Lin DY, Lai MZ, Ann DK, Shih HM. Promyelocytic leukemia protein (PML) functions as a glucocorticoid receptor co-activator by sequestering DAXX to the PML oncogenic domains (PODs) to enhance its transactivation potential. J Biol Chem. 2003;278:15958–65.
25. Zhao LY, Liu J, Sidhu GS, Niu Y, Liu Y, Wang R, Liao D. Negative regulation of p53 functions by DAXX and theinvolvement of MDM2. J Biol Chem. 2004;279:50566–79.
26. Salomoni P. The PML-Interacting Protein DAXX: Histone Loading Gets into the Picture. Front Oncol. 2013;3:152.
27. Yu P, Ye L, Wang H, Du G, Zhang J, Zhang J, Tian J. NSK-01105 inhibits proliferation and induces apoptosis of prostate cancer cells by blocking the Raf/MEK/ERK and PI3K/Akt/mTOR signal pathways. Tumour Biol. 2015;36: 2143–53.
28. Jiang M, Wen F, Cao J, Li P, She J, Chu Z. Genome-wide exploration of the molecularevolution and regulatory network of mitogen-activatedprotein kinase cascades uponmultiple stresses in *Brachypodium distachyon*. BMC Genomics. 2015;16:228.
29. Knight T, Irving JA. Ras/Raf/MEK/ERK pathway activation in childhood acute lymphoblastic leukemia and its therapeutic targeting. Front Oncol. 2014;4:160.
30. Lee S, Yoon S, Kim DH. A high nuclear basal level of ERK2 phosphorylation contributes to the resistance of cisplatin-resistant human ovarian cancer cells. Gynecol Oncol. 2007;104:338–44.
31. Goncharenko-Khaider N, Matte I, Lane D, Rancourt C, Piche A. Ovarian cancer ascites increase Mcl-1 expression in tumor cells through ERK1/2-Elk-1 signaling to attenuate TRAIL-induced apoptosis. Mol Cancer. 2012;11:84.
32. Correa RJ, Peart T, Valdes YR, DiMattia GE, Shepherd TG. Modulation of AKT activity is associated with reversibledormancy in ascites-derived epithelial ovarian cancer spheroids. Carcinogenesis. 2011;33:49–58.
33. Zhu S, Yoon K, Sterneck E, Johnson PF, Smart RC. CCAAT/enhancer binding protein-β is a mediator of keratinocyte survival and skin tumorigenesis involving oncogenic Ras signaling. Proc Natl Acad Sci U S A. 2002;99:207–12.
34. Lee HG, Minematsu H, Kim KO, Celil Aydemir AB, Shin MJ, Nizami SA, Chung KJ, Hsu AC, Jacobs CR, Lee FY. Actin and ERK1/2-CEBPβ signaling mediates phagocytosis-induced innate immune response of osteoprogenitor cells. Biomaterials. 2011;32:9197–206.
35. Mäuser W, Perwitz N, Meier B, Fasshauer M, Klein J. Direct adipotropic actions of atorvastatin: differentiation state-dependent induction of apoptosis, modulation of endocrine function, and inhibition of glucose uptake. Eur J Pharmacol. 2007;564:37–46.

25

Isolated ovarian tuberculosis in an Immuno-competent woman in the post partum period

Wondimu Gudu

Abstract

Background: Pelvic tuberculosis is a rare form of extrapulmonary tuberculosis. It commonly involves the fallopian tubes and the uterus from a lympho-hematogeneous spread. The presentation of pelvic tuberculosis as an isolated ovarian abscess is extremely rare and is reported only twice.

Case presentation: a 25 yrs. old para III mother in the post partum period undergone laparotomy for suspected tuboovarian abscess/ovarian tumor after presenting with abdominal pain, pelvic mass and fever. Intra-operatively, Isolated right ovarian mass with caseation in the cavity but no significant pelvic adhesions was detected and right oophorectomy was done. Post operative Histopathology of surgical specimens revealed tuberculous leision and patient recovered well after anti-tuberculosis treatment.

Conclusion: Isolated ovarian tuberculosis is a very rare form of Genital Tuberculosis which should always be considered in the evaluation of a woman presenting with any adnexal mass in highly prevalent areas.

Keywords: Ovary, Tuberculosis, Abscess, Pelvic, Isolated

Introduction

Tuberculosis (TB) is one of the top 10 causes of death worldwide. There were 1.4 million TB deaths and estimated 10.4 million new TB cases in 2015 [1]. Although pulmonary TB is the commonest clinical form, the incidence of extra-pulmonary Tuberculosis (EPTB), particularly abdomino-pelvic TB, is progressively increasing especially in developing countries due to the emergence of HIV/AIDS) [2]. It is estimated that Genital Tb affects about 12% of women with pulmonary Tuberculosis (PTB) and 15 to 20% of women with EPTB [3].

Genital TB is almost always secondary to TB elsewhere in the body, the commonest primary site being the lungs [4]. Lympho-hematogenous dissemination is most common, followed by intra-luminal and neighborhood spread [4, 5].

The commonest sites of involvement are the fallopian tubes in 90–100% and the endometrium in 50–80% of the cases while the ovaries are involved in 20–30% of cases genital Tb [5]. The classical presentation of Female genital tuberculosis is with a triad of infertility, menstrual irregularity & chronic pelvic pain. But isolated ovarian tuberculosis presenting as an adnexal mass and mimicking ovarian tumor is an extremely rare clinical variety and is reported only twice in the literature [6]. In here, a very rare case of an isolated unilateral ovarian tuberculosis in a woman in the postpartum period is presented.

Correspondence: wondgu@yahoo.com
Department of Obstetrics & Gynecology, Saint Paul's Hospital Millennium Medical College, P.O.Box 1271, Addis Ababa, Ethiopia

Case presentation

A 25 years old, married, para III, Ethiopian Somali woman presented with an insidious onset of lower abdominal pain, offensive vaginal discharge and intermittent fever of 1 month duration. She had associated anorexia, vomiting & episodic diarrhoea which were followed by progressive weight loss and drenching night sweats. Two weeks prior to her presentation she developed progressively increasing abdominal distension with urgency, frequency, dysuria and straining at micturition. The woman had smooth vaginal delivery at a health centre 2 months back and claimed to have uneventful pregnancy. She was lactating & didn't see any menses after delivery. She had no cough and didn't report any known medical illnesses. She lived with 2 relatives in the same room who were being treated for pulmonary tuberculosis 2 years ago. All her previous pregnancies and deliveries were uneventful. She was repeatedly treated with unspecified antibiotics at local health facilities with no improvement.

On Physical examination the woman was acutely sick looking. The pulse rate was 112 per minute; temperature 38 °c and she had pale conjunctive. The remarkable findings were on abdominal and pelvic examinations. Abdominal examination revealed distended abdomen with lower abdominal tenderness and rebound tenderness. There was a 14 cm by 12 cm sized, firm, tender, pelvic mass with limited mobility. Shifting dullness & fluid thrill were negative and bowel sounds were normal. Speculum examination showed hyperaemic otherwise normal looking cervix. Digital vaginal examination findings were: smooth & firm cervix; bulging pouch of Douglas; firm 18 cm by 18 cm sized pelvic right adnexal mass with adnexal and cervical motion tenderness.

Laboratory tests revealed anemia (Hgb = 9 g/dl), leukocytosis with left shift, raised ESR and Pyuria. Organ function tests, chest x-ray & plain abdominal films were normal. Ultrasound showed a hypoechoic, well outlined, thick-walled pelvic mass in the right adnexa extending to the pouch of Douglas with internal echoes (Fig. 1). Doppler revealed normal flow & resistance pattern of ovarian vessels. The uterus was normal sized with thin endometrial slit. The conclusion was a right adnexal (ovarian) tumor with possible differential diagnosis of tubo-ovarian abscess.

The mother was counselled on the presumptive diagnosis and informed consent was obtained for emergency laparotomy which revealed matted omentum obscuring the pelvic cavity & filmy adhesions (involving the uterus, right adnexa, intestines and bladder). Careful dissection and adhesiolysis, revealed thin offensive fluid extruding from the right adnexa; right ovarian 14 cm by 14 cm sized cystic to firm mass located between the ovarian fossa & pouch of Douglas (Figs. 2 and 3). There was no grossly identifiable ovarian tissue. Both tubes appeared normal except for presumably oedematous serosal surface of the right fallopian tube. The uterus and appendix were normal in size & appearance. Procedure was completed after performing right oophorectomy (complete excision of the mass) and securing omental & peritoneal biopsies. Incision of the wall of the mass revealed thick (caseating) pus with no mass in the cavity of the sac. Postoperatively she was having recurrent high grade fever for more than 1 week despite potent antibiotics administration.

The histopathology examination revealed chronic inflammation with caseation and histocytes granuloma formation which was consistent with tuberculous lesion. But culture and immune-histologic analysis were not done because of facility constraints The woman was then put on anti-Tb regimen (category-I) containing INH, Rifampicin, Pyrazinamide and Ethambutol and showed dramatic improvement at her follow up visit after completing the intensive phase.

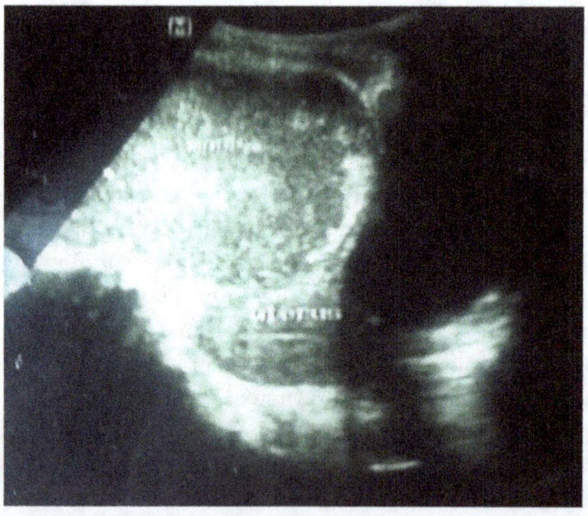

Fig. 1 Ultrasound image of the hypo-echoic right adnexal mass

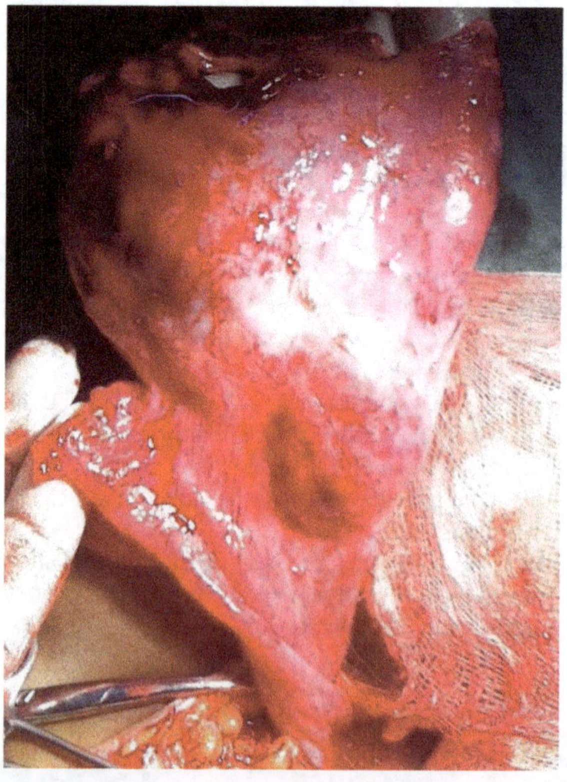

Fig. 2 The right ovarian mass after incision made at upper boarder and normal appearing right fallopian tube

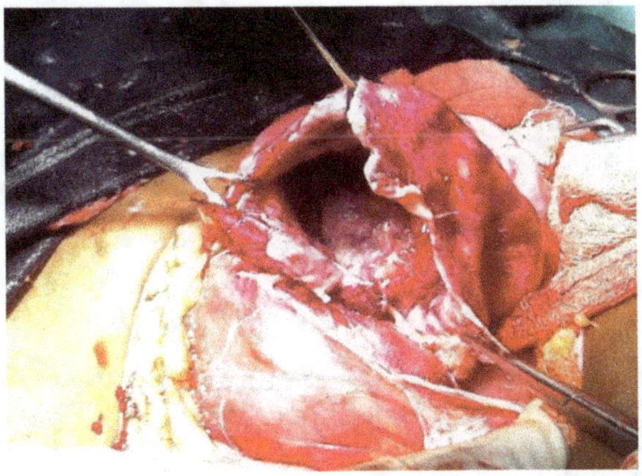

Fig. 3 The ovarian sac of abscess and the empty cavity after drainage

Discussion

Female genital tuberculosis (FGTB) is an important cause of significant morbidity especially infertility and chronic pelvic pain. The actual incidence of Genital Tb cannot be determined accurately because at least 11% of patients are asymptomatic and may remain undiagnosed [4, 5].

Several risk factors exist for EPTB and TB of the female genital tract. Most are host factors causing impaired immunity [7, 8]. Increased exposure to the infection is another factor and about 20% of patients with genital TB give a history of TB in their immediate family [4]. This was evident in our case who had prolonged exposure with diagnosed cases of tuberculosis.

Genital tract is vulnerable to tuberculous disease after puberty, and most cases occur during the childbearing period [4]. The focus in the lung often heals, and the lesion may lie dormant in the genital tract for years, only to reactivate at a later time [2, 4]. Although postpartum period is generally a risk factor for ascending infections (PID), we couldn't find any literature evidence explaining why there was reactivation of genital Tb in the immediate post-partum period in our case that had primarily ovarian involvement with grossly unaffected uterus and tubes. But it is reported that in those 15% of patients who didn't have infertility, symptoms of genital TB develop in one third to one half within one year after their last pregnancy was completed [4] which was evident in our case.

The clinical presentation of genital TB depends upon the site of involvement of genital tract [4, 5]. The age of presentation in 80% of women is 20–40 years, especially in developing countries [5]. Systemic symptoms tend to be relatively mild, if present, and may include weight loss, fatigue, and mild nocturnal fever. The four major presenting complaints in symptomatic patients are: infertility, abnormal uterine bleeding, pelvic pain, and amenorrhea [4].

Physical examination can be normal in up to 50% of cases of female genital Tb [5]. There is little correlation between presenting complaints and physical findings in genital TB [4]. When abnormal findings are present, they usually consist of adnexal masses or signs of ascites [4, 9].

In the case of Ovarian Tuberculosis, Two clinicopathological patterns of involvement are described: perio-ophoritis and ooporitis [4]. Peri-ooophorits is the most common form of tuberculous involvement of the ovary in which the tuberculous process starts from the tube and involves the ovary with extension of the lesion from the periphery (tunica) toward the center (parenchyma). This results in a tubo-ovarian mass, which is frequently adherent to omentum and intestines [4]. Oophoritis is a relatively rare condition in which infection starts in the stroma of the ovary, presumably from a hematogenous source that produces a caseating granuloma within the parenchyma. In Tb Oophoritis, typical tubercles or larger foci with caseous centers may be recognized on cross section in the hilum of the ovary [4].

In tubo-ovarian TB, patients usually present with adnexal mass and/or ascites [4, 7, 9]. Tuberculous tubo-ovarian masses are less tender than those due to pyogenic infection, although secondary infection and acute exacerbation may produce sharp pain and tenderness [5, 8]. Fixation of pelvic organs on bimanual examination may be appreciated. In our case, the abdominal and adnexal tenderness can be explained by superinfection of the ovarian mass which was witnessed during laparotomy as there was offensive exudate extruding from the right adnexa.

The clinical findings in most previous case reports of ovarian tuberculosis included: extensive pelvic adhesions; peritoneal seedlings; ascites or multi-septated masses. But the fact that our case presented with an apparent homogenous cystic solitary mass with no adhesions, ascites or peritoneal seedlings and that the presentation was in the postpartum makes it peculiar.

The absence of specific symptoms and conclusive signs during physical examination may delay a proper diagnosis [5, 7]. In ovarian Tb, the clinical presentation cam mimic ovarian malignancy which was also evident in our case in whom a diagnosis of ovarian tumor was made based on clinical and US findings. It should be noted that diagnostic imaging tests are non specific and both US and CT/MRI scan appearances are similar in both ovarian tuberculous abscess and other neoplastic ovarian masses [6]. An elevated CA-125 level is also found in some of the patients with ovarian Tb which further increases the diagnostic dilemma [5, 6, 9].

Laparoscopy and laparotomy are important in the diagnosis of ovarian/tubo-ovarian Tb. Intraoperative frozen sections (if available) are valuable to rule out the possibility of pelvic Tb in patients undergoing surgery for tubo-ovarian masses, especially in highly prevalent areas [6]. Hence keeping in mind the possibility of tubo-ovarian TB is crucial as it will avoid radical/extensive surgery and unnecessary removal of the ovaries for suspected ovarian malignancy in reproductive age women who desire to retain/preserve fertility. In areas with no frozen section, we believe retaining otherwise normal appearing ovaries during laparotomy for suspected ovarian malignancy is advisable.

The definitive diagnosis of pelvic Tb lies in identifying the tubercle bacilli by microbiologic examinations including culture or PCR which can still be negative despite the presence of tuberculous infection [7–9].

The management of pelvic tuberculosis is in general medical (6 to 9 months of anti-tuberculous therapy). Surgery is limited only for those cases that are unresponsive to treatment. Drainage of pyosalpinx and removal of large tubo-ovarian abscesses can be performed followed by anti Tb for better results [10].

In our case the removal of the diseased ovary was justified as it had gross caseation in the parenchyma and as this will decrease the risk of reactivation post operatively. Even though confirmation of the definitive diagnosis by culture could not be made, Postoperative anti Tb was initiated considering the exposure history of the patient, the histopathologic granulomatous lesion, and the high Tb endemicity of the area.

Conclusions

Isolated ovarian tuberculosis is a very rare form of female genital tuberculosis. It usually presents with adnexal mass and can mimic ovarian tumor. In highly prevalent areas, ovarian tuberculosis should be considered in the evaluation of women with adnexal masses.

Consent

Written informed consent was obtained from the patient for publication of this case report and any accompanying images.

Abbreviations

Anti-Tb: Anti-tuberculosis; HIV: Human Immuno-deficiency Virus; PCR: Polymerase Chain Reactions; Tb: Tuberculosis

Acknowledgements

I thank my wife, Gete Sorsa, for her continuous encouragement and the OR staff of the hospital for taking the pictures during the surgical procedure.

Funding

There were no any funding sources for all activities related with the preparation of the case report.

Authors' contributions

WG was directly involved in the evaluation and management of the case and inception and write up of the case report. All authors read and approved the final manuscript.

Competing interests

The author declares that he has no any competing interests.

References

1. World Health Organization. Global Tuberculosis Report, 2016. Geneva, Switzerland:http://www.who.int/tb/publications/global_report/en/ [Accessed March 12, 2017].
2. Uygur-Bayramicli O, Dabak G, Dabak R. A clinical dilemma: abdominal tuberculosis. World J Gastroenterol. 2003;9:1098–101.
3. Gatongi DK, Gitau G, Kay V, Ngwenya S, Lafong C, Hasan A. Female genital tuberculosis. Obstet Gynaecol. 2005;7:75–9.
4. Varma, T, Tuberculosis of the Female Genital Tract. Glob. libr. women's med., (ISSN: 1756–2228) 2008; DOI https://doi.org/10.3843/GLOWM.10034
5. Sharma JB. Current diagnosis and management of female genital tuberculosis. J Obstet Gynaecol India. 2015;65(6):362–71. https://www.ncbi.nlm.nih.gov/pmc/articles/PMC4666212/
6. Rabesalama S, et al. Isolated ovarian tuberculosis mimicking ovarian carcinoma: case report and literature review. Afr J Infect Dis. 2011;5(1):7–10.
7. Akbulut S, et al. Tubercular tubo-ovarian cystic mass mimicking acute appendicitis: a case report. J Med Case Rep. 2011;5:363.
8. M. Ilmer, F. Bergauer, K. Friese, and I. Mylonas. Case Report Genital Tuberculsis as the cause of Tubo ovarian Abscess in an Immunosuppressed Patient. Hindawi Publishing Corporation, Infectious Diseases in Obstetrics and Gynecology, 2009, 745060, 4 pages doi:https://doi.org/10.1155/2009/745060.
9. Ilhan AH, Durmuşoğlu F. Case report of a pelvic-peritoneal tuberculosis presenting as an adnexial mass and mimicking ovarian cancer, and a review of the literature. Infect Dis Obstet Gynecol. 2004;12:87–9.
10. Sharma JB. Tuberculosis and obstetric and gynecological practice. In: Studd J, Tan SL, Chervenak FA, editors. Progress in obstetric and gynaecology, vol. 18. Philadephia: Elsevier; 2008. p. 395–427.

26

The effects of probiotic and selenium co-supplementation on parameters of mental health, hormonal profiles, and biomarkers of inflammation and oxidative stress in women with polycystic ovary syndrome

Mehri Jamilian[1], Shirin Mansury[1], Fereshteh Bahmani[2], Zahra Heidar[3], Elaheh Amirani[2] and Zatollah Asemi[2*]

Abstract

Background: The aim of this study was to evaluate the effect of the co-administration of probiotic and selenium on parameters of mental health, hormonal profiles, and biomarkers of inflammation and oxidative stress in women with PCOS. Data on the effects of selenium and probiotic co-supplementation on mental health, hormonal and inflammatory parameters of patients with polycystic ovary syndrome (PCOS) are scarce. This investigation was carried out to evaluate the effects of selenium and probiotic co-supplementation on mental health, hormonal and inflammatory parameters in women with PCOS.

Methods: This randomized, double-blinded, placebo-controlled clinical trial was conducted on 60 subjects, aged 18–40 years old. Participants were randomly allocated into two groups to intake 8×10^9 CFU/day probiotic plus 200 μg/day selenium supplements ($n = 30$) or placebo ($n = 30$) for 12 weeks. Hormonal and inflammatory parameters were measured at baseline and after the 12-week intervention.

Results: Probiotic and selenium co-supplementation resulted in a significant improvement in beck depression inventory (β − 0.76; 95% CI, − 1.26, − 0.26; $P = 0.003$), general health questionnaire scores (β − 1.15; 95% CI, − 1.97, − 0.32; $P = 0.007$) and depression anxiety and stress scale scores (β − 1.49; 95% CI, − 2.59, − 0.39; $P = 0.009$) compared with the placebo. Furthermore, probiotic and selenium co-supplementation significantly reduced total testosterone (β − 0.26 ng/mL; 95% CI, − 0.51, − 0.02; $P = 0.03$), hirsutism (β − 0.43; 95% CI, − 0.74, − 0.11; $P = 0.008$), high-sensitivity C-reactive protein (hs-CRP) (β − 0.58 mg/L; 95% CI, − 0.97, − 0.19; $P = 0.004$) and *malondialdehyde (MDA)* levels (β − 0.29 μmol/L; 95% CI, − 0.56, − 0.02; P = 0.03), and significantly increased total antioxidant capacity (TAC) (β + 84.76 mmol/L; 95% CI, + 48.08, + 121.44; $P < 0.001$) and total glutathione (GSH) levels (β + 26.78 μmol/L; 95% CI, + 4.33, + 49.23; $P = 0.02$) compared with the placebo.

Conclusions: Overall, the co-administration of probiotic and selenium for 12 weeks to women with PCOS had beneficial effects on mental health parameters, serum total testosterone, hirsutism, hs-CRP, TAC, GSH and MDA levels.
This study was prospectively registered in the Iranian website (www.irct.ir) for registration of clinical trials (http://www.irct.ir: IRCT20170513033941N22).

Keywords: Probiotic, Selenium, Mental health, Hormonal profiles, Inflammatory markers, Polycystic ovary syndrome

* Correspondence: asemi_r@yahoo.com
[2]Research Center for Biochemistry and Nutrition in Metabolic Diseases, Kashan University of Medical Sciences, Kashan, I.R., Iran
Full list of author information is available at the end of the article

Background

Polycystic ovary syndrome (PCOS) is an endocrine disturbances accompanied by a lot of conditions as well as economic burden [1]. Excess of androgens and related consequences including hirsutism and acne are notable clinical features of this disorder [2]. Prior evidence indicated that defected antioxidant defense and elevated inflammatory status contribute to the progression of PCOS [3, 4]. In addition, it has been stated that the gut microbiota dysbiosis is involved in the pathogenesis of PCOS [5, 6]. A lower concentration of selenium is also reported in women with PCOS and a negative correlation is illustrated between selenium and testosterone levels [7]. In these patients, life style modification, as the first line of treatment, is associated with improvement in body composition, insulin resistance, hyperandrogenism and clinical manifestations [8].

Previous studies have shown several beneficial effects of probiotic supplementation on glycemic control in PCOS patients [9, 10]. Moreover, some researchers have demonstrated that probiotic consumption in patients with osteoarthritis [11], type 2 diabetes mellitus (T2DM) [12], and gestational diabetes mellitus (GDM) [13] was associated with decreased inflammatory markers. On the other hand, selenium supplementation has been reported to improve antioxidant parameters in patients with metabolic syndrome [14]. In addition, in a study by Abedelahi et al. [15], it was seen that sodium selenite improved the in vitro follicular development by increasing total antioxidant capacity (TAC) levels. Selenium supplementation is thought to confer protective effects against oxidative stress and inflammation through reducing the formation of reactive oxygen species (ROS) and modulating of cellular signaling pathways [16]. Probiotic may affect antioxidant status and hormonal profiles by alleviating insulin resistance and anti-inflammatory properties [17, 18]. Recently, it is stated that probiotic plus selenium co-administration in animal models give better effects on metabolic responses and reproductive performance thorough additive actions [19, 20]. Combined probiotic and selenium supplementation may ameliorate clinical symptoms of patients with PCOS by improving their metabolic profiles and attenuating oxidative stress and inflammation. Therefore, we conducted this study to determine the effects of probiotic and selenium co-supplementation on parameters of mental health, hormonal profiles, and biomarkers of inflammation and oxidative stress in women with PCOS.

Methods

This randomized double-blinded, placebo-controlled trial registered in the Iranian website for registration of clinical trials (http://www.irct.ir: IRCT20170513033941N22) and followed the Declaration of Helsinki and Good Clinical Practice guidelines. This trial was conducted among 60 women with PCOS, diagnosed based on the Rotterdam criteria [21], aged 18–40 years old whom referred to the Kosar Clinic in Arak, Iran, between December and March 2018. The study protocol was approved by the Ethics Committee of Arak University of Medical Sciences (AUMS). Written informed consent was obtained from all participants prior to the intervention. Exclusion criteria were as follows: pregnancy, adrenal hyperplasia, androgen-secreting tumors, hyperprolactinemia, thyroid dysfunction, diabetes at enrollment.

Supplementation

Sixty PCOS women were randomized into two groups to intake either 8×10^9 CFU/day probiotic containing *Lactobacillus acidophilus, Lactobacillus reuteri, Lactobacillus fermentum* and *Bifidobacterium bifidum* (2×10^9 CFU/g each) plus 200 μg/day selenium ($n = 30$) or placebo ($n = 30$) for 12 weeks. Shape and size of supplements and placebos capsules were similar and manufactured by Familact (Tehran, Iran) and Barij Essence Pharmaceuticals (Kashan, Iran), respectively. Compliance with probiotic and selenium supplements and the placebos was examined by asking subjects to return the medication containers and through brief daily cell phone reminders to take the supplements. All subjects completed 3-day diet recall at weeks 0, 3, 6, 9 and 12 of the intervention. Daily macro- and micro-nutrient intakes were calculated by nutritionist IV software (First Databank, San Bruno, CA).

Assessment of outcomes

Hormonal profiles were considered as the primary outcomes. Mental health parameters, biomarkers of inflammation and oxidative stress were recognized as the secondary outcomes.

Clinical measures

Mental health was judged with beck depression inventory (BDI), general health questionnaire-28 (GHQ-28) and depression anxiety and stress scale (DASS) at baseline and week 12 of the intervention. BDI is a self-compiled questionnaire of 21 items in multiple choice format [22]. The GHQ-28 comprises 28-item consisting of 4 subscales [23]. DASS questionnaire consists of three 14-item self-report scales that measure depression, anxiety and stress [24].

Biochemical assessment

Fasting blood samples (15 ml) were collected at baseline and the end of the intervention at Arak reference laboratory. Serum total testosterone and sex hormone-binding globulin (SHBG) with inter- and intra-assay with inter- and intra-assay CVs of lower than 7%% were measured using commercial validated kits (DiaMetra, Milano, Italy).

Free androgen index (FAI) was calculated as the percentage of total testosterone/SHBG. Serum high sensitivity C-reactive protein (hs-CRP) concentrations were quantified using commercial ELISA kit (LDN, Nordhorn, Germany) with inter- and intra-assay CVs of lower than 7%. The plasma NO using Griess method [25], TAC concentrations using Benzie and Strain method [26], total glutathione (GSH) using Beutler method [27] and malondialdehyde (MDA) concentrations thiobarbituric acid reactive substances spectrophotometric test [28] were quantified with CVs less than 5%.

Statistical analyses

The Kolmogorov-Smirnov test was done to determine the normality of data. Differences in dietary intakes between treatment groups were detected with independent-sample *t*-tests. Multiple linear regression models were used to assess the treatment effects on study outcomes after adjusting for confounding parameters including; age, and BMI. Significance of the treatment effects was presented as the mean differences with 95% confidence interval. Bootstrapping was also used as a sensitivity analysis of confidence interval. *P*-values < 0.05 were considered statistically significant. All statistical analyses were done using the Statistical Package for Social Science version 18 (SPSS Inc., Chicago, Illinois, USA).

Results

As demonstrated in the study flow diagram (Fig. 1), during the enrollment phase of the study, there were 68 women with PCOS; however, 8 participants did not meet the inclusion criteria and thus were excluded. During the follow-up, 60 participants [placebo ($n = 30$) and probiotic and selenium co-supplementation ($n = 30$)] completed the trial.

Mean age, height, weight and BMI at baseline and after the 12-week intervention were not statistically different between the two groups (Table 1).

There was no statistically significant difference in terms of dietary macro- and micro-nutrient intakes between probiotic plus selenium, and placebo groups (Data not shown).

Probiotic and selenium co-supplementation resulted in a significant improvement in BDI (β – 0.76; 95% CI, – 1.26, – 0.26; $P = 0.003$), GHQ (β – 1.15; 95% CI, – 1.97, – 0.32; $P = 0.007$) and DASS (β – 1.49; 95% CI, – 2.59, – 0.39; $P = 0.009$) compared with the placebo (Table 2). Furthermore, probiotic and selenium co-supplementation significantly reduced total testosterone (β – 0.26 ng/mL; 95% CI, – 0.51, – 0.02; $P = 0.03$), hirsutism (β – 0.43; 95% CI, – 0.74, – 0.11; $P = 0.008$), hs-CRP (β – 0.58 mg/L; 95% CI, – 0.97, – 0.19; $P = 0.004$) and *MDA* levels (β – 0.29 μmol/L; 95% CI, – 0.56, – 0.02; P = 0.03), and significantly increased TAC (β + 84.76 mmol/L; 95% CI, + 48.08, + 121.44; $P < 0.001$) and GSH levels (β + 26.78 μmol/L; 95% CI, + 4.33, + 49.23; $P = 0.02$) compared with the placebo.

Discussion

In the present study, for the first time, we evaluated the effects of combined probiotic and selenium

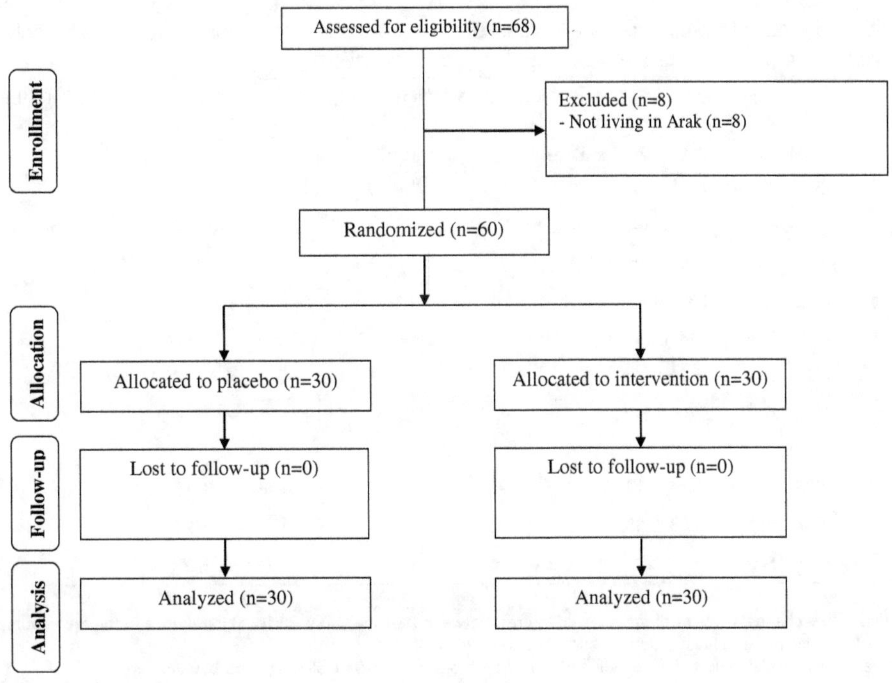

Fig. 1 Summary of patient flow diagram

Table 1 General characteristics of study participants

	Placebo group ($n = 30$)	Probiotic plus selenium group ($n = 30$)	P[a]
Age (y)	25.6 ± 3.8	26.0 ± 5.3	0.71
Height (cm)	161.6 ± 4.7	161.0 ± 4.4	0.63
Weight at study baseline (kg)	63.4 ± 7.7	63.9 ± 9.3	0.79
Weight at end-of-trial (kg)	63.2 ± 7.6	63.5 ± 9.2	0.86
Weight change (kg)	−0.2 ± 0.7	−0.4 ± 0.5	0.23
BMI at study baseline (kg/m^2)	24.0 ± 3.0	24.6 ± 3.3	0.67
BMI at end-of-trial (kg/m^2)	24.2 ± 3.0	24.5 ± 3.3	0.73
BMI change (kg/m^2)	−0.1 ± 0.3	−0.2 ± 0.2	0.23

Data are means± SDs
[a]Obtained from independent-samples *t*-test

supplementation on hormonal responses, biomarkers of inflammation and oxidative stress in women with PCOS. We found that the co-administration of probiotic and selenium for 12 weeks to women with PCOS had beneficial effects on mental health parameters, serum total testosterone, hirsutism, hs-CRP, TAC, GSH and MDA levels.

Effects on hormonal profiles

Previous evidence showed that total- free testosterone, and other androgens are significantly increased in women with PCOS [29], which associate with further consequences including hirsutism, acne, and alopcia and predisposing to infertility in long term [30, 31]. Androgen excess also increases obesity, insulin resistance and blood pressure, which in turn contributes to developing cardiovascular disease [32]. In addition, it is stated that the reduction of testosterone levels improves endothelial dysfunction, body weight, and dyslipidemia and insulin sensitivity in these patients [33]. Our findings demonstrated that probiotic and selenium co-administration to women with PCOS decreased mF-G scores and total testosterone, but did not affect SHBG concentrations. In addition, co-supplementation significantly improved mental health parameters. There are few studies investigating the effects of only probiotic or selenium supplementation on hormonal features of women with PCOS. In line with the present study, our previous research indicated that 12-week synbiotic supplementation decreased mF-G scores and increased SHBG levels in women with PCOS [34]. Moreover, probiotic supplementation for 12 weeks to women with PCOS led to a significant improvement in hirsutism, total testosterone and SHBG values [35]. In addition, it is reported that an

Table 2 Mental health and metabolic profiles at baseline and after the 12-week intervention in women with polycystic ovary syndrome that received either probiotic plus selenium supplements or placebo[a]

Variables	Placebo group ($n = 30$)		Probiotic plus selenium group ($n = 30$)		Difference in outcome measures between probiotic plus selenium and placebo groups[a]	
	Baseline	Week 12	Baseline	Week 12	β (95% CI)	P[b]
BDI total scores	15.6 ± 4.4	15.3 ± 4.7	15.5 ± 4.0	14.4 ± 3.7	−0.76 (−1.26, − 0.26)	0.003
GHQ scores	45.4 ± 8.1	44.6 ± 8.2	44.2 ± 7.3	42.4 ± 6.7	−1.15 (− 1.97, −0.32)	0.007
DASS scores	86.3 ± 13.1	85.1 ± 12.9	85.1 ± 11.2	82.5 ± 10.9	−1.49 (−2.59, −0.39)	0.009
Total testosterone (ng/mL)	1.3 ± 0.5	1.3 ± 0.4	1.4 ± 0.7	1.1 ± 0.6	−0.26 (− 0.51, − 0.02)	0.03
SHBG (nmol/L)	40.3 ± 17.5	40.4 ± 18.3	47.1 ± 19.7	49.5 ± 22.1	1.82 (−1.77, 5.42)	0.31
mF-G scores	13.0 ± 3.7	13.0 ± 3.6	14.5 ± 3.2	14.0 ± 2.9	−0.43 (−0.74, − 0.11)	0.008
hs-CRP (mg/L)	2.5 ± 1.6	2.7 ± 1.5	2.4 ± 1.5	2.0 ± 1.5	−0.58 (− 0.97, − 0.19)	0.004
NO (μmol/L)	36.5 ± 3.8	36.8 ± 4.0	36.6 ± 2.3	37.8 ± 3.5	0.94 (−0.65, 2.54)	0.24
TAC (mmol/L)	909.9 ± 110.8	909.4 ± 122.7	933.3 ± 59.8	1012.9 ± 69.4	84.76 (48.08, 121.44)	< 0.001
GSH (μmol/L)	496.4 ± 88.1	497.8 ± 88.3	528.3 ± 88.3	552.9 ± 83.1	26.78 (4.33, 49.23)	0.02
MDA (μmol/L)	2.4 ± 0.5	2.6 ± 0.7	2.8 ± 0.2	2.5 ± 0.2	−0.29 (−0.56, −0.02)	0.03

Data are mean ± SDs
[a]"Outcome measures" refers to the change in values of measures of interest between baseline and week 12. β [difference in the mean outcomes measures between treatment groups (probiotic plus selenium group = 1 and placebo group = 0)]
[b]Obtained from multiple regression model (adjusted for baseline values of each biochemical variables, age and baseline BMI)
BDI beck depression inventory, *DASS* depression anxiety and stress scale, *GHQ* general health questionnaire, *GSH* total glutathione, *hs-CRP* high-sensitivity C-reactive protein, *mF-G* modified Ferriman Gallwey, *MDA* malondialdehyde, *NO* nitric oxide, *SHBG* sex hormone-binding globulin, *TAC* total antioxidant capacity

8-week selenium supplementation in women with PCOS decreased mF-G scores, but did not affect free testosterone concentrations [36]. Although, selenium supplementation for 12 weeks did not affect total testosterone and SHBG levels in women with PCOS [37]. In contrast to our findings, probiotic supplementation to postmenopausal women did not enhance testosterone and SHBG levels [38]. The speculated mechanisms by which probiotic may improve hormonal profiles result from the balance of intestinal microbiota, enhancement of digestion and absorption of dietary nutrients [20], increasing insulin sensitivity [39], and interaction with the gut-brain axis [40]. In addition, induced oxidative stress involves in the development of hyperandrogenoism in PCOS [41]. The potential impacts of selenium supplementation on hormonal parameters may be explained by decreasing ROS production and elevating enzymatic anti oxidant activity [42].

Effects on biomarkers of inflammation and oxidative stress

Previous studies indicated that PCOS subjects are at risk for elevated inflammatory markers and abnormal antioxidant defense [43, 44]. In addition, it is demonstrated that in women with PCOS, inflammation involves in pancreatic beta cell dysfunction, insulin resistance, atherogenesis and ovarian disturbance [45], which accelerated by anti-oxidant imbalance [46]. The correction of oxidative stress and inflammatory status lead to alleviated hyperandrogenemia and atherogenic profiles [47, 48]. Our study indicated that probiotic and selenium co-supplementation to patients with PCOS resulted in a significant reduction in hs-CRP and MDA levels, and a significant increase in TAC and NO, but unchanged GSH concentrations. Similarly, selenium enriched probiotic in few animal studies enhanced antioxidant status. For instance, it is observed that a 4-week probiotic and selenium co-administration to mice fed a high-fat diet led to a significant decrease in MDA levels [19]. Similar results were observed in piglets grown in high ambient temperature after 6 weeks taking probiotic and selenium combination [49]. The findings of the present study are in agreement with our previous study indicated that a 10-week selenium supplementation to pregnant women at risk for intrauterine growth restriction resulted in decreased hs-CRP and elevated TAC levels [2]. Furthermore, an 8-week probiotic intervention in women with GDM significantly improved inflammation and oxidative stress biomarkers [50]. Although, Shoaei et al. [10] did not find any significant change in hs-CRP levels among women with PCOS receiving probiotic supplements for 8 weeks. In contrast to our study, 3-month selenium supplementation in patients with T2DM did not affect TAC levels [51]. Probiotic may attenuate inflammation and oxidative stress through metal ion chelating ability, modification of inflammatory signaling pathways, producing antioxidant metabolites, upregulating the antioxidant activity of the host and downregulating ROS producing enzymes [52]. Moreover, selenium involves in antioxidant defense system and play important roles in the increasing of glutathione peroxidase (GPx) activity, decreasing nuclear factor-kappaB (NF-κB) activation, inhibiting MAP kinase pathways and altering the metabolism of arachidonic acid, which in turn result in anti-inflammatory effects [53].

The current study had few limitations. Due to limited funding, we were unable to determine the effects of probiotic and selenium co-supplementation on circulating selenium levels. In the current study, sample size was low and did not meet our expectation. Future studies with longer duration of intervention, and large sample size are required to confirm the validity of our findings. The other limitation of this study was that the group of women surveyed was highly heterogeneous (18–40 years). As we recruited patients with PCOS from a referral center, all patients were received similar treatments based on available guidelines. However, we believe that age range would not influence our findings because mean age was not significantly different between intervention and non-intervention groups. This should be taken into account in the interpretation of our findings.

Conclusions

Overall, the co-administration of probiotic and selenium for 12 weeks to women with PCOS had beneficial effects on mental health parameters, serum total testosterone, hirsutism, hs-CRP, TAC, GSH and MDA levels.

Abbreviations

BDI: Beck depression inventory; DASS: Depression anxiety and stress scale; GHQ: General health questionnaire; GSH: Total glutathione; hs-CRP: High-sensitivity C-reactive protein; MDA: Malondialdehyde; mF-G: modified Ferriman Gallwey; NO: nitric oxide; SHBG: sex hormone-binding globulin; TAC: total antioxidant capacity

Acknowledgements

The present study was supported by a grant from the Vice-chancellor for Research, AUMS, Arak, and Iran.

Funding

The research grant provided by Research Deputy of Arak University of Medical Sciences (AUMS).

Authors' contributions

ZA contributed in conception, design, statistical analysis and drafting of the manuscript. MJ, SM, FB, ZH and EA contributed in data collection and manuscript drafting. All authors approved the final version for submission. ZA supervised the study.

Competing interests
The authors declare that they have no competing interests.

Author details
[1]Department of Gynecology and Obstetrics, Endocrinology and Metabolism Research Center, School of Medicine, Arak University of Medical Sciences, Arak, Iran. [2]Research Center for Biochemistry and Nutrition in Metabolic Diseases, Kashan University of Medical Sciences, Kashan, I.R., Iran. [3]Infertility and Reproductive Health Research Center, Shahid Beheshti University of Medical Sciences, Tehran, Iran.

References
1. Escobar-Morreale HF. Polycystic ovary syndrome: definition, aetiology, diagnosis and treatment. Nat Rev Endocrinol. 2018;14:270–84.
2. Mesdaghinia E, Rahavi A, Bahmani F, Sharifi N, Asemi Z. Clinical and metabolic response to selenium supplementation in pregnant women at risk for intrauterine growth restriction: randomized, double-blind, placebo-controlled trial. Biol Trace Elem Res. 2017;178:14–21.
3. Hyderali BN, Mala K. Oxidative stress and cardiovascular complications in polycystic ovarian syndrome. Eur J Obstet Gynecol Reprod Biol. 2015; 191:15–22.
4. Gonzalez F. Inflammation in polycystic ovary syndrome: underpinning of insulin resistance and ovarian dysfunction. Steroids. 2012;77:300–5.
5. Guo Y, Qi Y, Yang X, Zhao L, Wen S, Liu Y, et al. Association between polycystic ovary syndrome and gut microbiota. PLoS One. 2016;11: e0153196.
6. Liu R, Zhang C, Shi Y, Zhang F, Li L, Wang X, et al. Dysbiosis of gut microbiota associated with clinical parameters in polycystic ovary syndrome. Front Microbiol. 2017;8:324.
7. Coskun A, Arikan T, Kilinc M, Arikan DC, Ekerbicer HC. Plasma selenium levels in Turkish women with polycystic ovary syndrome. Eur J Obstet Gynecol Reprod Biol. 2013;168:183–6.
8. Moran LJ, Hutchison SK, Norman RJ, Teede HJ. Lifestyle changes in women with polycystic ovary syndrome. Cochrane Database Syst Rev. 2011: CD007506. https://doi.org/10.1002/14651858.CD007506.pub2.
9. Ahmadi S, Jamilian M, Karamali M, Tajabadi-Ebrahimi M, Jafari P, Taghizadeh M, et al. Probiotic supplementation and the effects on weight loss, glycaemia and lipid profiles in women with polycystic ovary syndrome: a randomized, double-blind, placebo-controlled trial. Hum Fertil (Camb). 2017; 20:254–61.
10. Shoaei T, Heidari-Beni M, Tehrani HG, Feizi A, Esmaillzadeh A, Askari G. Effects of probiotic supplementation on pancreatic beta-cell function and c-reactive protein in women with polycystic ovary syndrome: a randomized double-blind placebo-controlled clinical trial. Int J Prev Med. 2015;6:27. https://doi.org/10.4103/2008-7802.153866.
11. Lei M, Guo C, Wang D, Zhang C, Hua L. The effect of probiotic *Lactobacillus casei* Shirota on knee osteoarthritis: a randomised double-blind, placebo-controlled clinical trial. Benef Microbes. 2017;8:697–703.
12. Mohamadshahi M, Veissi M, Haidari F, Shahbazian H, Kaydani GA, Mohammadi F. Effects of probiotic yogurt consumption on inflammatory biomarkers in patients with type 2 diabetes. Bioimpacts. 2014;4:83–8.
13. Jafarnejad S, Saremi S, Jafarnejad F, Arab A. Effects of a multispecies probiotic mixture on glycemic control and inflammatory status in women with gestational diabetes: a randomized controlled clinical trial. J Nutr Metab. 2016;2016:5190846.
14. Ju W, Li X, Li Z, Wu GR, Fu XF, Yang XM, et al. The effect of selenium supplementation on coronary heart disease: a systematic review and meta-analysis of randomized controlled trials. J Trace Elem Med Biol. 2017;44:8–16.
15. Abedelahi A, Salehnia M, Allameh AA, Davoodi D. Sodium selenite improves the in vitro follicular development by reducing the reactive oxygen species level and increasing the total antioxidant capacity and glutathione peroxide activity. Hum Reprod. 2010;25:977–85.
16. Mattmiller SA, Carlson BA, Sordillo LM. Regulation of inflammation by selenium and selenoproteins: impact on eicosanoid biosynthesis. J Nutr Sci. 2013;2:e28.
17. Ghoneim MA, Moselhy SS. Antioxidant status and hormonal profile reflected by experimental feeding of probiotics. Toxicol Ind Health. 2016;32:741–50.
18. Carvalho BM, Saad MJ. Influence of gut microbiota on subclinical inflammation and insulin resistance. Mediat Inflamm. 2013;2013:986734.
19. Nido SA, Shituleni SA, Mengistu BM, Liu Y, Khan AZ, Gan F, et al. Effects of selenium-enriched probiotics on lipid metabolism, Antioxidative status, histopathological lesions, and related gene expression in mice fed a high-fat diet. Biol Trace Elem Res. 2016;171:399–409.
20. Pan C, Zhao Y, Liao SF, Chen F, Qin S, Wu X, et al. Effect of selenium-enriched probiotics on laying performance, egg quality, egg selenium content, and egg glutathione peroxidase activity. J Agric Food Chem. 2011; 59:11424–31.
21. Rotterdam ESHRE/ASRM-Sponsored PCOS Consensus Workshop Group. Revised 2003 consensus on diagnostic criteria and long-term health risks related to polycystic ovary syndrome. Fertil Steril. 2004;81:19–25.
22. Beck AT, Ward CH, Mendelson M, Mock J, Erbaugh J. An inventory for measuring depression. Arch Gen Psychiatry. 1961;4:561–71.
23. Goldberg DP, Hillier VF. A scaled version of the general health questionnaire. Psychol Med. 1979;9:139–45.
24. Crawford JR, Henry JD. The positive and negative affect schedule (PANAS): construct validity, measurement properties and normative data in a large non-clinical sample. Br J Clin Psychol. 2004;43:245–65.
25. Tatsch E, Bochi GV, Pereira Rda S, Kober H, Agertt VA, de Campos MM, et al. A simple and inexpensive automated technique for measurement of serum nitrite/nitrate. Clin Biochem. 2011;44:348–50.
26. Benzie IF, Strain JJ. The ferric reducing ability of plasma (FRAP) as a measure of "antioxidant power": the FRAP assay. Anal Biochem. 1996;239:70–6.
27. Beutler E, Gelbart T. Plasma glutathione in health and in patients with malignant disease. J Lab Clin Med. 1985;105:581–4.
28. Janero DR. Malondialdehyde and thiobarbituric acid-reactivity as diagnostic indices of lipid peroxidation and peroxidative tissue injury. Free Radic Biol Med. 1990;9:515–40.
29. Huang A, Brennan K, Azziz R. Prevalence of hyperandrogenemia in the polycystic ovary syndrome diagnosed by the National Institutes of Health 1990 criteria. Fertil Steril. 2010;93:1938–41.
30. Wehr E, Moller R, Horejsi R, Giuliani A, Kopera D, Schweighofer N, et al. Subcutaneous adipose tissue topography and metabolic disturbances in polycystic ovary syndrome. Wien Klin Wochenschr. 2009;121:262–9.
31. West S, Lashen H, Bloigu A, Franks S, Puukka K, Ruokonen A, et al. Irregular menstruation and hyperandrogenaemia in adolescence are associated with polycystic ovary syndrome and infertility in later life: northern Finland birth cohort 1986 study. Hum Reprod. 2014;29:2339–51.
32. Yanes Cardozo LL, Romero DG, Reckelhoff JF. Cardiometabolic features of polycystic ovary syndrome: role of androgens. Physiology (Bethesda). 2017; 32:357–66.
33. Amiri M, Golsorkhtabaramiri M, Esmaeilzadeh S, Ghofrani F, Bijani A, Ghorbani L, et al. Effect of metformin and flutamide on anthropometric indices and laboratory tests in obese/overweight PCOS women under hypocaloric diet. J Reprod Infertil. 2014;15:205–13.
34. Nasri K, Jamilian M, Rahmani E, Bahmani F, Tajabadi-Ebrahimi M, Asemi Z. The effects of synbiotic supplementation on hormonal status, biomarkers of inflammation and oxidative stress in subjects with polycystic ovary syndrome: a randomized, double-blind, placebo-controlled trial. BMC Endocr Disord. 2018;18:21.
35. Karamali M, Eghbalpour S, Rajabi S, Jamilian M, Bahmani F, Tajabadi-Ebrahimi M, et al. Effects of probiotic supplementation on hormonal profiles, biomarkers of inflammation and oxidative stress in women with polycystic ovary syndrome: a randomized, double-blind, placebo-controlled trial. Arch Iran Med. 2018;21:1–7.
36. Razavi M, Jamilian M, Kashan ZF, Heidar Z, Mohseni M, Ghandi Y, et al. Selenium supplementation and the effects on reproductive outcomes, biomarkers of inflammation, and oxidative stress in women with polycystic ovary syndrome. Horm Metab Res. 2016;48:185–90.

37. Mohammad Hosseinzadeh F, Hosseinzadeh-Attar MJ, Yekaninejad MS, Rashidi B. Effects of selenium supplementation on glucose homeostasis and free androgen index in women with polycystic ovary syndrome: a randomized, double blinded, placebo controlled clinical trial. J Trace Elem Med Biol. 2016;34:56–61.
38. Nettleton JA, Greany KA, Thomas W, Wangen KE, Adlercreutz H, Kurzer MS. Short-term soy and probiotic supplementation does not markedly affect concentrations of reproductive hormones in postmenopausal women with and without histories of breast cancer. J Altern Complement Med. 2005;11: 1067–74.
39. Crommen S, Simon MC. Microbial regulation of glucose metabolism and insulin resistance. Genes. 2017;9. https://doi.org/10.3390/genes9010010.
40. Saydam BO, Yildiz BO. Gut-brain axis and metabolism in polycystic ovary syndrome. Curr Pharm Des. 2016;22:5572–87.
41. Gonzalez F, Sia CL, Shepard MK, Rote NS, Minium J. Hyperglycemia-induced oxidative stress is independent of excess abdominal adiposity in normal-weight women with polycystic ovary syndrome. Hum Reprod. 2012;27:3560–8.
42. Wang S, He G, Chen M, Zuo T, Xu W, Liu X. The role of antioxidant enzymes in the ovaries. Oxidative Med Cell Longev. 2017;2017:4371714.
43. Murri M, Luque-Ramirez M, Insenser M, Ojeda-Ojeda M, Escobar-Morreale HF. Circulating markers of oxidative stress and polycystic ovary syndrome (PCOS): a systematic review and meta-analysis. Hum Reprod Update. 2013; 19:268–88.
44. Escobar-Morreale HF, Luque-Ramirez M, Gonzalez F. Circulating inflammatory markers in polycystic ovary syndrome: a systematic review and metaanalysis. Fertil Steril. 2011;95:1048–58.e1–2.
45. Gonzalez F. Nutrient-induced inflammation in polycystic ovary syndrome: role in the development of metabolic aberration and ovarian dysfunction. Semin Reprod Med. 2015;33:276–86.
46. Zuo T, Zhu M, Xu W. Roles of oxidative stress in polycystic ovary syndrome and cancers. Oxidative Med Cell Longev. 2016;2016:8589318.
47. Sathyapalan T, Shepherd J, Coady AM, Kilpatrick ES, Atkin SL. Atorvastatin reduces malondialdehyde concentrations in patients with polycystic ovary syndrome. J Clin Endocrinol Metab. 2012;97:3951–5.
48. Diamanti-Kandarakis E, Paterakis T, Alexandraki K, Piperi C, Aessopos A, Katsikis I, et al. Indices of low-grade chronic inflammation in polycystic ovary syndrome and the beneficial effect of metformin. Hum Reprod. 2006; 21:1426–31.
49. Gan F, Chen X, Liao SF, Lv C, Ren F, Ye G, et al. Selenium-enriched probiotics improve antioxidant status, immune function, and selenoprotein gene expression of piglets raised under high ambient temperature. J Agric Food Chem. 2014;62:4502–8.
50. Hajifaraji M, Jahanjou F, Abbasalizadeh F, Aghamohammadzadeh N, Abbasi MM, Dolatkhah N. Effect of probiotic supplements in women with gestational diabetes mellitus on inflammation and oxidative stress biomarkers: a randomized clinical trial. Asia Pac J Clin Nutr. 2018;27:581–91.
51. Faghihi T, Radfar M, Barmal M, Amini P, Qorbani M, Abdollahi M, et al. A randomized, placebo-controlled trial of selenium supplementation in patients with type 2 diabetes: effects on glucose homeostasis, oxidative stress, and lipid profile. Am J Ther. 2014;21:491–5.
52. Wang Y, Wu Y, Wang Y, Xu H, Mei X, Yu D, et al. Antioxidant properties of probiotic bacteria. Nutrients. 2017;9. https://doi.org/10.3390/nu9050521.
53. Duntas LH. Selenium and inflammation: underlying anti-inflammatory mechanisms. Horm Metab Res. 2009;41:443–7.

Permissions

All chapters in this book were first published in JOR, by BioMed Central; hereby published with permission under the Creative Commons Attribution License or equivalent. Every chapter published in this book has been scrutinized by our experts. Their significance has been extensively debated. The topics covered herein carry significant findings which will fuel the growth of the discipline. They may even be implemented as practical applications or may be referred to as a beginning point for another development.

The contributors of this book come from diverse backgrounds, making this book a truly international effort. This book will bring forth new frontiers with its revolutionizing research information and detailed analysis of the nascent developments around the world.

We would like to thank all the contributing authors for lending their expertise to make the book truly unique. They have played a crucial role in the development of this book. Without their invaluable contributions this book wouldn't have been possible. They have made vital efforts to compile up to date information on the varied aspects of this subject to make this book a valuable addition to the collection of many professionals and students.

This book was conceptualized with the vision of imparting up-to-date information and advanced data in this field. To ensure the same, a matchless editorial board was set up. Every individual on the board went through rigorous rounds of assessment to prove their worth. After which they invested a large part of their time researching and compiling the most relevant data for our readers.

The editorial board has been involved in producing this book since its inception. They have spent rigorous hours researching and exploring the diverse topics which have resulted in the successful publishing of this book. They have passed on their knowledge of decades through this book. To expedite this challenging task, the publisher supported the team at every step. A small team of assistant editors was also appointed to further simplify the editing procedure and attain best results for the readers.

Apart from the editorial board, the designing team has also invested a significant amount of their time in understanding the subject and creating the most relevant covers. They scrutinized every image to scout for the most suitable representation of the subject and create an appropriate cover for the book.

The publishing team has been an ardent support to the editorial, designing and production team. Their endless efforts to recruit the best for this project, has resulted in the accomplishment of this book. They are a veteran in the field of academics and their pool of knowledge is as vast as their experience in printing. Their expertise and guidance has proved useful at every step. Their uncompromising quality standards have made this book an exceptional effort. Their encouragement from time to time has been an inspiration for everyone.

The publisher and the editorial board hope that this book will prove to be a valuable piece of knowledge for researchers, students, practitioners and scholars across the globe.

List of Contributors

Wei-Ting Chao
Faculty of Medicine, College of Medicine, Fu-Jen Catholic University, Taipei, Taiwan
Section of Gynecologic Oncology, Department of Obstetrics and Gynecology, Taipei Veterans General Hospital, No. 201, Section 2, Shih-Pai Road, Taipei 112, Taiwan

Chia-Hao Liu, Yi-Jen Chen and Hua-Hsi Wu
Faculty of Medicine, School of Medicine, National Yang-Ming University, Taipei, Taiwan
Section of Gynecologic Oncology, Department of Obstetrics and Gynecology, Taipei Veterans General Hospital, No. 201, Section 2, Shih-Pai Road, Taipei 112, Taiwan

Chi-Mu Chuang
Faculty of Medicine, School of Medicine, National Yang-Ming University, Taipei, Taiwan
Section of Gynecologic Oncology, Department of Obstetrics and Gynecology, Taipei Veterans General Hospital, No. 201, Section 2, Shih-Pai Road, Taipei 112, Taiwan
Department of Midwifery and Women Health Care, National Taipei University of Nursing and Health Sciences, Taipei, Taiwan

Peng-Hui Wang
Faculty of Medicine, School of Medicine, National Yang-Ming University, Taipei, Taiwan
Section of Gynecologic Oncology, Department of Obstetrics and Gynecology, Taipei Veterans General Hospital, No. 201, Section 2, Shih-Pai Road, Taipei 112, Taiwan
Department of Medical Research, China Medical University Hospital, Taichung, Taiwan

Lei Li, Xiaoning Bi, Hengzi Sun, Simiao Liu, Mei Yu, Ying Zhang and Keng Shen
Department of Obstetrics and Gynecology, Peking Union Medical College Hospital, Chinese Academy of Medical Sciences and Peking Union Medical College, No. 1 Shuai Fu Yuan, Eastern District, Beijing 100730, China

Shifu Weng, Yanan Bao, Jinguang Wu and Yizhuang Xu
Beijing National Laboratory for Molecular Sciences, State Key Laboratory for Rare Earth Materials Chemistry and Applications, College of Chemistry and Molecular Engineering, Peking University, No. 202 Chengfu Road, Haidian District, Beijing 100871, China

Limin Yang
State Key Laboratory of Nuclear Physics and Technology, Institute of Heavy Ion Physics, School of Physics, Peking University, No. 202 Chengfu Road, Haidian District, Beijing 100871, China

Shuang-zheng Jia, Jun-ji Zhang, Jun-jun Yang, Yang Xiang and Jin-hua Leng
Department of Obstetrics and Gynecology, Peking Union Medical College Hospital, Chinese Academy of Medical Science and Peking Union Medical College, Beijing 100730, People's Republic of China

Zhiyong Liang
Department of Pathology, Peking Union Medical College Hospital, Chinese Academy of Medical Science and Peking Union Medical College, Beijing, People's Republic of China

Lu Qin, Huming Huang, Mengjie Chen, Yuejuan Liang and He Wang
Department of Gynecologic Oncology, Affiliated Tumor Hospital of Guangxi Medical University, 71 Hedi Road, Qingxiu District, Nanning, Guangxi 530021, People's Republic of China

Wei Jiang, Shuang Ye, Libing Xiang, Tiancong He, Xuan Pei and Huijuan Yang
Department of Gynecologic Oncology, Fudan University Shanghai Cancer Center, Shanghai 200032, China
Department of Oncology, Shanghai Medical College, Fudan University, Shanghai 200032, China

Wentao Yang
Department of Pathology, Fudan University Shanghai Cancer Center, Shanghai 200032, China Department of Oncology, Shanghai Medical College, Fudan University, Shanghai 200032, China

Lin Guo
Department of Oncology, Shanghai Medical College, Fudan University, Shanghai 200032, China Department of Clinical Laboratory, Fudan University Shanghai Cancer Center, Shanghai 200032, China

Cindy M. Yamamoto, Melanie L. Oakes and Taku Murakami
Hitachi Chemical Co. America, Ltd. R and D Center, 1003 Health Sciences Rd, Irvine, CA 92617, USA

Michael G. Muto and Ross S. Berkowitz
Department of Obstetrics, Gynecology and Reproductive Biology, Gynecologic Oncology Division, Brigham and Women's Hospital, Harvard Medical School, 75 Francis Street, Boston, MA 02115, USA

Shu-Wing Ng
Department of Obstetrics, Gynecology and Reproductive Biology, Gynecologic Oncology Division, Brigham and Women's Hospital, Harvard Medical School, 75 Francis Street, Boston, MA 02115, USA Department of Obstetrics and Gynecology, Tuft Medical Center, 800 Washington Street, Boston, MA 02111, USA

Soheila Aref
Avicenna Research Institute, ACECR, Tehran, Iran
Bahman Hospital Infertility Center, North Iran Zamin St, Shahrak Gharb, Tehran, Iran
Givar Infertility Center, Tehran, Iran

Gholamreza Khalili
Department of Epidemiology and Reproductive Health, Reproductive Research Center, Royan Institute for Reproductive Biomedicine, ACECR, Tehran, Iran

Homa Iranmanesh
Sarem Infertility Center, Sarem Women's Hospital, Shahrak Ekbatan, Tehran, Iran

Fattaneh Farifteh and Ahmad Hosseini
Cellular and Molecular Biology Research Center, Shahid Beheshti University of Medical science, Arabi Ave, Daneshjoo Blvd, Velenjak, Tehran, Iran

Human M. Fatemi
IVF department, IVI RMA Middle-East Fertility Clinic, Abu Dhabi, UAE

Barbara Lawrenz
IVF department, IVI RMA Middle-East Fertility Clinic, Abu Dhabi, UAE
Women's university hospital Tuebingen, Tuebingen, Germany

Zahra Faraahi
Division of Cancer Sciences, Faculty of Biology, Medicine and Health, University of Manchester, St Mary's Hospital, Manchester, UK

Mary Ellen Gee and Richard J. Edmondson
Division of Cancer Sciences, Faculty of Biology, Medicine and Health, University of Manchester, St Mary's Hospital, Manchester, UK
Department of Obstetrics and Gynaecology, Manchester Academic Health Science Centre, St Mary's Hospital, Central Manchester NHS Foundation Trust, Manchester Academic Health Science Centre, Level 5, Research, Oxford Road, Manchester, UK

Aiste McCormick
Northern Institute for Cancer Research, Newcastle University, Framlington Place, Newcastle upon Tyne NE2 4AD, UK

Allison R. Grover
Center for Reproductive Science, Northwestern University, Chicago, IL 60611, USA

Bruce F. Kimler
Department of Radiation Oncology, Kansas University Medical Center, Kansas City, KS 66160, USA

Francesca E. Duncan
Center for Reproductive Science, Northwestern University, Chicago, IL 60611, USA
Department of Obstetrics and Gynecology, Feinberg School of Medicine, Northwestern University, 303 E. Superior Street, Lurie 7-117, Chicago, IL 60611, USA

Mustafa A. El Sherbini, Amal A. Mansour, Maha M. Sallam and Emtiaz A. Shaban
Medical Biochemistry Department, Faculty of Medicine, Ain Shams University, Cairo, Egypt

Zeinab A. Shehab ElDin and Amr H. El-Shalakany
Gynecologic Oncology Unit, Ain Shams University Maternity Hospital, Cairo, Egypt

Spencer Keene
Department of Medicine, Division of Epidemiology, Vanderbilt Epidemiology Center, Institute for Medicine and Public Health, Vanderbilt University Medical Center, Nashville, TN, USA

Alicia Beeghly-Fadiel
Department of Medicine, Division of Epidemiology, Vanderbilt Epidemiology Center, Institute for Medicine and Public Health, Vanderbilt University Medical Center, Nashville, TN, USA
Vanderbilt-Ingram Cancer Center, Nashville, TN, USA

Marta A. Crispens
Vanderbilt-Ingram Cancer Center, Nashville, TN, USA
Department of Obstetrics and Gynecology, Division of Gynecologic Oncology, Vanderbilt University Medical Center, Nashville, TN, USA

Andrew J. Wilson and Meral El Ramahi
Department of Obstetrics and Gynecology, Division of Gynecologic Oncology, Vanderbilt University Medical Center, Nashville, TN, USA

Shu Xu
Department of Biochemistry, Vanderbilt University Medical Center, Nashville, TN, USA

Lawrence J. Marnett
Department of Biochemistry, Vanderbilt University Medical Center, Nashville, TN, USA
Vanderbilt Institute of Chemical Biology, Vanderbilt University Medical Center, Nashville, TN, USA

Oluwole Fadare
Department of Pathology, School of Medicine, University of California, San Diego, La Jolla, CA, USA

Dineo Khabele
Department of Obstetrics and Gynecology, Division of Gynecologic Oncology, The University of Kansas Medical Center, MS 2028, 3901 Rainbow Boulevard, Kansas City, KS 66160, USA

Lingqin Yuan
Department of Gynecologic Oncology, Shandong Cancer Hospital Affiliated to Shandong University, Shandong Academy of Medical Sciences, Jinan, Shandong, China

Hui Guo and Jing Guo
Department of Gynecologic Oncology, Shandong Cancer Hospital Affiliated to Shandong University, Shandong Academy of Medical Sciences, Jinan, Shandong, China
School of Medicine and Life Sciences, University of Jinan, Shandong Academy of Medical Sciences, Jinan, Shandong, China

Wenli Xie
Department of Gynecologic Oncology, Shandong Cancer Hospital Affiliated to Shandong University, Shandong Academy of Medical Sciences, Jinan, Shandong, China
Shandong University, Jinan, Shandong, China

Xiugui Sheng
Department of Gynecologic Oncology, Shandong Cancer Hospital Affiliated to Shandong University, Shandong Academy of Medical Sciences, Jinan, Shandong, China
Cancer Hospital Chinese Academy of Medical Sciences, Shenzhen Center, Guangdong, China

Tong Ren, Ting-Ting Sun, Shu Wang, Yang Xiang, Keng Shen and Jing-He Lang
Department of Obstetrics and Gynecology, Peking Union Medical College Hospital, Chinese Academy of Medical Science and Peking Union Medical College, 1 ShuaiFuYuan, DongCheng District, Beijing 100730, China

Jian Sun
Department of Pathology, Peking Union Medical College Hospital, Chinese Academy of Medical Science and Peking Union Medical College, Beijing, People's Republic of China

Ji Pang, Ying Wang, Lu Jiang, Hai Qian, Yan Tao, Yongchang Chen and Yan Wu
Department of Physiology, School of Medicine, Jiangsu University, Zhenjiang City, Jiangsu Province 212013, People's Republic of China.

Pengcheng Jiang and Ruxia Shi
Department of Obstetrics and Gynecology, Changzhou Second People's Hospital Affiliated to Nanjing Medical University, Changzhou City, Jiangsu Province, China

Jizong Gao
R and D Department, Changzhou BioRegen Biomedical (Changzhou) Co., Ltd., Changzhou City, Jiangsu Province, China

José de Jesús Zermeño-Nava and Ana Laura Rámirez-de-Ávila
División de Gineco-Obstetricia, Hospital Central Dr. Ignacio Morones Prieto, Ave. Venustiano Carranza 2395, Zona Universitaria, 78290 San Luis Potosí, SLP, Mexico

Aida Catalina Hernández-Arteaga, Ma. Guadalupe García-Valdivieso, Alondra Hernández-Cedillo and Hugo Ricardo Navarro-Contreras
Coordinación para la Innovación y Aplicación de la Ciencia y la Tecnología (CIACYT), Universidad Autónoma de San Luís Potosí, Álvaro Obregón 64, 78000 San Luis Potosí, SLP, Mexico

Miguel José-Yacamán
Coordinación para la Innovación y Aplicación de la Ciencia y la Tecnología (CIACYT), Universidad Autónoma de San Luís Potosí, Álvaro Obregón 64, 78000 San Luis Potosí, SLP, Mexico
Department of Physics and Astronomy, University of Texas at San Antonio, San Antonio, TX 78249, USA

Marco Ulises Martínez-Martínez
División de Gineco-Obstetricia, Hospital Central Dr. Ignacio Morones Prieto, Ave. Venustiano Carranza 2395, Zona Universitaria, 78290 San Luis Potosí, SLP, Mexico
Hospital General de Zona No.1, Instituto Mexicano del Seguro Social (IMSS), San Luis Potosí, SLP, Mexico

Anna Roberto, Silvia Radrezza and Paola Mosconi
Laboratory for medical research and consumer involvement, IRCCS Istituto di Ricerche Farmacologiche Mario Negri, Via G. La Masa 19, 20156 Milan, Italy

Justyna Łuczak and Maciej Bagłaj
Pediatric Surgery and Urology Department, Wroclaw Medical University, 52 M. Sklodowskiej - Curie ST, 50-369 Wroclaw, Poland

Zeliha Firat Cuylan, Murat OZ, Mehmet M. Meydanli, Mustafa Erkan Sari, Hanifi Sahin and Tayfun Gungor
Department of Gynecologic Oncology, Zekai Tahir Burak Women's Health Training and Research Hospital, Faculty of Medicine, University of Health Sciences, Ankara, Turkey

Emine Karabuk and Mehmet F. Kose
Faculty of Health Sciences, Department of Obstetrics and Gynecology, Acibadem University, Istanbul, Turkey

Ahmet Taner Turan
Department of Gynecologic Oncology, Etlik Zubeyde Hanim Women's Health Training and Research Hospital, Faculty of Medicine, University of Health Sciences, Ankara, Turkey

Salih Taskin
Division of Gynecologic Oncology, Department of Obstetrics and Gynecology, School of Medicine, AnkaraUniversity, Ankara, Turkey

Suat C. Ulukent
Department of General Surgery, Kanuni Sultan Suleyman Teaching and Research Hospital, Faculty of Medicine, University of Health Sciences, Istanbul, Turkey

Ozgur Akbayir
Department of Gynecologic Oncology, Kanuni Sultan Suleyman Teaching and Research Hospital, Faculty of Medicine, University of Health Sciences, Istanbul, Turkey

Kemal Gungorduk
Department of Gynecologic Oncology, Tepecik Education and Research Hospital, Faculty of Medicine, University of Health Sciences, Izmir, Turkey

Ali Ayhan
Division of Gynecologic Oncology, Department of Obstetrics and Gynecology, Faculty of Medicine, BaskentUniversity, Ankara, Turkey

Jeimy Pedraza and Ginna Ortiz
Laboratorio de Investigación y Diagnóstico Molecular, Instituto de Infertilidad y Genética, Ingenes México, Av. IPN 2508, 07360 CDMX, México

Esther López-Bayghen
Laboratorio de Investigación y Diagnóstico Molecular, Instituto de Infertilidad y Genética, Ingenes México, Av. IPN 2508, 07360 CDMX, México
Departamento de Toxicología, Centro de Investigación y de Estudios Avanzados del Instituto Politécnico Nacional, Av. IPN 2508, 07360 CDMX, México

Leonardo Porchia
Departamento de Toxicología, Centro de Investigación y de Estudios Avanzados del Instituto Politécnico Nacional, Av. IPN 2508, 07360 CDMX, México

Azucena Ocampo
Laboratorio de Investigación y Diagnóstico Molecular, Instituto de Infertilidad y Genética, Ingenes México, Av. IPN 2508, 07360 CDMX, México
Programa de Doctorado en Ciencias Biológicas y de la Salud, División de Ciencias Biológicas y de la Salud, Universidad Autónoma Metropolitana-Iztapalapa, Av. IPN 2508, 07360 CDMX, México

Elizabeth Hernández-Pérez
Programa de Doctorado en Ciencias Biológicas y de la Salud, División de Ciencias Biológicas y de la Salud, Universidad Autónoma Metropolitana-Iztapalapa, Av. IPN 2508, 07360 CDMX, México

Katarina Kalavska
2nd Department of Oncology, Faculty of Medicine, Comenius University and National Cancer Institute, Klenova 1, 833 10 Bratislava, Slovak Republic
Translational Research Unit, Faculty of Medicine, Comenius University, Bratislava, Slovakia

Michal Mego
2nd Department of Oncology, Faculty of Medicine, Comenius University and National Cancer Institute, Klenova 1, 833 10 Bratislava, Slovak Republic
Translational Research Unit, Faculty of Medicine, Comenius University, Bratislava, Slovakia
National Cancer Institute, Bratislava, Slovakia

Denisa Manasova
Translational Research Unit, Faculty of Medicine, Comenius University, Bratislava, Slovakia

Jozef Mardiak and Jozef Sufliarsky
2nd Department of Oncology, Faculty of Medicine, Comenius University and National Cancer Institute, Klenova 1, 833 10 Bratislava, Slovak Republic
National Cancer Institute, Bratislava, Slovakia

Tomas Minarik, Michaela Kubickova and Andrej Jurik
National Cancer Institute, Bratislava, Slovakia

Peter Celec and Barbora Vlkova
Institute of Molecular Biomedicine, Faculty of Medicine, Comenius University, Bratislava, Slovakia

Julie A. MacDonald, Niharika Kura, Carleigh Sussman and Dori C. Woods
Laboratory for Aging and Infertility Research, Northeastern University, Boston, MA 02115, USA

Jiaheng Li, Mingze Du, Zhan Zhang, Yichun Guan, Xingling Wang, Jing Liu, Zhouhui Pan, Bijun Wang and Wenxia Liu
The Reproduction Center, The Third Affiliated Hospital of Zhengzhou University, 7 Kangfuqian Road, Zhengzhou 450052, Henan, People's Republic of China

Xiao Zhang
Waterstone Clinic, Lotamore House, Tivoli, Cork, Ireland

Wenyu Li, Lulu Le and Fen Fu
The Second Affiliated Hospital of Nanchang University, Nanchang, Jiangxi 330031, People's Republic of China

Zheran Liu
Queen Mary School, Medical College of Nanchang University, Nanchang, Jiangxi 330031, People's Republic of China

Bowen Liang, Siyang Chen, Xinping Zhang, Xiaoqin Tong and Weiming Lou
School of Public Health, Nanchang University, Nanchang, Jiangxi 330031, People's Republic of China

Xiaoli Tang
School of Basic Medical Science, Nanchang University, Nanchang, Jiangxi 330031, People's Republic of China

Sheng-Bing Liu, Xue-Ping Lin, Ying Xu, Zhong-Fei Shen and Wei-Wei Pan
College of Medicine, Jiaxing University, Jiaxing 314001, China

Wondimu Gudu
Department of Obstetrics and Gynecology, Saint Paul's Hospital Millennium Medical College, Addis Ababa, Ethiopia

Mehri Jamilian and Shirin Mansury
Department of Gynecology and Obstetrics, Endocrinology and Metabolism Research Center, School of Medicine, Arak University of Medical Sciences, Arak, Iran

Fereshteh Bahmani, Elaheh Amirani and Zatollah Asemi
Research Center for Biochemistry and Nutrition in Metabolic Diseases, Kashan University of Medical Sciences, Kashan, I.R., Iran

Zahra Heidar
Infertility and Reproductive Health Research Center, Shahid Beheshti University of Medical Sciences, Tehran, Iran

Index

www.ingramcontent.com/pod-product-compliance
Lightning Source LLC
LaVergne TN
LVHW060940220926
848485LV00015B/1196
9781632429452